Clinical Studies in Medical Biochemistry

CLINICAL STUDIES
IN MEDICAL BIOCHEMISTRY

Third Edition

Edited by

Robert H. Glew

and

Miriam D. Rosenthal

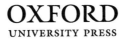

OXFORD

UNIVERSITY PRESS

2007

OXFORD
UNIVERSITY PRESS

Oxford University Press, Inc., publishes works that further
Oxford University's objective of excellence
in research, scholarship, and education.

Oxford New York
Auckland   Bangkok   Bogotá   Buenos Aires   Cape Town   Chennai
Dar es Salaam   Delhi   Hong Kong   Istanbul   Karachi   Kolkata
Kuala Lumpur   Madrid   Melbourne   Mexico City   Mumbai   Nairobi
São Paulo   Shanghai   Singapore   Taipei   Tokyo   Toronto

With offices in
Argentina   Austria   Brazil   Chile   Czech Republic   France   Greece
Guatemala   Hungary   Italy   Japan   Poland   Portugal   Singapore
South Korea   Switzerland   Thailand   Turkey   Ukraine   Vietnam

Copyright © 2007 by Oxford University Press

Published by Oxford University Press, Inc.
198 Madison Avenue, New York, New York, 10016
www.oup.com

Oxford is a registered trademark of Oxford University Press

Library of Congress Cataloging-in-Publication Data
Clinical studies in medical biochemistry / edited by Robert H. Glew and Miriam D. Rosenthal.—3rd ed.
p. ; cm.
Includes bibliographical references and index.
ISBN-13: 978-0-19-517687-2 (cloth)
ISBN-13: 978-0-19-517688-9 (paper)

1. Clinical biochemistry—Case studies.   I. Glew, Robert H.   II. Rosenthal, Miriam D.
[DNLM: 1. Biochemistry—Case Reports.   2. Laboratory Techniques and Procedures—Case Reports.
3. Metabolic Diseases—Case Reports. QU 4 C641 2006]
RB112.5.C57 2006
612'.015—dc22   2005054659

3 5 7 9 8 6 4 2

Printed in the United States of America
on acid-free paper

Contents

The Biochemical Perspectives section forms the heart of each chapter and is the longest section; it goes into considerable detail in explaining the fundamental defect that lies at the core of this case. Incorporating recent advances in molecular biology and human genetics, this section provides molecular biological as well as classic biochemical-enzymological explanations of pertinent physiological mechanisms. The fourth section of each chapter, Therapy, provides a concise account of how the disease in question is treated. If applicable, this section also incorporates discussion of current and experimental therapies based on molecular approaches.

Each chapter ends with a list of key primary and perhaps secondary references and a set of questions designed to test the reader's comprehension of the case in all its dimensions. The questions also serve to stimulate group discussions if the book is used in a small group or tutorial setting.

The diseases and disorders chosen for discussion and the order of presentation parallel subject matter taught in most first-year medical biochemistry. Chapters in the first part of the book, Nucleic Acids and Protein Structure, illustrate the relationships of protein structure and function with respect to collagen (Osteogenesis Imperfecta) and hemoglobin (Sickle Cell Anemia). The chapters Fragile X Syndrome and Hereditary Spherocytosis discuss key aspects of DNA and protein structure and their respective role in chromosomal and cytoskeletal structure. The chapter cardiac troponin and myocardial infarction provides an up-to-date demonstration of the usefulness of both structural proteins and enzymes as markers of cardiovascular disease, while the chapter α_1-Antitrypsin Deficiency discusses the important role of endogenous enzyme inhibitors.

The second section of the book is Fuel Metabolism and Energetics. Important pathways and enzymes involved in fuel utilization are discussed in the chapters Pyruvate Dehydrogenase Complex Deficiency, Mitochondrial Encephalomyopathy, and Systemic Carnitine Deficiency. The role of gluconeogenesis in glucose homeostasis is illustrated by a discussion in the chapter Neonatal Hypoglycemia.

An expanded section, Intermediary Metabolism, constitutes the third part of the book. Disorders of glucose and fatty acid metabolism are discussed in the chapters Glucose 6-Phosphate Dehydrogenase Deficiency, Biotinidase Deficiency, and Adrenoleukodystrophy. Catabolism of essential amino acid skeletons is discussed in the chapters Phenylketonuria and HMG-CoA Lyase Deficiency. The chapters Inborn Errors of Urea Synthesis and Neonatal Hyperbilirubinemia discuss the detoxification and excretion of amino acid nitrogen and of heme. The chapter Gaucher Disease provides an illustration of the range of catabolic problems that result in lysosomal storage diseases. Several additional chapters deal with key aspects of intracellular transport of enzymes and metabolic intermediates: the targeting of enzymes to lysosomes (I-Cell Disease), receptor-mediated endocytosis (Low-Density Lipoprotein Receptors and Familial Hypercholesterolemia) and the role of ABC transporters in export of cholesterol from the cell (Tangier disease).

The fourth section deals with various aspects: Digestion, Absorption, and Nutritional Biochemistry. The chapter Obesity considers current problems with respect to the ever-increasing incidence of imbalance between energy intake and utilization. Key problems of undernutrition are discussed in the chapters Protein-Energy Malnutrition and Vitamin A Deficiency in Children. The chapters Lactose Intolerance, Pancreatic Insufficiency, and Abetalipoproteinemia focus on the biochemical processes underlying food digestion and absorption. Calcium Deficiency Rickets, Vitamin B_{12} Deficiency, and Hemochromatosis provide discussions of absorption and utilization of vitamin D, vitamin B_{12}, and iron, respectively.

The last section, Endocrinology and Integration of Metabolism, includes chapters on hormonal regulation of energy metabolism (Type I Diabetes) and steroid hormone metabolism (Congenital Adrenal Hyperplasia).

This book could not have been put together without the assistance of the skilled and patient investigators who contributed chapters to this third edition of *Clinical Studies in Medical Biochemistry*; many have first-hand experience with the clinical disorders they describe. Furthermore, most of the authors of these chapters are themselves engaged in educating medical students. Whatever success this book enjoys, we owe to these contributors and to our skilled editors at Oxford, Jeffrey House and at Byteway Publishing, Kim Hoag.

Preface

During the last 25 years, medical schools have extensively integrated the teaching of basic science, including biochemistry, into the clinical world. It is now rare to find a medical school curriculum in which biochemistry is taught in isolation as a vast array of reactions, chemical mechanisms, and metabolic pathways dissociated from the normal and pathophysiological processes involved in human health and disease. Despite the current diversity in form of medical curricula—which range from traditional lectures, through various mixtures of lectures and small group formats, to the "new pathway," which relies primarily on small group, problem-based learning—the content is now solidly oriented in a clinical context. As such, many courses in biochemistry, particularly those located in or associated with medical schools, have a need for teaching materials in which biochemical concepts and particulars are articulated and developed through presentations of specific examples of human disease.

From its inception, this book was designed to meet this growing need. Both the first edition, published in 1987, and the expanded, revised 1997 edition have served effectively as companion texts to many of the standard textbooks of biochemistry, particularly at institutions that have retained much of the traditional lecture format. At the same time, experience has shown that the 8- to 14-page chapters that constitute this collection of actual case reports are sufficiently comprehensive and self-contained to stand on their own. As such, the book has been and can be used as the primary resource in "biochemistry of disease" courses at the advanced undergraduate level or in masters or doctorate graduate programs.

The chapters in the current edition have been substantially revised to incorporate new advances, particularly in molecular biology and in gene therapy, and to integrate more coherently into a comprehensive presentation of medical biochemistry. In addition, new chapters have been developed to expand the scope of the book, including collagen structure (osteogenesis imperfecta) and mitochondrial metabolism (mitochondrial myopathy) and reverse cholesterol transport (Tangier disease). A new chapter on hyperhomocystinemia provides discussion of recent insights on the effects of impaired metabolism of sulfur-containing amino acid metabolism on vascular disease. There is also more coverage of nutritional biochemistry, including new chapters on protein-calorie malnutrition, obesity, vitamin A deficiency, calcium deficiency rickets, and iron metabolism (hemochromatosis.)

Each chapter begins with a detailed case report that includes the relevant history, pertinent clinical laboratory data, and physical findings. In some cases, the patient about whom the chapter is developed was the same case that was the first of its kind described in the medical literature; in others, a more recent case is utilized to discuss advances in our understanding of the pathophysiology underlying enhanced diagnosis or therapy. The contributors to this book have been careful to define medical terms with which the readers might be unfamiliar and to minimize their need to resort to a medical dictionary. The case presentation is followed by a brief Diagnosis section, which includes a brief discussion of differential diagnosis and criteria needed for establishing the diagnosis. In addition, this section of each chapter usually explains the principles behind key laboratory and diagnostic tests.

Part V   Endocrinology and Integration of Metabolism

Contributors

WILLIAM L. ANDERSON, PH.D.
Department of Biochemistry and Molecular
  Biology
School of Medicine
University of New Mexico
Albuquerque, New Mexico

FRED S. APPLE, PH.D.
Department of Laboratory Medicine and
  Pathology
Hennepin County Medical Center
Minneapolis, Minnesota

WILLIAM S. BLANER, PH.D.
Department of Medicine
College of Physicians and Surgeons
Columbia University
New York, New York

ERIC P. BRASS, M.D., PH.D.
Department of Medicine
Center for Clinical Pharmacology
Harbor-UCLA Medical Center
Los Angeles, California

MARK R. BURGE, M.D.
Department of Internal Medicine
School of Medicine
University of New Mexico
Albuquerque, New Mexico

CATHERINE BURTON, M.A., MRCP
Department of Haematology
University College
London, United Kingdom

FRANK J. CASTORA, PH.D.
Division of Biochemistry
Department of Physiological Sciences
Eastern Virginia Medical School
Norfolk, Virginia

PRANESH CHAKRABORTY, M.D.,
FRCPSC, FCCMG
Children's Hospital of Eastern Ontario
University of Ottawa
Ottawa, Ontario, Canada

JAMES CHAMBERS, PH.D.
The Brain Research Laboratory of
  Biochemistry
Division of Life Sciences
University of Texas at San Antonio
San Antonio, Texas

ARUNA CHELLIAH, M.D.
University of New Mexico Health Sciences
  Center
Albuquerque, New Mexico

RAYMOND T. CHUNG, M.D.
Hepatology Center
Massachusetts General Hospital
Boston, Massachusetts

MARINA CUCHEL, M.D., PH.D.
Department of Medicine
University of Pennsylvania
Philadelphia, Pennsylvania

ANGELA M. DEVLIN, PH.D.
Department of Pediatrics
British Columbia Research Institute for
 Child and Women's Health
University of British Columbia
Vancouver, British Columbia, Canada

JEFFREY C. FAHL
Department of Pediatrics
School of Medicine
University of New Mexico
Albuquerque, New Mexico

SCOTT A. FINK, M.D., M.P.H.
Division of Gastroenterology
Department of Medicine
Brigham and Women's Hospital
Boston, Massachusetts

ARMANDO FLOR-CISNEROS, M.D.
Bone and Extracellular Matrix Branch
National Institute of Child Health and
 Human Development
National Institutes of Health
Bethesda, Maryland

MICHAEL T. GERAGHTY, M.B., MRCPI,
 FACMG, FRCPSC, FCCMG
Children's Hospital of Eastern Ontario
University of Ottawa
Ottawa, Ontario, Canada

LESA R. GILBERT, R.N.
Department of Medicine
University of Florida
Gainesville, Florida

ROBERT H. GLEW, PH.D.
Department of Biochemistry and
 Molecular Biology
School of Medicine
University of New Mexico
Albuquerque, New Mexico

VENKAT GOPALAN, PH.D.
Department of Biochemistry
College of Biological Sciences
Ohio State University
Columbus, Ohio

VIJAYAPRASAD GOPICHANDRAN, MBBS
Department of Biochemistry
College of Biological Sciences
Ohio State University
Columbus, Ohio

PAUL HARMATZ, M.D.
Clinical Research Center
Children's Hospital and Research Center
 at Oakland
Oakland, California

WILLIAM C. HINES
Department of Biochemistry and Molecular
 Biology
School of Medicine
University of New Mexico
Albuquerque, New Mexico

IAN R. HOLZMAN, M.D.
Department of Pediatrics
Mount Sinai School of Medicine
New York, New York

M. MAHMOOD HUSSAIN, PH.D.
Departments of Anatomy, Cell Biology,
 and Pediatrics
State University of New York Downstate
Medical Center
Brooklyn, New York

HIROSHI IDEGUCHI, M.D.
Department of Laboratory Medicine
School of Medicine
Fukuoka University
Fukuoka, Japan

ALLAN S. JAFFE, M.D.
Cardiovascular Division
Department of Internal Medicine and
Department of Laboratory Medicine
 and Cardiology
Mayo Clinic
Rochester, Minnesota

ABIODUN O. JOHNSON, M.B., B.S., M.D.
Department of Pediatrics
Texas Tech University Health Sciences
 Center
Amarillo, Texas

RICHARD KACZMARSKI, M.D., FRCP,
FRCPATH
Department of Haematology
Hillingdon Hospital
Uxbridge, United Kingdom

JUTTA KELLER, M.D.
Department of Medicine
Israelitic Hospital
Hamburg, Germany

LIEN B. LAI, PH.D.
Department of Biochemistry
College of Biological Sciences
Ohio State University
Columbus, Ohio

PETER LAYER, M.D., PH.D.
Department of Medicine
Israelitic Hospital
Hamburg, Germany

SERGEY LEIKIN, PH.D.
Section on Physical Biochemistry
National Institute of Child Health and
*   Human Development*
National Institutes of Health
Bethesda, Maryland

STEVEN R. LENTZ, M.D., PH.D.
Department of Internal Medicine
Carver College of Medicine
University of Iowa
Iowa City, Iowa

DENIS M. MCCARTHY
Department of Internal Medicine
School of Medicine
University of New Mexico
Albuquerque, New Mexico

MARGARET M. MCGOVERN, M.D., PH.D.
Department of Human Genetics
Mount Sinai School of Medicine
New York, New York

J. ROSS MILLEY, M.D., PH.D.
Division of Neonatology
Department of Pediatrics
University of Utah School of Medicine

STEVEN M. MITCHELL
School of Medicine
University of New Mexico
Albuquerque, New Mexico

KOJI NARAHARA
Department of Pediatrics
Okayama Red Cross Hospital
Okayama, Japan

SHINSUKE NINOMIYA
Department of Pediatrics
Okayama University Medical School
Okayama, Japan

MARCY P. OSGOOD, PH.D.
Department of Biochemistry and
*   Molecular Biology*
School of Medicine
University of New Mexico
Albuquerque, New Mexico

SRINIVAS PANJA, M.D.
School of Medicine
University of New Mexico
Albuquerque, New Mexico

LAWRENCE M. PASQUINELLI, M.D.
Department of Pediatrics
Eastern Virginia Medical School
Norfolk, Virginia

HARBHAJAN S. PAUL, PH.D.
Biomed Research & Technologies, Inc.
Wexford, Pennsylvania

GERALD J. PEPE, PH.D.
Department of Physiological Sciences
Eastern Virginia Medical School
Norfolk, Virginia

VIRGINIA K. PROUD, M.D.
Department of Pediatrics
Eastern Virginia Medical School
Norfolk, Virginia

KEITH QUIROLO, M.D.
Department of Hematology
Northern California Sickle Cell Center
Children's Hospital and Research Center
*   at Oakland*
Oakland, California

DANIEL J. RADER, M.D.
*University of Pennsylvania
   Medical Center
Philadelphia, Pennsylvania*

PAUL RAVA, B.S.
*Departments of Anatomy, Cell Biology,
   and Pediatrics
State University of New York Downstate
Medical Center
Brooklyn, New York*

MIRIAM D. ROSENTHAL, PH.D.
*Department of Physiological Sciences
Eastern Virginia Medical School
Norfolk, Virginia*

SARAH JANE SCHWARZENBERG, M.D.
*Department of Pediatrics
University of Minnesota School
   of Medicine
Minneapolis, Minnesota*

GAIL SEKAS
*Biomed Research & Technologies, Inc.
Wexford, Pennsylvania*

HARVEY L. SHARP
*Department of Pediatrics
University of Minnesota School
   of Medicine
Minneapolis, Minnesota*

PETER W. STACPOOLE, M.D., PH.D.
*General Clinical Research Center
University of Florida
Gainesville, Florida*

DAVID L. VANDERJAGT, PH.D.
*Department of Biochemistry and Molecular
   Biology
School of Medicine
University of New Mexico
Albuquerque, New Mexico*

DOROTHY J. VANDERJAGT, PH.D.
*Department of Biochemistry and Molecular
   Biology
School of Medicine
University of New Mexico
Albuquerque, New Mexico*

ELLIOTT VICHINSKY, M.D.
*Northern California Sickle Cell Center
Children's Hospital and Research Center
   at Oakland
Oakland, California*

EMORN WASANTWISUT, PH.D.
*Institute of Nutrition
Mahidol University
Bangkok, Thailand*

BARRY WOLF, M.D., PH.D.
*Connecticut Children's Medical Center
University of Connecticut School of
   Medicine
Hartford, Connecticut*

NUTTAPORN WONGSIRIROJ, M.A.
*Institute of Human Nutrition
College of Physicians and Surgeons
Columbia University
New York, New York*

YUJI YOKOYAMA, M.D.
*Department of Pediatrics
Okayama University Medical School
Okayama, Japan*

Part I

Nucleic Acids and Protein Structure and Function

Fragile X Syndrome

YUJI YOKOYAMA, SHINSUKE NINOMIYA, and KOJI NARAHARA

CASE REPORT

The patients were brothers, aged 2 years 9 months and 1 year 8 months, and were referred to our hospital for evaluation of developmental delay.

The Elder Brother

The elder brother was born at term when his mother was 22 years old and his father 33. Pregnancy and delivery were uneventful, and birth weight was 3260 g. Neonatal screening for metabolic diseases and hypothyroidism was unremarkable. However, gross psychomotor retardation became apparent; head control was achieved at the age of 5 months, sitting unaided at 12 months, and walking began at 20 months, but the child had not acquired any meaningful words at the time of examination (2 years 9 months).

Physical examination revealed a hyperactive boy with a height of 94.5 cm, weight of 13.2 kg, and head circumference of 47.8 cm (Fig. 1-1a). His face was somewhat long and square with a high forehead and large, prominent ears. The left lower incisor was absent, and the testes were not enlarged. Psychometric testing revealed developmental quotient to be 38% that of a normal child of the same age. The child exhibited unique behavioral abnormalities characterized by hyperactivity, short attention span, poor eye contact, and excessive withdrawal response to strange people or environments; however, these behaviors did not meet the *Diagnostic and Statistical Manual of Mental Disorders, Fourth Edition (DSM-IV)*

criteria for childhood autistic disorders. Electroencephalography (EEG) and acoustic brainstem response were normal.

The Younger Brother

The younger brother was born at the 36th week of gestation with a birth weight of 2780 g. Moderate psychomotor retardation was noted; he achieved head control at the age of 4 months, sat unaided at 10 months, and could stand up holding onto furniture at 20 months but had not acquired any meaningful words at the time of examination (1 year 8 months).

Physical examination revealed a hyperactive boy with normal height and head circumference. His face was somewhat square with a prominent forehead, everted ears, and absent left lower incisor, like his elder brother (Fig. 1-1b). Developmental quotient was assessed as 47% of normal. He had a short attention span but no social aversion or hand mannerisms. At the age of 20 months, EEG and acoustic brainstem response were unremarkable; however, from 18 months, massive epileptic discharges had become evident in the bilateral parieto-occipital regions during sleep.

The Family

Investigation of the patients' family (Fig. 1-2) revealed the presence of mental retardation in one maternal aunt (II-6, closed circle). She had been born at term with a birth weight of 3080 g. The pregnancy had been complicated by upper gastrointestinal radiographic exposure in the first trimester. While her motor

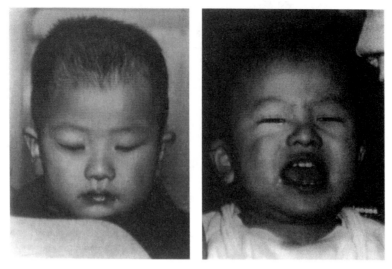

Figure 1-1. The two patients, the older brother, aged 2 years 9 months (left), and the younger brother, aged 1 year 8 months (right), showing the square faces, high forehead, and large everted ears.

development was reported to be almost normal, speech was grossly delayed, and she had attended special educational schools. Anticonvulsant drugs were administered for EEG abnormalities. Menstruation started at the age of 13 years and remained regular. Physical examination at age 20 years revealed a shy girl with mental retardation. Height and head circumference were normal although she had a somewhat long face with prognathism; however, her ears were not malformed. Speech disturbance was characterized by lack of fluency, echolalia, and inappropriate grammar. Psychometric testing demonstrated an intelligence

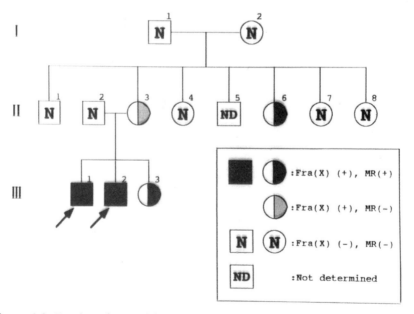

Figure 1-2. Family pedigree of the patients. Solid squares and circles indicate subjects with mental retardation, and circle with hatched lines denotes a person with borderline intelligence.

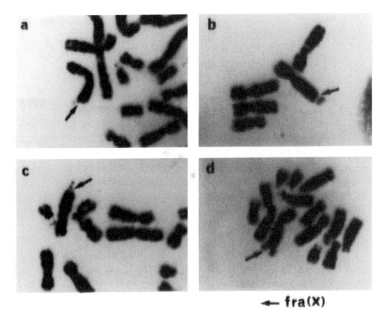

← fra(X)

Figure 1-3. Partial karyotypes of Giemsa-stained human chromosomes showing various manifestations of the fragile X site (arrows): a chromatid break (*a*), an isochromatid gap (*b*), a chromosome break (*c*), and endoreduplication (*d*).

quotient (IQ) of 45 (normal range, 77–124). The remaining maternal siblings appeared to be intellectually normal, although psychometric tests were not performed. Other than for one uncle (II-1) who left high school to work as a truck driver, no family history of education problems was reported. The mother's IQ was assessed at 92 on the Wechsler Adult Intelligence Scale. The maternal grandmother (I-2) was the sixth of a seven sibship and denied the presence of mental retardation in her brothers and sisters.

The mother became pregnant again 6 months after the first visit regarding her two sons. She refused prenatal fetal diagnosis on religious grounds, and a female infant weighing 3462 g was delivered at term by cesarean section. Psychomotor development of this infant was almost normal with the exception of speech; she began to speak a few meaningful words at 2 years 10 months. Examination revealed normal height and head circumference. She had a somewhat square face but otherwise appeared normal. Her intelligence was assessed at 85% that of a normal child.

DIAGNOSIS

The two probands presented with moderate-to-severe developmental retardation not associated with any recognizable malformation syndromes. Dysmorphic features included a long, square face, large prominent ears, and prominent forehead. The elder brother exhibited unique behavioral abnormalities and appeared to display autistic traits. Borderline mental retardation was also evident in the younger sister. Although the existence of mental retardation in one maternal aunt was difficult to explain, the familial disease was thought to be consistent with X-linked inheritance with low *penetrance* (the frequency with which a heritable trait is manifested by those carrying the affected gene) in females. Because fragile X syndrome represents about 40% to 50% of all forms of X-linked familial mental retardation, a diagnostic workup was initiated.

Cytogenetic studies have indicated that fragile X syndrome is associated with a rare fragile site at Xq27.3 (Fig. 1-3) and is caused by a mutation in the fragile X mental retardation 1 (*FMR1*) gene. Although diagnosis of the disorder should be based on molecular studies, cytogenetic studies are useful to exclude subtle abnormalities of sex and autosomal chromosomes frequently associated with nonspecific mental retardation. The fragile site, fra(X) (q27.3), can be induced under specific culture conditions (e.g., use of a medium deficient in folate or supplemented with methotrexate,

Table 1-1. Cytogenetic Studies of the Family

Subject	Sex	Age (yr)	Intelligence Quotient	Fra(X)(q27.3) Expression (%)	Ratio of Inactivated fra(X) Positive X (%)
I-1	M	59	Normal*	0	ND
I-2	F	53	Normal	0	ND
II-1	M	27	Normal	0	ND
II-2	M	35	Normal	0	ND
II-3	F	25	92	9	48
II-4	F	23	Normal	0	ND
II-5	M	21	Normal	ND	ND
II-6	F	20	45	19	53
II-7	F	18	Normal	0	ND
II-8	F	16	Normal	0	ND
III-1	M	2	38	28	ND
III-2	M	1	47	32	ND
III-3	F	2	85	18	58

ND, not determined.

*Normal range: 77–124.

fluorodeoxyuridine, or excess thymidine during the final 24 hours of culture to disturb folate metabolism). As shown in Table 1-1, the two patients (III-1 and III-2), sister (III-3), mother (II-3), and aunt (II-6) all expressed fra(X)(q27.3), whereas the remaining family members did not demonstrate this fragile site.

To determine whether selective inactivation of X chromosomes could be related to phenotypic differences in the female carriers with fra(X)(q27.3), we studied DNA replication patterns of the X chromosome using bromodeoxyuridine (thymidine analogue) incorporation during the final 7 hours of incubation. These studies demonstrated that the ratio of inactivated late-replicating X chromosomes (those incorporating large amounts of bromodeoxyuridine into DNA_s) carrying fra(X)(q27.3) did not differ significantly among the three female carriers.

The fragile X mutation involves expression of a CGG repeat stretch in the 5' encoding region of *FMR1*. *Hypermethylation* (a chemical alteration of DNA induced by methylation of deoxycytidine to 5-methyldeoxycytidine in the CG sequence where cellular regulation of gene expression or X inactivation is believed to occur) of a regulatory CpG island (a DNA region of high deoxycytidine and deoxyguanosine content linked by a phosphodiester bond located near the protein-coding region of a gene and related to its regulation of gene expression) just upstream of the CGG repeat segment and nonexpression of *FMR1* protein.

We investigated the length of the CGG repeat segment and the methylation status of the CpG island in the patients' family using Southern blot hybridization with pPCRFX1 (a kind of Pfxa3) as a DNA probe that detects restriction fragments containing the CGG repeat (Fig. 1-4). Digestion with a methylation-insensitive restriction enzyme, *EcoRI* generates a 5.2-kilobase (kb) fragment containing the mutable region. This fragment may be further digested by a methylation-sensitive restriction enzyme *EagI* into 2.4-kb and 2.8-kb fragments if the *EagI* site is not methylated. Normal males demonstrate a 2.8-kb band, whereas normal females will have a 2.8-kb band and a 5.2-kb band. The two patients (III-1 and III-2) exhibited an indistinct smear band (i.e., a dispersed expansion) ranging from 6 to 9 kb (0.7- to 4-kb expansion of the CGG repeat segment), and the aunt (II-6) also had an indistinct smear band ranging from 6 to 9 kb in addition to the 2.8- and 5.2-kb normal bands. The grandmother (I-2) and mother displayed additional 2.9-kb and 3.8-kb bands, respectively. Furthermore, the maternal uncle (II-1) had a 3.1-kb band instead of a normal 2.8-kb band. Intriguingly, the sister (III-3) exhibited an additional 4.0-kb band. The other family members showed normal blotting patterns. From the results of this analysis, the two patients and the aunt were diagnosed as having fragile X syndrome, and the mother, sister, uncle, and maternal grandmother as fragile X premutation carriers.

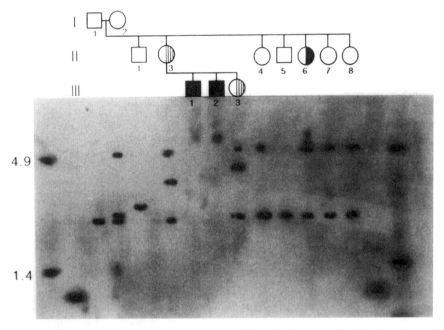

Figure 1-4. Southern hybridization analysis of the family using double digestion of DNAs with *EcoRI* and *EagI*.

MOLECULAR PERSPECTIVES

Fragile X Syndrome

The incidence of mental retardation is well known to be higher in males than in females. In 1943, Martin and Bell (1943) reported a familial mental retardation consistent with X-linked inheritance, and this family has now been demonstrated to be the first example of individuals with fragile X syndrome. Increasing interest in the etiological and biological mechanisms of mental retardation has stimulated much research in this area in the decades since the late 1960s. In 1969, Lubs (1969) described a *marker X* (a constriction in the distal long arm of the X chromosome) present in affected males and obligate carrier females of a family with X-linked mental retardation; however, this finding was not readily reproduced by standard cytogenetic techniques. It was not until 1977 that Sutherland (1977) reported that the induction of rare fragile sites, including marker X, is dependent on the composition of medium used for culturing peripheral blood lymphocytes. This condition was termed *fragile X syndrome* because, among all rare fragile sites, only the expression of the fragile in band Xq27.3 (FRAXA) is associated with clinical disease (Sutherland and Richards, 1994).

The establishment of cytogenetic methods for detecting fragile X syndrome prompted epidemiologic studies of its prevalence in various populations. The syndrome occurs in all ethnic groups and affects approximately 1 in 1250 males and 1 in 2500 females, accounting for around 20% of all familial mental retardation. This estimated prevalence is comparable to that of Down syndrome (1 in 800–1000) as a cause of mental retardation. However, determination of frequency in these studies has been based on cytogenetic detection, and the true prevalence may be even higher using a newly available molecular test for population screening.

The phenotypic features of fragile X syndrome in relation to puberty are summarized in Table 1-2. Although the syndrome is apparent from birth in affected patients, it is difficult to diagnose during early infancy. Prepubertal males tend to exhibit only nonspecific clinical findings, and characteristic physical features become obvious with age. Typical postpubertal males with fragile X syndrome exhibit a clinical triad of the so-called Martin-Bell syndrome: mental retardation, long face with large everted ears, and *macro-orchidism* (abnormally large testes). Other craniofacial features include prominent jaw, large forehead, and relative macrocephaly. Additional features are suggestive of connective

Table 1-2. Clinical Features in Males with Fragile X Syndrome

Prepubertal

    Birth weight: a mean at approximately the 70th percentile

    Height: mostly between 50th and 97th percentiles

    Head circumference: slightly increased

    Developmental delay: sit alone at 10 months, walk at 20.6 months, first meaningful words at 20 months

    Abnormal behavior: hyperactivity, hand mannerisms, excessive shyness, tantrum, autism

Postpubertal

    Mental retardation

    Craniofacial features: prominent forehead, prominent jaw, large prominent ears, long face

    Macro-orchidism

Additional features

    Orthopedic: joint hyperextensibility, flat feet, torticollis (a contracted state of the neck), kyphoscoliosis (backward and lateral curvature of the spinal column)

    Ophthalmologic: myopia and strabismus

    Cardiac: mitral valve prolapse and dilatation of ascending aorta

    Dermatologic: fine velvety skin with striae

    Genitourinary: cryptorchidism (failure of the testes to descend into the scrotum) and inguinal hernia

    Others: epilpsy, hyperreflexia, gynecomastia (excessive development of the male mammary glands)

tissue dysplasia: hyperextensible joints, mitral valve prolapse (allowing retrograde flow into the left atrium), and dilatation of the ascending aorta (aortic root dilatation). Developmental delay and mental retardation are the most significant and prominent symptoms of fragile X syndrome. Most male patients have IQ scores in the 20 to 60 range, with an average of 30 to 45. In particular, prepubertal boys with fragile X exhibit characteristic behavioral abnormalities, including hyperactivity, short attention span, emotional instability, hand mannerisms, and autistic features.

The physical and behavioral features of the disease in female patients are usually milder than in affected males. Somatic features may be absent or mild, although the faces of mentally retarded females tend to resemble those of male patients with advancing age. The intelligence deficit of female patients is less severe, with most patients having mild-to-borderline mental impairment. There is evidence of an increase in psychological and psychiatric problems among female patients.

The inheritance pattern of fragile X syndrome is unusual. While about 80% of males who inherit the mutation exhibit mental retardation and a more or less definitive phenotype, the remaining 20% of carrier males are phenotypically normal. Such clinically normal hemizygous males are termed *transmitting males* because the mutation is transmitted through their unaffected daughters to grandchildren, who often manifest this syndrome. The risk of mental retardation in grandchildren is 74% for males and 32% for females but is much lower among siblings of transmitting males (18% for males and 10% for females). Male offspring of mentally impaired carrier mothers have a higher risk of mental retardation (100%) than do female offspring (76%). The large variation in risk of mental retardation in fragile X families containing transmitting males cannot be explained by classic genetics and is termed the *Sherman paradox* after its discoverer (Sherman et al., 1985).

Because the cytogenetic approach is of limited value in detecting transmitting males and carrier females, efforts to identify and characterize a putative fragile X gene were undertaken in many molecular genetic laboratories. The association of the fragile site Xq27.3 with this form of X-linked mental retardation suggested the putative gene is located at or near the fragile X site. Tarleton and Saul (1993) described how positional cloning of the fragile X site was achieved. In addition to conventional analysis of restriction fragment length polymorphisms, new molecular tools, such as pulsed field gel electrophoresis and the yeast artificial chromosome, were used to define and isolate this region. The yeast artificial chromosome can accommodate large DNA fragments from species other than yeasts, facilitating the cloning of a gene of interest, while restriction fragment length polymorphisms provide useful molecular landmarks on chromosomes, thereby

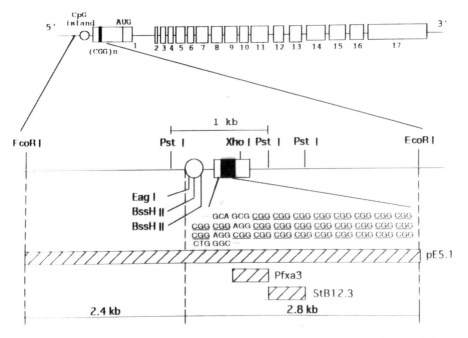

Figure 1-5. Diagram of the fragile X mental retardation (*FMR1*) gene with restriction map and *FMR1* probes used for diagnostic Southern blots. The circle indicates the CpG island, and the box represents the first exon. The dark region shows the location of triplet repeats.

enabling segregation analysis and risk assessment of the probability of inheriting a disease (linkage analysis).

The *FMR1* Gene

In 1991, several groups of investigators reported almost simultaneously that the mutation responsible for fragile X syndrome was an expansion of the trinucleotide sequence CGG (or CCG) within a gene termed fragile X mental retardation 1 (*FMR1*) (Oberle et al., 1991; Verkerk et al., 1991; Yu et al., 1991). The *FMR1* gene encompasses 38 kb on the X chromosome at the position of the fragile site and it comprises 17 exons. The triplet repeat of sequence CGG lies within the 5' untranslated region of the first exon, 69 base pairs (bp) upstream from the initiation codon and 250 bp downstream from the CpG island regulatory gene (Fig. 1-5).

This microsatellite repeat is polymorphic in normal humans, ranging from 6 to 52 repeats, with a mean of 30. In affected patients with fragile X syndrome, however, this repeat contains many times the normal number of triplet repeats: between 230 and several thousand copies of CGG. When the trinucleotide repeats exceed 230 copies, they are chemically modified in such a way that the *FMR1* gene will no longer function. The deoxycytidines within the repeats become methylated, producing 5-methyldeoxycytidines. These methylation events extend upstream into the regulatory CpG island, which is normally unmethylated, and prevent the gene from being expressed. Virtually all affected patients lack detectable *FMR1* mRNA, and the loss of *FMR1* function as a result of the suppression of transcription is believed to be the cause of fragile X syndrome. Three instances of non-CGG mutations of the *FMR1* gene, including deletions of the *FMR1* locus and a missense mutation involving the critical domain of *FMR1* in patients with apparent fragile X syndrome, have provided further supporting evidence for this hypothesis. It should be emphasized that a mutation resulting from triplet expansion has not been recognized as a cause of human genetic disease.

Although its complete sequence is known, the exact function of the *FMR1* gene has not yet been defined. The *FMR1* gene has properties of a housekeeping gene; it is expressed in diverse tissues and exhibits DNA sequences that are highly conserved in other species. Alternate splicing produces a considerable number of mRNA molecules. As would be expected, the gene is most intensely transcribed in both the brain and testes. Its protein product (fragile X mental retardation protein), which is predominantly cytoplasmic, has multiple functional domains, including two types of RNA-binding domain, a nuclear export signal, and a nuclear localization signal (Eberhart et al., 1996; Siomi et al., 1993). Extinction of an interaction between fragile X mental retardation protein and a subset of brain mRNA in neurons is thought potentially to play an important role in the neurological manifestation of fragile X syndrome. Moreover, autopsies of patients with fragile X have revealed defects in neurite density and morphology (Irwin et al., 2001), suggesting that *FMR1* may play a role in neurite branching.

Drosophila has proven to be a good model of fragile X syndrome since this species contains a single homolog of *FMR1*, *dfxr* (also called *dfmr1*). DFXR, the protein product of the *dfxr* gene, is expressed in brain neurons but not in glia. Loss of DFXR function results in marked loss of neurite extension, and irregular branching, and axon guidance defects in dorsal cluster neurons. The lateral neurons show variable defects in extension and guidance (Morales et al., 2002). The *dfxr* mutant alleles were found to cause failure of adult eclosion and disordered circadian rhythm (Dockendorff et al., 2002). DFXR constructs a complex that includes two ribosomal proteins, L5 and L11, along with 5S RNA, and Argonaute 2 (AGO2), which is an essential component of the RNA-induced silencing complex that mediates RNA interference (RNA$_i$) in *Drosophila* (Hammond et al., 2001) and a *Drosophila* homolog of p68 RNA helicase (Dmp 68) (Ishizuka et al., 2002). It is possible that RNA$_i$ and DFXR-mediated translational control pathways intersect, and that RNA$_i$-related machinery plays an important role in the control of neural function.

Fragile X families exhibit two types of *FMR1* gene mutation. The repeat expansion of more than 230 copies with subsequent methylation of the CpG island is referred to as a *full mutation*. All males and about half of the females who carry full mutations have mental retardation. Mosaic males with full mutations are almost always affected to the same extent as fully affected males, while mosaic females vary in clinical phenotype. The mosaic state is thought to reflect different degrees of expansion or DNA methylation in somatic cells. The other mutation, in which the repeat ranges from 50 to 230 copies, is termed a *premutation*. Because premutations are not methylated and are transcriptionally active, phenotypic abnormalities do not occur in any male or female carriers with this type of mutation. However, it should be understood that no precise number of copies marks the transition from the normal chromosome to premutation or from premutation to full mutation. In general, geneticists have agreed to define a copy number between 50 and 230 as premutation and one of more than 230 as full mutation.

The most prominent characteristic of the CGG repeat is the variation in its length. Because expansion occurs after conception, the range of repeat expansion varies in different cells from the same tissue in the same affected person. This variation is particularly prominent when the expanded repeat is transmitted from mother to child. When women transmit the repeat to offspring of either sex, the sequence usually increases in size (although it has been known to decrease); however, when transmitted by males, sequence size either remains constant or decreases. As males do not transmit more than 230 copies of the repeat, their daughters do not have fragile X syndrome. This means that even an affected male with a full mutation in nearly all of his cells may be essentially within the premutation range with respect to the repeat number in his sperm. No new mutation from the normal number of repeats has been seen in fragile X syndrome, and a complete family investigation always identifies a premutation in one of the ancestral generations. It is likely that small premutations may have segregated through many generations before a further repeat expansion occurred.

The Sherman paradox (Sherman, 1991; Sherman et al., 1985) was resolved by analyzing the *FMR1* gene in fragile X families with transmitting males (Fu et al., 1991). Transmitting males always have premutations, and the daughters of transmitting males inherit about the same number of CGG repeats as found in their fathers. The premutations become unstable after oogenesis (the process of gamete formation) in the daughters, leading to full mutations with over several hundred CGG repeats in their offspring.

Table 1-3. RFLP Patterns by Southern Blot Analysis from Normal Individuals, Premutation Carriers, and Patients Affected with Fragile X Syndrome*

| | DNA Digestion With EcoRI + EagI or BssHII Hybridization With | | PstI |
	pE5.1	Pfxa3 or StB12.3	Pfxa3
Normal (6–50 repeats)			
Male	2.4 + 2.8	2.8	1.0
Female	2.4 + 2.8 + 5.2	2.8 + 5.2	1.0
Premutation carriers (50-230 repeats)			
Male	2.4 + (2.9-3.3)	(2.9-3.3)	(1.1-1.6)
Female	2.4 + 2.8 + (2.9-3.3) + 5.2	2.8 + (2.9-3.3) + 5.2	1.0 + (1.1-1.6)
Patients with full mutations (> 230 repeats)			
Male	>5.7	>5.7	>1.6
Female	2.4 + 2.8 + 5.2 + >5.7	2.8 + 5.2 + >5.7	1.0 + > 1.6
Mosaic patients			
Male	(2.9-3.3) + >5.7	(2.9-3.3) + >5.7	(1.1-1.6) + >1.6
Female	2.4 + 2.8 + (2.9-3.3) + 5.2 + >5.7	2.8 + (2.9-3.3) + 5.2 + >5.7	1.0 + (1.1-1.6) + >1.6

RFLP, restriction fragment length polymorphism.

*Sizes of bands are expressed in kilobases.

Because the mothers of transmitting males have copy numbers of CGG repeats in the lower end of the carrier range (50–70), brothers of transmitting males are much less likely to have full mutations than premutations. Premutations larger than 80 CGG repeats, however, almost always expand into the full mutation range when passed through mothers. Therefore, the Sherman paradox indicates that the variation in the propensity of premutations to become full mutations may be related to the size of the premutation and the gender of the carrier.

The fragile X site is expressed when the CGG repeat is expanded to a copy number higher than 230. The expression of the fragile site is thought to be the result of an incomplete DNA replication in the expanded region caused by depletion of intracellular pools of dCTP and dGTP under specific culture conditions. However, the enormous expansion of CTG triplets in myotonic dystrophy, another genetic disease characterized by trinucleotide repeat expansion, has never been associated with any visible fragile site, suggesting that the nucleotide composition of the amplified repeats is also crucial to the expression of the fragile site. Unlike CTG repeats, CGG repeats undergo methylation, which might stabilize tetraplex DNAs formed by CGG tracts. These stable tetrahelical structures could suppress transcription, replication,

and chromatin condensation, leading to generation of the fragile site.

Now that the molecular basis of the fragile X syndrome has been defined and characterized, exclusion of this disorder on clinical or cytogenetic grounds is no longer warranted. Once a child is identified with this syndrome, family members should be evaluated to detect individuals at risk of having affected children and to facilitate decisions about future reproduction.

Southern Blotting

Molecular diagnosis of fragile X syndrome is now possible using Southern hybridization and PCR methods (Brown et al., 1993; Rousseau et al., 1991). Southern hybridization is the diagnostic method of choice because it can determine the extent of CGG repeat expansion as well as the methylation status of the CpG island. The choice between restriction enzyme and probe depends on the diagnostic information expected (Table 1-3). Cleavage with *PstI* and hybridization with a Pfxa3 probe is suitable for detecting small premutation alleles. To examine the methylation status and CGG repeat length simultaneously, double digestion with a methylation-sensitive enzyme, such as *BssHII* or *EagI*, can be used (see Fig. 1-5). A 5.2-kb band is observed from the inactive X, and two smaller bands (2.8 and 2.4 kb) are observed from the active X of the female and the single X of a normal male. As the CGG repeat lies in the 2.8-kb band, males with premutations show a band slightly larger than 2.8 kb, corresponding to an increase in the repeat length. Males with full mutations demonstrate a band larger than 5.2 kb, reflecting the methylated and expanded *FMR1* mutation. Females with premutations exhibit the three bands seen in the normal female pattern (unmethylated active state of 2.4 and 2.8 kb and methylated, inactive state of 5.2 kb) plus one additional premutation band, which sometimes merges into the normal bands. In full-mutation females, the expanded CGG repeat is always overmethylated, and a smear band in excess of 5.7 kb can be seen in addition to the normal female bands. The interpretation of data in mosaic female patients is more complex because the pattern of bands reflects the methylated and unmethylated states of both normal and abnormal X chromosome alleles.

Polymerase Chain Reaction

The PCR approach is particularly useful when a more accurate determination of CGG repeat numbers is necessary in normal or premutation carriers. Initial attempts to analyze the fragile X mutation by PCR were not successful owing to the difficulty in amplifying DNA regions with a high CG content, the preferential amplification of the smallest allele in females, and the failure to amplify full mutations. These disadvantages have been partially overcome by the substitution of 7-deaza-dGTP for dGTP, the use of improved primers, and the introduction of sequencing acrylamide gels. The advantages of PCR are that it is rapid and requires only minimal amounts of DNA. It will likely become the technique of choice in the diagnosis of fragile X syndrome if a method that can reliably amplify full mutations is devised.

PRENATAL DIAGNOSIS

Because no effective therapy is available, prenatal diagnosis of fragile X is of prime importance in pregnancies of female carriers who are at risk of having affected children. Cytogenetic analysis no longer has a place in the prenatal diagnosis of fragile X syndrome. Prenatal diagnosis can be accomplished by analyzing DNA

obtained by chorionic villus (a villus on the external surface of the chorion:fetal tissue) sampling using Southern blot analysis or, more recently, using PCR, which can detect the number of CGG repeats.

Male fetuses with 50 to 230 copies of the repeat should be asymptomatic, whereas those with more than 230 copies will have fragile X syndrome. Female fetuses with 50 to 230 copies also will be asymptomatic; however, it is difficult to predict the extent of mental retardation in female fetuses with more than 230 copies of the repeat. Although hypermethylation of the CpG island is a poor prognostic indicator, it is not always present in DNA extracted from chorionic villus samples (Sutherland et al., 1991). Empiric data showing that female carriers with full mutations have nearly a 50% risk of mental impairment should be considered reliable.

GENETIC DISEASES ASSOCIATED WITH DYNAMIC MUTATIONS

Fragile X syndrome was the first of 12 human genetic diseases in which dynamic mutation of the trinucleotide repeat was identified as the cause (Table 1-4). In these diseases, the sequence of the trinucleotide repeat and the effect of the expansion on the function of the gene in which it resides can differ. *Genetic anticipation* (a phenomenon in which the disease has an earlier age of onset and becomes increasingly severe in succeeding generations) is a common feature in these diseases and can be explained by the expansion of the repeat when transmitted from parent to child. Gender bias regarding the parent contributing the most severe form of the disease is evident in some of these disorders. For example, the form of myotonic dystrophy that is apparent from birth occurs only in children who have inherited the mutation from their mother. In contrast, the juvenile-onset forms of Huntington disease and spinocerebellar ataxia type I develop primarily when the mutation is transmitted from the father. It should be noted that expression of another fragile site, FRAXE (fragile site, X chromosome, E site), has a similar genetic mechanism to fragile X syndrome: an expansion of the CGG repeat and methylation of the CpG island, resulting in mental retardation. In contrast to fragile X syndrome, the repeat number in the FRAXE can expand or

Table 1-4. Genetic Diseases Associated with Dynamic Mutations

Disease	Chromosome Location	Repeated Sequence	Sex Bias of Parent Contributing Severe Form	Normal No. of Copies	No. of Copies Associated with the Diseases	Gene Product
Fragile X syndrome	Xq27.3	CGG	Maternal	6–50	Premutation: 50–230 Full mutation: 230–2000	FMR1
Fragile XE syndrome	Xq28	CGG	(—)	6–25	Premutation: 25–200 Full mutation: >200	FMR2
Spinobulbar muscular atrophy	Xq11-12	CAG	?	11–31	40–62	Androgen receptor
Huntington disease	4p16.3	CAG	Paternal	9–37	Premutation: 30–38 Full mutation: 37–121	Huntingtin
SCA1	6p22-23	CAG	Paternal	25–36	43–81	Ataxin 1
SCA2	12q24.1	CAG	Paternal	15–24	35–59	Ataxin 2
Machado-Joseph disease	14q32.1	CAG	Paternal	13–36	68–79	Ataxin 3
SCA6	19p13	CAG	?	5–20	21–30	Ataxin 6
SCA7	3p12-21.1	CAG	?	7–18	37–200	Ataxin 7
DRPLA	12p13.31	CAG	Paternal (mainly)	7–23	49–75	Atrophin
Friedreich's ataxia	9q13	GAA	Maternal	30–40	200–900	Frataxin
Myotonic dystrophy	19q13.3	CTG	Maternal	5–35	Premutation: 50–80 Full mutation: 80–2000	Myotonin protein kinase

DRPLA, dentatorubral-pallidoluysian atrophy; SCA, spinocerebellar ataxia.

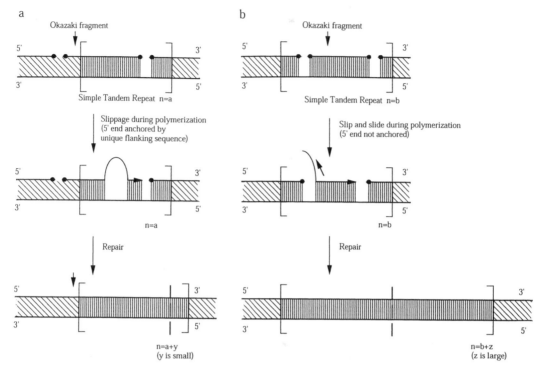

Figure 1-6. Models for instability and hyperexpansion involving Okazaki fragment slippage. For copy number below 80 (n = a), only one single-stranded break is likely to occur within the repeat during replication (*a*). Slippage of the elongated strand during polymerization can result in the addition or deletion of a few copies (y). For copy number above 80 (n = b), it is possible that two single-stranded breaks occur within the repeat in the process of replication (*b*). The strand between these breaks is not anchored at either end by unique sequence and is therefore free to slide during polymerization, enabling the addition of many more copies (z) than were present in the original sequence (b) pending the outcome of the repair process. From Richards and Sutherland (1994).

contract and is equally unstable when passed through the mother or father.

The molecular mechanism of repeat expansion in fragile X syndrome is not known. Linkage analyses of microsatellite markers flanking the CGG repeat have suggested a founder effect in fragile X syndrome: Numerous full fragile X mutations are derived from a few ancestral premutations that could increase in the genetic pool due to their relative stability and selective neutrality. There is other evidence that the CGG repeat of the *FMR1* gene in normal individuals exhibits AGG interruptions, and that repeats with documented unstable transmission have lost AGG interruptions (Eichler et al., 1994). This suggests that either DNA sequences flanking the repeat or variations in the repeat itself are involved in the mutation mechanism. The massive expansion of triplet repeats associated with

fragile X syndrome, when transmitted from a parent with more than approximately 80 copies of the repeat, cannot be explained by simple recombination. *Okazaki fragment slippage* (the tendency for a single-strand DNA with free ends caused by two breaks slides along a template strand, resulting in a greater likelihood of mutation after DNA replication) has been proposed as a possible mechanism for such rapid expansion (Fig. 1-6) (Richards and Sutherland, 1994).

THERAPY

Because no specific treatment for fragile X syndrome is available, medical, physical, and occupational interventions are directed toward alleviating neurological and behavioral manifestations of the disorder (Hagerman, 1989). It is also important for parents to have contact with other fragile X families for further support and information. Medical management of fragile X syndrome includes pharmacological treatment for specific behavioral problems and follow-up of frequently encountered complications. Folic acid supplementation is no longer recommended for treatment of the intellectual and behavioral deficits in fragile X syndrome since several studies have found that it is of no benefit. Central nervous system stimulants, such as methylphenidate and dextroamphetamine, have proved to be effective in improving the attention span and learning performance of some hyperactive fragile X children.

Educational interventions can be instituted after diagnosis of the disorder have been made and extensive genetic counseling of the family has been initiated. Teachers and therapists should create an educational program in keeping with neuropsychological characteristics of fragile X patients. Fragile X patients have more difficulty with auditory processing than with visual processing, which relates to their attentional problems, impulsivity, and distractibility, thereby validating the use of central nervous system stimulants in fragile X patients. Calming techniques, such as deep breathing, relaxation, and music therapy, are sometimes effective in avoiding emotional upsets and outbursts in new situations or confusing circumstances. The goal of speech and occupational therapies is to help fragile X patients reach their intellectual potentials.

QUESTIONS

1. What clinical features do prepubertal male patients affected with fragile X syndrome have?
2. Why is it important for medical personnel and scientists to understand the molecular basis of fragile X syndrome?
3. What is the Sherman paradox in fragile X syndrome, and how can this paradox be resolved on a molecular basis?
4. How would you go about informing the mother (II-3) and the uncle (II-1) of the patients regarding their risk of having children affected with fragile X syndrome in a future pregnancy?
5. Both the aunt (II-6) and the sister (III-3) of the patients had fragile X expression and apparent full mutation. Why was the phenotype of the sister much milder than that of the aunt?
6. What other human genetic diseases have been attributed to dynamic mutation of a trinucleotide repeat?

Acknowledgment: We would like to thank Dr. Grant R. Sutherland (Center for Medical Genetics, Department of Cytogenetics and Molecular Genetics, Women's and Children's Hospital, Adelaide, South Australia) for reading the manuscript and for permission to use Figure 1-6.

BIBLIOGRAPHY

Brown WT, Houck GE, Jeziorowska A, et al.: Rapid fragile X carrier screening and prenatal diagnosis using a non-radioactive PCR test. *JAMA* **270:**1569-1575, 1993.

Dockendorff TC, Su HS, McBride SMJ, et al.: *Drosophila* lacking dfmr1 activity show defects in circadian output and fail to maintain courtship interest. *Neuron* **34:**973-984, 2002.

Eberhart DE, Malter HE, Feng Y, et al.: The fragile X mental retardation protein is a ribonucleoprotein containing both nuclear localization and nuclear export signals. *Hum Mol Genet* **5:**1083-1091, 1996.

Eichler EE, Holden JJA, Popovich BW, et al.: Length of uninterrupted CGG repeats determines instability in the FMR1 gene. *Nature Genet* **8:**88-94, 1994.

Fu YH, Kuhl DPA, Pizzuti A, et al.: Variation of the CGG repeat at the fragile X site results in genetic instability: resolution of the Sherman paradox. *Cell* **67:**1047-1058, 1991.

Hagerman R: Behaviour and treatment of the fragile X syndrome, *in* Davies KE (ed): *The Fragile X Syndrome.* Oxford, UK, Oxford University Press, 1989, pp. 56-75.

Hammond SM, Boettcher S, Caudy AA, et al.: Argonaute 2, a link between genetic and biochemical analyses of RNAi. *Science* **293:**1146-1150, 2001.

Irwin SA, Patel B, Idupulapati M, et al.: Abnormal dendritic spine characteristics in the temporal and visual cortices of patients with fragile-X syndrome: a quantitative examination. *Am J Med Genet* **98:**161-167, 2001.

Ishizuka A, Siomi M, Siomi H: A *Drosophila* fragile X protein interacts with components of RNA$_i$ and ribosomal proteins. *Genes Dev* **16:**2497-2508, 2002.

Lubs HA: A marker X chromosome. *Am J Hum Genet* **21:**231-244, 1969.

Martin JP, Bell J: A pedigree of a mental defect showing sex-linkage. *J Neurol Psychiatry* **6:**151-154, 1943.

Morales J, Hiesinger PR, Schroeder AJ, et al.: *Drosophila* fragile X protein, DFXR, regulates neuronal morphology and function in the brain. *Neuron* **34:**961–972, 2002.

Oberle I, Rousseau F, Heitz D, et al.: Instability of a 550-base pair DNA segment and abnormal methylation in fragile X syndrome. *Science* **252:** 1097–1102, 1991.

Richards RI, Sutherland GR: Simple repeat DNA is not replicated simply. *Nature Genet* **6:**114–116, 1994.

Rousseau F, Heitz D, Biancalana V, et al.: Direct diagnosis by DNA analysis of the fragile X syndrome of mental retardation. *N Engl J Med* **325:**1673–1681, 1991.

Sherman S: Epidemiology, *in* Hagerman RJ, Silverman AC (eds): *Fragile X Syndrome: Diagnosis, Treatment, and Research.* Baltimore, MD, Johns Hopkins Press, 1991, pp. 69–97.

Sherman SL, Jacobs PA, Morton NE, et al.: Further segregation analysis of the fragile X syndrome with special reference to transmitting males. *Hum Genet* **69:**289–299, 1985.

Siomi H, Siomi MC, Nussbaum RL, et al.: The protein product of the fragile X gene, FMR1, has characteristics of an RNA-binding protein. *Cell* **74:**291–298, 1993.

Sutherland GR: Fragile sites on human chromosomes: demonstration of their dependence on the type tissue culture medium. *Science* **197:** 265–266, 1977.

Sutherland GR, Gedeon A, Kornman L, et al.: Prenatal diagnosis of fragile X syndrome by direct detection of the unstable DNA sequence. *N Engl J Med* **325:**1720–1722, 1991.

Sutherland GR, Richards RI: Dynamic mutations. *Am Sci* **82:**157–163, 1994.

Tarleton JC, Saul RA: Molecular genetic advances in fragile X syndrome. *J Pediatr* **122:**169–185, 1993.

Verkerk AJMH, Pieretti M, Sutcliffe JS, et al.: Identification of a gene (FMR-1) containing a CGG repeat coincident with a break-point cluster region exhibiting length variation in fragile X syndrome. *Cell* **65:**905–914, 1991.

Yu S, Pritchard M, Kremer EJ, et al.: Fragile X genotype characterized by an unstable region of DNA. *Science* **252:**1179–1181, 1991.

Sickle Cell Anemia

KEITH QUIROLO

CASE HISTORY

The patient was an 11-year-old girl diagnosed at birth by newborn screening as having hemoglobin F and hemoglobin S. She was subsequently determined to be hemoglobin SS. She had a long history of complications of her sickle cell disease, beginning with splenic sequestration at 6 months of age. At that time, she was treated with transfusions and eventually required a partial splenectomy. She was admitted to the hospital at 19 months of age with acute chest syndrome as a complication of respiratory syncytial viral infection.

Over the next several years, she had recurrent episodes of reactive airway disease. At the age of 4 years, she had a life-threatening episode of acute chest syndrome requiring admission to the intensive care unit and exchange transfusion. She was subsequently transfused with red blood cells monthly for 6 months to prevent recurrence. Two years later, she was again admitted to the intensive care unit with acute chest syndrome. During this admission, she was found to have *Streptococcus pneumoniae* sepsis and pneumonia. She again received RBC transfusions monthly for 6 months. Following this course of transfusion therapy, she was offered therapy with hydroxyurea, but this therapy was never instituted.

She had been well until the evening prior to admission, when she developed a fever without other symptoms. On admission to the emergency room, her parents gave a history of a cough, decreased physical activity, and fever at home of 38.8°C (normal is 37°C). She was admitted to the emergency room and seen immediately. Her only prescribed medications were 250 mg penicillin twice a day, 1 mg folic acid per day, and albuterol using a metered dose inhaler given as two inhalations on an as-needed basis.

Her admitting examination was performed at 1230 hours. Her examination revealed an alert but toxic-appearing young girl with slightly labored and rapid breathing, decreased activity, and intermittent sleepiness. She was asking for food and drink. Her initial temperature was 38°C orally, her heart rate was 158 beats per minute, her respiratory rate was 24 to 28 breaths per minute (normal is 12–20 breaths per minute), and her blood pressure was 90/40 mmHg (normal for sickle cell disease is 104 to 110/60 to 74 mmHg). Her oxygen saturation on room air was 99% (normal is 98% to 100%).

On physical examination, she had icteric sclera, dry mucus membranes, shotty anterior cervical adenopathy, and an erythematous posterior pharynx. Her chest was clear to auscultation; her heart had a regular rate and rhythm with a grade II/VI systolic ejection murmur (a flow murmur is common in children, particularly in those who have anemia due to the required increase in blood flow to maintain normal tissue oxygenation). Her abdomen was diffusely tender with the liver edge palpable 2 cm below the right costal margin. Her skin had a fine scarlatiniform rash (an exanthem consisting of a generalized erythematous eruption of small bright red macules, commonly caused by infection with streptococcal organisms); she was pale and appeared slightly jaundiced. With the exception of her lethargy, her neurological examination was normal.

Her initial laboratory evaluation showed a

hematocrit of 17.5% (normal is 30%–43%) with hemoglobin of 62 g/L (normal for this patient was between 60 and 70 g/L; normal for children of her age is 115 to 135 g/L), with a reticulocyte count of 12.9% (normal for age is 1.18%–3.78%). Her total leukocyte count was 9.1×10^6/L (normal is 4.5–13.5×10^6/L). The differential included 46% neutrophils and 25% band forms (normal is 35%–54% neutrophils, 3%–5% bands). Her platelet count was 1860×10^9/L (normal is 1300 to 4000 10^9/L). She had normal electrolytes, a serum glucose of 2.8 mmol/L (normal is 4.1–5.9 mmol/L), bicarbonate of 15 mmol/L (normal is 22–29 mmol/L), serum urea nitrogen of 8.2 mmol/L (normal is 2.1–7.1 mmol/L), and a creatinine of 115 mmol/L (normal is 62–115 mmol/L). Her unfractionated (i.e., total) bilirubin was 32.5 mmol/L (normal is 3–22 mmol/L). A urinalysis revealed a specific gravity of 1.005 (normal is 1.002–1.030), trace bilirubin, and a normal microscopic examination. Additional laboratory tests included a type and crossmatch for 3 units of leukopoor (blood filtered after collection to remove white blood cells), phenotypically matched (blood matched for red cell antigens in addition to the usual ABO blood groups) packed red blood cells.

A chest radiograph was obtained; it revealed atelectasis (loss of lung volume due to collapse of the lung) of the right lung base and mild cardiomegaly. Due to her tender abdomen, she also had a radiograph of her abdomen, which revealed a mass in the right upper quadrant compatible with hepatomegaly.

She was treated with a 20-mL/kg bolus of lactated Ringer's solution for her hypotension and was given ceftriaxone (75 mg/kg) for presumed sepsis. She appeared so ill that she was also given vancomycin (10 mg/kg) in the event she had a bacterial infection resistant to the cephalosporin. Shortly after receiving antibiotics, she became more hypotensive and required further intravenous fluids; her oxygen saturation decreased to 92% on room air. An arterial blood gas was obtained that showed a pH of 7.29 (normal is 7.35–7.45), an arterial oxygen pressure (pO_2) of 6 kPa (normal is 11.1–14.4 kPa), a pCO_2 of 4.30 kPa (normal is 4.26–5.99 kPa), bicarbonate of 15 mmol/L (normal is 22–29 mmol/L), and an oxygen saturation of 76%. She was immediately placed on oxygen by nasal cannula and transferred to the intensive care unit. The time was now 1500 hours, which was 2.5 hours after her initial examination in the emergency department.

On arrival to the intensive care unit, she was lethargic but sitting up and able to cooperate with the staff. Her oxygen saturation suddenly decreased to 67%, and she became pale and unresponsive. A femoral access line was placed; she was intubated and placed on a ventilator with 100% oxygen. The packed red blood cells ordered in the emergency room were available, and she was given a blood transfusion as a rapid bolus to increase her perfusion and blood pressure; her hemoglobin was 17 g/L on the bedside blood-monitoring device. It was noted that she had an enlarging right upper quadrant mass. With the blood transfusions and 100% oxygen via endotracheal tube her arterial blood gas had a pH of 7.29, an O_2 of 6 kPa, a pCO_2 of 4.30 kPa, and bicarbonate of 15 mmol/L. After intubation, her blood gas improved, but she continued to become more acidotic: pH 7.22, a pO_2 of 70.4 kPa, a pCO_2 of 2.80 kPa, and a bicarbonate of 9 mmol/L. A blood count after transfusion revealed a hemoglobin of 81 g/L, a platelet count of 17,000, and a leukocyte count of 12.7%. Her glucose was 2.8 mmol/L, and her calcium was 2.00 mmol/L (normal is 2.15–2.50 mmol/L).

She began bleeding from all venipuncture sites, and bruising was noted on her trunk and lower extremities. Her blood pressure could not be maintained with intravenous fluids consisting of fresh frozen plasma, cryoprecipitate, platelet concentrates, and normal saline. She was begun on vasopressors along with volume support. She was noted to have no urine output after a Foley urinary catheter was placed. At 1800 hours, 6 hours after presenting in the emergency department, she expired from septic shock.

It was noted that she had gram-negative rods on her blood smear; her blood culture grew penicillin-sensitive *Streptococcus pneumoniae*, in 6 hours. At autopsy, she was noted to have *Streptococcus pneumoniae* endocarditis of the right ventricle, focal ischemia of the left ventricle, bilateral pleural effusions, hepatic congestion with thrombosis, renal congestion, bilateral adrenal hemorrhage, and necrosis. Death was due to septic shock from *Streptococcus pneumoniae*.

DIAGNOSIS

The diagnosis of sickle cell disease is based on the identification of the hemoglobin type found in the patient's red cells, usually determined at the time of newborn screening and subsequently confirmed by follow-up testing. Optimally, parental hemoglobin samples are used to establish the diagnosis with certainty. When only one parent is available, DNA methods can be used to establish the hemoglobin mutations present in the newborn.

Newborn screening for sickle cell disease was implemented on a large-scale basis in the United States in the early 1990s. In some states, ethnic groups were targeted for hemoglobin screening, historically missing about 20% of newborns with sickle cell disease. Prior to that time, an individual with sickle cell disease was diagnosed due to a symptom of the disease prompting the individual's physician to investigate sickle cell disease as a possible diagnosis. This is still the case in areas where newborn testing is not performed.

Currently, almost all states in the United States and some members of the European Union require newborn screening for hemoglobinopathies, including sickle cell disease. A blood spot is obtained by the Guthrie method of blood collection on filter paper from a newborn. The dried blood can be used for high-performance liquid chromatography (HPLC) or for isoelectric focusing as the initial screening test. Both of these methods use the molecular charge on the hemoglobin molecule to differentiate between normal and variant hemoglobins. States performing hemoglobinopathy screening require a second test to confirm and refine the initial diagnosis. This confirmatory testing includes hemoglobin electrophoresis, β-globin chain analysis by DNA testing such as reverse dot-blot, amplification refractory mutation system, DNA sequencing, or α-gene mapping as required to make an accurate diagnosis.

The separation of hemoglobin species depends not only on the net charge of the molecule but also on the ability of the hemoglobin species to migrate through the media with the application of an electric field. Therefore, use of varied pH and media will separate hemoglobins by charge and migration. Many hemoglobin species have similar net charge and size and migrate together. Generally, more than one method is needed for definitive identification of hemoglobin type. The two most useful solid media for hemoglobin electrophoresis are cellulose acetate at a pH of 8.2 to 8.6 and citrate agar at a pH of 6.0 to 6.2 (Fig. 2-1).

Isoelectric focusing uses a pH gradient to separate hemoglobins at their isoelectric points. The *isoelectric point* is the point at which the hemoglobin molecule has no net charge. There are polyacrylamide or cellulose acetate gels embedded with amphoteric molecules with varied isoelectric points that create a pH gradient across the gel. When hemoglobins are migrated across the gel in an electric field, they are held at their isoelectric points. The hemoglobins are then stained and can be read with respect to standard hemoglobins as well as quantitated using a densitometer. Although most hemoglobins are sharply separated using this method, there are some hemoglobins that comigrate together even in this system.

HPLC consists of a negatively charged stationary absorbent column over which the hemoglobin solution is passed. Within the column, the different hemoglobin species are separated by charge. The hemoglobin is then eluted by an increasingly positive buffer competing with the hemoglobin for sites on the absorbent. The net charge on the hemoglobin molecule determines the elution time. The system is automated and computerized, and the hemoglobin can be identified and quantitated. This is the most commonly used method for mass screening of newborns in the United States. Variant hemoglobin species detected by HPLC are confirmed by other methods.

BIOCHEMICAL PERSPECTIVES

Sickle cell disease was first diagnosed in Western medicine in 1904 when a medical intern, Ernest Irons, observed "pear shaped elongated forms" on the blood smear while investigating a patient who had pneumonia. Dr. Irons was serving at the Presbyterian Hospital in Chicago. The patient was Walter Clement Noel, a dental student from Barbados, who had been ill for a month with respiratory symptoms. The attending physician, James Herrick, had an interest in blood and cardiovascular diseases. Dr. Herrick followed this patient for the next 2.5 years. In 1910, he published a brief article describing the blood findings for Mr. Noel in the *Archives of Internal Medicine* (Herrick, 1910); it was the first characterization of sickle cell disease in a journal publication. After finishing dental school, Dr. Noel returned to Grenada and died 9 years later from acute chest syndrome. Serjeant (2001) has written a review of the history and medical advances in the treatment of sickle cell disease.

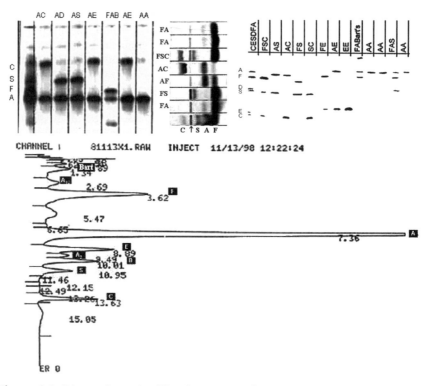

Figure 2-1. Diagnostic testing. The three upper figures are cellulose acetate, citrate agar, and isoelectric focusing; high-performance liquid chromatography is shown on the bottom. High-performance liquid chromatography is used in most states for newborn screening. The result is confirmed by a combination of electrophoretic methods and DNA studies.

In 1922, V. R. Mason (Mason, 1992) published a case review in the *Journal of the American Medical Association* entitled "Sickle Cell Anemia," and the homozygous condition has since then been referred to by the description of the shape of the red cells seen by Dr. Irons a decade earlier. In his review article, Dr. Mason promulgated the misconception that this disease was exclusively seen in persons of African origin. In 1923, Sydenstricked and colleagues reviewed the cases of two children with sickle cell disease and observed the blood smears of Caucasian and African Americans and concluded, with Mason, that sickle cell anemia was a condition peculiar to people of African descent. Neel (1949) reviewed blood smears of families with sickle cell disease over a 2-year period and correctly concluded that sickle cell anemia was a disease with Mendelian inheritance.

Also in 1949, Pauling, Itano, Singer, and Wells published a now-famous article in the journal *Science*: "Sickle Cell Anemia: A Molecular Disease." Itano, working in Pauling's laboratory, used electrophoresis to separate hemoglobins from individuals who had clinical evidence of sickle cell disease, related individuals who had abnormal hemoglobin electrophoresis without the disease, and individuals who had normal hemoglobin. He showed that there was a slight charge difference between these three hemoglobins. Pauling, who had a research interest in antigen–antibody reactions, deduced that there must be a conformational change in the hemoglobin molecule that caused the molecules to align and change the shape of the red cell. In 1956 Ingram was able to separate hemoglobin A from hemoglobin S and showed that hemoglobin S had a positive charge relative to hemoglobin A. In 1957, Ingram published a report showing that there was more valine and less glutamic acid in hemoglobin S. Twenty years later, Morotta showed that this was consistent with a one-nucleotide change of an adenine for a thymine, a residue in the β-globin gene: GAG to GTG, leading to the amino acid substitution predicted by Ingram. The mutation was shown to be at the position of the sixth amino acid on the β-globin chain.

In the late 1940s and 1950s, researchers in Africa searched for kindred having sickle cell disease but were unable to find evidence of a familial pattern of inheritance. In 1949 and again in 1956, Lehmann and Raper described a community in Uganda in which they predicted 10% of the population would have sickle cell anemia. However, they could find no children or adults with the disease. Other scientists studying populations in different areas of Africa confirmed this observation. Later, it became evident that these early studies in Africa sampled populations after young children, like the child in the case study, had died. The infant mortality rate and life expectancy of indigenous Africans was so short and infant death was so common that it was not immediately apparent that those affected by sickle cell disease had not survived childhood.

Although the homozygous condition for sickle cell disease leads to early mortality, the heterozygous condition confers a positive survival advantage. This is termed a *balanced polymorphism*. Many hemoglobinopathies, including sickle cell disease, occur in areas where *Plasmodium falciparum* malaria is common. Heterozygosity for sickle hemoglobin S with normal hemoglobin A confers a selective advantage to children living in these areas. These children have lower rates of infection and less parasitemia than children with normal hemoglobin. There have been many theories concerning this phenomenon, including one that contends that the dehydration and sickling of hemoglobin AS-containing red cells kills infecting trophozoites, changes adhesion molecules for *P. falciparum*, and changes cytokine production, leading to a moderation of malaria in AS individuals. However, a definitive pathophysiological mechanism for this effect has not been determined. The protective effect of the sickle gene is most compelling between the ages of 2 and 16 months, when parasitemia and anemia are most prevalent and when children have lost the protection of maternal antibodies but have not developed natural immunity.

The mutation for sickle hemoglobin occurred at least three times in Africa and once on the Indian subcontinent. The disease has spread from Africa to the Mediterranean, areas of Turkey, North and South America, the Caribbean, and the United Kingdom. The sickle hemoglobin combined with common hemoglobin variants in those areas: β-thalassemia in the Mediterranean, α-thalassemia and hemoglobin C in Africa, and hereditary persistence of fetal hemoglobin in North Africa and India. These combinations have created diverse presentations of this disease, the most severe being hemoglobin SS and hemoglobin Sβ zero thalassemia.

An understanding of sickle cell disease requires an understanding of the hemoglobin gene clusters occurring on chromosomes 11 and 16 and their expression, as well as the structure and function of the hemoglobin molecule. Max Perutz is most responsible for elucidating the structure and function of the hemoglobin molecule. Dr. Perutz together with Sir John Kndrew received the Noble Prize in 1962 for their research on hemoglobin.

Current understanding of the hemoglobin gene clusters required the work of so many scientists that there is not a readily identifiable scientist whose work brought understanding to their structure and function. In the 1970s, there was a burst of activity related to determining the structure of hemoglobin genes using Southern blotting and gene cloning. Pioneers in the hemoglobin field had characterized the structure of the hemoglobin protein and determined the function and organization of the hemoglobin genes without knowing the exact location or structure of the genes. This knowledge greatly facilitated the efforts of the later molecular biologists in their research on the β-globin gene structure and function. A historical review of this period of hemoglobin discovery was published by Weatherall (2001).

Two similar gene clusters code for the two globin proteins (Fig. 2-2). The β-globin gene cluster is found on the short arm of chromosome 11 (11p15.4), and the α-globin gene cluster is found on the short arm of chromosome 16 (16p13.3). The globin gene clusters are highly conserved, probably arising from duplication and unequal crossing over within these regions. The genes are similar all vertebrates, including humans.

In both the α- and β-genes there are three exons, or coding regions, and two introns or intervening sequences. Within the β-globin gene cluster, there are five functional genes and one pseudogene. Within the α-gene cluster, there are three functional genes and two pseudogenes. The α-gene mutations most commonly involve deletions, duplications, and triplications. In contrast, in the β-gene, point deletions predominate. In both gene clusters, the genes are arranged in

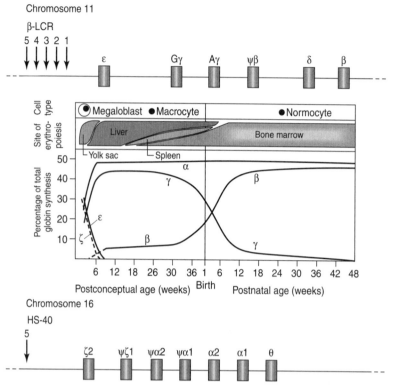

Figure 2-2. α- and β-globin gene clusters. Gene arrangement on the two clusters and their ontogenic order of expression. The regulatory locus control region (LCR) and the hypersensitive region (HSR) are 5' to the clusters. The middle graph shows relative levels of hemoglobin and hemoglobin switching. The second bar shows the sites of hematopoiesis through development. Not shown is hemoglobin A2, which appears near the 12th week after birth and plateaus soon after birth, reaching about 2.5% of the total hemoglobin. Reproduced with permission from Weatherall (2001).

the order of expression during fetal development from the 5' end to the 3' end. During fetal development, there are two β-like globin switches, epsilon to gamma and gamma to beta; and one α-like globin switch, zeta to alpha, in early fetal development. During these switches, the hemoglobin produced changes from the embryonic Gower 1 and 2 ($\zeta_2\varepsilon_2$ and $\zeta_2\alpha_2$) and Portland ($\zeta_2\gamma_2$) hemoglobins to fetal ($\alpha_2\gamma_2$) hemoglobin. After birth, hemoglobin switches to adult hemoglobin: A ($\alpha_2\beta_2$) and A2 ($\alpha_2\delta_2$) or, in the case of sickle cell disease, S ($\alpha_2\beta^s_2$).

Promoter regions control each globin gene. The globin gene promoter regions share conserved sequences that bind transcription factors. The entire β-globin cluster is controlled upstream by a locus control region consisting of five hypersensitive sites. The α-globin cluster is controlled by a similar hypersensitive region. There are numerous erythroid-specific and non-

specific *trans*-acting factors not coded on either chromosome 11 or chromosome 16 that regulate hemoglobin gene expression. An example of an erythroid-specific *trans*-acting transcription factor is the erythroid Krupple-like factor. This protein is a member of the zinc finger proteins and binds to CACC motifs in the promoter region of the β-globin gene. It is a specific activator of the β-globin gene and may be involved in the globin switch from γ- to β-globin expression during the transition from fetal to adult hemoglobin. The most important generalized regulator of gene function for hemoglobin F synthesis on *trans*-acting chromosomes is at Xp22.2 on the X chromosome.

A dominant theme in the treatment of sickle cell disease is the manipulation of the hemoglobin switch from fetal to adult hemoglobin. If the switch did not occur at all or if the γ-globin gene did not completely switch to β-globin after birth, then the symptoms of sickle cell disease would be greatly attenuated. An understanding of hemoglobin maturation has greatly advanced the search for treatment modalities and the basic science of hemoglobinopathies, including sickle cell disease.

Each individual globin chain envelopes and stabilizes the oxygen-binding heme moiety. The globin chains interact with each other under the influence of heterotophic ligands: hydrogen ions, carbon dioxide, chloride ions, and 2,3-bisphosphoglycerate. All of these ligands, all different (heterotrophic), have a stabilizing effect on the deoxyhemoglobin species, thereby decreasing oxygen affinity and shifting the oxygen equilibrium curve to the right. Oxygen and carbon monoxide (CO) are considered homotrophic ligands; the binding of oxygen or CO to one of the hemes in the hemoglobin molecule increases the affinity of the other three for oxygen, shifting the oxygen equilibrium to the left. Hemoglobin influences the solubility of carbon dioxide in plasma by the release of protons (Bohr effect) when hemoglobin is deoxygenated. Deoxyhemoglobin is also a carbon dioxide transporter. When carbon dioxide is bound covalently to α-amino groups on the globin chains, protons are released, and chloride ions are drawn into the cell. 2,3-bisphosphoglycerate is synthesized in the red cell and stabilizes deoxyhemoglobin.

The interaction between hemoglobin and these heterotrophic ligands changes hemoglobin affinity for oxygen and alters the shape of the molecule through what are called allosteric effects. *Allostery* refers to the ability of a ligand to change the structure of an enzyme by binding to a site distant from the active site of the enzyme, or in this case the heme moiety of hemoglobin. Most proteins that exhibit allostery also exhibit cooperativity. In the presence of these heterotropic ligands, the hemoglobin molecule is in the deoxygenated or "tense state" (T structure), whereas in the presence of oxygen the hemoglobin molecule is in the "relaxed state" (R structure). The cooperative effect of hemoglobin refers to the progressively increased oxygen affinity when the second or the third oxygen molecule is bound to the hemoglobin. It is at this point that the hemoglobin molecule switches from the T to the R structure (Fig. 2-3). The classic allosteric enzyme exhibiting cooperativity is described by the familiar sigmoid plot of the oxygen dissociation curve (Fig. 2-4).

The polymerization of sickle hemoglobin only occurs with the hemoglobin in the T, deoxygenated, state. Heterotrophic ligands increase polymerization of sickle hemoglobin. In the absence of oxygen, only 1 in 3 million molecules of hemoglobin are in the R state, a condition that greatly increases the probability of polymerization within the red cell.

Besides combining with oxygen, hemoglobin also binds CO and nitric oxide (NO). NO is a potent vasodilator. During hemolysis, there is an increased level of CO production. The role of CO and heme oxygenase in sickle cell disease has not been studied. However, NO has been studied extensively, and its effects in sickle cell disease are just being appreciated. The concentrations of both NO and its precursor, arginine, are low in patients with sickle cell disease. Replacing arginine has a beneficial effect in sickle cell disease.

The polymerization of deoxygenated sickle hemoglobin is the pathognomonic event in sickle cell disease (Fig. 2-5). The requisite features are hemoglobin in the deoxygenated T state and increased concentration of hemoglobin within the red cell. Other factors favoring polymerization are low pH, increased temperature, and decreased availability of oxygen.

Reflecting on the scenario of the case history, one can infer what was occurring at the molecular level during the child's illness. Our young patient presented with a history of fever, dehydration, metabolic acidosis, and relative hypoxia due to anemia and pneumonia. All of these factors contribute to an increase in sickle hemoglobin polymerization. Due to acidosis, her hemoglobin remained in the T state with a decreased ability to take up oxygen in the pulmonary capillaries. Regional hypoxia leads to V/Q mismatch, a condition in which areas of the lung with decreased oxygenation due to atelectasis or other disease process experience a reflexive decrease in blood flow in the pulmonary vasculature. She then developed hemoglobin polymerization in her lungs, a unique complication of sickle cell disease, namely the acute chest syndrome.

In dilute solutions, both hemoglobin A and hemoglobin S have identical oxygen-binding curves. At the concentrations of hemoglobin occurring within the red cell, the solubility of hemoglobin S is decreased. This decreased solubility increases the possibility of polymerization when the red cell enters the microcirculation and releases oxygen, increasing the hemoglobin

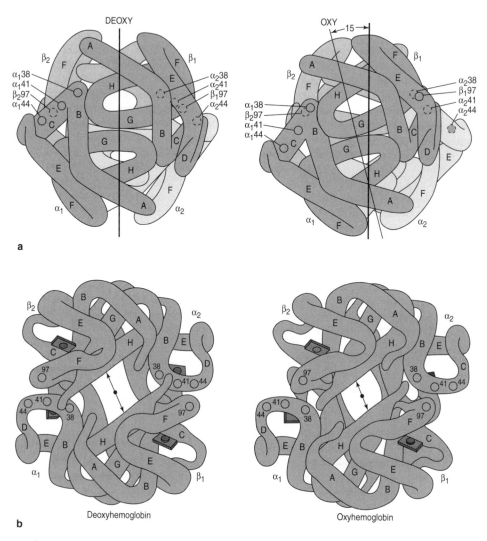

Figure 2-3. *Hemoglobin transition states* T (tense): deoxygenation state; R (relaxed): oxygenated state. (a) Viewed perpendicular to the axis showing rotation along this axis and sliding of the alpha and beta chains over each other. (b) Viewed from the top showing narrowing of the central cavity with oxygenation. Sickle hemoglobin polymerization can only occur in the T state. Reproduced with permission, Mathews, Van Holde, Ahern, 1999. © Irving Geis.

in the T state within the cell, therefore favoring polymerization. During the journey of red cells through the relatively hypoxic microcirculation, there is an increase in T-state hemoglobin and an increase in the possibility of nucleation formation of sickle hemoglobin. Polymerization begins with homogeneous nucleation of individual hemoglobin molecules with a uniform delay time. This nucleation progresses to a heterogeneous process with new nuclei for polymerization occurring on the surface of the

existing polymer, leading to a stochastic increase in growth of the polymers. At low oxygen tension, sickle hemoglobin and sickle hemoglobin polymers are in the T state, binding oxygen with low affinity. At low oxygen tension, cooperativity is lost, shifting the oxygen-binding curve to the right. This shift is actually beneficial to the patient since increased amounts of oxygen become available to the tissues.

Under normal conditions, only about 5% of

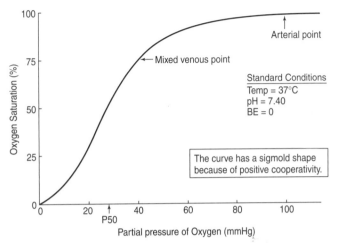

Figure 2-4. Oxygen dissociation curve for adult hemoglobin (HbA) demonstrating the characteristics of allosteric positive comparativity. Right shift of the curve caused by heterotrophic ligands and increased temperature leads to decreased oxygen affinity.

sickle red cells actually undergo polymer formation while traversing the microcirculation. Impeding polymer formation are the variability of transit time, the variability of hemoglobin concentration in individual red cells, and the heterogeneity of the concentration of hemoglobin F in the red cells. Many of the sickled cells regain their normal shape after reoxygenation; however, some cells become irreversibly sickled cells (ISC). These ISC can be those that are subjected to repeated cycles of polymer formation or can be formed after one cycle of polymerization. These ISC are dense cells with a mean hemoglobin concentration as high as 500 g/L. ISC tend to be younger red cells with a shortened life span. In the case history, our young patient had severe dehydration, leading to red cell dehydration, which resulted in increased polymerization of hemoglobin within the red cell.

The molecular contacts between hemoglobin S occur in axial and lateral planes. The β6 sickle mutation is involved in the lateral contacts between the β-globin chains. The unoccupied space is taken up by water, thereby giving rise to the formation of hydrogen bonds in the free space between the β-globin molecules. The axial contacts are much more complex. Seven double strands make up each hemoglobin fiber, which has a helical arrangement with a periodicity of 22 Å (Fig. 2-6). Both hemoglobin A and hemoglobin C can copolymerize with hemoglobin S due to the fact that these two hemoglobins have charged amino acids at the β6 site.

Neither hemoglobin F nor hemoglobin A2 copolymerize with sickle hemoglobin, and both inhibit sickling. Hemoglobin A2 differs from hemoglobin A by 12 amino acids, but only one change, at the amino acid site δ87 (Glu to Thr) on the β-chain, inhibits copolymerization. Hemoglobin F differs from hemoglobin A by 39 amino acids, at least 2 of which are involved in the inhibition of copolymerization, γ80 (Asp to Asn) and γ87 (Glu to Thr). The mechanism of hemoglobin F inhibition of polymerization is not completely understood since there may be other of the 39 amino acid changes involved in inhibition.

Polymerization and sickle hemoglobin affect the red cell membrane, which in turn interacts with the microvascular epithelium and molecular environment within the circulatory system to account for the pathognomonic changes of sickle cell disease. Sickle hemoglobin itself causes oxidative damage to the cell membrane by creating hemichrome (an oxidation product of methemoglobin) that can be seen microscopically within the red cell as Heinz bodies on the inner membrane. During polymerization, the hemoglobin fibers cause red cell membrane-cytoskeleton uncoupling, which results in the release of microvesicles of red cell membrane and free hemoglobin into the circulation. The altered membrane damages the proteins responsible for maintaining the asymmetry of the lipid membrane. This results in phosphatidylserine exposure to the circulation and activation of the coagulation cascade,

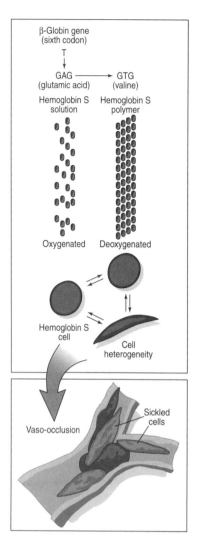

Figure 2-5. Pathologic changes in sickle cell diseases. Vaso-occlusion is a combination of exposure of phosphatidylserine on the red cell membrane, activation of vascular endothelial cells, activation of leukocytes, and a state of increased coagulability. From Steinberg, 1999. Copyright © 1999, Massachusetts Medical Society. All rights reserved.

measured by an increase in markers of fibrinolysis, and d-dimer formation.

In addition, vascular endothelial cells become activated in patients with sickle cell disease, resulting in the exposure of adhesion molecules, in particular, vascular cell adhesion molecule 1 (VCAM-1), which is present on the surface of the vascular endothelium in sickle cell disease. An integrin on the red cell, designated very late activation antigen 4, binds with

VCAM-1, causing upregulation of this adhesion molecule. Soluble VCAM-1 is found in increased amounts in plasma during inflammation and sickle vaso-occlusive episodes. VCAM-1, intercellular adhesion molecule-1 (ICAM-1), and E-selectin are all molecules found during inflammation and upregulated in sickle cell disease, and all these have been implicated in the vascular endothelial damage occurring during sickle cell vaso-occlusion.

Sickle cell disease can be characterized as a state of abnormally activated vascular endothelium that promotes increased adhesion of the red cells and leukocytes as well as a procoagulant state. The catastrophic events described in the case history were the direct result of sepsis, hepatic sequestration of red blood cells, and acute chest syndrome. Most of the chronic effects of sickle cell disease can be explained by inflammation, coagulopathy, and arteriolar obstruction. Membrane disruption and adhesion to endothelial surfaces disrupts the red cell membrane, leading to hemolysis and anemia. Vaso-occlusion is a complex event involving endothelial activation, leukocyte and red cell adhesion, hemoglobin polymerization, vessel occlusion, and tissue damage from necrosis. In this case, pain was not a feature of the child's presentation, illustrating that even without pain the effects of sickle cell disease can be severe. Had this child survived her infection and hepatic sequestration, she would have been at risk for vessel occlusion within the cerebral arteries and stroke. As the life span of patients with sickle cell disease increases, they become at risk for pulmonary hypertension, renal failure, bone necrosis and osteoporosis, brain injury, coagulopathy, red cell destruction, vessel obstruction, and the effects of inflammation.

THERAPY

Therapy for sickle cell disease has changed dramatically since the mid-1990s. Prior to the 1980s therapeutic interventions for sickle cell disease consisted of supportive care during acute illness, opioids for pain management, and occasional transfusions for severe anemia or life-threatening complications. At that time, sickle cell disease was considered a pediatric disease as there were few children who survived into adulthood. In 1986, the Penicillin Prophylaxis Study was conducted, providing evidence that early intervention with penicillin prevented

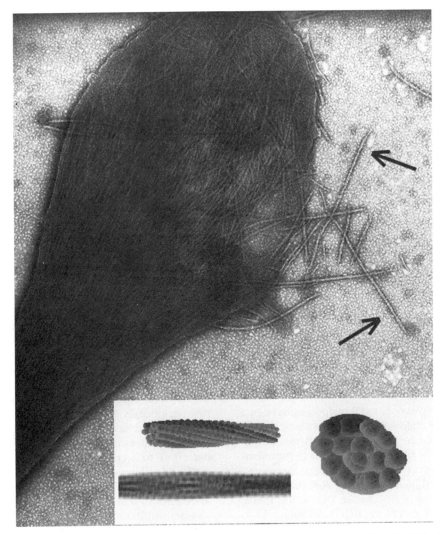

Figure 2-6. Electron micrograph of individual fibers of sickle hemoglobin. Individual strands of polymerized hemoglobin in red cell are shown. The inset shows an electron micrograph of an individual fiber with a periodicity of 22 Å. The model reveals the seven double strands making up each hemoglobin S fiber with one pair detailing the helical arrangement of the fibers. Adapted with permission from Josephs (1999).

80% of life-threatening infections by *Streptococcus pneumoniae*. Penicillin was subsequently established as a therapy for newborns and children with sickle cell disease. This intervention made sickle cell disease and, by default, all hemoglobinopathies eligible for inclusion in newborn screening programs. Penicillin therapy and newborn screening ushered in a new era of treatment for patients with sickle cell disease.

In 1984, hydroxyurea was shown to be effective in increasing fetal hemoglobin levels in patients with sickle cell disease and was the first accepted therapy to treat the basic patho-physiology of sickle cell disease, namely, hemoglobin polymerization. Hydroxyurea is a drug that inactivates ribonucleoside reductase and blocks the synthesis of deoxynucleotides, thus inhibiting DNA synthesis. Hydroxyurea is absorbed from the gastrointestinal tract and has a half-life of about 2 hours in the circulation. After trials were conducted in adults to determine efficacy and in children to determine safety it was found that this drug has numerous effects in addition to increasing fetal hemoglobin that were not generally appreciated in the early studies.

Hydroxyurea therapy results in a decreased leukocyte count, a decrease in markers of inflammation, a decrease in endothelial adhesion markers, an increase in NO, and with prolonged use, an increase in hemoglobin concentration. Hydroxyurea has been shown to decrease the incidence of most complications of sickle cell disease, with the possible exception of first stroke. Hydroxyurea therapy requires close monitoring because of the side effects that can occur with this therapy. Hydroxyurea therapy may increase the possibility of malignancy, birth defects or other complications; however, as of 2004, these effects were not reported in patients with sickle cell disease.

Other chemotherapeutic agents have been used in sickle cell disease and are currently in trials. These agents include magnesium, clotrimazole, and other novel inhibitors of membrane transport used to induce red cell hydration and decrease the concentration of hemoglobin; arginine-containing compounds to increase substrate for the production of NO; compounds that decrease cell adherence; and agents to increase fetal hemoglobin. Combination therapy is under investigation, such as with hydroxyurea and magnesium.

For many years, blood transfusion has been a therapy for children and adults with sickle cell disease. Prior to the 1980s, due to the lack of availability of blood products and the standard of care at that time, transfusion was used infrequently and generally only for catastrophic complications of this disease. During the 1980s, the risk of infection through transfusion was so high that transfusion continued to be used infrequently. When reliable testing for infectious diseases (e.g., HIV and hepatitis) in blood products became available, the use of red cell transfusion became standard of care for complications of sickle cell disease.

In 1988, transfusion to prevent stroke became the standard therapy after the Stroke Prevention Trial in Sickle Cell Disease (the STOP trial). Transfusion therapy decreases morbidity in acute chest syndrome and surgery, and decreases the recurrence of stroke in sickle cell disease. By reducing the red cells containing hemoglobin S to 30% or less of the total hemoglobin, stroke risk is decreased dramatically. Reducing hemoglobin S to 50% can decrease the morbidity of the disease. An emerging and severe complication of sickle cell disease, and of hemolytic anemias in general, is pulmonary hypertension. It is not clear that transfusion alone can reduce the incidence or severity of this complication.

An unavoidable complication of blood transfusion is iron accumulation in body tissues, called *transfusion-induced hemosiderosis*. There are no excretory pathways to eliminate excess iron, and accumulation results in organ damage and failure. The challenge in transfusion therapy is the reduction of iron overload in transfused patients with the administration of chelator drugs such as desferrioxamine. Chelating agents must be given daily by subcutaneous injection over hours. Exchange blood transfusion by erythrocytapheresis can delay or prevent the accumulation of iron in some patients and is the standard of care for transfusion in sickle cell disease. Blood donors and patients with sickle cell disease are generally ethnically diverse, and the red cell antigens (other than ABO and Rh) present on the majority of donor red cells occur at different frequencies than in most recipients. Patients with sickle cell disease are typed for these minor red cell antigens and receive antigen-compatible blood beyond the usual red cell ABO, Rh identification, decreasing antibody formation against the transfused red cells.

Stem cell transplantation using bone marrow, peripherally collected stem cells, or umbilical cord blood has been used to cure sickle cell disease (Walters et al., 2000). There is an ongoing effort to increase the availability of stem cells with sibling umbilical cord blood collection and unrelated cord blood banking. There are efforts to reduce the toxicity of bone marrow transplantation with the use of nonmyeloablative therapies and new therapies for graft-versus-host disease. Studies are ongoing to modify T-effector cells involved in graft-versus-host to make this complication less likely. There can be significant morbidity from this therapy, and it is generally reserved for those patients who have severe disease due to stroke, severe acute chest syndrome, or other chronic complications. The patients who have the best outcomes are those under the age of 2 years. Usually, these children have not declared themselves to be patients with severe disease meeting the criteria for stem cell transplant.

QUESTIONS

1. Patients who have hemoglobin SS as well as a mutation that produces hereditary persistence of fetal hemoglobin have few

symptoms of sickle cell disease. Explain why this is the case.

2. An infant has 96% hemoglobin F and 4% hemoglobin S at birth. What are the possible diagnoses? What tests can be done to confirm the newborn screening test?

3. Couples who each have sickle cell trait have three children; none of their children have sickle cell disease. They tell you they do not want to have another child because they know there is a one in four possibility for their children to have sickle cell disease, and they already have three unaffected children. What is the probability their next child will have sickle cell disease? If they have another child and this child has sickle cell disease, then what is the probability that one of the other children will be an HLA match?

4. Describe the concept of allostery as it applies to hemoglobin and to regulatory enzymes.

5. A mother complains to you at a clinic visit that her 10-year-old child, homozygous for hemoglobin S, still has enuresis at night. Can you explain to her, and to yourself, why this might be the case? What other organ dysfunction might be expected in a child this young?

6. Why does deoxygenated hemoglobin S polymerize? Besides polymerization, what are the causes of the clinical manifestations of sickle cell disease?

7. How could the child in the case study have died from pneumococcal sepsis if this bacterium was sensitive to penicillin?

8. If both hemoglobin A and hemoglobin S have the same oxygen-carrying capacity and exhibit the same oxygen saturation curves when at low hemoglobin concentrations, then why does hemoglobin S have a decreased oxygen-carrying capacity at the concentrations found in the red cell? Trace the path of a red cell in sickle cell disease from the lungs to the capillary bed and back to the lungs, noting the hemoglobin changes that are likely to occur during the journey.

BIBLIOGRAPHY

Bain BJ: *Haemoglobinopathy Diagnosis*. Blackwell Science, Oxford, UK, 2001.

Claster S, Vichinsky EP: Managing sickle cell disease. *Br Med J* **327**:1151-1155, 2003.

De Franceschi L, Corrocher R: Established and experimental treatments for sickle cell disease. *Haematologica* **89**:348-356, 2004.

Herrick JB: Peculiar elongated and sickle shaped red blood corpuscles in a case of severe anemia. *Arch Intern Med* **6**:517-521, 1910.

Jison ML, Munson PJ, Barb JJ, et al.: Blood mononuclear cell gene expression profiles characterize the oxidant, hemolytic and inflammatory stress of sickle cell disease. *Blood* **104**:270-280, 2004.

Josephs R: Research on sickle cell hemoglobin, virtual tour of sickle hemoglobin polymerization. Laboratory for Electron Microscopy at the University of Chicago, 1999. Available at: *http://gingi.uchicago.edu/sc2-tour1.htm*, 2004.

Lenfant C, National Institutes of Health, National Heart Lung and Blood Institute: The Management of Sickle Cell Disease. 2002. Publication No. 02-2117. Available at: *www.nhlbi.nih.gov/health/prof/blood/sickle/sc_mngt.pdf*, 2004.

Locatelli F, Stefano PD: New insights into haematopoietic stem cell transplantation for patients with haemoglobinopathies. *Br J Haematol* **125**:3-11, 2004.

Manci EA, Culberson DE, Yang YM, et al., and Investigators of the Cooperative Study of Sickle Cell Disease: Causes of death in sickle cell disease: an autopsy study. *Br J Haematol* **123**:359-365, 2003.

Mason VR: Sickle cell anemia. *JAMA* **79**:1318-1320; 1922.

Neel JV: The inheritance of sickle cell anemia. *Science* **110**:64-65, 1949.

Old JM: Screening and genetic diagnosis of haemoglobin disorders. *Blood Rev* **17**:43-53, 2003.

Roberts I: The role of hydroxyurea in sickle cell disease. *Br J Haematol.* **120**:177-186, 2003.

Serjeant GR: The emerging understanding of sickle cell disease. *Br J Haematol* **112**:3-18, 2001.

Serjeant GR, Serjeant BE: *Sickle Cell Disease*. 3rd ed. Oxford University Press, New York, 2001.

Steinberg MH, Forget BG, Higgs DR, et al.: *Disorders of Hemoglobin*. Cambridge University Press, Cambridge, UK, 2001.

Vichinsky EP, Neumayr LD, Earles AN, et al.: Causes and outcomes of the acute chest syndrome in sickle cell disease. National Acute Chest Syndrome Study Group. *N Engl J Med* **342**:1855-1865, 2000.

Walters MC, Storb R, Patience M, et al.: Impact of bone marrow transplantation for symptomatic sickle cell disease: an interim report. Multicenter investigation of bone marrow transplantation for sickle cell disease. *Blood* **95**:1918-1924, 2000.

Weatherall DJ: Towards molecular medicine: reminiscences of the haemoglobin field, 1960-2000. *Br J Haematol.* **115**:729-738, 2001.

Osteogenesis Imperfecta

ARMANDO FLOR-CISNEROS and SERGEY LEIKIN

CASE REPORTS

Patient 1

The patient is a 1.5-year-old white female admitted to the NIH Clinical Center for evaluation of bone deformities in the lower extremities, generalized osteopenia, and a recent left femur fracture. She was the product of an uncomplicated, full-term pregnancy delivered by cesarean section and was born with normal Apgar scores and a birth weight of 2954 g (normal for full-term newborns). A prenatal ultrasound done at 35 weeks of gestation suggested shortening and bowing of femurs, tibias, and fibulas and rhizomelic proportions (shortening of proximal limb segments) of the upper extremities. Her perinatal hospital course was uncomplicated. However, she was noted to have bilateral clavicle fractures at birth.

The past medical history was significant for a dislocated left elbow at 6 months of age that resolved spontaneously, left femur fracture at 16 months of age that occurred while she was trying to pull up to stand, and chronic sinusitis due to an underdeveloped ethmoidal-sphenoid sinus (air-filled cavity in the skull behind the bridge of the nose). Her psychosocial development appeared normal. She was able to crawl and scoot but could not cruise yet.

On physical examination, her height was 63.6 cm (<3rd percentile for chronological age and 50th percentile for a child aged 4 months). Her weight was 7.2 kg (<3rd percentile for chronological age and 50th percentile for a child aged 6 months), and head circumference was 46.2 cm (45th percentile). Her skull shape was normal with slightly triangular facies and a flattened midface. Her anterior fontanelle was open; measuring 3 × 2 cm. Sclera hue was light blue with normal reflexes and extraocular movements. Her ears were in normal position and shape, and her oral examination revealed seven erupted gray-translucent pointed teeth. Her heart, lungs, and abdominal examination were normal. Her spine was straight, and her upper extremities had no major deformities. Examination of her lower extremities revealed mild bowing of both femurs and anterior bowing of her tibias. Both upper and lower extremities had normal range of motion with no muscle contractures. Her neurological exam was entirely normal.

Her initial x-rays (babygram) revealed osteopenia (low bone mineral density) throughout the bony structures. There were deformities of multiple thoracolumbar vertebral bodies (bony segments of upper and lower spine), and her ribs appeared thin. The proximal left femur and distal right femur showed mild anterolateral bowing. Anterior bowing of both tibias and fibulas was also seen. A bone densitometry study of the L1–L4 spine done at 3 years of age was 6.66 standard deviations below the mean for children of the same age.

Patient 2

The second child was a 9-month-old white female admitted to the NIH Clinical Center for evaluation of multiple long-bone fractures. She was born to a 31-year-old mother with a previous spontaneous miscarriage. The patient was the product of a normal pregnancy born at 38 weeks of gestation with pronounced craniotabes (softening of the skull bones) and a large posterior fontanelle. The delivery was vaginal with normal Apgar scores and a birth weight of 2800 g. At 4 weeks of age, the baby was admitted to the local hospital for irritability and inconsolable crying. Physical examination at that time revealed an infant with swollen bilateral upper leg areas and a flaccid right arm. A bone survey revealed generalized osteopenia, bilateral femur and right tibia midshaft fracture, right humerus fracture, a right clavicle fracture with new callous formation, and an old posterior fifth rib fracture. Her past medical history was significant for poor weight gain and growth, constipation, and an umbilical hernia. At 5 months, she fractured her left humerus, and 3 months later she fractured both femurs again.

On physical examination, her weight was 5.8 kg (<3rd percentile for chronological age and 50th percentile for a child aged 4 months), her height was 63 cm (<3rd percentile for chronological age and 50th percentile for a child aged 4 months), and her head circumference was 45 cm (50th percentile). Her head showed a flattened occiput with frontal bossing, a triangular face with small chin and a wide-open anterior fontanelle measuring 4 × 6 cm (abnormally enlarged for age). Her sclerae were blue, and her ears were low set and posteriorly rotated. Her heart and lungs were normal. Her chest had a pectus carinatum shape (protruding chest), and her abdomen showed a small umbilical hernia. Examination of her upper extremities revealed moderate bowing of right and left humerus and left ulna. Her lower extremities showed pronounced bowing of right and left femurs and distal left tibia.

Her x-ray series revealed generalized undermineralization throughout the bony structures. Her ribs were thin, and the spine showed the presence of multiple compression fractures at the thoracolumbar level. There was marked bowing of all extremities with evidence of old fractures in femurs, humerus, and left ulna. A bone mineral density study of the lumbar vertebral bodies (L1–L4) performed at 5 years of age revealed a value of 6.57 standard deviations below the mean for children of the same age.

DIAGNOSIS

The clinical presentation and the radiological abnormalities seen in both patients suggested a moderately severe form of osteogenesis imperfecta (OI) with moderate bone fragility in patient 1 and a severe, progressively deforming form of OI in patient 2. OI—also known as brittle bone disease—is a relatively rare (~1 per 10,000 for all types of OI), heterogeneous group of heritable disorders (Table 3-1) characterized by bone fragility, usually accompanied by other connective tissue abnormalities (Byers and Cole, 2002).

Many epidemiological, clinical, genetic, and biochemical studies have been conducted since the first widely recognized descriptions of OI in the 18th century. The disease has been shown to be caused by defective synthesis of type I collagen, a triple helical protein made from two $\alpha1(I)$- and one $\alpha2(I)$-chains with fibers that form the structural frame of bone matrix.

Table 3-1. Clinical Heterogeneity and Inheritance of Osteogenesis Imperfecta

OI Type	Clinical Features	Inheritance
I	Normal stature; little or no deformity; blue sclerae; hearing loss in 50% of individuals; dentinogenesis imperfecta rare but may distinguish a subset	AD
II	Lethal in the perinatal period; minimal calvarial mineralization; thin beaded ribs; marked long bone deformity; platyspondyly	AD (new mutations) with parental mosaicism
III	Progressively deforming bones, usually with moderate deformity at birth; extreme short stature; sclerae variable in hue, often lighten with age; common dentinogenesis imperfecta and hearing loss	AD with parental mosaicism; autosomal recessive (rare)
IV	Mild-to-moderate bone deformity; variable short stature; white or blue sclerae; common dentinogenesis imperfecta; hearing loss in some patients	AD with parental mosaicism
V	Bone fragility; mild-to-moderate short stature; no dentinogenesis imperfecta; radioulnar synostosis; hyperplastic callus formation	Probably AD

AD, autosomal dominant.

Abnormal electrophoretic mobility confirmed the presence of defects in type I collagen from both patients (see next section). Subsequent DNA sequencing revealed a glycine-to-serine substitution at helical position 238 in the α2(I)-chain from patient 1 and a similar substitution at helical position 193 in the α1(I)-chain from patient 2.

Sillence Classification of Osteogenesis Imperfecta

Although the majority of OI cases are caused by type I collagen mutations, current approach to clinical diagnosis of different OI forms is still based on family history and physical and radiographic findings rather than biochemical analyses or underlying pathophysiological mechanisms. The original Sillence classification (Sillence et al., 1979) distinguishes four different types of OI.

OI type I is the mildest and most common form of the disease, with autosomal dominant mode of inheritance. Affected individuals usually have blue sclerae and mild-to-moderate bone fragility prior to puberty. Fractures rarely occur *in utero*. During infancy and childhood, the fractures are related to moderate trauma. The height of individuals with type I OI is usually normal or near normal. About half have early hearing loss that usually starts in the late teens and may progress to severe loss by adulthood. Type I OI is subdivided based on the absence (IA) or presence (IB) of dentinogenesis imperfecta. Additional clinical findings for OI type I are mitral valve prolapse, easy bruising, and hyperextensibility of large joints.

OI type II is the most severe form of the disease, leading to fetal demise or death in the perinatal period. It is caused mostly by new, dominant mutations. The small rate of recurrence of this phenotype among siblings is most consistent with parental mosaicism. Infants are usually stillborn or born prematurely with both weight and length small for their gestational age. If they survive birth, then affected infants usually die of respiratory failure within the first 2 months of life. Type II OI is characterized by triangular face, flat midface, small beaked nose, and bluish-gray sclerae. The head is large for body size with an extremely soft calvarium and a large anterior and posterior fontanelle. The thorax is deformed and small with a narrow apex. Radiographic examination reveals multiple *in utero* fractures in various stages of healing. The long bones are osteopenic, cylindrical, and deformed with very little cortex.

OI type III or progressively deforming OI (Fig. 3-1B, 3-1D) is the most severe form of the disease compatible with life beyond infancy. The majority of cases appear to result from dominant mutations, but rare autosomal recessive cases have also been reported. Affected individuals are recognized after birth because of long bone fractures and cranial abnormalities (as seen in patient 2). Many individuals with type III OI die in childhood or in adulthood due to respiratory, cardiac, or neurological complications. Those who survive exhibit gradual deformity of the long bones and spine with pronounced vertebral compression. Patients with type III OI have extreme growth deficiency; adults have the height of prepubertal children. Clinically, these individuals usually have macrocephaly (increased head circumference) and a triangular, flat midface. The sclera is initially bluish and whitens with age. Radiographically, there is generalized osteoporosis, wormian bones (irregular plates of bone interposed in the sutures between the large cranial bones), and "codfish" vertebra. As childhood progresses, a flared long bone metaphysis develops, and the long bones appear thin, twisted, and cylindrical.

OI type IV (Fig. 3-1A, 3-1C) envelops a large spectrum of moderately severe forms of dominantly inherited disorders characterized by mild-to-moderate bone fragility. Some children with type IV OI have prenatal fractures and deformity at birth, while others have mild-to-moderate bowing. During childhood, they may have several fractures per year. The fracture frequency usually declines after puberty. In addition to osteoporosis, these individuals have modeling abnormalities of the long bones, and about one third of patients develop progressive scoliosis. Clinically, these patients have variable short stature, grayish to normal sclerae, and macrocephaly. Similar to type I, OI type IV is also subdivided into type IVA and IV B based on dentinogenesis imperfecta (abnormal dentin formation). The clinical and radiological findings for patient 1 are most consistent with OI type IV.

Additional OI types

Since the original classification was proposed, 25 years of studies revealed difficulties in separating the wide and nearly continuum spectrum

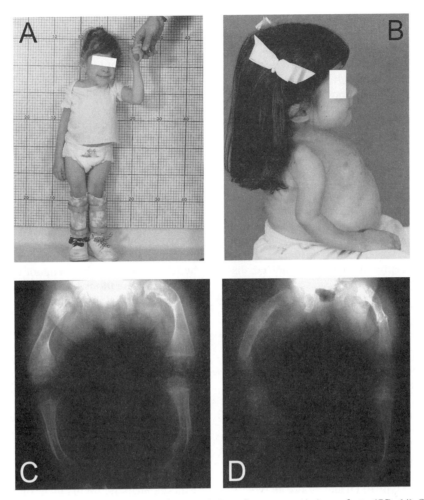

Figure 3-1. (*A*), (*B*) Phenotypic characteristics of osteogenesis imperfecta (OI): (*A*) OI type IV and (*B*) OI type III. (*C*), (*D*) Radiographs of the long bones of the lower limbs: (*C*) patient 1 with type IV OI and (*D*) patient 2 with the deforming type III OI.

of OI phenotypes into four distinct categories. Most commonly, patients not fitting more narrowly defined types I–III are diagnosed with type IV OI, resulting in a rather broad range of clinical and radiological findings within this category. However, several new OI types were proposed based on differences in bone histology observed within the Sillence type IV group (Rauch and Glorieux, 2004).

OI type V is now widely recognized as a distinct OI phenotype with characteristic clinical and radiological features, such as predisposition to formation of hypertrophic callus at sites of fractures or surgical interventions, early calcification of the interosseous membrane of the forearm, and appearance of dense metaphyseal bands in radiographs. Patients have moderate

bone fragility, white sclerae, and no dentinogenesis imperfecta. Their histological examination reveals a characteristic, meshlike bone lamellation pattern. Type V OI has an autosomal dominant inheritance pattern, but no evidence of type I collagen abnormalities has been found.

Unusual histological findings of increased osteoid formation and abnormal, "fish scale" bone lamellation pattern were used to suggest a new type VI OI (Rauch and Glorieux, 2004). So far, these findings were reported in fewer than a dozen patients, and the mode of inheritance of the disorder was not established. Another peculiar disorder with recessive inheritance (unusual for type IV OI) was observed in a community of Native Americans in northern Quebec (Rauch and Glorieux, 2004). In these patients, bone fragility was accompanied by prominent short-ening of proximal limb segments (rhizomelia) and a decrease in the femoral neck shaft angle (coxa vara). The mutation was localized to chromosome 3p22-24.1, outside the loci for type I collagen genes. The authors of this study proposed to classify this disorder as type VII OI. There is little doubt regarding the merits of grouping OI cases with distinct histological and genetic findings. However, so far these cases have not been demonstrated to have distinct clinical and radiological features common for many unrelated patients, which could be used as phenotype criteria following the tradition established by the original Sillence classification. Therefore, the available information is still not sufficient for determining whether these groups truly represent newly recognized distinct Sillence types of OI.

BIOCHEMICAL PERSPECTIVE

Since OI is a dominant genetic disorder, a cure for it would require repair, removal, or inactivation of the affected genes—a daunting task likely to require many years of research (Prockop, 2004). However, the same mutations often cause drastically different OI phenotypes, for instance, several patients with the same Gly238Ser substitution in $\alpha2$(I)-chain as patient 1 but different symptoms were described, including severe type III OI and moderate type IV OI. One case was even originally classified as mild type I OI. Large variation in the OI severity was also found in unrelated patients with identical mutations, within affected families, and in the *Brtl* mouse model of OI (Forlino et al., 1999). These observations suggest that better knowledge of OI biochemistry underlying the phenotype variability might lead to simpler pharmacological treatments, reducing severity of the disease. Some progress in understanding molecular origins of OI has been made, but much remains to be discovered before such treatments become a reality.

Osteogenesis Imperfecta Mutations

The overwhelming majority of OI cases are caused by mutations in COL1A1 and COL1A2 encoding the $\alpha1$(I)- and $\alpha2$(I)-chains of type I collagen, respectively. Several hundred different OI mutations were described (see, e.g., an online mutation database at *www.le.ac.uk/genetics/collagen/*; Dalgleish, 1998). Based on their effect on collagen synthesis, these mutations can be separated into three groups: COL1A1 and COL1A2 "null allele" and structural mutations.

COL1A1 null allele mutations do not produce mutant collagen. Instead, the affected allele fails to produce functional $\alpha1$(I)-chains, and cells make about half the normal amount of collagen. Insufficient synthesis of normal collagen is believed to be the primary cause of type I OI (Byers and Cole, 2002).

COL1A2 null allele mutations produce collagen that has three $\alpha1$(I)-chains rather than two $\alpha1$(I)- and one $\alpha2$(I)-chains (50% of all type I collagen in heterozygous and 100% in homozygous cases). The $\alpha1$(I)-homotrimer does have a "normal" role, but only as a minor collagen in fetal tissues. Mutations that result in exclusive synthesis of $\alpha1$(I)-homotrimers cause rare recessive forms of OI and Ehlers-Danlos syndrome (Schwarze et al., 2004).

Structural mutations in COL1A1 or COL1A2 produce abnormal type I collagen with substitutions, deletions, or insertions of amino acids. Mutations of this group usually cause type II, III, or IV OI (Byers and Cole, 2002). However, patients with phenotype closer to type I OI were also reported (e.g., one with the same Gly238Ser substitution as patient 1). By far the most common type of structural mutations (>80%) is substitutions of "obligatory" glycines as in patients 1 and 2; these mutations are the focus of this chapter.

Collagen Structure and Stability

The obligatory glycines are located in every third position of the collagen triple helix. They are required for maintaining the structural integrity of mature type I collagen molecule, which consists of a long triple helix (1014 amino acid) flanked by short (11–26 amino acids), nonhelical peptides. Preponderance of glycine substitutions indicates that disruptions of the triple helix structure are the primary cause of moderate, severe, and lethal OI. However, the relationship between structural defects and OI symptoms is not straightforward, as illustrated by studies of collagen thermal stability.

In particular, the triple helix irreversibly denatures within minutes at 41°C–42°C unless it is incorporated into fibers, where it becomes substantially more stable (Leikina et al., 2002). Structural defects caused by OI mutations reduce the denaturation temperature T_m, some by

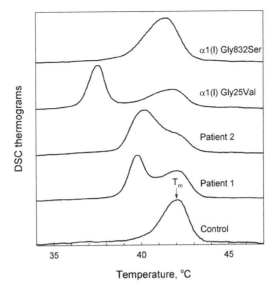

Figure 3-2. Analysis of collagen thermal stability by differential scanning calorimetry (DSC). DSC measures the heat of denaturation on temperature variation at a constant scanning rate (here 0.125°C/min). DSC thermogram of normal (control) collagen has a single denaturation peak with the apparent denaturation temperature $T_m \approx 42$°C. Additional peaks with lower T_m in DSC tracings from patients 1 and 2 are associated with mutant molecules. Patient 2 collagen molecules with one and two mutant α1(I)-chains have a similar T_m, so only one broadened mutant peak is observed. The fraction of mutant molecules can be estimated from the area under the corresponding peak (e.g., 45% ± 5% mutant in patient 1 and 70% ± 5% mutant in patient 2). Some mutations reduce the apparent T_m to normal core body temperature or even below it (e.g., $T_m \approx 37.5$°C for α1(I)-Gly25Val substitution). Other mutations have minimal effect on T_m (e.g., only a single broadened peak of mutant and normal collagen is observed for α1(I)-Gly832Ser).

as much as 5°C–6°C (Fig. 3-2). At least in model, collagenlike peptides, larger changes in T_m correlate with larger structural disruptions of the triple helix (Beck et al., 2000). The change in T_m might also directly affect fibrillogenesis and matrix formation (e.g., if T_m drops below normal body temperature and molecules denature before they have a chance to form fibers). Thus, one could expect T_m changes to correlate with the severity of OI, but no such correlations were found (Bachinger et al., 1993). It was argued that the T_m values traditionally measured by triple-helix susceptibility to proteolytic enzymes might be unreliable. However, our studies of several dozen mutations by differential scanning calorimetry (DSC) did not produce any correlations as well (DSC is widely accepted as the most reliable and accurate technique for T_m measurement). For instance, despite the phenotype differences, DSC tracings showed the same 2°C change in T_m for both of our patients (Fig. 3-2). A smaller T_m change (≤1°C) is observed in a

patient with an α1(I)-Gly832Ser substitution, and a much larger change (~5°C) is seen in a patient with an α1(I)-Gly25Val substitution, although both patients have type IV OI.

Chain Synthesis and Association

To understand how structural defects in collagen could cause OI, we need to follow the collagen fiber synthesis pathway (Fig. 3-3). It starts from synthesis of precursor (procollagen) chains. Association of two pro-α1(I)- and one pro-α2(I)-chains at their C-propeptides initiates procollagen folding, which proceeds in a zipperlike manner from C- to N-terminal end of the molecule (Engel and Prockop, 1991). These processes occur inside the endoplasmic reticulum (ER) and are assisted by a variety of ER chaperones and enzymes (Lamande and Bateman, 1999).

Substitutions of the obligatory glycines do not affect collagen chain synthesis and association. Thus, heterozygous substitutions in α2(I) should

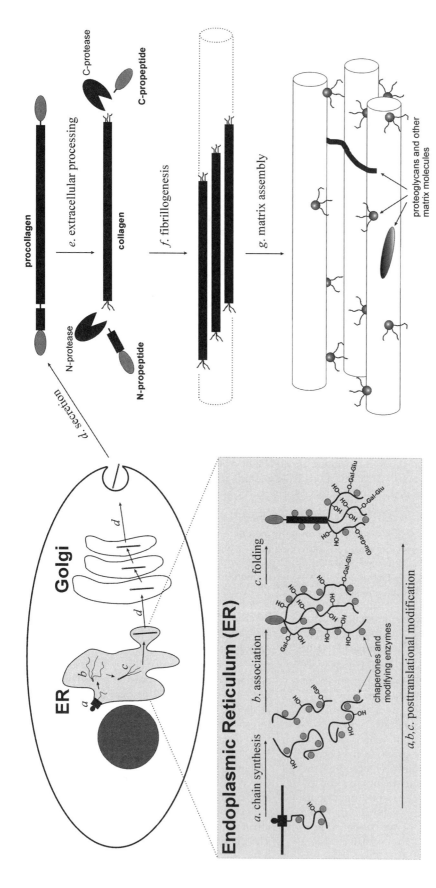

Figure 3-3. Collagen matrix synthesis pathway. Type I collagen precursor (procollagen) is a heterotrimer of two pro-α1(I)- and one pro-α2(I)-chains. It is synthesized and folded within endoplasmic reticulum (ER) (steps *a* through *c*). Procollagen folding is triggered by association of fully synthesized chains at C-propeptides (*b*). It proceeds in a zipperlike manner from C- to N-terminal end (*c*). Chain synthesis, association, and folding processes are assisted by chaperones and are accompanied by hydroxylation of proline residues within Xaa-Pro-Gly triplets, hydroxylation of some lysine residues, and glycosylation of hydroxylysine residues. Folded procollagen is transported from ER through Golgi and secreted from cells (*d*). Mature collagen is a 300-nm long triple helix flanked by short (11–26 amino acids) nonhelical peptides. It is formed by cleavage of C- and N-propeptides from procollagen by specialized proteases (*e*). Propeptide cleavage triggers self-assembly of collagen triple helices into fibrils (*f*). The fibrils bind proteoglycans and other molecules (*g*) and assemble into a complex fiber network, which serves as a matrix for bone and other connective tissues.

generate 50% molecules with one mutant chain and 50% normal molecules (assuming equal expression of both alleles). Mutations in α1(I) should also generate 50% molecules with one mutant chain, but only 25% normal molecules and 25% molecules with two mutant chains.

Interestingly, glycine substitutions in α1(I) generally lead to more severe OI than similar substitutions at the same site in α2(I). This effect might be caused by a larger amount of defective collagen produced by α1(I)-mutations and could explain the more severe phenotype of patient 2 compared to patient 1. However, it cannot explain the phenotype variation in cases with the same α2(I)-Gly238Ser substitution.

Procollagen Folding

Procollagen folding is preceded by hydroxylation of prolines in Y positions of sequential Gly-Xaa-Yaa triplets and is accompanied by hydroxylation and glycosylation of some lysines within unfolded regions of procollagen chains. Folding of collagen molecules with glycine substitutions proceeds normally from the C-terminus up to the mutation site, where it stops (Engel and Prockop, 1991). Folding resumes only after a conformation of the chains accommodating the mutation is found, and helix formation is renucleated. The resulting prolonged exposure of unfolded chains on the N-terminal side of the mutation to ER enzymes leads to excessive hydroxylation and glycosylation of lysine residues. This *posttranslational overmodification* is the hallmark of structural mutations. It is usually detected by slower migration of collagen chains and their CNBr fragments in gel electrophoresis (Fig. 3-4).

The overmodification of collagen from patients 1 and 2 is weak because it occurs only on the N-terminal side of the mutation. Mutations located closer to the C-terminal end lead to substantially larger overhydroxylation and overglycosylation. In principle, this overmodification gradient could explain milder OI symptoms observed for N-terminal glycine substitutions (e.g., almost no lethal substitutions in the N-terminal quarter of collagen were reported, and many of these cases were classified as type I OI). However, no consistent severity gradient and no correlations of symptoms with overmodification were found for mutations located further toward the C-terminal end. Thus, the role of overmodification in OI phenotype still remains unclear.

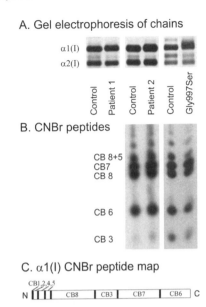

A. Gel electrophoresis of chains

B. CNBr peptides

C. α1(I) CNBr peptide map

Figure 3-4. Gel electrophoresis of (*A*) collagen chains and (*B*) α1(I) CNBr peptides (B) and (*C*) location of different cyanogen bromide (CNBr) fragments on α1(I)-chain. Posttranslational overmodification can be detected from slower migration of mutant chains in (*A*) or asymmetric shape of CB spots in (*B*). The spots correspond to peptides obtained by CNBr digestion of α1(I)-bands and electrophoresis in a second, perpendicular direction. Slower migration of overmodified, mutant α1(I)-chains is clearly visible in the Gly997Ser lane in (*A*) but barely detectable in patients 1 and 2 due to substantially weaker overmodification (typical for mutations in the first 200–300 amino acids from the N-terminal end). Correspondingly, all α1(I)-CNBr peptides from Gly997Ser collagen appear to be overmodified. In collagen from patient 2, only CB 8+5 has the characteristic asymmetric shape. Since only the fragments located on the N-terminal side of the mutation are overmodified, analysis of CNBr fragments allows estimation of approximate mutation location. For instance, Gly997Ser mutation at the C-terminal end of the molecule causes overmodification of all CNBr peptides, while Gly193Ser mutation in patient 2 causes overmodification of CB 8+5 but not CB 6, CB 7, CB 3, or CB 8.

Secretion

After completion of folding, procollagen is transferred from ER, transported through the Golgi system, and secreted from cell (Kadler, 1994). Abnormal protein is retained within ER and targeted for degradation. Some mutant molecules are recognized as abnormal and destroyed, while others escape the quality control system and are secreted. The outcome varies from significant retention to complete secretion depending on the mutation. The retention and degradation of mutant molecules puts an extra stress on collagen-producing cells, potentially explaining their reduced activity and viability commonly observed in OI.

Characterization of intracellular retention/degradation is important but often challenging. Unlike Gly → Cys substitutions, which can be selectively labeled by [^{35}S]-Cys, chains with Gly → Ser substitutions are difficult to distinguish by simple biochemical assays. Sometimes an increased ratio of type III/type I collagen in fibroblast culture media is used as an indicator of abnormal secretion of type I molecules, but the results should be confirmed by other methods. For patients 1 and 2, the type III/type I ratio was within the "normal" range of 10%–15%. To confirm the secretion and to estimate the retained/degraded fraction, we used the change in T_m of mutant molecules. From deconvolution of mutant and normal peaks in DSC thermograms, we found that more than 80% of mutant molecules were secreted (Fig. 3-2).

Extracellular Processing

Secreted procollagen undergoes additional processing by specialized enzymes that cleave N- and C-propeptides and convert some lysine and hydroxylysine residues into reactive allysyl aldehydes (Kadler, 1994). Most glycine substitutions do not affect these reactions. However, several cases with slow or incomplete cleavage of N-propeptides due to altered conformation of the cleavage site were reported. The conformational change can be caused by mutations in the adjacent N-terminal part of the triple helix as well as by long-range structural rearrangements (such as a chain register shift) induced by glycine substitutions located even several hundred residues away. Delayed or incomplete N-propeptide cleavage leads to incorporation of uncleaved molecules, limiting the thickness of collagen fibers. The resulting reduction in the fiber mechanical strength might cause more severe joint laxity and hyperextensibility than usually observed in OI (resembling type VII Ehlers-Danlos syndrome associated with N-propeptide cleavage site mutations).

In vitro testing of fibroblast procollagen from patients 1 and 2 showed normal cleavage by purified bovine N-proteinase, indicating that these mutations do not induce long-range structural changes propagating all the way to the N-terminal end of the triple helix.

Intermolecular Interactions and Fibrillogenesis

Propeptide cleavage triggers collagen self-assembly into fibers. The fibers are stabilized by cross-linking of allysyl aldehydes with lysine residues on adjacent collagen helices. They bind proteoglycans and other matrix molecules and organize into a complex three-dimensional network serving as a scaffold for bone mineralization (Kadler, 1994).

All information needed for fiber self-assembly is encoded within the collagen triple helix. For instance, a solution of purified helices in a physiological buffer forms nativelike fibers when heated to body temperature. Structural defects introduced by mutations might disrupt interactions that govern the self-assembly process, potentially explaining altered *in vitro* fiber formation observed for OI collagens. However, because collagens from only one control and one patient with a given mutation are typically compared in such studies, effects of different genetic background of the two individuals cannot be excluded (e.g., variations in the sites and the extent of posttranslational modification). A systematic study of interactions between mutant type I collagen helices has so far been performed only for the *Brtl* mouse model of OI with an α1(I)-Gly349 → Cys substitution (Kuznetsova et al., 2004). A wide variation of *in vitro* fibrillogenesis of tissue collagens from animals with the same genotype but different genetic background was observed, but no statistically significant difference between the mutant and wild type was found. The absence of changes in interactions between type I collagen molecules was confirmed by direct measurement of intermolecular forces. Still, it remains unclear whether this is just a peculiar feature of this particular mutation.

In vivo, type III, type V, and other collagens are also incorporated into fibers, although in smaller quantities (dependent on the tissue). Interactions of type I collagen with them appears to be important for formation and functional properties of the fibers. Glycine substitutions might affect these interactions directly as well as by altering the composition of the collagen mix secreted by collagen-producing cells. An elevated content of type III collagen was observed in tissues and cell cultures from OI patients, but no systematic studies of interactions between type III and type I collagens and their role in OI phenotype were reported. In the *Brtl* mice, we found substantial variations in the content of type III collagen in different tissues and fibroblast cultures, but no statistically significant correlations with the animal phenotype.

In addition to other collagens, at least several dozen matrix molecules are known to interact with type I helices. Some understanding of these interactions (e.g., likely locations of binding sites) has been developed (Di Lullo et al., 2002). Disruption of these interactions by OI mutations within the binding sites might explain, for instance, the appearance of distinct lethal and nonlethal regions of glycine substitutions in the $\alpha 2(I)$-chain (Forlino and Marini, 2000). However, no direct confirmation of this hypothesis has so far been reported. For instance, collagen-proteoglycan interactions are believed to play an important role in bone formation and mineralization. Based on the proposed binding site map (Di Lullo et al., 2002), the $\alpha 2(I)$-Gly238 → Ser mutation of patient 1 is located within a region where no sites have been discovered so far. The $\alpha 1(I)$-Gly193 is located within a proposed decorin-binding region. Its substitution might contribute to more severe symptoms of patient 2, but without corroborating evidence, this is just a speculation.

Molecular Mechanisms of Pathology

In summary, substitutions of obligatory glycine residues alter the structure of collagen triple helix. It has now been widely accepted that structural changes in type I collagen affect osteoblast function by causing reduced thermal stability, slower folding, posttranslational overmodification, and intracellular retention/degradation of procollagen molecules. These changes also affect interactions of type I collagen molecules with each other, with other collagens, and with other matrix molecules. Abnormal activity and viability of osteoblasts and abnormal extracellular interactions of secreted mutant collagens lead to abnormal bone matrix formation and bone fragility. This picture of molecular defects contributing to OI is reasonably clear. However, no consistent correlations of OI phenotype and severity with any specific defects have been found so far.

Animal Models

Probably one of the most important factors hindering studies of the phenotype-genotype relationship has been the lack of good animal models. Presently, only one nonlethal mouse OI model (the *Brtl* mouse) with a Gly349 → Cys substitution knocked into one col1a1 allele is available (Forlino et al., 1999). The initial biochemical and biophysical study of collagen from this model (Kuznetsova et al., 2004) revealed significant variations of posttranslational overmodification (hence, likely the rate of folding), intracellular retention and degradation, and intermolecular interactions of OI collagens within the same genotype. The properties of collagen purified from cell cultures and different tissues originating from the same animal were significantly different. For instance, femur collagen had substantially larger extent of posttranslational modification, higher T_m and different *in vitro* fibrillogenesis kinetics compared to skin or fibroblast collagen. Furthermore, a significant animal-to-animal variation, exceeding the difference between mutant and wild-type animals, was observed.

Thus, many of the biochemical abnormalities are tissue specific and are significantly affected by the genetic background of the animal, stressing the need for systematic biochemical analysis of collagen from many individuals (animals) with the same or similar mutations and different genetic background. Only then can we hope to understand the genotype-phenotype relationship, determine the molecular origins of phenotype variability within the same OI genotype, and rationally design effective pharmacological treatments.

THERAPY

In general, the mainstay conventional clinical management of OI is to facilitate the achievement of gross motor skills, including ambulation and head control, and to maximize skills for independent living. In patients with type III and IV, this is best accomplished by early intensive physical rehabilitation and by orthopedic intervention as needed. Gross motor skills are delayed in OI due to muscle weakness and joint laxity. Patients with moderate OI who have potential for independent walking should have protected ambulation with a combination of bracing, surgical correction, and physical therapy beginning as early as possible.

Patients with OI should be under the care of an orthopedic surgeon with experience in management of OI. Bone fractures and deformities can be managed by a combination of splinting, cast immobilization, and intramedullary rodding to provide anatomic positioning of extremities and to prevent loss of function. The aim of surgery is to correct bowing and interrupt the fracture and refracture cycle. The classical surgical approach is to perform multiple osteotomies with realignment of long bone sections and fixation with intramedullary rods (Byers and Cole, 2002).

The search for beneficial pharmacological treatment of OI with the goal to reduce the rate of fractures and promote longitudinal growth continues. Several uncontrolled studies of bisphosphonates as a potential monotherapy for OI have caused great excitement in the OI community (Glorieux et al., 1998). Cyclic pamindronate infusions have been widely used as an off-label treatment of OI. This drug is a potent nitrogen-containing bisphosphonate that is internalized by osteoclasts. It inhibits enzymes of the mevalonate pathway, thereby preventing the biosynthesis of isoprenoid compounds that are essential for the posttranslational modification of small GTP-binding proteins. The inhibition of protein prenylation and disruption of key regulatory proteins explain the loss of osteoclast activity. Most of the experience with these compounds is derived from studies in postmenopausal osteoporosis. When used in OI, this drug would not affect the synthesis and deposition of abnormal collagen. Thus, patients with OI might have quantitatively more bone after treatment, but their bone would not be expected to have better structural quality than before drug administration. Uncontrolled studies of pamindronate in children with OI reported increased vertebral height and bone mineral density, decreased fractures, and improved ambulation (Glorieux et al., 1998). Conversely, a recent 2-year placebo-controlled study using the oral bisphosphonate olpandronate reported an increase of spinal bone mineral content but no beneficial effects on the functional outcome in the olpandronate group compared to controls (Sakkers et al., 2004). Moreover, the long-term effects of this drug are still under investigation. Thus, the question of whether bisphosphonates will alter the natural history of OI remains unresolved. More controlled trials are essential to determine if increased bone density is associated with stronger bone, or if increased density correlates with increased brittleness.

QUESTIONS

1. A couple with a history of two pregnancies resulting in children with type II OI sought genetic counseling prior to subsequent pregnancy. Which is the most likely explanation of their pregnancy history?
2. What information and recommendations would you give to the couple described in question 1?
3. The blue coloration is an indication of abnormally thin sclerae. Why is it commonly observed in type I OI?
4. Examination of type I collagen from a patient with type IV OI revealed normal electrophoretic mobility but altered thermal stability. Which region of the molecule is likely to contain the mutation?
5. Why do mutations in C-propeptides cause significant posttranslational overmodification of type I collagen?
6. In 1984, a homozygous patient with a recessive type III OI was described. His cells synthesized nonfunctional α2(I)-chains, and his type I collagen secreted by cells consisted only of that from α1(I)-homotrimers. Recently, several patients with homozygous and compound heterozygous null allele mutations in COL1A2 were described. Their cells produced unstable COL1A2 transcripts and did not synthesize α2(I)-chains. Their cells also secreted only α1(I)-collagen homotrimers, but the phenotype of these patients had prevalent features of the Ehlers-Danlos syndrome rather than OI. What could be the molecular reason for this drastic phenotype difference?
7. Why does a reduction of collagen thermal stability by 6°C prevent incorporation of the corresponding mutant molecules into bone matrix?
8. A teenager with a history of fractures but no skeletal deformities and no acute distress was diagnosed with moderate type IV OI. After learning that radiographic analysis revealed low bone mineral density in their child, the parents inquired about a possibility of bisphosphonate therapy. How would you respond to their inquiry?

Acknowledgments: We are grateful to Joan C. Marini for stimulating discussions and critical comments. The gels in Figure 3-4 were kindly provided by Wayne A. Cabral.

BIBLIOGRAPHY

Bachinger HP, Morris NP, Davis JM: Thermal stability and folding of the collagen triple helix and the effects of mutations in osteogenesis imperfecta on the triple helix of type I collagen. *Am J Med Genet* **45:**152–162, 1993.

Beck K, Chan VC, Shenoy N, et al.: Destabilization of osteogenesis imperfecta collagen-like model peptides correlates with the identity of the residue replacing glycine. *Proc Natl Acad Sci USA* **97:**4273–4278, 2000.

Byers PH, Cole WG: Osteogenesis imperfecta, *in* Royce PM, Steinmann B (eds): *Connective Tissue and Its Heritable Disorders. Molecular, Genetic, and Medical Aspects,* 2nd edition. New York: Wiley-Liss, 2002, pp. 385–430.

Dalgleish R: The Human Collagen Mutation Database 1998. *Nucleic Acids Res* **26:**253–255, 1998.

Di Lullo GA, Sweeney SM, Korkko J, et al.: Mapping the ligand-binding sites and disease-associated mutations on the most abundant protein in the human, type I collagen. *J Biol Chem* **277:**4223–4231, 2002.

Engel J, Prockop DJ: The zipper-like folding of collagen triple helices and the effects of mutations that disrupt the zipper. *Annu Rev Biophys Biophys Chem* **20:**137–152, 1991.

Forlino A, Marini JC: Osteogenesis imperfecta: prospects for molecular therapeutics. *Mol Genet Metab* **71:**225–232, 2000.

Forlino A, Porter FD, Lee EJ, et al.: Use of the Cre/lox recombination system to develop a non-lethal knock-in murine model for osteogenesis imperfecta with an alpha1(I) G349C substitution. Variability in phenotype in BrtlIV mice. *J Biol Chem* **274:**37923–37931, 1999.

Glorieux FH, Bishop NJ, Plotkin H, et al.: Cyclic administration of pamindronate in children with severe osteogenesis imperfecta. *N Engl J Med* **339:**947–952, 1998.

Kadler K: Extracellular matrix 1: fibril-forming collagens. *Prot Profile* **1:**519–638, 1994.

Kuznetsova NV, Forlino A, Cabral WA, et al.: Structure, stability and interactions of type I collagen with GLY349-CYS substitution in α1(I)chain in a murine osteogenesis imperfecta model. *Matrix Biol* **23:**101–112, 2004.

Lamande SR, Bateman JF: Procollagen folding and assembly: the role of endoplasmic reticulum enzymes and molecular chaperones. *Semin Cell Dev Biol* **10:**455–464, 1999.

Leikina E, Mertts MV, Kuznetsova N, et al.: Type I collagen is thermally unstable at body temperature. *Proc Natl Acad Sci USA* **99:**1314–1318, 2002.

Prockop DJ: Targeting gene therapy for osteogenesis imperfecta. *N Engl J Med* **350:**2302–2304, 2004.

Rauch F, Glorieux FH: Osteogenesis imperfecta. *Lancet* **363:**1377–1385, 2004.

Sakkers R, Kok D, Engelberg R, et al.: Skeletal effects and functional outcome with olpadronate in children with osteogenesis imperfecta: a 2 year randomised placebo control study. *Lancet* **363:**1427–1431, 2004.

Schwarze U, Hata R, McKusick VA, et al.: Rare autosomal recessive cardiac valvular form of Ehlers-Danlos syndrome results from mutations in the COL1A2 gene that activate the nonsense-mediated RNA decay pathway. *Am J Hum Genet* **74:**917–930, 2004.

Sillence DO, Senn A, Danks DM: Genetic heterogeneity in osteogenesis imperfecta. *J Med Genet* **16:**101–116, 1979.

4

α_1-Antitrypsin Deficiency

SARAH JANE SCHWARZENBERG and HARVEY L. SHARP

CASE REPORT

The patient was a 35-year-old white male with α_1-antitrypsin deficiency. He received a combined liver-kidney transplant for cirrhosis complicated by portal hypertension, renal insufficiency secondary to membranoproliferative glomerulonephritis, and combined restrictive and obstructive pulmonary disease at age 18 years.

Jaundice and pruritus were observed at age 6 weeks and resolved spontaneously after approximately 2 months. He was hospitalized for pneumonia at age 20 months, and an enlarged liver was noted. A percutaneous needle biopsy specimen from the liver was interpreted to show postnecrotic cirrhosis, although reevaluation of the biopsy specimen showed the presence of globules that were periodic acid–Schiff (PAS) positive, diastase resistant (Fig. 4-1). He was then referred to our institution at age 2.5 years for liver transplantation.

At the time of the initial evaluation, the physical examination revealed a well-developed young boy in no acute distress. He was not jaundiced; however, it was notable that he had a protuberant abdomen with a liver edge palpable 3 cm below the right costal margin in the midclavicular line. The liver was nontender and hard. The spleen was palpable 6 cm below the left costal margin. No other physical abnormalities were noted.

The child's laboratory tests revealed a normal hematological picture except for a platelet count of 122,000/mm³ (below normal). He had normal liver enzymes except for a serum glutamic oxaloacetic transaminase level of 197

units/mL (mildly increased). Both his blood urea nitrogen (BUN) and creatinine levels were normal. The patient's serum protein electrophoresis was abnormal, with a low serum albumin of 2.9 g/dL (normal 3.3–4.6 g/dL) and an α_1-globulin band that was barely visible. Because of this last finding, protease inhibitor (PI) phenotyping was done on the child and his family. The child's phenotype was PIZZ, while both parents had the heterozygote, that is, the PIMZ phenotype. The nomenclature of the PI types is based on the electrophoretic mobility of the various PI types at pH 4.9. PiMM represents the homozygous normal allele; letters alphabetically before M designate anodal variants, and those after M designate cathodal variants.

The child's subsequent course was one of gradual hepatic deterioration. At age 3 years, he was noted to have ascites (intra-abdominal fluid accumulation). This progressed slowly until the age of 6 years, when severe ascites and peripheral edema necessitated the initiation of spironolactone (a potassium-sparing diuretic). Several admissions to the hospital were required over the next 6 years for ascites with scrotal edema. Serum albumin values were persistently low, less than 2.0 g/dL. During this time, the patient also had two episodes of primary peritonitis (intraperitoneal infection) and one episode of α-streptococcal sepsis.

By age 11 years his renal function decreased, as measured by a creatinine clearance of 71 mL/min (normal is 105 mL/min). He also developed protein-losing nephropathy with a 24-hour urinary protein excretion of 600 mg that increased to 14 g after albumin infusions

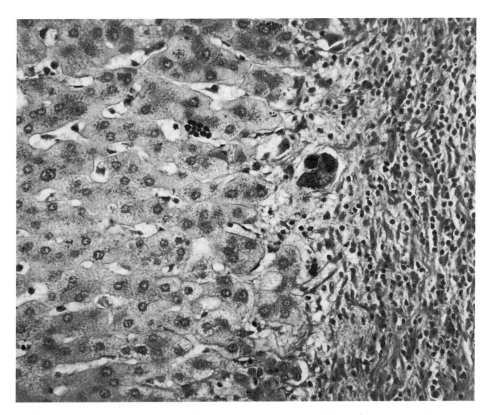

Figure 4-1. Photomicrograph of periportal hepatocytes of liver from patient in case report. Note variation in size and presence of cytoplasmic globules. The stain used is periodic acid–Schiff after diastase.

(normal urinary protein excretion is 100 mg/24 h). Because of abnormal coagulation studies, renal biopsy was deferred; however, the clinical picture was consistent with the membranoproliferative glomerulonephritis seen in α_1-antitrypsin deficiency.

At age 12, the patient was admitted with acute chest pain from a left spontaneous pneumothorax (air within the pleural cavity). This required hospitalization and chest tube insertion, but he recovered without sequelae. After the resolution of this problem, pulmonary function testing revealed findings of both severe airway obstruction and destruction of alveolar lung tissue, consistent with emphysema. No further pulmonary problems occurred until the patient was age 16 years, when he developed occasional episodes of bronchospasm (spasmodic contraction of the smooth muscles of the bronchus). Pulmonary function studies at that time, though improved from those immediately following his pneumothorax, still revealed combined obstructive and destructive lung disease.

Also at about age 12 years, the patient began

to experience episodes of acute hepatic encephalopathy (graded onset of coma brought on by circulating false neurotransmitters). The first of these episodes was the most severe. The patient entered the hospital in a confused and disoriented state and with an elevated ammonia level. The immediate problem was easily controlled with neomycin (a nonabsorbable antibiotic that kills intestinal, ammonia-forming bacteria) enemas. During this admission, gastrointestinal bleeding developed, exacerbating the hyperammonemia (plasma ammonia of 450 μmol/L; normal < 35 μmol/L). The patient gradually slipped into grade IV hepatic coma with fundoscopic changes consistent with increased intracranial pressure. Coagulopathy (increased bleeding tendency) prevented placement of an intracranial pressure monitor. He was treated empirically for presumed cerebral edema associated with acute hepatic encephalopathy with hyperventilation, a mannitol drip, and barbiturate coma. The patient recovered without neurological sequelae. Despite protein restriction (1.0 g protein per kilogram body weight per day), the patient had two other milder episodes of hyperammonemia over that year. He continued on limited protein intake, neomycin, and lactulose, with periodic monitoring for subclinical hepatic encephalopathy by electroencephalography.

Despite these complications of α_1-antitrypsin deficiency, he maintained an active life, attending school and camping with his parents. By the age of 16 years, his renal condition had deteriorated considerably, with a creatinine clearance of only 23 mL/min. He was therefore accepted as a candidate for a combined liver-kidney transplant. After a 2-year wait for an immunologically compatible donor, the transplant was successfully performed at age 18 years at the University of Minnesota Hospitals. He completed high school and was employed full time in good health for over a decade.

Seventeen years after his transplant, he was found to have cirrhosis from hepatitis C, likely acquired from the many blood transfusions he required prior to and during his transplantation. He died awaiting a second hepatic transplant.

DIAGNOSIS

This patient illustrates a complicated clinical course of α_1-antitrypsin deficiency. Our patient had liver disease that presented during infancy and developed into hepatic cirrhosis. He exhibited most of the complications of cirrhosis, including portal hypertension with ascites, hyperammonemia, malnutrition, and variceal hemorrhage. These complications of cirrhosis are not unique to α_1-antitrypsin deficiency, but it is important to note the potential severity of the liver disease associated with this condition.

α_1-Antitrypsin deficiency is suspected in three clinical situations:

1. Cholestasis in infancy (see Fig. 4-2).
2. Cirrhosis of undetermined etiology at any age.
3. Emphysema early in life, especially if predominantly basilar.

Liver disease is commonly associated with α_1-antitrypsin deficiency and may develop at any age. Approximately 10% to 20% of α_1-antitrypsin-deficient infants with the phenotype PIZZ are first seen for neonatal cholestatic liver disease, as was the child in this case report. Conjugated hyperbilirubinemia and he-

patomegaly are noted in the first month of life. The clinical course in the first year of life may be mild or severe. Most children improve with time and resolve their liver disease by 1-2 years of age. Jaundice after 6 months of age is usually an ominous finding, suggesting a significant deterioration in clinical status within 1 year. A decrease in hepatic synthetic capacity accompanies this deterioration, manifest by a decrease in coagulation factors synthesized by the liver.

Most children with α_1-antitrypsin deficiency are normal in the newborn period. Approximately 50% of people who are PIZZ do not ever manifest liver disease. In the other half, liver disease develops insidiously over many years, presenting at some point in adulthood as cirrhosis. Clinically, cirrhosis associated with α_1-antitrypsin deficiency is similar to that seen in other forms of childhood liver disease. Malnutrition, coagulopathy, and complications of portal hypertension, including splenomegaly, variceal hemorrhage, and ascites, develop to a varying degree. In the absence of infection or an episode of dehydration, both of which may precipitate hepatic deterioration, a patient may survive for years with cirrhosis and adequate hepatic function. Hepatocellular carcinoma is more common in individuals with PIZZ-associated α_1-antitrypsin deficiency. While it is often a complication of long-standing cirrhosis, carcinoma can develop in individuals with α_1-antitrypsin deficiency who do not have cirrhosis. It is most commonly seen in older adults with this disease.

While liver disease may become manifest at any age, from infancy to extreme old age, emphysema is extremely rare in childhood, presenting more commonly in the adult α_1-antitrypsin-deficient individual. Indeed, it represents the most common manifestation of the deficiency. The emphysema associated with α_1-antitrypsin deficiency (representing about 2% of all cases of emphysema) develops at a relatively early age (in the third or fourth decade of life) with an equal distribution between men and women. The majority of young symptomatic PIZZ individuals with emphysema have a history of cigarette smoking. Abstention from cigarettes may delay the disease onset by 20 years. In a study of 22 nonsmokers homozygous for α_1-antitrypsin deficiency living in areas free of urban air pollution, it was found that the onset of emphysema was later than in smokers (51.4 years for smokers compared to 71.0 years for nonsmokers).

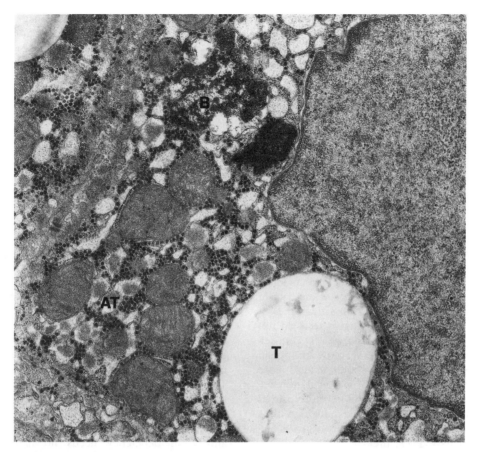

Figure 4-2. Photomicrograph of a portion of a hepatocyte from a cholestatic infant with PIZ phenotype. Amorphous α1-antitrypsin (AT) is in the transitional zone between rough and smooth endoplasmic reticulum. B, bile; T, triglyceride droplet.

More nonsmokers were completely free of symptoms or had only mild symptoms in their sixth or seventh decades.

Emphysema usually presents with shortness of breath, dyspnea, and chronic cough. Pneumothorax may result from the bursting of an emphysematous bleb. The emphysema associated with α_1-antitrypsin deficiency is indistinguishable from nonfamilial forms, although chronic bronchitis and the associated cough occur less frequently than in other forms of emphysema.

There is a wide range of disability associated with the pulmonary complications of α_1-antitrypsin deficiency, from completely asymptomatic individuals to chronic pulmonary cripples. Most patients develop chronic obstructive pulmonary disease. Unfortunately, once emphysema becomes symptomatic in the α_1-antitrypsin-deficient individual, it usually pursues a relentless course. A Danish registry study reported that the life expectancy of PIZZ smokers is 52 years and that of those who never smoked is 69 years.

Renal disease is seen in 17% of infants with α_1-antitrypsin deficiency. It causes massive protein loss, hypoalbuminemia, and renal failure. The kidney disease is an immunological disorder occurring only in patients with liver disease, resulting in a membranoproliferative glomerulonephritis with immunoreactive α_1-antitrypsin antigen present, as well as complement and immunoglobulins. It should not be confused with the nonspecific spotty asymptomatic glomerulonephritis or hepatorenal syndrome, commonly seen in cirrhosis.

Vascular conditions have been associated with α_1-antitrypsin deficiency, including panniculitis (an ulcerative, necrotizing skin condition) and cerebral aneurysm, among others.

It is controversial whether heterozygote (PIMZ) individuals are at risk for liver or lung disease. Some studies have suggested that PIMZ individuals are overrepresented among patients with chronic end-stage liver disease. PIMZ individuals are also overrepresented in diagnostic liver biopsies with cirrhosis as apposed to only mild fibrosis. It is equally unclear whether carriers of the Z allele are at increased risk of emphysema if they smoke. Large prospective studies of heterozygotes would solve these dilemmas.

The diagnosis of α_1-antitrypsin deficiency may be suspected during direct observation of the cellulose acetate serum protein electrophoresis, in which the α_1-globulin band is small or undetectable. As α_1-antitrypsin represents 90% of the total α_1-globulin peak, depression of this peak usually represents deficiency of that protein. Serum levels of α_1-antitrypsin are low in PIZZ individuals, less than 15% of normal levels. Serum quantitative tests do not permit accurate diagnosis and genetic counseling; therefore, abnormal levels of α_1-antitrypsin on screening examination should lead to more specific diagnostic tests. This is true of individuals with intermediate levels of α_1-antitrypsin as well. While it is likely that a patient with a serum α_1-antitrypsin level of 30%–80% is unlikely to have PIZZ, they may well have α_1-antitrypsin deficiency predisposing them to lung disease. Appropriate counseling and disease management requires knowledge of the patient's specific phenotype. The diagnostic test of choice is PI typing, in which isoelectric focusing is used to separate the various α_1-antitrypsin species in the individual's serum by charge differences. Comparison with sera of known PI type permits identification of the phenotype of the individual.

In patients with evidence of significant hepatic involvement, liver biopsy is important in the evaluation of α_1-antitrypsin-associated liver disease as it facilitates a more accurate prognosis. The patient with α_1-antitrypsin deficiency may have one of several histological pictures. In the neonate with α_1-antitrypsin deficiency, the liver may have evidence of fibrosis or cirrhosis, and some specimens will demonstrate paucity of the intrahepatic bile ducts. However, the usual histological finding in the neonate is proliferation of the intrahepatic bile ducts that simulates the histological picture of extrahepatic biliary atresia. There are usually few giant cells (multinucleated hepatocytes) seen. α_1-Antitrypsin deficiency is therefore an important diagnosis to exclude in the evaluation of the child suspected of extrahepatic biliary atresia since it may mimic this disease clinically and histologically. Patency of the extrahepatic biliary tree may be demonstrated by radionuclide scanning, detection of bile in duodenal contents, or cholangiography.

Periodic acid Schiff (PAS)-positive, diastase-resistant globules representing the retained α_1-antitrypsin protein are found in periportal hepatocytes on light microscopy. In the PAS/diastase study, periodic acid is used to oxidize bonds in sugars in liver tissue, allowing them to react with Schiff reagent to produce a magenta color. Glycogen is the material most commonly stained this way, but unsecreted α_1-antitrypsin will also stain with PAS. To allow the α_1-antitrypsin to be seen, the glycogen is first digested with diastase. The subsequent PAS test then stain magenta the globules of α_1-antitrypsin. These globules represent the abnormal α_1-antitrypsin not transported from the endoplasmic reticulum. These inclusions are fairly pathognomonic of the deficiency state. They can be verified with α_1-antitrypsin antibody stains and are also seen in heterozygote individuals (PIMZ).

Although the average child with α_1-antitrypsin deficiency needs no more pulmonary evaluation than careful periodic examinations, PIZZ adults with symptomatic pulmonary disease require more specific evaluation. The first step in evaluating patients suspected of having emphysema is the chest roentgenogram and pulmonary function testing. The chest x-ray film may show hyperinflation, flattened diaphragms, the presence of bullae, and narrowing of the pulmonary arteries. As basal emphysema is more common in α_1-antitrypsin deficiency, the lower zones of the lungs are more commonly involved. Even with normal x-ray findings, pulmonary function tests may reveal early emphysematous changes. The α_1-antitrypsin-deficient patient may have a decrease in forced expiratory volume in 1 second and forced expiratory flow with an increase in total lung capacity and functional residual capacity. These findings are probably the results of a combination of obstructive lung disease with a decrease in the elasticity of the lung. Computed tomography of the lung is more sensitive in demonstrating early evidence of lung destruction. Some authors suggest this modality provides the best prognostic information.

Hypercarbia on examination of arterial blood gases is nonspecific and generally a late finding.

Renal disease is detected through urinanalysis done yearly on PIZZ individuals with liver disease. Detection of proteinuria would lead to examination of a quantitative 24-hour urine for protein. If confirmation of the diagnosis is essential, then renal biopsy would be necessary.

BIOCHEMICAL PERSPECTIVES

α_1-Antitrypsin deficiency is an inborn error of metabolism predisposing to emphysema; it was identified in the early 1960s by Sten Eriksson and C.-B. Laurell (Laurell and Ericksson, 1963). In 1969, Harvey Sharp recognized the association of hepatic cirrhosis and α_1-antitrypsin deficiency. The natural course of the liver disease was difficult to define at first as most patients were referred because of serious liver disease. Several decades ago, Tomas Sveger and his associates (Sveger and Thelin, 2000) began an ongoing study of the natural history of this disease in 1976, identifying all deficient children in a 2-year cohort of Swedish infants. This difficult study has allowed a more thorough and balanced clinical picture of liver disease associated with α_1-antitrypsin deficiency. During the 1960s and 1970s, many investigators examined the lung disease of α_1-antitrypsin deficiency. A major contribution was made by C. Larsson in 1978, who convincingly showed that cigarette smoking was an independent risk factor in the development of lung disease.

Sequencing of the human α_1-antitrypsin gene in 1984 initiated an explosion in the study of this disease. Transgenic mice were created to study the effects of α_1-antitrypsin deficiency, and cell culture studies of the regulation of the gene became possible. In 1992, D. A. Lomas and colleagues (Lomas et al., 1992) showed that the accumulation of abnormal α_1-antitrypsin in the ER of the liver was the result of polymerization of α_1-antitrypsin. This discovery set the stage for the study of the effects of this polymerized material on the liver, which it is hoped will allow the mechanism of liver disease associated with α_1-antitrypsin deficiency to be determined.

α_1-Antitrypsin is a 52-kd glycoprotein produced primarily not only by the hepatocyte, but also by macrophages. Serum α_1-antitrypsin is derived almost exclusively from the liver. The function of this serine protease is to protect tissues from proteolytic enzymes released during the normal inflammatory response. Although α_1-antitrypsin has some activity against most serum proteases, its primary protease target is elastase, with some activity against cathepsin G and proteinase 3. The mechanism of inhibition is an irreversible reaction between α_1-antitrypsin and elastase at the reactive center of α_1-antitrypsin, a methionine residue at position 358. This residue is called the *reactive center*. Elastase, which cleaves proteins at methionyl residues, recognizes α_1-antitrypsin as a substrate and attempts to cleave it. In doing so, the protease is trapped by the α_1-antitrypsin molecule, and a drastic conformational change of the antiprotease crushes the protease, rendering it inactive and preparing it for clearance from the serum. α_1-Antitrypsin represents the primary regulating factor for elastase. Deficiency of this antiprotease results in excessive pulmonary elastase activity.

This antiprotease is encoded by a 12.2-kb (kilobase) gene located on the long arm of chromosome 14, the protease inhibitor or PI locus. The gene consists of seven exons and six introns, with the transcriptional start site varying depending on the cell type in which transcription occurs. The regulation of cell-specific expression is complex. Hepatocytes produce predominantly a single 1.6-kb transcript, although they can produce small amounts of transcripts characteristic of the monocyte cell line when stimulated by interleukin 6. Monocytes and macrophages use variable splicing of the first exon to produce four different transcripts, with lengths varying from 1.8 to 2.0 kb.

The α_1-antitrypsin promoter contains a consensus TATA box, a B-recognition element for transcription-activating factor IIB, a hepatocyte nuclear factor 1 site, and two non-tissue-specific regions that increase transcription. There is a 3' enhancer region with five potential binding sites for transcription factors. The specific factors that bind in this area remain to be described.

α_1-Antitrypsin is an acute phase reactant, which means that synthesis of the protein increases during inflammation, including malignancy, bacterial infections, and severe burns. It also rises during certain changes in hormonal conditions, as in pregnancy and during treatment with estrogen-containing birth control pills. The increase in serum α_1-antitrypsin in inflammation is regulated primarily at the level of gene transcription by cytokine mediators of inflammation, predominantly interleukin 6. Inflammatory-mediated increased transcription is regulated by an interaction (as yet unspecified) between the 3' enhancer and the promoter regions of the α_1-antitrypsin gene.

Sequence similarities to other serine PIs established the existence of a large evolutionarily related gene family, the SERPINs (serine protease inhibitors). Members of this gene family are found in plants and viruses as well as animals. Some examples of SERPINs include α_1-antichymotrypsin, antithrombin III, α_2-antiplasmin, thyroid- and corticosteroid-binding proteins, and ovalbumin. This gene family likely has a common ancestry, evolving through gene duplication and mutation. Functionally, there is broad diversity, from functional PIs to regulators of the clotting cascade and hormone-binding proteins.

During protein synthesis, the nascent translation product of the α_1-antitrypsin gene is co-translationally translocated to the ER, where the signal peptide is cleaved and high mannose glycosylation residues are added (Fig. 4-3). As the glycoprotein completes its transit through the ER to the Golgi apparatus, the terminal mannose residues of the oligosaccharide moiety are cleaved, and secondary glycosylation residues, including sialic acid, are added. The mature glycoprotein is packaged in the Golgi and secreted into the serum. The secreted protein contains variability in the secondary carbohydrate side chains, which produces a microheterogeneity, causing the glycoprotein to resolve into multiple bands when subjected to acid protein electrophoresis.

The mechanism by which Z-α_1-antitrypsin is transported out of the ER and degraded has been of interest to investigators. Since intracellular trapping of α_1-antitrypsin is a significant feature in the pathophysiology of the liver disease, understanding the degradation of the molecule might provide avenues to correct the defect. It appears that Z-α_1-antitrypsin is bound to calnexin (a chaperone molecule that transitions abnormally folded molecules to a degradation pathway) longer than it is to M-α_1-antitrypsin, which would increase degradation of the Z molecule. The Z-α_1-antitrypsin that is secreted has achieved a normal molecular conformation, suggesting that in the ER, chaperone molecules are achieving their role as mediators of correct conformation. It appears that the majority of Z-α_1-antitrypsin is degraded, probably by the proteasome, and that this requires retrograde transport of the protein back into the cytosol. Some investigators have suggested that

individuals who develop liver disease have a decreased capacity to clear Z-α_1-antitrypsin from the ER.

The PI locus is highly pleomorphic, with more than 75 allelic variants identified. The nomenclature of the PI locus is based on the electrophoretic mobility of the α_1-antitrypsin variants at pH 4.9. PIM represents the normal allele; it is actually composed of four M alleles, M1–M4. Letters alphabetically before M designate anodal variants, and those after M designate cathodal variants. The majority of these variant alleles produce no change in α_1-antitrypsin serum levels or function. Null alleles exist that produce no detectable serum α_1-antitrypsin. Since both alleles are expressed codominantly, heterozygosity for the PI locus may be identified electrophoretically. This is important for family studies of α_1-antitrypsin-deficient patients. Identity of unusual allelic variants may be confirmed by DNA sequencing.

Although many variant forms of the antiprotease exist, the most common alleles associated with its deficiency are the S and Z variants, both producing proteins that migrate cathodal to the normal protein. Homozygosity for these variants (PIZZ and PISS genotypes), as well as compound heterozygosity (PISZ), are all associated with deficient serum levels of α_1-antitrypsin. PIZZ individuals have approximately 10% to 20% of the normal level of α_1-antitrypsin, while PISZ individuals have approximately 35% of the normal level. The rare individual with homozygosity or compound heterozygosity of the null gene with one of these alleles has severe α_1-antitrypsin deficiency.

These abnormal PI alleles are most commonly found in individuals of European descent. Approximately 3% of Europeans are heterozygotes for the Z allele, while about 7% carry the S gene. The Z allele tends to be found more commonly in northern Europeans, while southern Europeans tend to have the S allele at a slightly higher frequency. The incidence of serious α_1-antitrypsin disease is about 1 in 2000 among individuals of northern European extraction. The Z variant, which has been studied most extensively, has a single base-pair mutation leading to the production of a protein in which lysine is substituted for glutamic acid at position 342. Primary glycosylation residues are added to the Z-variant polypeptide in the ER, but subsequent transport out of the ER is impaired. This trapping of the relatively insoluble Z-α_1-antitrypsin is the result of the tendency of

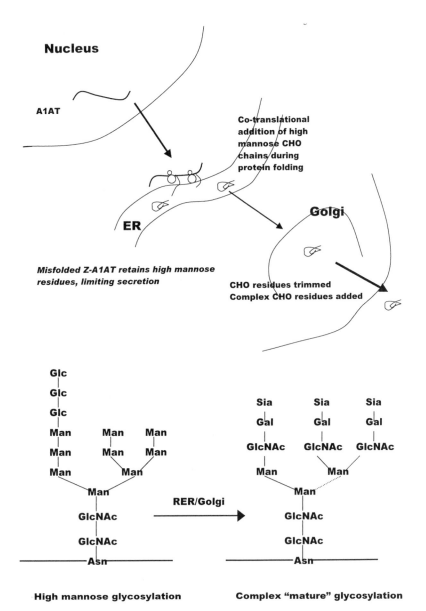

Figure 4-3. (Top) Synthetic pathway of α_1-antitrypsin diagramming the translocation of the nascent polypeptide chain into the endoplasmic reticulum (ER), with addition there of high-mannose glycosylation residues to the newly folded protein. The protein, carrying the "primitive" glycosylation residues, translocates to the Golgi apparatus, where the high-mannose residues are cleaved, and sialic acid residues are added. The protein, with mature glycosylation residues, is then secreted. CHO, carbohydrate. (Bottom) Processing of glycosylation residues. High-mannose residues (Man), attached to an oligosaccharide backbone consisting of N-acetylglucosamine residues (GlcNAc) and glucose residues (Glc) attached to the amino acid asparagine (Asn), comprise the initial glycosylated protein, on the left. In the Golgi, mannose residues are cleaved and further N-acetylglucosamine, galactose (Gal), and sialic acid (Sia) residues are added. The dotted line illustrates the alternative bi- and triantennary side-chain structures of α_1-antitrypsin.

Z-α_1-antitrypsin to undergo spontaneous polymerization when present in high concentrations in the ER. The main β-sheet of the Z-α_1-antitrypsin molecule can open spontaneously, allowing the reactive loop of a second Z-α_1-antitrypsin molecule to insert itself into the opening. Polymers of Z-α_1-antitrypsin are created with a stable structure that resists the normal degradative processes. Thus, the PIZZ individual accumulates large amounts of endoplasmic reticular α_1-antitrypsin protein that is not released into the circulation, thereby accounting for the markedly reduced serum levels of α_1-antitrypsin. The Z protein that is released into the serum has the ability to inhibit elastase and has a half-life similar to that of the M protein. Carriers for this allele (PIMZ) have serum α_1-antitrypsin levels approximately 60% of normal, with small α_1-antitrypsin-containing globules visible in their hepatocytes. Other rare phenotypes associated with both low serum levels of α_1-antitrypsin and hepatic globules include PIM$_{Malton}$ and PIM$_{Duarte}$.

The S variant has a mutation at amino acid position 264, where valine is substituted for glutamic acid. The S-α_1-antitrypsin appears to have normal protease-inhibitory activity but is degraded intracellularly prior to secretion. The null alleles (PIQ) produce no immunologically or functionally active protein; there are several such allelic variants described, generally involving deletion of large portions of the α_1-antitrypsin gene.

The pathogenesis of the lung disease in PIZZ individuals is fairly well established. Deficiency of α_1-antitrypsin produces an imbalance in the ratio of protease to PI, resulting in emphysema. Both alveolar macrophages and polymorphonuclear leukocytes contain proteases, including neutrophil elastase, cathepsin G, and proteinase 3. Neutrophil elastase is released in large quantities in the lung and has as its substrate elastin, a component of the extracellular matrix, as well as other proteins. During the normal inflammatory response in the lung, as might occur with infection or cigarette smoking, these phagocytic cells migrate to the lung alveoli, releasing their proteases. In the lungs of a normal individual, α_1-antitrypsin is the major inhibitor of neutrophil elastase and keeps elastase activity localized to the site of the inflammation, allowing it to scavenge damaged proteins and gram-negative bacterial cell walls, thereby protecting alveolar tissue. In the lungs of PIZZ individuals, an imbalance exists in the protease/PI ratio, allowing elastase uninhibited access to alveolar and pulmonary connective tissue, producing the emphysematous lesion.

Cigarette smoking markedly increases the risk of emphysema in PIZZ homozygotes. Cigarette smoke causes the release of neutrophil chemotactic factor, increasing the number of protease-containing neutrophils in the lung. Release of elastase from these cells is increased in the presence of cigarette smoke. Cigarette smoke oxidizes the reactive-site methionine in the small amount of Z-α_1-antitrypsin that escapes the liver, destroying its inhibitory capacity for elastase. Thus, emphysema associated with α_1-antitrypsin deficiency is not simply due to a genetic defect, but requires an environmental stimulus as well.

There remains controversy regarding the pathophysiology of liver disease associated with α_1-antitrypsin deficiency. Studies in transgenic animals and clinical analysis of human disease suggested that the globules of Z-α_1-antitrypsin trapped in the ER of the liver either directly damage the hepatocyte or facilitate damage by infection or toxins. The mechanism for this injury is unclear.

It has been shown in cell culture models of α_1-antitrypsin that Z-α_1-antitrypsin in the ER causes expression of a novel set of stress genes with products that have the role of restoring ER function to normal. Z-α_1-Antitrypsin induces two signal transduction pathways: the ER overload response and unfolded protein response pathways. Via these transduction pathways, the presence of Z-α_1-antitrypsin, as opposed to M-α_1-antitrypsin, induces an hepatic inflammatory response. It is thought that this ER-specific stress response results in hepatic injury.

An alternative hypothesis is that ER retention of Z-α_1-antitrypsin results in autophagy, specifically of hepatic mitochondria. The basis for this hypothesis is the increase in autophagosomes in cells engineered for inducible expression of Z-α_1-antitrypsin. The mutant protein, along with the chaperone molecule calnexin, can be found in these autophagosomes by immune electron microscopy. It is postulated that mitochondrial dysfunction results from the damage to the mitochondria in the PIZZ liver, leading to the hepatic injury.

THERAPY

Conventional medical management of emphysema consists of supportive care, including early antibiotic treatment of all pulmonary infections. Patients are immunized against influenza virus and *Streptococcus pneunoniae*. If, on pulmonary function testing, any reversibility of the airway obstruction can be effected with bronchodilators, these may be used. As the pathogenesis of emphysema associated with α_1-antitrypsin deficiency is related to cigarette smoking, it is important to counsel the patient to stop smoking. This is the only measure known to improve life expectancy for these patients.

Fractionation techniques have made it possible to recover active α_1-antitrypsin from blood. Use of this product for intravenous replacement therapy in deficient individuals has shown that it is possible to increase levels in the serum to those of PISZ heterozygotes who experience no increase in pulmonary disease over the general population. Pulmonary lavage of patients transfused with this product showed that functional α_1-antitrypsin reaches the alveolar structures. The Food and Drug Administration has approved weekly administration of purified serum-derived α_1-antitrypsin to PIZZ and PI null individuals with pulmonary disease. Although serum levels of α_1-antitrypsin increase to those believed to be protective, it has not been possible to show clinical improvement. Furthermore, viral transmission via blood products is a significant risk factor.

The use of recombinantly produced α_1-antitrypsin would reduce the risk of transfusion-related viral disease; however, its half-life is too short to produce adequate serum levels without daily infusion. Studies have shown that the recombinant product can be administered as an aerosol. It diffuses across the respiratory epithelium, enters the lung lymph, and eventually reaches the systemic circulation. Unfortunately, it is not known whether this therapy has any influence on the development or progression of emphysema. Further carefully controlled, multicenter trials are necessary.

Lung transplantation has been used in the treatment of lung disease associated with α_1-antitrypsin deficiency. Survival is the same as for patients undergoing the procedure for chronic obstructive pulmonary disease. As with any transplantation, lifelong immunosuppression is necessary.

Liver disease is managed conventionally, maintaining appropriate nutritional support and managing the complications of portal hypertension and hepatic failure as they occur. We counsel heterozygote parents of a PIZZ

child to stop cigarette smoking because of the danger passive cigarette smoke represents to the lungs of their PIZZ child. Definitive therapy of the liver disease is limited to successful liver transplantation. There is no evidence of recurrence of the liver disease after successful liver transplant. Theoretically, one would assume that liver transplantation, by providing normal serum levels of α_1-antitrypsin, would prevent development of the lung disease; however, studies necessary to prove this hypothesis have not been done. No data support a role for α_1-antitrypsin replacement therapy in liver disease.

Some investigators have speculated that it should be possible to solubilize intracellular Z-α_1-antitrypsin, allowing it to complete its secretory pathway. If achieved, this would ameliorate both the pulmonary and the hepatic disease associated with PIZZ phenotype. Phenylbutyrate was suggested as one possible therapy, but it has been ineffective for this purpose. Helen Parfrey and colleagues (Parfrey et al., 2004) have shown *in vitro* that an oligopeptide that specifically binds to Z-α_1-antitrypsin can inhibit its polymerization. The peptide can dissociate from the binary complex, allowing the Z-α_1-antitrypsin to have full antiprotease activity. This and other novel mechanisms of promoting secretion rather than degradation of the Z-α_1-antitrypsin may allow medical therapy of this condition.

Gene therapy offers the hope that the disease might eventually be completely cured. The human α_1-antitrypsin gene has been successfully introduced into rat hepatocytes, which when transplanted into a rat liver, expressed the protein in small quantities. This strategy would most likely be successful in preventing the development of emphysema. However, it is unclear whether it would cure the liver disease. If liver disease is dependent on the presence of unsecreted Z-α_1-antitrypsin, then adding the normal α_1-antitrypsin gene would not stop its development or progression. Investigators in this field are working to develop techniques of targeted homologous recombination to replace completely the α_1-antitrypsin exon containing the PIZ mutation. Patients thus treated would express only the M-α_1-antitrypsin.

There is a phase 1 trial (trials that examine the toxicity of the proposed treatment and determine an appropriate dose of the treatment) of an intramuscularly delivered α_1-antitrypsin gene in a modified adeno-associated virus vector. It will be some time before efficacy data are available;

however, studies using this vector in animals suggested that it may allow prolonged gene expression at levels sufficient to supply normal serum levels of α_1-antitrypsin. It also induces minimal levels of inflammation. This strategy may allow prevention and treatment of lung disease but is unlikely to affect liver disease.

We recommend that all relatives of a patient with α_1-antitrypsin deficiency be PI typed because relatives of the proband may have clinically unsuspected PIZZ liver or lung disease. For future counseling of the family, it is important to identify the PI type of the patient accurately and to identify heterozygotes. Although measurement of α_1-antitrypsin immunologically or functionally is accurate, there may be some difficulty identifying PIMZ heterozygotes with these methods since they have α_1-antitrypsin levels that may rise to normal levels during inflammation. One must therefore rely on PI typing, which should be done by an institution familiar with the many α_1-antitrypsin alleles.

Neonatal screening for α_1-antitrypsin deficiency has been debated for years. Sweden screened a cohort of 200,000 infants born in 1972-1974. Subsequent evaluation of these children has shown that there was little psychosocial impact on the family from the identification of a child as α_1-antitrypsin deficient through screening. A slight increase in maternal anxiety was the only negative impact found. Discrimination by insurance companies and employers remains a theoretical risk. Importantly, adolescents with α_1-antitrypsin deficiency identified through screening were significantly less likely to smoke than their peers. This finding, combined with the capacity to prevent passive smoke exposure in children with α_1-antitrypsin deficiency, has led many investigators to call for screening programs in countries with large numbers of affected births.

It is possible to offer parents who are known heterozygotes for the Z allele low risk early diagnosis of α_1-antitrypsin deficiency *in utero*. Prenatal diagnosis can be done on fibroblasts collected by amniocentesis or by chorionic villus biopsy using polymerase chain amplification and analysis of the mutated region of the gene. Counseling of the families of a PIZZ individual requires a careful explanation of the principles of codominant inheritance. Parents who are both PIMZ heterozygotes have a one-in-four risk of having a PIZZ child in any subsequent pregnancy. The risk of serious liver disease in a PIZZ child is small, and the risk of lung disease can be significantly modified by avoiding cigarette smoking. Thus, there are few medical reasons to recommend *in utero* diagnosis of α_1-antitrypsin deficiency, although ultimately the decision should be left to the family.

QUESTIONS

1. Describe the range of possible clinical signs and symptoms of α_1-antitrypsin deficiency in a newborn.
2. The mother of the child in the case report was PIMZ. Discuss the likely results of a serum α_1-antitrypsin level and a liver biopsy in the mother. If her serum α_1-antitrypsin level was found to be 75% of normal, then how would you explain it?
3. If the parents of the proband sought genetic counseling from you in a subsequent pregnancy, then what information would you give them?
4. If a drug existed that specifically stimulated the transcription of messenger ribonucleic acid for α_1-antitrypsin in the liver, then would this be a reasonable therapy for PIZZ individuals? Why or why not? Would your recommendation be different for the PISS patient?
5. As the patient described reaches maturity, what medical advice would you give him to help him protect his lungs?

BIBLIOGRAPHY

Carrell RW Lomas DA: α_1-antitrypsin deficiency—a model for conformational disease. *N Engl J Med* **346**:45-53, 2002.

Graziadei IW, Joseph JJ, Wiesner RH, et al.: Increased risk of chronic liver failure in adults with heterozygous α_1-antitrypsin deficiency. *Hepatology* **28**:1058-1063, 1998.

Ibarguen E, Gross CR, Savik SK, et al.: Liver disease in α_1-antitrypsin deficiency: prognostic indicators. *J Pediatr* **117**:864-870, 1990.

Kalsheker N, Morley S, Morgan K: Gene regulation of the serine proteinase inhibitors α_1-antitrypsin and α_1-antichymotrypsin. *Biochem Soc Trans* **30**:93-98, 2002.

Laurell CB, Ericksson, S: The electrophoretic α_1-globulin pattern of serum in α_1-antitrypsin deficiency. *Scand J Clin Lab Invest* **15**:132, 1963.

Lomas DA, Evans DL, Finch JT, et al.: The mechanism of Z α_1-antitrypsin accumulation in the liver. *Nature* **357**:605-07, 1992.

Needham M, Stockley RA: α_1-Antitrypsin deficiency. 3: Clinical manifestations and natural history. *Thorax* **59**:441-445, 2004.

Parfrey H, Dafforn TR, Belorgey D, et al.: Inhibiting polymerization: new therapeutic strategies for Z α_1-antitrypsin-related emphysema. *Am J Respir Cell Mol Biol* **31(2)**:133-9, 2004.

Perlmutter DH: α_1-Antitrypsin deficiency. *Semin Liver Dis* **18**:217-225, 1998.

Perlmutter DH: α_1-Antitrypsin deficiency: liver disease associated with retention of a mutant secretory glycoprotein in the endoplasmic reticulum. *Methods Mol Biol* **232**:39-56, 2003.

Seersholm N, Kok-Jensen A: Clinical features and prognosis of life time non-smokers with severe α_1-antitrypsin deficiency. *Thorax* **53**:265-268, 1998.

Silverman GA, Bird PI, Carrell RW, et al.: The serpins are an expanding superfamily of structurally similar but functionally diverse proteins. Evolution, mechanism of inhibition, novel functions, and a revised nomenclature. *J Biol Chem* **276**:33293-33296, 2001.

Stecenko AA, Brigham KL: Gene therapy progress and prospects: α_1-antitrypsin. *Gene Ther* **10**:95-99, 2003.

Sveger T, Thelin T: A future for neonatal α_1-antitrypsin screening? *Acta Paediatr* **89**:628-631, 2000.

5

Cardiac Troponin: Clinical Role in the Diagnosis of Myocardial Infarction

FRED S. APPLE and ALLAN S. JAFFE

CASE REPORT

The patient, a 63-year-old Caucasian female, was hospitalized on 4 April 2002 though 10 April 2002 for a non-ST segment elevation myocardial infarction (non-Q-wave MI per chart documentation). She had a negative adenosine stress test after the initial event. Her serum cardiac-specific troponin I (cTnI) concentration 24 hours after her onset of chest pain was 1.4 μg/L (upper limit of normal is 0.3 ng/mL), and her creatine kinase (CK) MB level was 12.5 μg/L (upper limit of normal 6.0 ng/mL). Three days post-event her cTnI level was 0.5 μg/L and her CK-MB level was 4.5 μg/L (Fig. 5-1). MB refers to one of the isoenzyme forms of CK found in serum. The form of the enzyme that occurs in brain (BB) does not usually get past the blood-brain barrier and therefore is not normally present in the serum. The MM and MB forms account for almost all of the CK in serum. Skeletal muscle contains mainly MM, with less than 2% of its CK in the MB form. MM is also the predominant myocardial creatine kinase and MB accounts for 10%–20% of creatine kinase in heart muscle.

At 72 hours after presentation, the patient experienced new-onset chest pain, described as a burning pain in the left shoulder, arm, and epigastrium. The electrocardiogram (ECG) demonstrated only nonspecific T-wave abnormalities and was not different from the one obtained at the time of her initial presentation. Normal sinus rhythm was now present. Nitroglycerin provided some relief. Based on new symptoms, along with recurring T-wave abnormalities and

an increasing cTnI, diagnosis of reinfarction (extension of her initial event) was made. The cTnI concentration on the day of her suspected reinfarction (day 4) was increased to 1.8 μg/L with a corresponding CK-MB value of 13.6 μg/L. Cardiac catheterization revealed a 95% distal left anterior descending stenosis, a 95% mid-right coronary artery narrowing, and a 90% occluded circumflex proximally. Stents were placed in both the distal and proximal right coronary artery. The rest of her hospital stay was uneventful, and she was discharged home on day 7. At 3-month follow-up, the patient was participating in a cardiac rehabilitation program and doing well.

DIAGNOSIS

The term *acute myocardial infarction* (AMI) is defined as an imbalance between myocardial oxygen supply and demand, resulting in injury to and the eventual death of myocytes. When the blood supply to the heart is interrupted, "gross necrosis" of the myocardium results. Abrupt and total loss of coronary blood flow usually results in a clinical syndrome known as ST segment elevation AMI (STE AMI or Q-wave MI; diagnostic by electrocardiogram) because of the characteristic electrocardiographic changes that occur. Partial loss of coronary perfusion, if severe, also can lead to necrosis, which is generally less extensive, and this type of infarction is usually termed non–ST elevation myocardial infarction (NSTEMI or

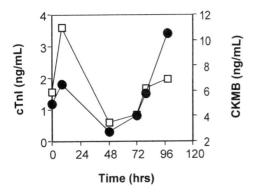

Figure 5-1. Time-course of changes in serum cardiac troponin I and creatine kinase MB (CK-MB) following myocardial infarction and subsequent reinfarction during hospitalization. Cardiac-specific troponin I (cTNI), open squares; CK-MB, filled circles. Reprinted from Apple and Murakami (2005).

non–Q-wave MI; not diagnostic by electrocardiogram). There is considerable overlap between the pathophysiology and the pattern of necrosis of the two entities. Other events of less severity may be missed entirely or if detected may be diagnosed as angina that can range from stable to unstable.

The term *acute coronary syndrome* (ACS) encompasses most of the patients defined so far in this chapter who present with unstable ischemic heart disease. Most of these syndromes occur in response to an acute event in the coronary artery when circulation to a region of the heart is obstructed. If the obstruction is high grade and persists, then necrosis usually ensues. Since necrosis takes some time to develop, it is apparent that therapy, including opening the blocked coronary artery in a timely fashion, often can prevent some of the death of myocardial tissue. These syndromes are usually, but not always, associated with chest discomfort.

Previously, the diagnosis of AMI established by the World Health Organization required at least two of the following criteria: a history of chest pain, evolutionary changes on the ECG, or elevations of serial cardiac biomarkers (initially defined as a twofold increase of total serum CK or CK-MB). However, it was rare for a diagnosis of AMI to be made in the absence of biochemical evidence of myocardial injury. A 2000 European Society of Cardiology/American College of Cardiology (ESC/ACC) consensus conference has codified the role of biomarkers, with specific focus on cardiac troponins, by advocating

that the diagnosis be based on evidence of myocardial injury based on biomarkers of cardiac injury in the appropriate clinical situation.

For these guidelines, either of the following criteria satisfies the diagnosis for an acute, evolving, or recent MI. The first is a typical rise or gradual fall of cardiac troponin, or more rapid rise and fall of CK-MB, with at least one of the following: (1) ischemic symptoms; (2) development of pathologic Q waves on the ECG; (3) ECG changes indicative of ischemia (ST segment elevation or depression); or (4) coronary artery intervention (e.g., coronary angioplasty). For the second, there should be pathologic findings of an AMI as identified at autopsy. The guidelines recognized the reality that neither the clinical presentation nor the ECG had adequate sensitivity and specificity, but that the troponin markers, in particular, could provide both. These guidelines do not suggest that all elevations of these biomarkers should elicit a diagnosis of AMI, only those associated with the appropriate clinical (ischemic presentation) and ECG findings. When elevations of cardiac troponin are observed that are not due to acute ischemia, the clinician is obligated to search for another etiology for the cardiac injury.

Patients with ACS can be categorized into four groups. First, there is the group of patients who present early to the emergency room, within 0 to 4 hours after the onset of chest pain, and who lack diagnostic ECG evidence of AMI. These patients require rapid laboratory testing for evidence of cardiac injury. Thus, useful laboratory markers of cardiac injury are those that are released rapidly from the heart and are highly specific for cardiac myoctye damage. These assays must be rapid and sensitive enough to detect even the small changes within the reference interval that can occur in blood early after the onset of symptoms.

The second patient group presents 4 to 48 hours after the onset of chest pain but without diagnostic evidence of AMI by ECG. This group of patients also requires serial monitoring of cardiac biomarkers and ECG changes.

The third group is patients who present still later, more than 48 hours after the onset of chest pain, and also lack diagnostic ECG changes. The ideal biomarker of myocardial injury for this group would have to be one that persists in the circulation for several days to provide a late diagnostic time window. The shortfall of such a marker might be its inability to distinguish recurrent injury from the prior, older injury.

The fourth group is those who present to the emergency department at any time after the onset of chest pain with clear ECG evidence of AMI. In this group, detection with serum biomarkers of myocardial injury is not necessary initially. Many of these patients may qualify for reperfusion therapy at a time before blood markers of cardiac injury have increased, and therapy should not be withheld if these criteria are met. Subsequently, specific and sensitive myocardial markers could be employed to monitor the success of reperfusion during the 60- to 90-minute period after therapy. Rapid assays providing early serial values followed by interpretation of the markers' patterns of appearance are often helpful in determining subsequent management.

BIOCHEMICAL PERSPECTIVES

Cardiac Troponin I and T

The contractile proteins of the myofibril include three troponin regulatory proteins. The troponin complex includes three protein subunits, troponin C (the calcium-binding component), troponin I (the inhibitory component), and troponin T (the tropomyosin-binding component). The subunits exist in a number of isoforms. The distribution of these isoforms varies between cardiac muscle and slow- and fast-twitch skeletal muscle. Only two major isoforms of troponin C are found in human heart and skeletal muscle. These are characteristic of slow- and fast-twitch skeletal muscle. The heart isoform is identical with the slow-twitch skeletal muscle isoform. Isoforms of cardiac-specific troponin T (cTnT) and cTnI also have been identified and are the products of unique genes. All cardiac troponins are localized primarily in the myofibrils (94%–97%), with a smaller cytoplasm fraction (3%–6%).

Cardiac troponin subunits I and T are encoded by different genes than the respective skeletal muscle isoforms and have different amino acid sequences, giving them unique cardiac specificity. cTnI has never been shown to be expressed in normal, regenerating, or diseased human or animal skeletal muscle. By contrast, small amounts of cTnT are expressed as one of four identified isoforms in skeletal muscle during human fetal development, in regenerating rat skeletal muscle, and in diseased human skeletal muscle. cTnT isoform expression has been demonstrated in skeletal muscle specimens

obtained from patients with muscular dystrophy, polymyositis, dermatomyositis, and end-stage renal disease. Thus, care is necessary to choose antibody pairs for cardiac assay use that do not detect the isoforms reexpressed in noncardiac tissue. The commercial assay used in clinical practice only detects the heart cTnT form.

Cardiac troponin I exists as a part of the troponin T-I-C ternary complex as a structural and regulatory component of the myofibril. Following myocardial injury, multiple forms of cardiac troponins are elaborated both in tissue and in blood (Fig. 5-2). These include the T-I-C ternary complex, IC binary complex, free I, and multiple modifications of these three forms resulting from oxidation, reduction, phosphorylation, and dephosphorylation, as well as both C- and N-terminal degradation. What is elaborated likely reflects the nature of the injurious stimulus, blood flow that determines how long the protein remains in the tissue prior to reaching the circulation, the timing of the insult (i.e., forms may change as the tissue damage evolves), and perhaps genetics. Depending on which fragments are elaborated, the selection of antibodies used to detect cTnI (i.e., different antibody configurations) can lead to substantially different recognition patterns. It is now clear that assays need to be developed with the antibodies that recognize epitopes in the stable region of cTnI and ideally demonstrate an equimolar response to the different cTnI forms that may circulate in the blood.

Creatine Kinase Isoenzymes and Isoforms

Three cytosolic isoenzymes (CK-MM, CK-MB, CK-BB) and one mitochondrial isoenzyme (CK-Mt) of CK have been identified. Three different genes have been identified that encode for and are specific for CK-M, CK-B, and CK-Mt subunits. Although CK-MM is predominant in both heart and skeletal muscle, CK-MB has been shown to be more specific for the myocardium, which contains 10% to 20% of its total CK activity as CK-MB, compared to amounts varying from 0% to 7% in skeletal muscle.

Early studies involving animal hearts or specimens obtained at autopsy from human hearts suggested a uniform distribution of CK-MB ranging from 5% to 50% of the total CK activity. However, it has been shown by Ingwall and colleagues (1985) that the proportion of CK-MB was 6% to 15% lower in the surrounding normal areas of tissue than in infarcted myocardium in

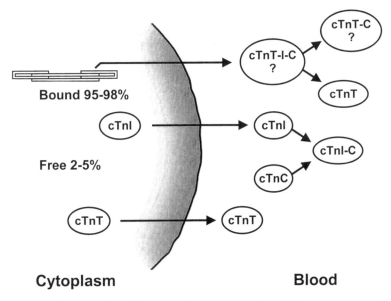

Figure 5-2. Schematic of cardiac troponin I and T release following myocardial cell necrosis into the circulation, demonstrating the multiple forms that exist in the blood. cTnI, cardiac-specific troponin I; cTnT, cardiac-specific troponin T.

humans. When studied more completely in humans, CK-MB concentrations ranged from 15% to 24% of total CK in myocardial tissue obtained from patients with left ventricular hypertrophy (LVH) due to aortic stenosis, from patients with coronary artery disease (CAD) without LVH, and from patients with CAD and LVH due to aortic stenosis. In contrast, patients with normal left ventricular tissue had a low percentage of CK-MB (<2%). These data suggest that changes in the CK isoenzyme distribution are dynamic and occur in hypertrophied and diseased human myocardium. Diseased cells also have less total CK per cell.

Normal skeletal muscle usually contains very little CK-MB. Levels as high as 5%–7% have been reported in some muscles, but less than 2% is much more common. Severe skeletal muscle injury following trauma or surgery can lead to absolute elevations of CK-MB above the upper reference (normal) limit of CK-MB in serum. Increases in serum total CK and CK-MB in several patient groups often present a diagnostic challenge to the clinician. Persistent elevations of serum CK-MB resulting from chronic muscle disease occur in patients with muscular dystrophy, end-stage renal disease, and polymyositis (a generative disease of skeletal muscle) as well as in healthy subjects who undergo extreme exercise or physical activities. The increase in serum CK-MB in runners, for example, may be related

to the adaptation by the skeletal muscle during regular training and after acute exercise, resulting in increased CK-MB tissue concentrations. The mechanism responsible for increased CK-MB in skeletal muscle following chronic muscle disease or injury is thought to be due to the regeneration process of muscle, with reexpression of CK-B genes similar to those found in the heart, thus giving rise to increased CK-MB levels in skeletal muscle. Thus, skeletal muscle can become like heart muscle in its CK isoenzyme composition, with up to 50% CK-MB in some patients with severe polymyositis.

IMMUNOASSAY PERSPECTIVES FOR MONITORING CARDIAC BIOMARKERS

Cardiac Troponins

The first assay (a radioimmunoassay) that measured cTnI used polyclonal anti-cTnI antibodies. The first monoclonal enzyme-linked immunosorbent assay, anti-cTnI antibody-based immunoassay, was described by Bodor and co-workers (1992). Numerous manufacturers have now developed monoclonal antibody-based diagnostic immunoassays for the measurement of cTnI in serum. Assay times range from 5 to 30 minutes.

Table 5-1. Cardiac Troponin Assays Cleared by the Food and Drug Administration

	Assay	LLD	99th	ROC	10% CV
Abbott	AxSYM ADV*	0.02	0.04	0.4	0.16
	Architect*	0.009	0.012	0.3	0.032
Bayer	ACS	0.03	0.1	1.0	0.35
	Centaur	0.02	0.1	1.0	0.35
Beckman	Access*	0.01	0.04	0.5	0.06
Biosite	Triage*	0.19	0.19	0.4	0.5
Dade	RxL*	0.04	0.07	0.6–1.5	0.14
	CS*	0.03	0.05	0.6–1.5	0.06
DPC	Immulite	0.1	0.2	1.0	0.6
i-STAT	i-STAT	0.03	0.08	ND	0.1
Ortho	Vitros	0.02	0.08	0.4	0.12
Roche	Elecsys†	0.01	0.01	0.1	0.03
	Reader	0.05	<0.05	0.1	NA
Tosoh	AIA*	0.06	0.06	0.31–0.64	0.06

LLD, lower limit of detection; 99th, 99th percentile reference limit; ROC, receiver operator characteristic curve optimized cutoff; 10% CV, lowest concentration to provide a total imprecision of 10%.

*Second generation.

†Third generation

NA, not available

As shown in Table 5-1, over a dozen assays have been cleared by the Food and Drug Administration (FDA) for patient testing within the United States on central laboratory and point-of-care (POC) or near-bedside testing platforms. In addition to these quantitative assays, several assays have been FDA-cleared for the qualitative determination of cTnI.

In practice, two obstacles limit the ease for switching from one cTnI or cTnT assay to another. First, there is currently no primary reference cTnI material available for manufacturers to use for standardizing their assays. Second, because of the different epitopes recognized by the different antibodies used, assay concentrations fail to agree. While standardization of assays remains elusive, harmonization of cTnI concentrations by different assays has been narrowed from a 20-fold difference to a 2- to 3-fold difference.

Several adaptations of the Roche Diagnostics cTnT immunoassay have been described, resulting in an FDA-cleared third-generation assay available worldwide. Two monoclonal anticardiac troponin T antibodies are used in the third-generation assay. Skeletal muscle TnT is no longer a potential interferent, as was found in the first-generation enzyme-linked immunosorbent cTnT assay. In contrast to cTnI, no standardization bias exists for cTnT because the same antibodies (M11, M7) are used in both the

central laboratory and POC quantitative and POC qualitative assay systems.

In 2001, quality specifications for cardiac troponin assays were published. These specifications were intended for use by the manufacturers of commercial assays and by clinical laboratories utilizing troponin assays. The overall goal was to attempt to establish uniform criteria so all assays could objectively be evaluated for their analytical qualities and clinical performance. Both analytical and preanalytical factors were addressed. The following recommendations have been proposed:

1. The antibody specificity (which epitope locations are identified) needs to be delineated. Epitopes located on the stable part of the cTnI molecule should be a priority.
2. Assays need to clarify whether different cTnI forms (i.e., binary vs. ternary complex) are recognized in an equimolar fashion by the antibodies used in the assay. Specific relative responses need to be described for the following cTnI forms: free cTnI; the I-C binary complex; the T-I-C ternary complex; and oxidized, reduced, and phosphorylated isoforms of the three cTnI forms.
3. The effects of different anticoagulants on binding of cTnI need to be addressed.

4. The source of material used to calibrate cTn assays, specifically for cTnI, should be traceable.

While clinicians and laboratorians continue to publish guidelines supporting turnaround times (TATs; defined as the time from blood draw to reporting of the result to a health care provider) of less than 60 minutes for cardiac biomarkers, the largest TAT study published to date demonstrated that TAT expectations are not being met in a large proportion of hospitals. A survey study of 7020 cardiac troponin and 4368 CK-MB determinations in 159 hospitals demonstrated that the median and 90th percentile TATs for troponin and CK-MB were as follows, respectively: 74.5 min, 129 min; 82 min, 131 min. Less than 25% of hospitals were able to meet the TAT in less than 60 minutes. Preliminary data has shown that implementation of POC cardiac troponin testing can decrease TATs to less than 30 minutes in cardiology critical care and short-stay units. These data highlight the continued need for laboratory services and health care providers to work together to develop better processes to meet a TAT that is less than 60 minutes as requested by physicians.

Reference Intervals for Cardiac Troponins and Creatine Kinase Isoenzymes

If possible, each laboratory should determine a 99th percentile of a reference group for cardiac troponin assays using the specific assay used in clinical practice or validate the assay based on findings in the literature. Further, acceptable imprecision (coefficient of variation, %CV) of each cardiac troponin assay (as well as for CK-MB mass assay) has been defined as 10% or lower CV at the 99th percentile reference limit. Unfortunately, the majority of laboratories do not have the resources to perform adequately powered reference interval studies. Therefore, clinical laboratories have to rely on the peer-reviewed published literature to establish reference intervals. When reviewing reference studies, caution must be taken when comparing the findings reported in the manufacturer's approved package inserts with the findings reported in journals because of differences in total sample size, distributions by gender and ethnicity, age ranges, and the statistic used to calculate the 99th percentile given.

There is no established guideline set to mandate a consistent evaluation of the 99th percentile reference limit for cardiac troponins. The largest and most diverse reported reference interval study to date showed plasma (heparin; used for anticoagulation of blood) 99th percentile reference limits for eight cardiac troponin assays (seven cTnI, one cTnT) and seven CK-MB mass assays (Table 5-2). These studies were performed in 696 healthy adults (age range 18 to 84 years) stratified by gender and ethnicity. The data demonstrate several issues. First, two cTnI assays showed a 1.2- to 2.5-fold higher 99th percentile for males versus females. Second, two cTnI assays demonstrated a 1.1- to 2.8-fold higher 99th percentile for African Americans versus Caucasians. Third, there was a 13-fold difference between the lowest versus the highest measured cTnI 99th percentile limit. The lack of cardiac troponin assay standardization (there is no primary reference material available) and the differences in antibody epitope recognition between assays (different assays use different antibodies) give rise to substantially discrepant results.

Although many studies have addressed the total imprecision of cTn assays, the manufacturers' package inserts prefer to publish imprecision data primarily based on within-run or within-day precision. Again, there is no consistent specification regarding the precision value that should be reported in the package insert. Published findings demonstrating the total imprecision for 13 commercial assays have indicated none of the assays were able experimentally to achieve a 10% CV (total imprecision) at their 99th percentile cutoff.

Therefore, to avoid the potential for false-positive diagnostic criteria based on cTn monitoring at the 99th percentile, a group of experts in both the laboratory medicine and cardiology communities has endorsed the concept that until cardiac troponin assay imprecision improves at the low concentrations, the lowest concentrations to attain a 10% CV (CV is the same as precision) should be used as a modified ESC/ACC diagnostic cutoff for detection of myocardial injury. This concept has been endorsed by several cardiology and laboratory medicine groups. The ultimate goal will be to have all cTn assays attain a 10% CV at the 99th percentile reference limit. This approach should reduce false-positive analytic results from lack of imprecision values between the 10% CV cutoff and the 99th percentile. However, all biomarker increases above the 99th percentile should be interpreted cautiously, especially in the high-risk patient, and

Table 5-2. Heparin-Plasma 99th Percentile Reference Limits (µg/L) by Gender and Race for Cardiac Troponin Assays Cleared by the Food and Drug Administration

	n^*	Abbott	Beckman	Dade	OCD	Roche[†]	$n^‡$	Tosoh	$n^§$	Bayer	$n^\|$	DPC
All	696	0.8	0.08	0.06	0.10	<0.01	473	0.07	403	0.15	281	0.21
Male	315	0.8	0.10	0.06	0.11	<0.01	223	0.07	187	0.17	115	0.21
Female	381	0.7	0.04	0.06	0.09	<0.01	250	<0.06	216	0.14	166	<0.2
P	—	.739	.034	.985	.017	.534	—	.521	—	.441	—	.21
Caucasian	400	0.8	0.07	0.04	0.11	<0.01	215	<0.06	193	0.17	166	0.21
African-American	218	0.5	0.08[¶]	0.03	0.10	<0.01	196	0.17	156	0.17	91	<0.2

*Number of samples tested in the Abbott, Beckman, Dade-Behring, OCD, and Roche assays.

[†]The Roche assay is the only Cardiac-Specific troponin T assay on the market; all other assays are for Cardiac-Specific troponin I.

[‡]Number of samples tested in the Tosoh assay.

[§]Number of samples tested in the Bayer assay.

[‖]Number of samples tested in the DPC assay.

[¶]Significantly different ($P = .05$) from Caucasians based on mean concentrations.

DPC = Diagnostics Products Corporation

OCD = Ortho-Clinical Diagnostics

followed with serial samples over a 6- to 12-hour period after presentation.

Myocardial Infarction Detection Rates and Cardiac Troponins

Advances in diagnostic technology for the development of improved low-end analytical detection of cardiac troponins have impacted the prevalence of AMI detection. Accumulating data suggest that the more sensitive cardiac troponin tests result in greater rates of MI diagnosis and greater rates of cardiac troponin positivity, compared to CK-MB. Smaller MIs will be detected. Clinical cases that were earlier classified as unstable angina will be given a diagnosis of MI (due to an increased cTn), and now procedure-related troponin increases (i.e., following angioplasty) will be labeled MI.

The importance of small troponin increases has been confirmed by their association with a poor prognosis. Based on several studies that compared CK-MB and cardiac troponin assays in patients with ACS, a substantial increase in rate of MIs ranging from 12% to 127% was detected. In one study of 1719 patients with ACS presenting to rule in/rule out MI, a subset (5%) of cTnI-negative but CK-MB-positive patients revealed the potentially underlying false-positive MI rate when using CK-MB as a standard for MI detection. This was likely due to release of CK-MB from skeletal muscle, in the absence of myocardial injury. Further, a subset (12%) of

cTnI-positive, CK-MB-negative patients demonstrated a subset of MIs that would not have been detected without cardiac troponin monitoring. All these data taken together support the implementation of cardiac troponin in place of, not in combination with, CK-MB. This fact will then have an impact on the prognosis of AMI overall.

Creatine Kinase MB

CK-MB can be measured in numerous ways. Immunoassays developed in recent years have improved on the analytical and clinical sensitivity and specificity of the earlier immunoinhibition and immunoprecipitation assays. These assays now: (1) measure CK-MB directly and provide mass measurements, (2) are easily automated, and (3) provide rapid results (≤30 minutes). Mass assays reliably measure low CK-MB concentrations in both samples with low total enzyme activity (<100 U/L) and with high total enzyme activity (>10,000 U/L). Furthermore, no interferences from other proteins have been documented. The majority of commercially available immunoassays that use monoclonal anti-CK-MB antibodies are the same as those listed in Table 5-2 for cardiac troponin assays. Excellent concordance has been shown between mass concentration and activity assays. A primary reference material is commercially available to assist in harmonization. If used for assay standardization, then this material allows concentrations to be reported within 20% of each other.

As has been recognized for years for total CK, all CK-MB assays demonstrate a significant 1.2- to 2.6-fold higher 99th percentile for males versus females. Several assays showed higher, up to 2.7-fold, concentrations for African-Americans versus Caucasians. These data demonstrate that clinical laboratories must consider establishing different CK-MB reference cutoffs for at least men versus women.

CLINICAL UTILIZATION OF CARDIAC BIOMARKERS

Use in Patients with Acute Coronary Syndrome

The ideal marker of myocardial injury should: (1) provide early detection of injury, (2) allow rapid diagnosis of cardiac injury, (3) serve as a risk stratification tool in patients with ACS, (4) assess the success of reperfusion after thrombolytic therapy, (5) detect reocclusion and reinfarction, (6) determine the timing of an infarction as well as infarct size, and (7) detect procedural-related perioperative MI during cardiac or noncardiac surgery. At present, the perfect biomarker to satisfy all these needs does not exist. It is the function of the laboratory to provide advice to physicians about cardiac biomarker characteristics.

Patients present to emergency departments or other primary care providers with a multitude of clinical signs and symptoms for which the differential diagnosis of AMI (heart attack) is considered. Figure 5-3 demonstrates the complete spectrum of clinical presentations of such a patient. This entire spectrum of clinical presentations has been designated ACS. The cornerstone of the redefinition of MI is predicated on cardiac biomarkers, specifically cTnI or cTnT. The following are designated as biochemical indicators for detecting myocardial necrosis:

1. A maximal concentration of cTnI or cTnI exceeding the decision limit, defined as the 99th percentile of values for a reference control group, on at least one occasion during the first 24 hours after the index clinical event.
2. A maximal value of CK-MB (preferably mass) exceeding the 99th percentile of values for a reference control group on two successive samples or a maximal

value exceeding twice the upper reference limit during the first hours after the index clinical event. Although the consensus document states values for troponin and CK-MB should rise and fall, either a rising or a falling pattern should be considered diagnostic. Values that remain elevated without change are rarely due to MI.
3. In the absence of availability of a cardiac troponin or CK-MB assay, total CK greater than two times the upper reference limit may be employed.

In addition to the ESC/ACC consensus document for redefining MI, the ACC/American Heart Association guidelines for management of unstable angina recommend monitoring cardiac troponin in patients with ACS as a way of differentiating unstable angina (defined as when cardiac troponin is within the 99th percentile reference limit) and non–ST segment-elevation MI (defined as when cardiac troponin is increased above the 99th percentile reference limit).

Several markers should no longer be used to evaluate cardiac disease, including aspartate aminotransferase, total CK, total lactate dehydrogenase (LDH), and LDH isoenzymes. Due to their wide tissue distribution, these markers have poor specificity for the detection of cardiac injury. Because total CK and CK-MB have served as standards for so many years, some laboratories may continue to measure them to allow for comparisons to cardiac troponin over time, before discontinuing use of CK and CK-MB. In addition, the use of total CK in developing countries may be the preferred or only alternative for financial reasons. However, it should be clear that, for monitoring ACS patients to assist in clinical classification, cardiac troponin is the preferred biomarker.

For the majority of patients, blood should be obtained for testing at hospital admission (0 hours), at 6 to 9 hours, and again at 12 to 24 hours if the earlier specimens are normal and the clinical index of suspicion is high. For patients in need of an early diagnosis that would parallel a rapid triage protocol, a rapidly appearing biomarker such as myoglobin has been suggested to be added to serial cardiac troponin monitoring. In practice, it appears that the majority of hospitals throughout the world do not use these markers.

Several general clinical impressions can be made regarding cTnI and cTnT. First, the early

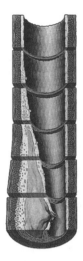

Stages of Vascular Inflammation
- Proinflammatory Cytokines
  - IL-6
- Plaque Destabilization
  - MPO
- Plaque Rupture
  - sCD40l
- Acute Phase Reactants
  - hs-CRP
- Ischemia
  - IMA
- Necrosis
  - cTnT
  - cTNi
- Myocardial Dysfunction
  - BNP
  - NT-proBNP

Figure 5-3. Complete spectrum of acute coronary pathophysiological process from initiation of atherosclerosis to cell death. Biomarkers released at different stages include interleukin 6 (IL-6), myeloperoxidase (MPO), soluble CD40 ligand (sCD40L), high-sensitivity C-reactive protein (Hs-CRP), ischemia-modified albumin (IMA), cardiac troponins I and T (cTnT and cTnI, respectively), B-type natriuretic peptide (BNP), and N-terminal proBNP (NT-proBNP). Of these, only the troponins and BMPs are myocardial specific.

release kinetics of both cTnI and cTnT are similar to those of CK-MB after AMI, with increases above the upper reference limit seen at 2 to 6 hours. The initial increase is due to the 3% to 6% cytoplasm fraction of troponin (CK-MB is 100% cytoplasmic). Second, cTnI and cTnT can remain increased up to 4 to 14 days after AMI. The mechanism is likely the ongoing release of troponin from the 94% to 97% myofibril-bound fraction since the half-life in clearance studies of either the native protein or of complexes is in the range of 2 hours. The long interval of cardiac troponin increase has resulted in its utilization in place of the LDH isoenzyme assay in the detection of late-presenting AMI patients. Third, the very low to undetectable cardiac troponin values in serum from patients without cardiac disease (normal, healthy reference population) permits use of lower discriminator concentrations compared to CK-MB for the determination of myocardial injury. Finally, cardiac tissue specificity of cTnI and cTnT should eliminate false clinical impression of AMI in patients with increased CK-MB concentrations following skeletal muscle injuries.

Clinical use of the percentage relative index [%RI; %RI = (CK-MB mass/Total CK activity × 100)] or %CK-MB (CK-MB activity/Total CK × 100) aids in the interpretation of CK-MB concentrations for the detection of AMI. While not absolute, an increased %CK-MB or %RI points to the heart as the source of CK-MB in serum. However, the %RI and %CK-MB should not be used for interpretation when the total CK activity remains within the reference interval. Any concomitant skeletal muscle injury will decrease the sensitivity of the relative index for the detection of cardiac events.

As increases in cardiac troponin detect any form of myocardial injury, nonischemic mechanisms of injury are also responsible for cardiac troponin release from the heart, causing increases in circulating troponin. Table 5-3 shows a list of potential etiologies that have been responsible for increases in non-ischemic damage to the heart. Thus, whenever cardiac troponin is monitored, it is important to follow the serial pattern of a rising or a falling pattern of the biomarker. An increased cTn pattern that remains relatively unchanged and is not indicative of this serial trend is likely not an MI.

Strategies for the Role of Cardiac Troponin for Risk Assessment

Numerous prospective and retrospective clinical studies have evaluated and compared the utility of measurements of cTnI and cTnT for risk stratification or clinical outcomes assessment of patients with ACS with possible myocardial

Table 5-3. Elevations of Troponins without Overt Ischemic Heart Disease

Trauma (including contusion, ablation, pacing, cardioversion)

Congestive heart failure, acute and chronic*

Aortic valve disease and hypertrophic obstructive cardiomyopathy with significant left ventricular hypertrophy*

Hypertension

Hypotension, often with arrhythmias

Postoperative noncardiac surgery patients who seem to do well*

Renal failure*

Critically ill patients, especially with diabetes, respiratory failure*

Drug toxicity, such as adriamycin, 5-fluorouracil, herceptin, snake venoms*

Hypothyroidism

Coronary vasospasm, including apical ballooning syndrome

Inflammatory diseases such as myocarditis (e.g., with parvovirus B19, Kawasaki disease, sarcoidosis, smallpox vaccination, or myocardial extension of bacterial endocarditis)

Postpercutaneous coronary intervention patients who appear without complication*

Pulmonary embolism, severe pulmonary hypertension*

Sepsis*

Burns, especially if total burn surface area >30%*

Infiltrative diseases, including amyloidosis, hemochromatosis, sarcoidosis, and scleroderma*

Acute neurological disease, including cerebrovascular accident, subarachnoid bleeds*

Rhabdomyolysis with cardiac injury

Transplant vasculopathy

Vital exhaustion

*Designations imply prognostic information has been reported.

ischemia in the emergency department. Patients presenting with a complaint of chest pain or other symptoms suggesting ACS have been assigned to blood-sampling protocols including only a single draw at presentation as well as to several serial blood samplings over a 12- to 24-hour period following presentation. Overall, in the approximately 18,000 patients studied, at 30 days the odds ratio for an adverse outcome was 3.4 for increased troponin. As both cTnT and cTnI offer powerful risk assessment, cTn monitoring needs to be included in current practice guidelines not only regarding diagnosis and management of ACS patients, but also as useful risk stratification tools. It is recommended to draw two samples on patients with ACS who do not rule in for AMI: one at presentation and one at 6 to 9 hours following presentation. This will allow for an increase in either cardiac troponin to occur above baseline in a patient presenting with a very recent acute coronary lesion. However, it should be noted that a normal cardiac troponin does not remove all risk.

Several studies have now documented that assays with lower limits of detection are able to identify more patients with ACS with poor prognosis who may be candidates for early invasive procedures. In one representative study (Venge et al., 2000), two assays were compared to assess clinical performance in unstable patients with CAD. While both assays showed patients with normal cTnI levels had a significantly better prognosis than patients with increased levels, a cohort of 11% of patients (n = 98) with a poor prognosis was identified only by the second-generation assay with a lower limit of detection. Invasive treatment only reduced clinical events in the group of patients with increased cTnI. Thus, each troponin assay, I or T, needs to evaluate the stratification of patients at low-end concentrations to avoid the potential of analytical inaccuracies leading to inappropriate management decisions and therapy. These high-risk patients have been shown to benefit from aggressive therapies, including low molecular weight heparin, IIb/IIIa glycoprotein platelet inhibitors, and an early interventional strategy.

Clinicians are often confronted with a clinical history of a patient without overt CAD and a low probability of myocardial ischemia. However, as a precautionary reflex, serial cardiac biomarkers, specifically cTn, are ordered. The 20% of suspected ACS patients who clinically do not rule in for MI but display an increased cTn represent those nonischemic pathologies such as myocarditis, blunt chest trauma, or chemotherapeutic agents for which the mechanisms of injury are well defined (Table 5-3) as well as the unexpected finding of myocardial injury, for which patients have been shown to have increased cTn, but the mechanism of release is not clear. These observations have led to important and novel investigations involving patients with nonischemic heart disease and the role for cardiac troponin as a diagnostic and prognostic tool. The conditions shown in Table 5-3 that are indicated by an asterisk demonstrate that, in addition to cardiac troponin being indicative of cardiac injury, the data have also indicated that increased cardiac troponin is useful as a prognostic tool for assessing risk of death and MI.

Monitoring Reperfusion Following Thrombolytic Therapy

Release of cTnI or cTnT from myocardium into the blood following AMI and after the washout that accompanies successful reperfusion generates an excellent signal compared to no detectable baseline levels prior to myocardial damage. The initial rapid release of cardiac troponin subunits I and T following successful reperfusion is most likely derived from the soluble cytosolic myocardial fraction (6% cTnT, 3% cTnI). The clinical utility of cardiac biomarkers for monitoring reperfusion following thrombolytic therapy has not gained favor as a routine form of testing for determining the success or failure of reperfusion therapy because it cannot distinguish TIMI 2 from TIMI 3 flow, which is a critical issue in regard to prognosis. (TIMI is the timed intervention in myocardial infarction. TIMI 2 and 3 refer to the extent of flow through coronary vessels, with TIMI 2 referring to partial flow and TIMI 3 to complete flow.)

It is accepted that the kinetics of myocardial protein appearance in the circulation depends on infarct perfusion. Early reperfusion causes an earlier increase above the upper reference limit and an earlier and greater enzyme peak after reperfusion. However, once the peak has occurred, there is no difference in the time of clearance of enzymes. In addition, enhanced washout identifies whether an artery is patent or closed but cannot distinguish between normal and abnormal coronary perfusion, which is another key prognostic parameter. Further, it is difficult to assess the amount of irreversible myocardial injury by infarct sizing because of the large variability in the amount of enzyme washout that appears after reperfusion.

Strategies Using Multimarkers

There is a growing body of evidence suggesting that different cardiac biomarkers provide independent and complementary information about pathophysiology, diagnostics, prognostics, and response to therapy in patients with ACS. Thus, it is probable that multimarker strategies or biochemical profiling may be used to characterize individual patients presenting with ACS. For example, in one multicenter study, cTnI, CK-MB, and myoglobin multimarker analysis identified positive patients earlier and provided a better risk stratification for 30-day mortality than central laboratory analysis of CK-MB alone (20% vs. 3%, respectively).

Estimation of Infarct Size

Older studies have shown that one can use the integrated values for total or CK-MB to estimate the biochemical extent of infarction. Further studies verified that the amount of cardiac damage is the primary determinant of prognosis. Such determinations have been correlated with morphological infarct size. Some have used the peak CK-MB value as a surrogate for the integrated data. Reperfusion changes the release ratio (the percentage of marker that appears in the blood relative to the amount depleted from myocardium), making infarct sizing problematic in the modern era. Additional data from both experimental and patient-related data have suggested that the 72-hour troponin measurement correlates with scintigraphically-determined infract size. The data are stronger for troponin T than for I, although the principles are probably similar for both analytes. At present, it is not recommended that serial monitoring of cardiac troponin or CK-MB be used for infarct sizing.

Reinfarction

Figure 5-1 demonstrates the serial patterns for cardiac troponin I and CK-MB both during the initial infarct and reinfarction, as described for the initial case presentation. Although the number of reinfarction cases presented in the literature is fewer than 20, the findings demonstrate that CK-MB analysis is no longer clinically relevant, or cost-effective, in the differential diagnosis of myocardial reinfarction in patients with ACS when cardiac troponin monitoring is available. We encourage others to test this hypothesis to be able to dispel the theoretical rationale for use of CK-MB testing in addition to cTn testing, expediting the cost-effective adaptation favoring only cTn monitoring in testing for MI or reinfarction.

QUESTIONS

1. Diagram the rising and falling serial biomarker profiles for cardiac troponins compared to CK-MB.
2. Define the ESC/ACC consensus guidelines for the redefinition of AMI.
3. Review the role of cardiac biomarkers for infarct sizing and monitoring the success of reperfusion following therapy.
4. List the multiple forms of cardiac troponin I that may exist in the circulation.
5. Define the two major concerns that have been responsible for substantial concentration differences when measuring cardiac troponin I by different commercial immunoassays.
6. Explain how the determination of reference intervals can have an impact on the number of MI cases that are defined in a given population of patients with chest pain.
7. Explain the role of cardiac troponin determinations in risk-stratifying patients who present with ACS.

BIBLIOGRAPHY

Alpert JS, Thygesen K, Antman E, et al.: Myocardial infarction redefined—a consensus document of the Joint European Society of Cardiology/American College of Cardiology Committee for the redefinition of myocardial infarction. *J Am Coll Cardiol* **36**:959-959, 2000.

Apple FS: Tissue specificity of cardiac troponin I, cardiac troponin T, and creatine kinase MB. *Clin Chim Acta* **284**:151-159, 1999.

Apple FS, Falahati A, Paulsen PR, et al.: Improved detection of minor ischemic myocardial injury with measurement of serum cardiac troponin I. *Clin Chem* **43**:2047-2051, 1997.

Apple FS, Murakami MM: Cardiac troponin and creatine kinase MB monitoring during in-hospital myocardial reinfarction. *Clin Chem* **51**:460-463, 2005.

Apple FS, Quist HE, Doyle PJ, et al.: Plasma 99th percentile reference limits for cardiac troponin and creatine kinase MB mass for use with European Society of Cardiology/American College of Cardiology consensus recommendations. *Clin Chem* **49**:1331-1336, 2003.

Apple FS, Wu AHB, Jaffe AS: European Society of Cardiology and American College of Cardiology guidelines for redefinition of myocardial infarction: how to use existing assays clinically and for clinical trials. *Am Heart J* **144**:981-986, 2002.

Bodor GS, Porter S, Landt Y, et al.: Development of monoclonal antibodies for an assay of cardiac troponin-I and preliminary results in suspected cases of myocardial infarction. *Clin Chem* **38**:2203-2214, 1992.

Fishbein MC, Wang T, Matijasevic M, et al.: Myocardial tissue troponins T and I: an immunohistochemical study in experimental models of myocardial ischemia. *Cardiovasc Pathol* **12**:65-71, 2003.

Ingwall JS, Kramer MF, Fifer MA, et al.: The creatine kinase system in normal and diseased human myocardium. *N Engl J Med* **313**:1050-1054, 1985.

Jaffe AS, Landt Y, Parvin CA, et al.: Comparative sensitivity of cardiac troponin I and lactate dehydrogenase isoenzymes for diagnosing acute myocardial infarction. *Clin Chem* **42**:1770-1776, 1996.

Jaffe AS, Ravkilde J, Roberts R, et al.: It's time for a change to a troponin standard. *Circulation* **102**:1216-1220, 2000.

Katrukha AG, Bereznikova AV, Filtaov VL, et al.: Degradation of cardiac troponin I: implication for reliable immunodetection. *Clin Chem* **44**:2433-2440, 1998

Katus HA, Looser S, Hallermayer K, et al.: Development and *in vitro* characterization of a new immunoassay of cardiac troponin T. *Clin Chem* **38**:386-393, 1992

Lin JC, Apple FS, Murakami MM, et al.: Rates of positive cardiac troponin I and creatine kinase MB among patients hospitalized for suspected acute coronary syndromes. *Clin Chem* **50**:333-338, 2004.

Ottani F, Galvani M, Nicolini A, et al.: Elevated cardiac troponin levels predict the risk of adverse outcome in patients with acute coronary syndromes. *Am Heart J* **40**:917-927, 2000.

Panteghini M, Gerhardt W, Apple FS, et al.: Quality specifications for cardiac troponin assays. *Clin Chem Lab Med* **39**:174-178, 2001.

Venge P, Lagerquist B, Diderholm E, et al. on behalf of the FRISC II Study Group: Clinical performance of three cardiac troponin assays in patients with unstable coronary artery disease (a FRISC II Substudy). *Am J Cardiol* **89**:1035-1041, 2000.

6

Hereditary Spherocytosis

HIROSHI IDEGUCHI

CASE REPORT

A 25-year-old Japanese man was admitted to the hospital because of fever, sore throat, and general malaise. He had been febrile for several days and had noticed that the color of his urine was unusually dark. On admission, his temperature was 37.8°C. The physician noted anemic conjunctiva (delicate membrane lining the eyelids and covering the eyeballs), injected pharyngeal mucosa (mucous membrane), cervical lymphadenopathy (swelling of the lymph nodes), and mild splenomegaly (enlargement of the spleen).

Hematological data showed moderate anemia (hemoglobin 95 g/L; normal is 136–172 g/L), increased reticulocytes (7.8%; normal is <2.4%), and leukocytosis (leukocytes 12×10^9/L; normal is 3.2–9.8×10^9/L) with increased lymphocytes (62% of total leukocytes). The blood film showed moderate anisocytosis (variability of size of erythrocytes), increased spherocytes (small, globular erythrocytes without the usual central pallor), and a scatter of atypical lymphocytes.

The urine examination revealed no abnormality except an increase of urobilinogen. The erythrocyte sedimentation rate was increased (45 mm per hour; normal is <20 mm per hour).

Biochemical data for his serum were as follows: total bilirubin 99.2 μmol/L (normal is 3.4–20.5 μmol/L); conjugated bilirubin 15.4 μmol/L (normal is 0–6.8 μmol/L); alanine aminotransferase 125 U/L (normal is 0–40 U/L); and lactate dehydrogenase 570 U/L (normal is 120–250 U/L).

The serological examinations for Epstein-Barr virus confirmed that he had infectious mononucleosis. He was kept in bed for 2 weeks, by which time the signs of inflammation and hepatocellular damage entirely disappeared. However, mild anemia (hemoglobin 110–120 g/L) with reticulocytosis (5.0%–6.0%), increased serum unconjugated bilirubin, and splenomegaly still remained, suggesting the presence of persistent hemolysis. The physician therefore performed further examinations to confirm the diagnosis of hemolytic anemia.

Bone marrow aspirates from the sternum showed marked erythroid hyperplasia, with a granuloid to erythroid ratio of 1:1.5. The antiglobulin (Coombs) test failed to detect autoantibodies to red blood cells. The sugar-water test and Ham test, the diagnostic tests for paroxysmal nocturnal hemoglobinuria, were negative. The levels of both hemoglobin F and hemoglobin A_2 were normal, and hemoglobin electrophoresis showed no abnormally migrating hemoglobins. The isopropanol test did not reveal any unstable hemoglobins. In contrast, the osmotic fragility of the patient's erythrocytes was increased, and it was enhanced by incubating the cells at 37°C for 24 hours. These results were consistent with a diagnosis of hereditary spherocytosis (HS).

Abdominal ultrasound revealed moderate splenomegaly and gallstones. The patient had an episode of transient jaundice of unknown etiology at the age of 22 years. His parents had been in apparent good health. However, his father had also experienced repeated episodes of mild jaundice since childhood. His father's erythrocytes were also spherical and osmotically fragile.

(a) **(b)**

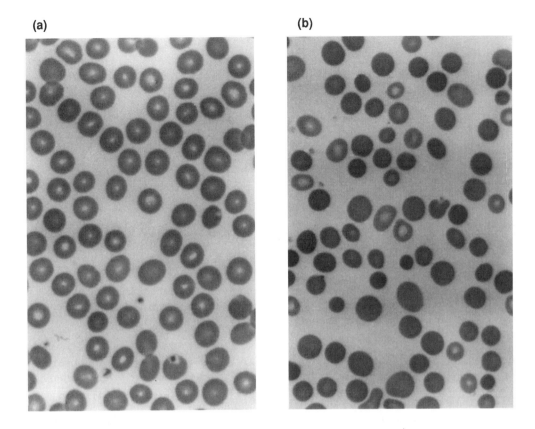

Figure 6-1. Photomicrographs of blood films of a normal subject (*a*) and a patient with HS (*b*). Small, densely staining microspherocytes can be seen in (*b*).

From these findings, he was finally diagnosed as having (1) HS with gallstones and (2) infectious mononucleosis. The patient underwent splenectomy and cholecystectomy at the age of 26 years. An enlarged spleen weighing 530 g and a gallbladder containing numerous small stones were removed. Two months after the operation, all previous findings reflecting accelerated hemolysis disappeared.

DIAGNOSIS

The most important diagnostic features of HS are as follows: (1) congenital hemolytic anemia; (2) microspherocytosis on the peripheral blood film; (3) increased osmotic fragility, particularly in incubated red cells; and (4) negative antiglobulin (Coombs) test.

A typical HS patient is relatively asymptomatic, and mild jaundice may be the only symptom of the disease. Anemia is usually mild or even absent owing to compensatory erythroid hyperplasia in bone marrow. Spherocytosis, or more correctly microspherocytosis, is a characteristic feature of the stained blood films (Fig. 6-1). The microspherocytes are small cells, usually with perfectly round contours, that stain relatively densely with May-Grunwald-Giemsa stain. The reticulocyte count is usually increased (5%–20%) and remains high throughout the patient's life unless splenectomy has been carried out.

The osmotic fragility test is the most sensitive and useful test for the diagnosis of HS (Fig. 6-2). Although the fresh red cells of about 20% of HS patients have a normal or near-normal osmotic fragility, the test performed in cells incubated at 37°C for 24 hours is more often positive in association with an increased rate of spontaneous hemolysis (autohemolysis).

Patients with HS are occasionally subject to "crises," a sudden exaggeration of their anemia. Two types of crises, hemolytic and aplastic, are

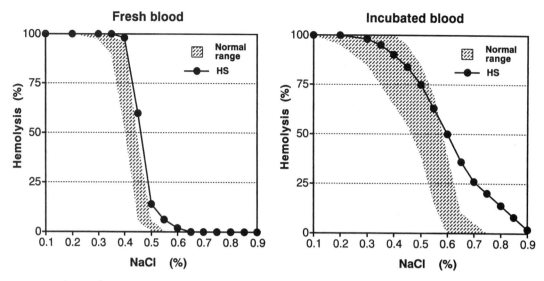

Figure 6-2. Osmotic fragility test (Parpart method). A typical osmotic fragility curve of fresh (left) or 24-hour incubated (right) erythrocytes from a patient with HS is shown. The hatched area represents the normal range.

known. As in the patient described in the case report, hemolytic crises usually occur with common viral syndromes and are characterized by a manifestation of accelerated destruction of red cells, such as a transient increase in jaundice, anemia, reticulocytosis, and splenomegaly. On the other hand, aplastic crises are brought about by a temporary failure of erythropoiesis, mostly caused by human parvovirus B19 infection (erythema infectiosum). During the aplastic phase, the counts of red cells and reticulocytes rapidly fall, and marrow erythroblasts disappear.

Aplastic crises are less frequent but are usually more serious, and severe life-threatening anemia can result.

Gallstones are a common complication of HS, and most patients eventually develop them; they are rarely found in children, and their incidence increases with age. Since gallstone colic (severe convulsive abdominal pain) and cholecystitis (inflammation of the gall bladder) are quite common, it is desirable that patients with HS should be periodically examined by abdominal ultrasound.

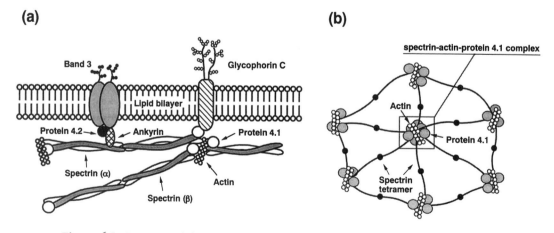

Figure 6-3. Structure of the red cell membrane (*a*) and the hexagonal lattice structure of the membrane skeleton (*b*).

BIOCHEMICAL PERSPECTIVES

History

HS was first described in 1871 by Vanlair and Masius (Vanlair and Masius, 1871). They reported a young woman who had repeated attacks of abdominal pain and jaundice and found that some of her erythrocytes were spherical and much smaller than normal. In 1907, Chauffard (Chauffard, 1907) demonstrated increased osmotic fragility of erythrocytes as the hallmark of the disease. A membrane lesion was first suggested by the observation of Bertles in 1957 (Bertles, 1957) that HS red cells are unusually permeable to sodium ions. Since then, many abnormalities have been reported in HS red cells, but it is now clear that HS is a consequence of heterogeneous defects in the red cell membrane proteins.

Red Cell Membrane Organization

The red cell membrane has been well characterized biochemically, and the topological organization of various lipids and proteins has been delineated (Fig. 6-3a). The major lipid components are phospholipids and cholesterol, and their composition is responsible for the fluidity of the membrane matrix in which transmembrane proteins reside. The membrane proteins are conventionally separated in the laboratory by sodium dodecyl sulfate-polyacrylamide gel electrophoresis (Fig. 6-4; Table 6-1). They are classified into two groups, integral and peripheral proteins. The integral proteins, such as band 3 and glycophorin C (Fig. 6-3), penetrate into or are embedded in the lipid bilayer and are tightly bound to the membrane lipids through hydrophobic interactions. In contrast, the peripheral proteins such as spectrin are located on the cytoplasmic surface of the lipid bilayer and associated with each other to form a flexible, filamentous network, generally referred to as the *membrane skeleton*; they are responsible for red cell shape and deformability.

The major components of the membrane skeleton are spectrin, actin, and protein 4.1. Spectrin is a highly flexible, rodlike molecule composed of two nonidentical polypeptides: α-spectrin and β-spectrin. These chains are aligned side by side in the form of a αβ-heterodimer, and spectrin heterodimers in turn join head to head to form (αβ)$_2$-tetramers. The tail ends of spec-

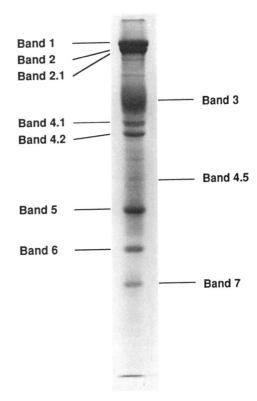

Peripheral — **Integral**

Band 1
Band 2
Band 2.1
Band 3
Band 4.1
Band 4.2
Band 4.5
Band 5
Band 6
Band 7

Figure 6-4. Sodium dodecyl sulfate polyacrylamide gel electrophoresis pattern of normal red cell membrane proteins with Coomassie blue staining.

trin tetramers are associated with short actin filaments. Although the spectrin–actin interaction is itself weak, each spectrin–actin junction is greatly stabilized by the formation of a ternary complex with the protein 4.1. Thus, six spectrin termini complex with each actin oligomer to form a network with an approximately hexagonal lattice (Fig. 6-3b).

The major integral proteins include band 3 (anion exchanger 1) and the glycophorins (Fig. 6-3). These proteins span the membrane and have distinct structural and functional domains. The two clearly established functions of band 3 are: the (1) mediation of the Cl^-–HCO_3^- exchange across the membrane, which is essential for the transport of CO_2 from the tissues to the lungs; and (2) anchorage of the underlying membrane skeleton to the membrane by binding to ankyrin (band 2.1) and possibly protein 4.2.

Table 6-1. Major Red Cell Membrane Proteins

Band	Designation	Molecular Weight	Peripheral (P) or Integral (I)	Function
Band 1	Spectrin-α	240 K	P	Membrane skeleton
Band 2	Spectrin-β	220 K	P	Membrane skeleton
Band 2.1	Ankyrin	210 K	P	Anchoring skeleton to bilayer
Band 3	Anion exchanger	95 K	I	Anion transport; binding sites for ankyrin, protein 4.2
Band 4.1	Protein 4.1	80 K	P	Membrane skeleton; association with GPC
Band 4.2	Protein 4.2	72 K	P	Stabilizing ankyrin–band 3 interaction (?)
Band 5	Actin	43 K	P	Membrane skeleton
Band 6	G3PD	35 K	P	Glyceraldehyde 3-phosphate dehydrogenase
Band 7	Stomatin	31 K	I	Regulating monovalent cation transport (?)
GPA	Glycophorin A	36 K	I	MNSs blood group*
GPB	Glycophorin B	20 K	I	
GPC	Glycophorin C	32 K	I	Gerbich blood group; association with protein 4.1
GPD	Glycophorin D	23 K	I	

*MN and Ss are antigens on human red blood cells. Each of the antigens M,N,S, and s are identifiable by reaction with specific antisera: anti-M, anti-N, anti-S, and anti-s. These glycophorin A and glycophorin B antigens are polypeptides are coded by genes on chromosome 4.

The four sialic acid-rich glycoproteins (glycophorins A, B, C, and D) also belong to the class of integral proteins. The presence of sialic acids imparts a strong net negative charge to the erythrocyte surface; this is functionally important in reducing the interaction of red cells with one another as well as with other blood cells or the vascular endothelium.

Molecular Lesions in Hereditary Spherocytosis Erythrocytes

As knowledge of the membrane skeleton and its contribution to red cell shape and stability emerged during the 1970s, investigators sought evidence of a skeletal protein defect in HS. The search was given impetus by the finding of a marked spectrin deficiency in the common house mouse. The red cells of these mice were spherocytic and osmotically fragile, and they spontaneously vesiculated in the circulation. Thus, investigators have focused on spectrin as the possible primary lesion of HS.

In 1982, Agre and coworkers (Agre et al., 1982) first described two patients with severe HS inherited autosomal recessively and whose red cells had only about half of the normal spectrin content. However, in the majority of HS patients, spectrin deficiency may not represent the primary molecular defect since recent cytogenetic studies and subsequent biochemical studies have led to the identification of dis-

tinct molecular defects in other membrane proteins (Table 6-2).

It is now clear that a deficiency or dysfunction of ankyrin, the protein that anchors the spectrin-based skeleton to band 3 (Fig. 6-3), may represent a common membrane lesion in HS. The synthesis of ankyrin and its assembly on the membrane were reduced, and as a consequence, assembly of spectrin was also impaired despite normal spectrin synthesis. In 1996, Jarolim et al. showed that a deficiency of ankyrin (and its related spectrins) was present in 60% of 166 unrelated patients with HS.

Partial deficiency of band 3 was reported in about 25% of patients with HS who presented with a phenotype of a mild-to-moderate dominantly inherited HS. Nearly 50 different band 3 mutations associated with HS have been reported.

A deficiency of protein 4.2 has also been noted in several patients with recessively inherited HS, particularly in the Japanese population. Although the physiological role of protein 4.2 remains to be established, this protein is thought to stabilize the binding of band 3 to spectrin mediated by ankyrin.

Because of the heterogeneous molecular nature of HS (Table 6-2), the "HS genes" can be assigned to several chromosomes: chromosome 1 (α-spectrin), chromosome 8 (ankyrin), chromosome 14 (β-spectrin), chromosome 15 (protein 4.2), and chromosome 17 (band 3). The

Table 6-2. Molecular Basis of Hereditary Spherocytosis

Responsible Gene	Chromosome Locus	Phenotype and Molecular Lesion	Inheritance	Clinical Expression	Prevalence
Spectrin-α	1	Spectrin deficiency	AR	Severe	Rare
Spectrin-β	14	Defective binding to protein 4.1 Spectrin Kissimmee (202Trp→Arg) Others	AD	Mild to moderate	~10%
Ankyrin	8	Ankyrin and spectrin deficiency Ankyrin gene deletion Promoter region mutations Ankyrin Stuttgart (329: 2-nt deletion) Ankyrin Einbeck (572: 1-nt Insertion) Ankyrin Marburg (797/798: 4-nt deletion) Ankyrin Bovenden (1436Arg→ter) Others	AD or AR	Mild to severe	50%–60%
Band 3	17	Band 3 deficiency Band 3 Boston (285Ala→Asp) Band 3 Coimbra (488Val→Met) Band 3 Kyoto (490Arg→Cys) (Bicêtre I) Band 3 Prague II (760Arg→Gln) Band 3 Birmingham (834His→Pro) Band 3 Philadelphia (837Thr→Met) Others	AD	Mild to moderate	20%–30%
Protein 4.2	15	Protein 4.2 deficiency Protein 4.2 Nippon (142Ala→Thr) Protein 4.2 Fukuoka (119Trp→ter) Protein 4.2 Tozeur (310Arg→Gln) Protein 4.2 Shiga (317Arg→Cys) Others	AR	Mild to moderate	Rare; more common in Japan

AD, autosomal dominant; AR, autosomal recessive.

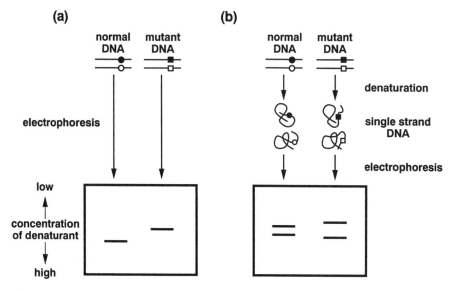

Figure 6-5. Rapid and sensitive methods for detecting mutations in DNA. (*a*) Denaturing gradient gel electrophoresis. (*b*) Single-strand conformation polymorphism.

inheritance is both autosomal dominant (in the majority of patients with HS) and autosomal recessive.

Several rapid and sensitive methods have been developed to detect mutations in cDNA and genomic DNA. These include ribonuclease (RNase) protection analysis, denaturing gradient gel electrophoresis, and single-strand conformation polymorphism analysis. These methods can be used in conjunction with the PCR technique to detect small deletions or insertions and single base substitutions.

RNase protection is used to detect the RNase-sensitive site in a synthetic RNA probe that has been hybridized with the DNA fragment to be examined. If a particular mutation lies within the DNA fragment, then the RNA probe is mismatched at the site of the mutation where RNase digestion occurs.

Denaturing gradient gel electrophoresis is used to detect the change in mobility of DNA fragments run on a polyacrylamide gel formed with an increasing gradient of the denaturant (urea, formamide). It is based on the principle that different DNA fragments have different points in the gradient where they begin to undergo regional denaturation, and the rate of migration is markedly slowed (Fig. 6-5a).

Single-strand conformation polymorphism analysis is the more popular method because of its simplicity and wide applicability to many different genes. This method makes use of

sequence-dependent folding of single-stranded DNA, which alters the electrophoretic mobility of the fragments, to detect sequence differences between closely related molecules. In brief, regions of DNA thought to contain mutations are amplified using the PCR technique and rendered single stranded by heating in a denaturing buffer. The separated strands are then fractionated on polyacrylamide gels under conditions that may resolve two molecules differing by a single base (Fig. 6-5b). If by one of these methods the DNA fragment appears to be abnormal, then the specific change can be determined by subsequent nucleotide sequence analysis.

Pathophysiology of Hemolysis in Hereditary Spherocytosis Erythrocytes

The importance of the spleen in the pathophysiology of the hemolysis of HS has been substantiated. Two factors determine the selective destruction of the HS cells in the spleen: (1) poor HS red cell deformability, which is a reflection of a decreased surface-to-volume ratio resulting from the loss of membrane; and (2) the unique anatomy of the splenic vasculature, which acts as a "microcirculation filter." As shown in Table 6-2, the underlying molecular basis of HS is heterogeneous, and the primary molecular lesion in HS is likely to involve several membrane proteins, including spectrin, ankyrin,

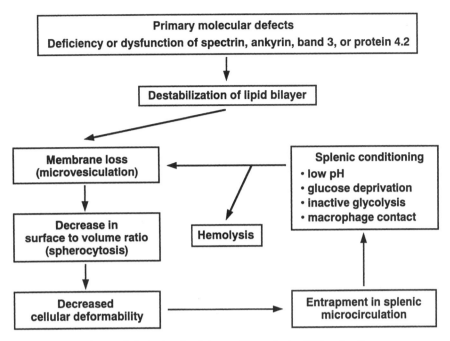

Figure 6-6. Pathophysiology of hemolysis of HS red cells.

band 3, and protein 4.2. These molecular lesions may finally lead to lipid bilayer destabilization and microvesiculation, resulting in surface area deficiency and formation of poorly deformable spherocytes (Fig. 6-6).

The principal sites of red cell entrapment in the spleen are openings in the endothelial wall of splenic sinuses, where blood enters the venous circulation. In contrast to normal discocytes, which have an abundant surface that allows red cells to deform and pass through narrow slits, the HS red cells lack the extra surface needed to permit deformation. Consequently, the nondeformable spherocytes accumulate in the red pulp and become grossly engorged. Once entrapped by the spleen, HS red cells incur additional damage. Because of the stagnant circulation, lactic acid accumulates, and the extracellular pH falls, probably to between 6.5 and 7.0. The intracellular pH also declines, inhibiting hexokinase and phosphofructokinase, the rate-limiting enzymes of glycolysis and thereby retarding glucose utilization and ATP production.

Contact of red cells with macrophages may inflict additional damage on the red cell membrane. Thus, the spherocytes in the splenic cords are severely stressed by detaining in a metabolically threatening environment and are subject to further loss of surface area and an increase in

the density of the cells. This process is known as *splenic conditioning* (Fig. 6-6). The conditioning effect of the spleen is likely to represent a cumulative injury. Conditioned red cells appear as microspherocytes in the peripheral circulation and are particularly susceptible to recapture and destruction in the spleen and other parts of the reticuloendothelial system.

THERAPY

Patients with mild cases of HS often do not need any treatment. However, these patients should be watched carefully for the development of hemolytic or aplastic crisis. Splenectomy is the treatment of choice in moderate-to-severe HS cases. In general, splenectomy is indicated in patients who are continuously anemic or who have a history of gallstone colic or repeated crises. The clinical results of splenectomy for HS are almost uniformly excellent. However, splenectomy in very young children should be postponed to later in childhood because splenectomized infants are more susceptible to serious and potentially lethal infections than are older children and adults. At the time of splenectomy, it is important to identify and remove any accessory spleen; otherwise, the operation will result in an unfavorable outcome. Patients who experience an episode of gallstone colic or cholecystitis may have to undergo simultaneous cholecystectomy.

Within days following splenectomy, jaundice fades, the hemoglobin concentration rises, and red cell survival usually returns to near normal. Although the number of peripheral blood microspherocytes remains unchanged, the morphological features of accelerated erythropoiesis are not observed. Blood transfusion is rarely indicated except during aplastic crisis. At such times, red cell replacement may be lifesaving.

QUESTIONS

1. What are the essential findings for the clinical diagnosis of HS?
2. Patients with HS may occasionally undergo two types of crises. Describe the mechanisms causing these crises.
3. Explain why HS red cells are hemolyzed *in vivo* principally in spleen.
4. Describe the structural organization of the membrane skeleton that is a major determinant of red cell shape and deformability.
5. Hereditary spherocytosis is a group of disorders caused by heterogeneous intrinsic defects of the red cell membrane proteins. Describe the rapid and sensitive methods to detect mutations in genomic DNA and complementary DNA.

BIBLIOGRAPHY

Agre P, Orringer EP, Bennett V: Deficient red-cell spectrin in severe recessively inherited spherocytosis. *N Engl J Med* **306**:1155-1161, 1982.

Becker PS, Lux SE: Hereditary spherocytosis and hereditary elliptocytosis, *in* Scriver CR, Beaudet AL, Sly WS, Valle D (eds): *The Metabolic and Molecular Basis of Inherited Disease*. 7th ed., Vol. 3. McGraw-Hill, New York, 1995, pp. 3513-3560.

Bertles JF: Sodium transport across the surface membrane of red cells in hereditary spherocytosis. *J Clin Invest* **36**:816-824, 1957.

Chauffard A: Pathogéne de l'ictére congenital de l'adulte. *Semin méd (Paris)* **27**:25-29, 1907.

Dacie J: Hereditary spherocytosis (HS), *in* Dacie J (ed): *The Haemolytic Anaemias*. 3rd ed., Vol. 1. Churchill Livingstone, Edinburg, Scotland, 1985, pp. 134-215.

Gallagher PG, Jarolim P: Red cell membrane disorders, *in* Hoffman R, Benz EJ, Shattil SJ, et al. (eds): *Hematology Basic Principles and Practice*. 3rd ed. Churchill Livingstone, 2000, pp. 576-610.

Hassoun H, Palek J: Hereditary spherocytosis: a review of the clinical and molecular aspects of the disease. *Blood Rev* **10**:129-147, 1996.

Jarolim P, Murray JL, Rubin HL, et al.: Characterization of 13 novel band 3 gene defects in hereditary spherocytosis with band 3 deficiency. *Blood* **88**:4366-4374, 1996.

Palek J, Sahr KE: Mutations of the red cell membrane proteins: from clinical evaluation to detection of the underlying genetic defect. *Blood* **80**:308-330, 1992.

Vanlair CF, Masius JB: De la microcythémie. *Bull Acad R Méd Belg* **5**, 3rd series:515-613, 1871.

Part II

Fuel Metabolism and Energetics

7

Pyruvate Dehydrogenase Complex Deficiency

PETER W. STACPOOLE and LESA R. GILBERT

CASE REPORT

Identical twins with the fictitious names Ann and Elizabeth were born 6 weeks prematurely to a healthy 26-year-old mother whose pregnancy was uneventful. The family history was noteworthy for epilepsy in a paternal aunt, congenital deafness in another paternal aunt, and possible mental retardation in a maternal cousin. The twins' sister was a healthy 3-year-old girl with the same biological father. The birth weight was 3 pounds 9 ounces for Ann and 3 pounds 12 ounces for Elizabeth. Apgar scores (numerical expressions of the condition of a newborn infant; based on assessment of heart rate, respiratory effort, muscle tone, reflex irritability, and color) 1 and 5 minutes after birth were 8 and 9 for both girls (maximum score is 10). Other than prematurity, neither child evidenced physical or laboratory abnormalities, and they were discharged home within 2 weeks (for Ann) and 3 weeks (for Elizabeth), both apparently in good health. The mother subsequently remarried and gave birth to a son, who has remained well through age 6 years.

During the 3 months following their birth, both sisters sustained recurrent upper respiratory illnesses. These were more severe in Elizabeth, who required frequent hospitalizations. Physical examination of both infants during this period disclosed poor feeding habits, failure to thrive, floppiness, microcephaly (small head size), and delayed developmental milestones. They were below the fifth percentile for weight and height. These findings were more pro-

nounced in Elizabeth, who also demonstrated ocular hypertelorism (abnormal increase in intraorbital distance) and pseudoathetosis (involuntary movements) of the lower face and hands. Magnetic resonance imaging (MRI) of Elizabeth's head revealed mild frontal atrophy and increased T2 signals in the periventricular and subcortical white matter. These signals are indicative of scarring or abnormalities in myelination. A pediatric neurologist diagnosed probable cerebral palsy in Elizabeth at age 1.5 years.

Formal neurobehavioral evaluation of both children at age 3 years 10 months generated the results summarized in Table 7-1. Further testing of Elizabeth showed profound hypotonia (decreased muscle tone), electrophysiological evidence of peripheral neuropathy, normal somatosensory evoked potentials, and a normal electroencephalogram recorded during sleep.

At age 2 years, the twins were placed on a diet comprised of approximately 60% total calories as (mainly saturated) long-chain fatty acids (see "Therapy" section). They tolerated this "ketogenic diet" well, gained weight, and showed mild psychomotor improvement. At age 3 years 9 months, they enrolled in a controlled clinical trial of oral dichloroacetate (DCA), an activator of the pyruvate dehydrogenase complex (PDC). Venous blood concentrations of lactate, obtained initially after an overnight fast and then 2 hours after a liquid meal containing 40% of calories as carbohydrate, were 1.2 mmol/L and 2.8 mmol/L, respectively, in Ann and 1.6 mmol/L and 5.7 mmol/L, respectively, in Elizabeth (normal venous blood lactate after

Table 7-1. Neurobehavioral Examination of Twins (Aged 3 years 10 months)

| Test | Developmental Age (months) | |
	Ann	Elizabeth
Vineland*	13–21	6–11
Bayley[†] mental	19	7
Bayley[†] motor	24	8

*Based on parental assessment of skills of communication, daily living, socialization, and motor function.

[†]From Black and Matula, (2000).

fasting 0.4–1.0 mmol/L). The cerebrospinal fluid lactate concentration, obtained prior to carbohydrate ingestion, was approximately 5.6 mmol/L (normal approximately 1 mmol/L) in both children.

DIAGNOSIS

The twins were referred subsequently to a metabolic specialist because of the suspicion of an inborn error of metabolism. Biochemical testing revealed each had a hyperchloremic (increased blood chloride concentration) metabolic acidosis that was more profound in Elizabeth. Serum levels of glucose and liver transaminases were normal. Urinary organic acids revealed modestly increased concentrations of lactate and ketone bodies. Blood samples and fibroblasts from skin biopsies from both girls were sent to an established diagnostic laboratory for genetic mitochondrial diseases. Tests of respiratory chain complex enzymatic activities were normal.

Results of the measurement of PDC enzyme activity are summarized in Table 7-2. These data revealed severely reduced PDC activities in both freshly isolated peripheral blood lymphocytes and cultured fibroblasts in Ann and an even more striking reduction in enzyme activities in cells from Elizabeth. In each case, the defect in PDC activity could be traced to

a deficiency in the α-subunit of the first (E1) enzyme (pyruvate dehydrogenase; pyruvate decarboxylase) of the complex.

BIOCHEMICAL PERSPECTIVES

Pyruvate Dehydrogenase Complex

PDC is a multienzyme complex located in the inner mitochondrial membrane. Under aerobic conditions, PDC catalyzes the rate-determining reaction for the oxidative removal of glucose, pyruvate, and lactate and helps sustain the tricarboxylic acid cycle by providing acetyl-CoA (Fig. 7-1). Reducing equivalents, in the form of NADH and $FADH_2$, are generated by reactions catalyzed by the PDC and by various dehydrogenases in the tricarboxylic acid cycle and provide electrons to the respiratory chain for eventual reduction of molecular oxygen to water and synthesis of ATP.

The PDCs of eukaryotes are the largest ($M_r \sim 10^7$) multienzyme complexes known. They are distinguished not only by size, but also by their morphology and unusual structural biology features. The complex is entirely nuclear encoded and consists of three basic functional types of catalytic protein (Fig. 7-2), a property shared with the other two mammalian α-ketoacid dehydrogenases that use α-ketoglutarate or branched-chain ketoacids as substrates, respectively. Pyruvate dehydrogenase (E1; EC 1.2.4.1) is a heterotetrameric (α2β2) α-ketoacid decarboxylase that irreversibly oxidizes pyruvate to acetyl-CoA in the presence of thiamine pyrophosphate (TPP) and catalyzes the subsequent reductive acetylation of the lipoyl moiety of dihydrolipoamide transacetylase (E2; EC 2.3.1.12). Lipoyl groups (Lip) that are covalently linked to E2 facilitate transfer of both protons and acetyl groups between the different component enzymes of the PDC. The resulting acetyl-lipoamide intermediate reacts with

Table 7-2. Residual Activity of the Pyruvate Dehydrogenase Complex (PDC) in Blood Lymphocytes or Cultured Skin Fibroblasts

| Enzyme Component | Residual Activity (% of normal) | |
	Ann	Elizabeth
PDC (total activity)	55% (lymphocytes)	18% (lymphocytes)
	28% (fibroblasts)	14% (fibroblasts)
E1 (pyruvate dehydrogenase)	34% (fibroblasts)	10% (fibroblasts)
E2 (dihydrolipoyl transacetylase)	Normal	Normal
E3 (dihydrolipoyl dehydrogenase)	Normal	Normal

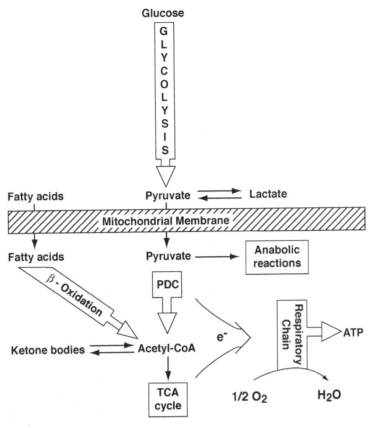

Figure 7-1. Pathways of fuel metabolism and oxidative phosphorylation. Pyruvate may be reduced to lactate in the cytoplasm or may be transported into the mitochondria for anabolic reactions, such as gluconeogenesis, or for oxidation to acetyl-CoA by the pyruvate dehydrogenase complex (PDC). Long-chain fatty acids are transported into mitochondria, where they undergo β-oxidation to ketone bodies (liver) or to acetyl-CoA (liver and other tissues). Reducing equivalents (NADH, FADH$_2$) are generated by reactions catalyzed by the PDC and the tricarboxylic acid (TCA) cycle and donate electrons (e$^-$) that enter the respiratory chain at NADH ubiquinone oxidoreductase (Complex I) or at succinate ubiquinone oxidoreductase (Complex II). Cytochrome c oxidase (Complex IV) catalyzes the reduction of molecular oxygen to water, and ATP synthase (Complex V) generates ATP from ADP. Reprinted with permission from Stacpoole et al. (1997).

coenzyme A (CoASH) to form acetyl-CoA and reduced lipoamide [Lip(SH)$_2$]. NAD$^+$ is the final electron acceptor, and reducing equivalents are transferred to the respiratory chain via NADH.

The central feature of the complex in eukaryotic cells is the 60-mer E2 core, which is highly conserved among species. The core is arranged as a pentagonal dodecahedron, a cagelike structure that serves as a scaffold about which the other components are organized (Fig. 7-3). Mammalian PDCs require a binding protein (BP; previously termed protein X) to anchor the dehydrolipoyl dehydrogenase dimer (E3; EC 1.8.1.4) to the core. The relative stochiometry for the structural components of bovine kidney PDC is approximately 22 molecules of E1, about 6 molecules of E2, and about 6 molecules of E3. Thus, each multienzyme complex contains potentially 60 centers for acetyl-CoA synthesis. Highly flexible structural domains in the PDC promote the channeling of intermediates of catalysis between the active sites and contribute to the remarkable structural and functional organization of the complex.

The PDC is a "junction box" for cellular metabolism and energetics in which substrates may be diverted toward anabolic pathways (e.g., carbohydrate synthesis) or catabolic reactions and

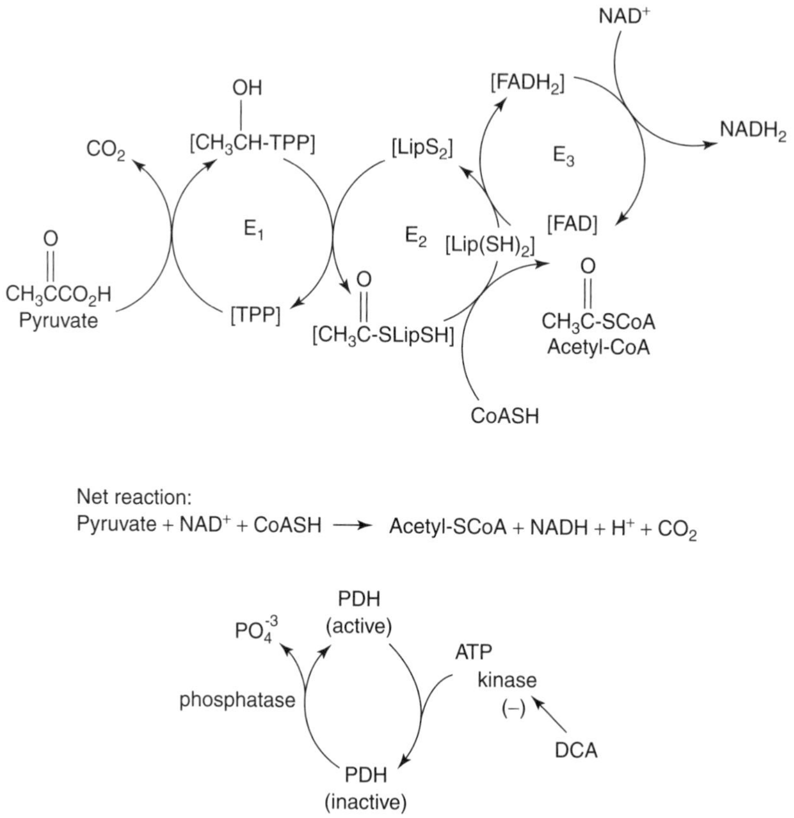

Figure 7-2. Reactions of the pyruvate dehydrogenase (PDH) multienzyme complex (PDC). Pyruvate is decarboxylated by the PDH subunit (E_1) in the presence of thiamine pyrophosphate (TPP). The resulting hydroxyethyl-TPP complex reacts with oxidized lipoamide (LipS$_2$), the prosthetic group of dehydrolipoamide transacetylase (E_2), to form acetyl lipoamide. In turn, this intermediate reacts with coenzyme A (CoASH) to yield acetyl-CoA and reduced lipoamide [Lip(SH)$_2$]. The cycle of reaction is completed when reduced lipoamide is reoxidized by the flavoprotein, dehydrolipoamide dehydrogenase (E_3). Finally, the reduced flavoprotein is oxidized by NAD$^+$ and transfers reducing equivalents to the respiratory chain via reduced NADH. PDC is regulated in part by reversible phosphorylation, in which the phosphorylated enzyme is inactive. Increases in the intramitochondrial ratios of NADH/NAD$^+$ and acetyl-CoA/CoASH also stimulate kinase-mediated phosphorylation of PDC. The drug dichloroacetate (DCA) inhibits the kinase responsible for phosphorylating PDC, thus "locking" the enzyme in its unphosphorylated, catalytically active state. Reprinted with permission from Stacpoole et al. (2003).

ATP synthesis (oxidative phosphorylation). It is not surprising, therefore, that the complex is highly regulated (Fig. 7-2). The PDC undergoes rapid posttranslational changes in catalytic activity by reversible phosphorylation of up to three serine residues on the E1α protein, rendering the complex inactive. Phosphorylation is mediated by pyruvate dehydrogenase kinase (PDK), a dimeric protein. In mammals, at least four isoenzymes (PDK1–PDK4) are expressed in a tissue-specific manner. PDK2 is expressed

ubiquitously, whereas tissue expression of the other isoforms is more restricted. It is noteworthy that PDK4 is highly expressed in tissues (e.g., heart, skeletal muscle, liver, kidney, and pancreatic islets) involved in fuel homeostasis.

PDK activity is enhanced by increases in the ratios of NADH/NAD$^+$ or acetyl-CoA/CoA and is inhibited by pyruvate or ADP. Pyruvate dehydrogenase phosphatase (PDP) catalyzes the dephosphorylation of E1α and activates the PDC.

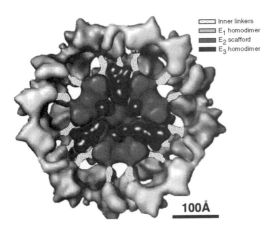

Inner linkers
E_1 homodimer
E_2 scafford
E_3 homodimer

100Å

Figure 7-3. Cutaway model of the fully assembled pyruvate dehydrogenase complex (PDC) viewed on its threefold axis. The dehydrolipoyl dehydrogenase (E_3) homodimer (black) is docked into the pentagonal opening of the core (gray). The binding protein (BP)-E_3 components associated with the core are not revealed in this model. The inner linkers (dotted) bind pyruvate dehydrogenase (E_1) (light gray) to the dihydrolipoyl transacetylase (E_2) scaffold (gray). The E_1-binding site of the E_2 inner linker is located about 50 Å above the scaffold, as indicated by the asterisk and serves as the anchor for the lipoyl domains to pivot. The swinging arm pivots about a position that is approximately 50 Å from the E_1, E_2, and E_3 active sites. Reprinted with permission from Zhou et al. (2001). Copyright 2001, National Academy of Sciences, U.S.A.

PDP is stimulated by calcium and magnesium. Like PDK, PDP is a dimer, but it is more loosely bound than the kinase to the complex. Mammals have two PDP isoforms, each of which contains both regulatory and catalytic subunits. PDP1 is highly expressed in cardiac and, to a lesser degree, skeletal muscle. PDP2 is present in both oxidative (heart, kidney) and lipogenic (liver, adipose) tissues.

From this discussion, it follows that the activity of the PDC tends to be directly associated with high rates of ATP turnover or high concentrations of pyruvate, that is, conditions during which the oxidative removal of glucose, lactate, and pyruvate is accelerated. In contrast, PDC activity tends to be inversely associated with diversion of these substrates toward gluconeogenesis. A reciprocal relationship exists in some tissues between the oxidation of carbohydrate and long-chain fatty acids that is mediated, in part, by the ratio of phosphorylated/unphosphorylated PDC. This phenomenon, termed the *glucose–fatty acid cycle*, is best demonstrable

in tissues that normally exhibit high rates of oxidative metabolism. An exception is the central nervous system (CNS), which cannot metabolize fatty acids and relies almost exclusively on the oxidation of glucose or lactate for energy under fed conditions or on the combination of carbohydrate and ketone bodies (acetoacetate, β-hydroxybutyrate) during fasting.

It is not surprising, therefore, that the activity of the PDC is high in brain, where the complex exists predominantly in its unphosphorylated form. In contrast, the PDC is more highly regulated in many other tissues to meet fluctuating metabolic demands. For example, enzyme activity in liver is highest in the fed state, during which acetyl-CoA can be utilized for lipogenesis. In contrast, hepatic PDC activity is suppressed during fasting, and pyruvate is diverted toward gluconeogenesis via oxaloacetate formation. In the resting state, myocardial cells preferentially oxidize long-chain fatty acids, and the PDC is mainly phosphorylated and inactive. However, during myocardial work, the ratio of unphosphorylated to phosphorylated PDC is increased, as is the proportion of energy derived from aerobic glucose metabolism.

Congenital Disorders of the Pyruvate Dehydrogenase Complex

The PDC is the subject of intense scrutiny because of its pivotal role in fuel metabolism and its association with numerous acquired and congenital disorders. Descriptions of proven or putative acquired deficiencies of the complex may be found elsewhere; this chapter focuses on the genetics, biochemistry, clinical presentation, and course of congenital defects in the PDC. Over 200 cases of PDC deficiency have been reported, and many other cases have been diagnosed but remain unpublished. The diagnosis in most patients has been based on demonstrating reduced total catalytic activity of the complex or in one of its component enzymes.

For diagnostic purposes, these assays are applied most commonly to freshly isolated peripheral blood lymphocytes, fresh or frozen skeletal muscle (usually quadriceps), or primary cultures of skin fibroblasts. The procedure is based on the TPP/NAD$^+$/CoASH-dependent decarboxylation of 1-^{14}C-pyruvate, with residual activity of total PDC, E1, E2, and E3 expressed individually as nanomoles product/minute incubation at 37°C/milligram total cell protein. Preincubation of cells with DCA (which inhibits PDK) or fluoride (which inhibits PDP) can be used to examine activation/inactivation of the complex. Results obtained in patient cells should be interpreted relative to clinical presentation and to enzyme activities obtained in both concurrently assayed and previously measured (historical) control cell samples. In many cases, a definitive diagnosis requires repeated assay of cells from a single tissue sample or from different tissue types (e.g., lymphocytes and fibroblasts).

Several additional strategies have been employed as aids in the diagnosis of PDC deficiency. These include: (1) mutational analysis, based on sequencing of genomic DNA, complementary DNA, or both; (2) visualization of the proteins of the complex by electrophoresis/ immunoprecipitation or electrophoresis/immunoblotting techniques; and (3) most recently, an immunocytochemical method for assaying the content of E1α protein in individual patient cells.

E1 Defects

Approximately 90 percent of biochemically proven causes of PDC deficiency are due to defects in the E1α subunit, which is on the X chromosome. Both hemizygous males and heterozygous females are affected by this condition, such that E1α deficiency is represented equally between the sexes. Most cases appear to be new mutations. In other cases, the mother may exhibit little or no clinical phenotype. Three general classes of mutations in the E1α gene have been identified (Okajima et al., 2005):

1. *Missense point mutations,* resulting in loss of PDC catalytic activity without reduction of E1α protein or mRNA (stable, immunoreactive, catalytically impaired enzyme).
2. *Deletions or exon-skipping mutations,* resulting in significant loss of E1α mRNA and protein (diminished E1α synthesis). These cells will likely also exhibit loss of immunoreactive E1β protein since it has been shown that the presence of both subunits is required for stability of their normal heterotetrameric structure.
3. *Deletions, missense, or nonsense mutations,* resulting in loss of immunoreactive E1α and, consequently, E1β without loss of E1α mRNA (unstable E1α).

In general, the clinical manifestations of E1α deficiency are more severe in boys than in girls.

Greater variability of expression of the defect in females is due to random inactivation (lyonization) of one X chromosome during early embryonic development. Although all tissues from affected females contain cells that express the mutant gene, the relative distribution of normal and mutated cells among tissues is stochastic. Therefore, the clinical phenotype reflects primarily the combined effects of three independent factors:

1. The severity of the particular mutation, meaning the level of residual PDC activity, if any, that is retained by cells harboring the mutant allele
2. The degree to which X inactivation (in females) involves the mutant allele in a given tissue or organ
3. The susceptibility of a particular tissue to factors 1 and 2 above, meaning the dependency of that tissue on the PDC for supporting its energy needs

This concept helps rationalize the clinical, biochemical, and anatomical heterogeneity of patients with PDC deficiency (Table 7-3) and the fact that the reported frequency of this X-linked disease is similar between genders. It also explains the particular vulnerability of the CNS to E1α mutations, given the rate-limiting quality of PDC for fuel metabolism in nerve tissue and experimental evidence that the complex must operate at near capacityi.e., predominantly unphosphorylated) for normal brain function. In heterozygous female individuals, even a modest reduction of PDC activity in brain cells may limit normal function, whereas more severe mutations or a pattern of X inactivation favoring expression of the mutant allele will cause more severe CNS consequences. Such variable expression of the defect within the brain may also account for the anatomical location and extent of CNS structural abnormalities associated with PDC deficiency and observed by brain imaging, although this hypothesis has not been addressed experimentally.

The qualitatively and quantitatively variable impact of the mutation also helps us to appreciate the challenge in establishing an unequivocal biochemical diagnosis, in which variability within tissues (e.g., cultured fibroblast lines derived from separate biopsies) and among tissues (e.g., skin, muscle, leukocytes) of the enzyme deficiency is common. Although an individual may exhibit striking lactic acidosis and CNS clinical and neuroimaging findings

Table 7-3. Reported Clinical, Metabolic, and Anatomical Manifestations of Pyruvate Dehydrogenase Complex Deficiency

Finding	Comment
Clinical	
Failure to thrive	
Developmental delay	Most common early manifestations
Hypotonia	
Mental retardation	Almost universal
Seizures	Common; includes West syndrome
Choreoathetosis	
Myoclonic jerks	
Decerebrate posturing	
Ataxia	
Diminished deep tendon reflexes	
Peripheral neuropathy	Formal nerve conduction testing required
Cortical blindness	
Ophthalmoloplegia	
Ptosis	
Dysphagia	
Abnormal electrocardiogram	Tachycardia, conduction abnormalities
Respiratory disturbances	Tachypnea; awake or sleep apnea
Cyanosis	
Metabolic	
Serum or plasma	
↑ Lactate*	Highly variable
↑ Pyruvate	Highly variable
↓ pH (venous)	Common, but usually mild
↓ pH (arterial)	Uncommon, unless in metabolic crisis
↑ β-Hydroxybutyrate	From poor feeding or ketogenic diet
↓ Bicarbonate	
↑ Chloride	Mild hyperchloremic, metabolic acidosis common
Anion gap	
↓ Creatinine	Low muscle mass
↑ Ammonia	
↑ Alanine	From block in pyruvate oxidation
↓ Protein	
↑ Uric acid	
Urine	
↑ Lactate	Most common abnormalities
↑ Ketones	
↓ Creatine clearance	
↑ Calcium	
↑ Protein	
↑ Amino acids	
↑ Uric acids	
↓ Fe_{Na} and Fe_{PO_4}†	
Fanconi syndrome‡	
Cerebrospinal fluid	
↑ Lactate	Often higher than corresponding blood level
Anatomic	
Cephalic	
Microcephaly	
Facial dysmorphysim§	Many features
Optic atrophy	
Brain dysgenesis‖	Many features

(Continued)

Table 7-3. (*Continued*)

Finding	Comment
Other	
Short stature	Almost universal
Short fingers/arms	
Simian creases	
Renal dysmorphysim	Variable

*Persistently or intermitantly normal or moderately elevated (≤ 5 mmol/L) in stably ill patients.

†Fractional excretion of sodium and phosphorus.

‡Based on the presence of at least three of the following findings: generalized aminoaciduria, glucosuria, increased Fe_{PO4}, decreased blood bicarbonate concentration.

§May include narrow head, frontal bossing, low anterior hairline, upslanting eyes, wide nasal bridge, upturned nose, long philtrum, flared nostrils, low set ears, micrognathia.

‖May include Leigh's syndrome; hypogenesis/agenesis of corpus callosum; cerebral atrophy; ventriculomegaly; ectopic olivary nuclei; hypoplasia of basal ganglia, cerebellum, and brainstem; cystic changes in cerebrum, basal ganglia, and brainstem.

consistent with PDC deficiency, the inability to biopsy the most affected tissues leads to a dependence on measuring enzyme activity in alternative cell types in which PDC activity is in the normal range. For similar reasons, it may be extremely difficult to prove biochemically whether an apparently healthy female is a carrier of the mutation. Furthermore, the antenatal diagnosis of E1α deficiency in male fetuses can be performed using currently available measurements of enzymatic activity and immuno(cyto)chemical analyses described in the "Diagnosis" section. However, in the case of female fetuses, normal enzymatic or immunochemical findings do *not* exclude a diagnosis of E1α deficiency.

It might be assumed that the amount of residual E1α activity measured in cells (fibroblasts, leukocytes) would correlate more closely with clinical phenotype in males who are hemizygous for a mutation than in females, in whom the biochemical expression of the defect depends on the degree of lyonization. However, there is generally poor correlation between measured enzyme activity and clinical presentation and course, except for newborns of either sex with marginal residual activity, in whom fulminant lactic acidosis usually portends death within days or a few weeks of birth. Affected patients who survive the neonatal period may still exhibit early clinical manifestations (Table 7-4), intermittent or persistent hyperlactatemia, and

Table 7-4. Naturally Occurring Compounds of Unproven Efficacy Administered Singly or in Combination to Patients with Pyruvate Dehydrogenase Complex (PDC) Deficiency

Compound	Purported Mechanism
Carnitine	Raises CoASH/acetyl-CoA ratio
Lipoic acid	Antioxidant and PDC cofactor
Coenzyme Q	Antioxidant and respiratory chain component
Vitamins C and K	Facilitate electron transport by respiratory chain
Thiamine*	PDC cofactor
Riboflavin	Precursor of FAD (PDC cofactor)
Biotin†	Pyruvate carboxylase cofactor
Vitamin E	Antioxidant

CoA, coenzyme A.

*Rare cases of thiamine-responsive PDC deficiency have been well documented.

†Biotin is a cofactor of various carboxylases, but its effectiveness in pyruvate carboxylase deficiency is unproven. However, it has been used effectively in cases of biotinidase deficiency, a vary rare cause of congenital lactic acidosis.

CNS structural abnormalities, but their illness tends to be more protracted, and the measured biochemical defect tends to be less severe.

It is important to emphasize that the concentration of blood lactate is a relatively insensitive indicator of disease severity. Basal (postprandial, resting) lactate levels may be normal or only minimally elevated in clinically severely affected patients unless a secondary stress (i.e., energy demand) such as a respiratory infection or an asthmatic attack precipitates life-threatening acid–base decompensation. Other patients with similar measurable degrees of residual PDC activity and symptomatology may have persistent moderate (2–5 mmol/L) hyperlactatemia, often in association with decreased blood bicarbonate and increased blood chloride levels, a mildly increased anion gap (usually defined as the difference, in mmol/L, between the sum of the serum concentrations of sodium and potassium minus the serum concentrations of chloride and bicarbonate; the normal anion gap range is 12–14 mmol/L) and a modestly depressed venous pH. In stably ill patients, the circulating concentration of pyruvate usually mirrors that of blood lactate, so the lactate/pyruvate ratio remains normal. The CSF lactate level is often higher than the corresponding blood concentration and probably reflects the extreme vulnerability of the CNS to PDC deficiency. Urinary lactate is frequently present and is the principal organic acid anion excreted in PDC deficiency.

Three cases of defects in E1β have been reported. This condition is inherited in an autosomal recessive manner.

E2, E3 and Binding Protein Defects

A small number of patients have been described in whom there is good evidence for a defect in the E2 (dihydrolipoyl transacetylase) or E3 (dihydrolipyl dehydrogenase) gene or in the HsPDX1 gene encoding the PDC binding protein (BP). Clinical phenotype varies widely and includes intermittent or persistent hyperlactatemia and a spectrum of cognitive function from normal to profound psychomotor retardation with Leigh syndrome (a genetically heterogeneous condition characterized by developmental delay or regression, lactic acidosis, and focal, symmetrical, necrotic, and demyelinating lesions of the basal ganglia of the brain; also called subacute necrotizing encephalomyelopathy).

No clinical signs distinguish patients with these defects from each other or from patients with E1α deficiency. The diagnosis is based on determination first of a decrease in overall PDC activity, followed by enzymatic evidence of a deficiency in E2 or E3 or reduced expression of E2, E3, or BP on immunoblotting, with normal amounts of the other proteins, including E1α. Patients with E3 mutations manifest combined α-keto acid deficiency, with elevated concentrations of pyruvate, lactate, α-ketoglutarate, and branched-chain amino acids (valine, leucine, isoleucine) in blood and increased excretion of pyruvate, lactate, α-hydroxybutyrate, α-ketoglutarate, and α-hydroxyisovalerate in urine. Chorionic villus sampling was employed to diagnose a female fetus with a large homozygous deletion found at the 5' end of the HsPDX1 coding sequence. This and other cases of defective BP result in low residual activity of PDC and illustrate the essential role of the BP in preserving the overall structural and functional integrity of the complex.

Pyruvate Dehydrogenase Phosphatase Defects

At least four cases of PDC deficiency have been described in which the intrinsic defect lay not in the complex *per se* but in one of the two genetically distinct isozymes required to dephosphorylate the serine residues of the E1α subunit. The clinical signs of PDP deficiency do not distinguish it from primary defects of E1α, E1β, E2, E3, or BP. The most telling biochemical abnormality reported to date has been the inability to activate PDC in cells cultured with DCA. However, neither direct measurements of PDP activity nor mutations in the PDP gene have been reported for any published case of phosphatase deficiency.

THERAPY

Treatment of most patients with genetic mitochondrial diseases has been disappointing and has usually been approached in a sporadic, uncontrolled manner. There is no proven therapy for patients with PDC deficiency. Current strategies rely on nutritional or pharmacological interventions or both to improve patient quality of life. Recent studies have also begun to address the potential role of gene transfer for E1α defects.

Nutritional "cocktails" are commonly provided patients with PDC deficiency or other mitochondrial diseases (Table 7-4). While these vary in composition, they are generally predicated on the belief that (1) the components are safe and (2) they may interdict at various points in the process of oxidative phosphorylation to enhance energy production or mitigate the accumulation of reactive oxygen species generated in abnormal amounts by a compromised respiratory chain. However, use of two nutritional interventions, so-called ketogenic diets and high doses of thiamine (vitamin B_1), are more strongly anchored to sound biochemical rationales and have been investigated widely, albeit anecdotally.

Ketogenic Diets

Ketogenic diets have been used for almost a century in the treatment of epilepsy in children. Although a compelling biochemical rationale for this intervention has never been well defined, the usual ketogenic diet for epileptics consists of a 4:1 caloric ratio of fats to carbohydrates and proteins. Ketogenic diets have also been employed to treat certain severe acquired or congenital errors of intermediary metabolism. Patients with PDC deficiency do not oxidize carbohydrates efficiently; hence, the pyruvate derived from glycolysis is more likely to be reduced in the cytoplasm to lactate. Indeed, carbohydrate-containing meals may exacerbate or precipitate life-threatening lactic acidosis in patients with severe PDC deficiency. This has led to the widespread use of high-fat diets that induce ketosis and provide an alternative source of acetyl-CoA, particularly for the CNS, which can utilize ketone bodies for energy metabolism (Fig. 7-1). Case reports of a few children with PDC deficiency whose clinical course improved dramatically while following a high-fat diet are consistent with this postulate.

Unfortunately, ketogenic diets have never been applied in a consistent or controlled manner to patients with PDC deficiency, leading to considerable variation in both the quality and quantity of fat calories provided to patients. In general, however, published reports in which the dietary composition has been specified typically include a caloric distribution of 55% to 80% fat, up to 25% carbohydrate, and 10% to 20% protein. Strong proponents of ketogenic diets for PDC deficiency advocate a fat intake of

at least 75% of total calories. Traditionally, a high proportion of the fatty acids provided by such a regimen has been saturated fatty acids.

Despite the logic of ketogenic diets for PDC deficiency on biochemical grounds, there are several theoretical concerns regarding their long-term use. For example, diets in which the fat intake is relatively low ($\leq$65%) may contain an amount of protein (to accommodate caloric needs) that exceeds the age-adjusted recommended dietary allowance. The acid load from such diets could exacerbate the congenital acid–base disorder in PDC-defective individuals and could contribute to the renal hyperfiltration reported to occur in some patients. Ketogenic diets may also cause hypercalciuria and increase the risk of bone demineralization in PDC deficiency.

Last, diets habitually high in fat can exert profound effects on both carbohydrate and lipid metabolism. Oxidation of long-chain saturated fatty acids increases the intramitochondrial ratios of acetyl-CoA/CoASH and NADH/NAD$^+$ and consequently the activity of PDKs that reversibly phosphorylate and inhibit the PDC (Table 7-3). Therefore, diets high in saturated fats might further dampen any residual PDC activity in affected patients. In contrast, polyunsaturated fatty acids, particularly those of the omega-3 class, are reported to have opposite effects on PDC activity. Moreover, investigations in animals and humans have demonstrated that consumption of diets enriched in saturated fat provoke deleterious effects on circulating concentrations of lipids and lipoproteins and inhibit the action of insulin on peripheral tissues. In comparison, diets high in mono- or polyunsaturated fatty acids tend to improve lipid metabolism and insulin action.

In summary, cogent reasons exist for incorporating ketogenic diets into the standard of care for PDC deficiency. Equally compelling reasons exist for undertaking a prospective, rigorously controlled evaluation of the long-term benefits and risks of such regimens, particularly regarding their nutrient composition.

Thiamine

Very high doses of thiamine, sometimes exceeding 2 g/day, are reported to benefit some patients with PDC deficiency. TPP is an obligate cofactor for the E1 component of the PDC, and two molecules are bound to each

$\alpha_2\beta_2$ tetramer. According to a model of the TPP-binding site for E1, the pyrophosphate moiety of TPP is bound by means of a single calcium ion to a site formed by closure of a flexible loop of the α-subunit, whereas the thiazolium ring of TPP is bound to a site located on the β-subunit.

Most early clinical descriptions of apparent thiamine-responsive PDC deficiency were not characterized biochemically to ascertain true thiamine dependence. In subsequent reports, immunochemical analyses have demonstrated varied patterns of α- and β-subunit expression, and *in vitro* studies of cultured cells have sometimes found altered E1 enzyme kinetics (high K_m, low V_{max}) for TPP. When molecular genetic analyses have been undertaken, different mutations have been identified within the conserved TPP-binding motif that are considered to lead to diminished binding affinity for TPP or to decreased stability of the $\alpha_2\beta_2$ tetramer.

Dichloroacetate

DCA is the only drug that has been investigated in detail for the treatment of PDC deficiency. It inhibits PDKs and thus maintains E1α in its unphosphorylated, catalytically active form. DCA is a potent lactate-lowering agent, primarily by virtue of its effect on the PDC. The rationale for its use in PDC deficiency is based on the expectation it would stimulate residual enzyme activity in patients with either partial PDC activity or enzyme heterozygosity. In the latter case, activation of E1 by DCA in normal cells might help decrease lactate accumulation in adjacent defective cells and improve overall tissue or organ energy metabolism.

Based on promising anecdotal reports, a randomized, double-blind, placebo-controlled trial of DCA was conducted in 43 children with congenital lactic acidosis due to deficiencies in PDC or one or more respiratory chain complexes or to a mutation in mitochondrial DNA (mtDNA). Comparisons were made after 6 months of 12.5 mg/kg DCA, administered twice daily by mouth or feeding tube, or placebo. All patients received thiamine (1 mg/kg/day). DCA was well tolerated and significantly decreased blood lactate concentrations following carbohydrate meal challenges but did not alter various clinical indices of neurological or neurobehavioral function or the frequency or severity of intercurrent illnesses or hospitalizations. Although DCA may cause reversible peripheral neuropathy and hepatotoxicity, the frequency of these adverse events did not differ between treatment groups. Following the double-blind phase of this trial, 6 patients have continued receiving open-label DCA for up to 7 years without toxicity. Four subjects have PDC E1α deficiency, and their clinical course has remained stable. It is unknown whether DCA may be particularly effective in this or other subgroups of patients with congenital lactic acidosis.

Gene Transfer

Human gene therapy for genetic mitochondrial diseases is in its preclinical infancy and has focused mainly on overcoming defects in mtDNA. However, the central role of the PDC in cellular energetics and the relatively high frequency of PDC deficiency as a cause of congenital lactic acidosis make the complex an attractive target for gene therapy. Furthermore, since all the PDC components are nuclear encoded, evolutionary mechanisms already exist for their importation from the cytoplasm into the mitochondria, unlike proteins normally encoded by mtDNA.

Studies using recombinant adeno-associated virus as a vector to deliver full-length E1α with its own mitochondrial targeting presequence have demonstrated the potential utility of this strategy for defects in PDC. Transduction of cells with the recombinant adeno-associated virus E1α vector resulted in its localization in mitochondria and in partial restoration of PDC activity in cultured fibroblasts from a male patient with E1α deficiency. It is unknown whether effective gene transfer of wild-type E1α will depend on the type of mutation harbored by defective cells or whether enhancement of enzyme activity can be achieved *in vivo*, initially in an animal model of the disease. This last goal is particularly challenging due to the difficulty in generating viable offspring from animals with targeted inactivation of the E1α gene. Resolving these problems raises the intriguing possibility of eventually combining gene and pharmacological therapy for E1α deficiency, in which successful gene transfer would be followed by administration of DCA in the hope of maximally dephosphorylating the transgene.

QUESTIONS

1. Based on the genetics of PDC, how could the phenotypic heterogeneity between identical twins Ann and Elizabeth be explained?
2. Why are some tissues more vulnerable to inhibition of PDC activity, and how does this selective tissue vulnerability explain the cardinal clinical manifestations of the disease?
3. What are the common classes of mutations in the PDCA1 gene that give rise to PDC deficiency?
4. Why might the measurement of PDC activity vary markedly among cells from the same patient?
5. What is the biochemical rationale for ketogenic diets in treating PDC deficiency, and what are the potential caveats associated with their use?
6. What is the primary mechanism of action of dichloroacetate, and why might patients with E1α deficiency be responsive to this drug?

BIBLIOGRAPHY

Black MM, Matula K: Essentials of Bayley Scales of infant development. II Assessment. New York, NY, Wiley, 2000.

Brown RM, Fraser NJ, Brown GK: Differential methylation of the hypervariable locus DXS255 on active and inactive X chromosomes correlates with the expression of a human X-linked gene. *Genomics* **7**:215-221, 1990.

Fuerhlein BS, Rutenberg MS, Silver JN, et al.: Differential metabolic effects of saturated versus polyunsaturated fats in ketogenic diets. *J Clin Endocrinol Metab* **89**:1641-1645, 2004.

Holness MJ, Sugden MC: Regulation of pyruvate dehydrogenase complex activity by reversible phosphorylation. *Biochem Soc Trans* **31**:1143-1151, 2003.

Kerr DS: Treatment of congenital lactic acidosis: review. *Intern Pediatr* **10**:75-81, 1995.

Lib MY, Brown RM, Brown GK, et al.: Detection of pyruvate dehydrogenase E1α subunit deficiencies in females by immunohistochemical demonstration of mosaicism in cultured fibroblasts. *J Histochem Cytochem* **50**:877-884, 2002.

Lissens W, De Meirleir L, Seneca S, et al.: Mutations in the X-linked pyruvate dehydrogenase (E1)α subunit gene (PDHA1) in patients with a pyruvate dehydrogenase complex deficiency. *Hum Mutat* **15**:202-219, 2000.

Okajima K, Mewhort LZ, Lusk MM, et al.: Relationships of clinical and biochemical manifestations to genotype analysis in patients with pyruvate dehydrogenase complex deficiency. *Molecular Genetics and Metabolism* **84**:232-33, 2005.

Robinson BH: Lactic academia: disorders of pyruvate carboxylase and pyruvate dehydrogenase, *in* Scriver CR, Beaudet AL, Sly WS, Valle D (eds), *The Metabolic and Molecular Bases of Inherited Disease*. 8th ed. McGraw-Hill, New York, 2001, pp. 2275-2296.

Stacpoole PW, Barnes CL, Hurbanis MD, et al.: Treatment of congenital lactic acidosis with dichloroacetate: a review. *Arch Dis Child* **77**:535-541, 1997.

Stacpoole PW, Owen R, Flotte TR: The pyruvate dehydrogenase complex as a target for gene therapy. *Cur Gene Ther* **3**:239-245, 2003.

Weber TA, Antognetti MR, Stacpoole PW: Caveats when considering ketogenic diets for the treatment of pyruvate dehydrogenase complex deficiency. *J Pediatr* **138**:390-395, 2001.

Wexler ID, Hemalatha SG, McConnell J, et al.: Outcome of pyruvate dehydrogenase deficiency treated with ketogenic diets: studies in patients with identical mutations. *Neurology* **49**:1655-1661, 1997.

Zhou ZH, McCarthy DB, O'Connor CM, et al.: The remarkable structural and functional organization of the eukaryotic pyruvate dehydrogenase complexes. *Proc Natl Acad Sci USA* **98**:14802-14807, 2001.

Mitochondrial Encephalomyopathy, Lactic Acidosis, and Strokelike Episodes (MELAS): A Case of Mitochondrial Disease

FRANK J. CASTORA

CASE REPORT

A 17-year-old Caucasian female was referred to a neurologist following a 3-day episode of severe headache accompanied by repeated vomiting. She complained of weakness in her arms and legs and of a general feeling of fatigue, especially after minor amounts of exercise, which left her "feeling exhausted." She indicated that she had suffered from migraine headaches "since she was little," and during her recent episodes she had auditory and visual hallucinations. Her speech was slurred, and she had slight paralysis of the right side (hemiparesis).

Her birth history was normal. She was the product of a nonconsanguineous marriage and weighed 3850 gm after an unremarkable pregnancy, labor, and delivery. However, several motor and mental developmental milestones were abnormal. She was of short stature (<25th percentile) and low weight (<15th percentile). Since age 8 years, she had been identified as learning impaired and had attended special education classes throughout elementary and secondary school.

On physical examination, the patient was slightly febrile (38.4°C). Serum concentrations of lactate (24.6 mg/dL) and pyruvate (3.8 mg/dL) were elevated (normal values are 5-18 mg/dL and 0.55-1.0 mg/dL, respectively). Her lactate:pyruvate ratio was elevated as well (34:1; normal range 10:1 to 20:1). Analysis of lumbar cerebrospinal fluid (CSF) showed an abnormally high protein concentration of 0.66 mg/dL (normal range 0.18-0.58 mg/dL) and increased lactate (3.7 mmol/L; normal is < 2.8 mmol/L) and pyruvate (284 µmol/L; normal is 8-150 µmol/L). An electroencephalogram indicated moderate slowing of conduction in the right hemisphere, and a computed tomographic (CT) scan showed a hypodensity in the right temporoparietal and occipital cortices. On audiometric examination, she was found to have decreased perception of high tones and moderate bilateral sensorineural hearing loss. Several of her maternal relatives (mother, grandmother, and maternal uncle) also had some degree of hearing loss.

In addition to ptosis of the left eye (Fig. 8-1), bilateral external ophthalmoplegia (paralysis of some or all of the muscles of the eye) and proximal muscle weakness were observed during the neurological examination. Magnetic resonance imaging (MRI) of the brain revealed signal intensity and diffusion coefficient changes compatible with acute ischemic infarct as well as some degree of cerebellar and cerebral atrophy.

The presence of lactic acidosis, bilateral hearing loss, progressive muscle weakness, and strokelike episodes was suggestive of a mitochondrial disorder. DNA extracted from peripheral blood cells from the patient, her mother, grandmother, mother's brother, and symptomless younger sister was positive for a mutation

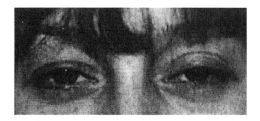

Figure 8-1. Ptosis (droopy eyelids). The patient shown here has left eye ptosis, a drooping of the left upper eyelid, most likely due to paralysis of the third nerve or to loss of sympathetic innervation.

at nucleotide position 3243 of the mitochondrial DNA (mtDNA) genome.

DIAGNOSIS

Mitochondrial encephalomyopathy, lactic acidosis, and strokelike episodes (MELAS) is a progressive neurodegenerative disorder with high morbidity and mortality. Early death is a common outcome. The reported ages of patients with MELAS at the time of death range from 10 to 35 years, but patients alive in their 50s also have been described. Most deaths are due to medical complications; a few are a result of status epilepticus (an epileptic seizure that lasts more than 30 minutes or a constant or near-constant state of having seizures without gaining consciousness between them).

The typical presentation of patients with MELAS includes mitochondrial encephalomyopathy (a disorder causing both brain and muscle cells to function abnormally), lactic acidosis, and strokelike episodes. In addition, neurosensory hearing loss and diabetes mellitus are sometimes present as part of this syndrome. It is also not unusual to find multiple organ systems involved, including the central nervous system, skeletal muscle, eye, cardiac muscle, and, more rarely, the gastrointestinal system. The physical examination will often include an assortment of nonspecific findings such as short stature, muscle weakness, and cognitive and psychiatric problems (e.g., learning difficulties, dementia, psychosis, personality disorders). Cardiomyopathy with signs of congestive heart failure may also be observed in the physical examination. On ophthalmologic examination, some patients may present with ophthalmoplegia, ptosis, and pigmentary retinopathy (hereditary, progressive degenerative disease of the eye marked by atrophy and pigment changes in the

retina, constriction of the visual field, and eventual blindness).

Strokelike episodes are the hallmark feature of this disorder. In many patients with MELAS, presentation occurs with the first stroke-like episode, usually when an individual is aged 4–15 years. Episodes initially may manifest with vomiting and headache that may last up to several days. These patients also may be affected with episodes of seizures and visual abnormalities followed by hemiplegia (total or partial paralysis of one side of the body). Seizure types may be tonic-clonic or myoclonic. Migraine or migrainelike headaches observed in these patients also may reflect the strokelike episodes. Pedigrees of patients with classic MELAS identify many members whose only manifestations are migraine headaches.

Some patients may experience hearing loss, which may accompany diabetes. Usually, type 2 diabetes is described in individuals with MELAS, although type 1 or insulin-dependent diabetes also may be observed. Palpitations and shortness of breath may be present in some patients with MELAS secondary to cardiac conduction abnormalities such as Wolff-Parkinson-White syndrome. Acute onset of gastrointestinal manifestations (e.g., acute onset of abdominal pain) may reflect pancreatitis, ischemic colitis, and intestinal obstruction. Numbness, tingling sensation, and pain in the extremities can be manifestations of peripheral neuropathy. Some patients may have the presentation of Leigh syndrome (i.e., subacute necrotizing encephalopathy).

A CT scan or MRI of the brain following a strokelike episode reveals a lucency (an area of luminosity) that is consistent with infarction. Later, cerebral atrophy and calcifications may be observed on brain imaging studies. The vascular territories of focal brain lesions and the prior medical history of these patients differ substantially from those of typical patients with stroke. Serial MRI studies often demonstrate lesion resolution, differentiating these lesions from typical ischemic strokes. An electroencephalogram is often performed when seizures are a concern. This is especially necessary in MELAS since patients occasionally have intractable status epilepticus as a terminal condition. Mental deterioration usually progresses after repeated episodic attacks. Psychiatric abnormalities (e.g., altered mental status, schizophrenia) may accompany the strokelike episodes. The encephalopathy may progress to dementia, and eventually the patient may become cachectic and die. Another cause of high mortality is the less-common feature of cardiac involvement. Causes can be a hypertrophic cardiomyopathy and conduction abnormalities, such as atrioventricular blocks or Wolff-Parkinson-White syndrome.

When a patient is suspected of having a mitochondrial disorder such as MELAS, the physician will usually combine clinical, biochemical, and morphological information to establish a diagnosis. Often, the diagnosis of a mitochondrial disorder is obtained by a three-tiered testing approach. The initial, noninvasive screening will include basic glucose and electrolyte analysis, and blood counts. In addition, screening for a variety of metabolic disorders that could give rise to similar symptoms will be performed. These include: thyroid and parathyroid disorders, Cushing syndrome, inflammatory myopathies (immune cells invading muscle tissue), endocrinopathies (diabetes), and collagen vascular diseases. Blood and urine ammonia, ketones, and lactic acid levels will also be determined.

If the history, physical findings, and laboratory results are suggestive but not conclusive of a particular mitochondrial disease (e.g., MELAS), then a second tier of tests is performed. These include: blood and CSF lactate and pyruvate, as well as the lactate/pyruvate ratio; timed or random measurement of amino acids in blood, urine, and CSF; organic acids in urine and CSF; and ketones and free and total carnitine in blood and urine.

Lactic acidosis is a very important feature of this disorder. After first eliminating the more common causes of lactic acidosis, such as tissue hypoxic-ischemic injury, hyperglycemia, and hypoglycemia, the assessment of lactic acidosis in MELAS patients can be critically important in reaching the correct diagnosis of this disorder. In general, lactic acidosis does not lead to systemic metabolic acidosis, and it may be absent in patients with significant CNS involvement. In some individuals with MELAS, acid levels may be normal in blood but elevated in CSF. In respiratory chain defects, the ratio between lactate and pyruvate is high. Characteristics of lactic acidosis in MELAS are unique. Arterial lactate and pyruvate are high, and CSF lactate also may be high. Lactate and pyruvate may increase substantially with exercise. In concert with the absolute increases in lactate and pyruvate, the lactate/pyruvate ratio usually is increased as well. Unlike tissue-injury lactic acidosis where

an increased ratio is coincident with decreased O_2 saturation, the increased lactate/pyruvate ratio of MELAS patients is observed at normal O_2 saturation.

Positron emission tomographic (PET) studies may reveal a reduced cerebral metabolic rate for oxygen utilization, while single-photon emission computed tomographic (SPECT) studies can ascertain strokes in individuals with MELAS by using a tracer, *N*-isopropyl-p-[123-I]-iodoamphetamine. The tracer accumulates in the parieto-occipital region, and it can delineate the extent of the lesion. SPECT studies are used to monitor the evolution of the disease.

At this point, if the results have suggested a specific mitochondrial disorder (e.g., MELAS), then mtDNA isolated from blood cells can be tested for any known mutations associated with the suspected disorder. Unfortunately, many disease-causing mutations are not detectable in mtDNA isolated from blood cells (because of the rapid turnover in these cells, defective mitochondria are often lost). Therefore, inconclusive results may warrant further testing.

This third tier of diagnostic tests includes repeat testing for some of the same compounds as before but now under different conditions (e.g., after a fast or during an illness). In addition, a skin or muscle biopsy will be performed. As these last procedures are very invasive, the costs and risks must be compared to the benefits gained from establishing the diagnosis. Furthermore, although most hospitals can perform many of the basic diagnostic tests, few are equipped to perform all the metabolic or molecular genetic tests required. Therefore, material from the skin or muscle biopsy must be appropriately prepared and shipped to the performing laboratory to maintain the integrity of the sample.

The biopsy material is used to obtain biochemical, morphological, and genetic information to establish a diagnosis. Mitochondria isolated from the fresh muscle biopsy or from cells (fibroblasts) cultured from the skin biopsy can be used to measure respiratory chain activity by polarography. This procedure measures O_2 consumption as different respiratory chain substrates are added to the mitochondrial suspension.

A recurring feature of MELAS and many other mitochondrial disorders is the presence of ragged red fibers that are demonstrable after treating the muscle cells with modified Gomori trichome stain (Fig. 8-2). The muscle biopsy is positive for ragged red fibers in at least 85% of

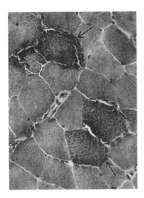

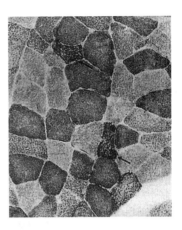

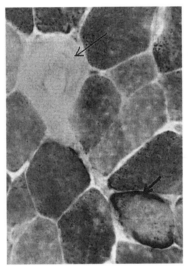

Figure 8-2. Histochemical staining of muscle fibers. Left: Gomori trichome stain showing abnormally proliferating ragged red fibers (arrows). Center: Cytochrome oxidase (respiratory Complex IV) staining showing fibers with reduced or absent staining (long, thin arrow) and fibers with increased cytochrome oxidase staining (short, thick arrow). Right: Succinate dehydrogenase (respiratory Complex II) staining with arrows indicating fibers with increased succinate dehydrogenase.

MELAS cases. Ragged red fibers, common to MELAS, myoclonic epilepsy with ragged red fibers, Kearns-Sayre, and overlap syndromes, reflect proliferation of abnormal mitochondria under the sarcolemma. However, some patients with MELAS do not develop such a proliferation of abnormal subsarcolemmal mitochondria, so a negative muscle biopsy finding, particularly early in the course of disease progression, does not preclude consideration of this syndrome.

Enzyme histochemical staining of muscle fibers can identify abnormal levels of respiratory Complexes II, IV, and V, while specific immunohistochemical stains can be used to evaluate specific respiratory chain subunits (e.g., subunit I or II of cytochrome c oxidase). Muscle fibers from patients with MELAS will often show significantly increased staining for succinate dehydrogenase (respiratory Complex II) as well as reduced staining for cytochrome c oxidase (respiratory Complex IV), although normal or excessively positive staining for cytochrome oxidase can be seen in some ragged red fibers (Fig. 8-2).

Fresh or even frozen muscle can be used to determine electron transport chain (ETC) activity by spectrophotometric assays. Patients with MELAS have been found to have marked deficiency in the activity of complex I of the respiratory chain. Some patients with the disorder have a combined deficiency of Complex I and Complex IV. Morphologically abnormal mitochondria, some with paracrystalline bodies, as well as abnormally proliferating mitochondria can also be visualized by electron microscopy.

Molecular analysis of mtDNA from muscle biopsies often provides a definitive diagnosis of MELAS. Individuals with more severe clinical manifestations of MELAS generally have greater than 80% mutant mtDNA in postmitotic tissues such as muscle. In approximately 80% of MELAS cases, the responsible mutation is an $A \rightarrow G$ base substitution at nucleotide position 3243. A smaller subset of MELAS patients (7.5%) possesses a different point mutation, a $T \rightarrow C$ transition at nucleotide position 3271. At least eight additional point mutations and one four-base pair deletion mutation also have been described.

BIOCHEMICAL PERSPECTIVES

Mitochondrial myopathies are a heterogeneous group of disorders that usually involve multiple organ systems and that display a wide variety of symptoms, including muscle weakness, retinopathy, deafness, seizure, cardiac conduction defects, cardiomyopathy, and lactic acidosis. The earliest report of a mitochondrial disorder can be traced to Theodur Leber's description in 1871 of a patient suffering from bilateral vision loss and retinopathy (Howell, 1999), although at that time it was not known to be a mitochondrial disease. The first disease proposed to be a mitochondrial disorder was reported in 1962 when Luft and coworkers described a female with polydipsia (abnormal thirst), polyphasia (extreme talkativeness), excessive sweating, and a basal metabolic rate twice the norm. It was 26 years later that the first reports of evidence associating mtDNA mutations with two mitochondrial diseases, Leber's hereditary optic neuropathy (Wallace et al., 1988) and Kearns-Sayre syndrome (Lestienne and Ponsot, 1988), were published.

The mitochondrion, in addition to being the "powerhouse of the cell" (because it generates more than 90% of the ATP used by the cell), is also the site of fatty acid oxidation, the tricarboxylic acid (TCA) cycle, electron transport, and amino acid metabolism. Central to the utilization of fuel molecules—carbohydrates, pro-

tein, and fats—is the catabolism of these large macromolecules into smaller molecules that serve as substrates for the TCA cycle. Carbohydrates and fats are metabolized to acetyl-CoA, which is also used in the TCA cycle to condense with oxaloacetate to form citrate. Protein degradation also results in the generation of acetyl-CoA (from metabolism of 11 of the amino acids) as well as in amino acids that serve as precursors for several of the TCA cycle intermediates.

In addition to the obvious role in the catabolism of macromolecules, the TCA cycle provides numerous intermediates for anabolic reactions, such as the synthesis of porphyrins from succinyl-CoA, purines from α-ketoglutarate, pyrimidines from fumarate and oxaloacetate, and proteins from amino acids derived from oxaloacetate, fumarate, and α-ketoglutarate.

The oxidation of the fuel molecules that enter the TCA cycle results in the release of carbon dioxide and the formation of the reduced electron carriers NADH and $FADH_2$. To maximize the recovery of energy (in the form of ATP) from these fuel molecules, the electrons carried by NADH and $FADH_2$ are transferred to the electron transport chain (ETC), a series of five complexes embedded in the inner mitochondrial membrane. The ETC is designed to recover the energy of the various fuel molecules by coupling the transfer of electrons down the ETC to the synthesis of ATP, the energy currency of the cell, in a process termed oxidative phosphorylation (OXPHOS). A diagram of the components of the OXPHOS system is shown in Figure 8-3.

Electrons enter the ETC at respiratory Complexes I and II. The electrons from NADH enter at respiratory Complex I (RC I, NADH dehydrogenase) with the concomitant oxidation of NADH to NAD^+. The electrons carried by $FADH_2$ are transferred to RC II (succinate dehydrogenase) as the $FADH_2$ is oxidized to FAD and succinate is reduced to fumarate. These electrons from RC I and II are transferred to the quinone form of coenzyme Q (CoQ), which delivers them to RC III (UQ-cytochrome c reductase). Cytochrome c then accepts the electrons from RC III, and the reduced cytochrome c is reoxidized as it delivers the electrons to RC IV, cytochrome c oxidase. The electrons are then used by RC IV to reduce molecular oxygen to water.

At RC I, III, and IV, the transfer of electrons is accompanied by the pumping, by these complexes, of H^+ in the mitochondrial matrix across

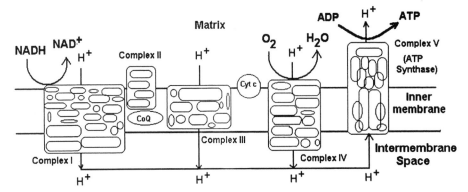

Figure 8-3. The components of oxidative phosphorylation located in the inner membrane of the mitochondria. ADP, adenosine diphosphate; ATP, adenosine triphosphate; NADH, nicotinamide adenine dinucleotide.

the impermeable mitochondrial inner membrane into the intermembrane space. The increased accumulation of H$^+$ on the cytosolic side of the inner membrane establishes both a proton and electrical gradient. Ultimately, the gradient potential is used to drive H$^+$ back into the mitochondrial matrix through a channel in the ATP synthase (RC V). This flow through the synthase provides the energy necessary for the synthesis of ATP by the condensation of inorganic phosphate with ADP.

As seen in Figure 8-4, disruption in the flow of electrons through the ETC can lead to an increase in NADH depending on the location of the block in electron transport. The increase in NADH will shut down the TCA cycle via specific inhibition of key TCA enzymes by NADH. The buildup of NADH will thus result in depletion of NAD$^+$ stores. How are the NAD$^+$ levels restored? The NADH is used to reduce pyruvate to lactate, as indicated in the following diagram:

$$CH_3-\overset{\overset{\textstyle O}{\|}}{C}-\overset{\overset{\textstyle O}{\|}}{C}\diagdown_{O^-} \ + \ NADH \ + \ H^+ \ \longrightarrow$$

Pyruvate

$$CH_3-\overset{\overset{\textstyle OH}{|}}{C}H-\overset{\overset{\textstyle O}{\|}}{C}\diagdown_{O^-} \ + \ NAD^+$$

Lactate

For patients with MELAS and other mitochondrial disorders, this reaction can result in

development of lactic acidosis as elevated levels of lactate create lower pH in the cell.

Another consequence of the failure of electrons to move completely through the ETC is the increased release of reactive oxygen species (ROS) such as superoxide anion (O$_2^-$) in the mitochondrion. Such ROS are produced as oxygen molecules react with electrons at the CoQ or RC I stage. The superoxide and other ROS derived from it (H$_2$O$_2$ and OH•) cause damage to nearby proteins, membranes, and nucleic acids.

Approximately 1000 proteins comprise the mitochondrion; the majority are encoded on genes located on nuclear DNA. In fact, as seen in Figure 8-5, the mtDNA encodes only 13 proteins. These mtDNA-encoded proteins are the seven subunits (ND1, 2, 3, 4, 4L, 5, and 6) of the NADH-dehydrogenase (RC I); one subunit (cytochrome b) of RC III; three subunits (CO I, II, and III) of cytochrome c oxidase (RC IV); and two subunits (A6 and A8) of the ATP synthase (RC V). All of these proteins are components of the ETC or the ATP synthase involved in OXPHOS. In addition to these 13 protein-coding genes, the mtDNA encodes 22 mitochondrial transfer ribonucleic acids (tRNAs) and two ribosomal RNA (rRNA) molecules (the large 16S rRNA and the small 12S rRNA).

As can be seen in Table 8-1, the respiratory complexes of the OXPHOS system are multi-subunit complexes, all except RC II having subunits encoded by both nuclear and mitochondrial genes.

Mutations in the nuclear genes that specify mitochondrial proteins can lead to mitochondrial disorders that obey Mendelian genetics. For

$$NADH \xrightarrow{e^-} RC\ I \xrightarrow{e^-}\!\!/ CoQ \xrightarrow{e^-} RC\ III \xrightarrow{e^-} RC\ IV \xrightarrow{e^-}\!\!/ O_2 \longrightarrow H_2O$$

MELAS

NADH ⬆

Lactate

MELAS

NADH ⬆

Lactate

Figure 8-4. The effect of the MELAS mutation on mitochondrial function is to interfere with function of respiratory Complex I or I and IV, leading to increased levels of NADH and thus also of lactate. CoQ, coenzyme Q; MELAS, mitochondrial encephalomyopathy, lactic acidosis, and strokelike episodes; RC, respiratory complex.

example, some mitochondrial disorders resulting from large and or multiple deletions in mtDNA, such as Kearns-Sayre syndrome and chronic progressive external ophthalmoplegia, are found in some cases to be autosomal dominant, indicating a nuclear-encoded gene as the defect responsible for the production of deleted mtDNA. On the other hand, a number of mitochondrial disorders resulting from mutations in mtDNA will usually appear sporadic or follow

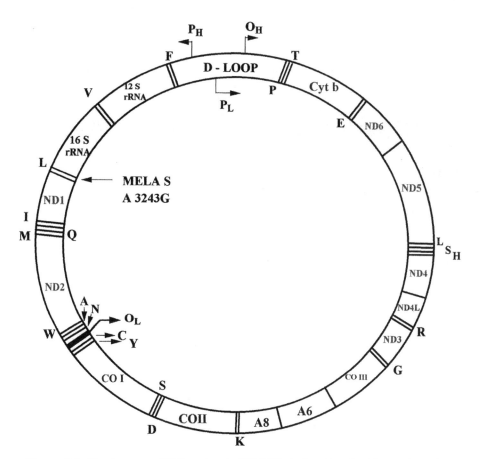

Figure 8-5. The human mtDNA molecule (16,569 bp) showing the 13 protein-coding genes, 2 rRNA genes, and the 22 tRNA genes as well as the D-loop region containing the heavy strand and light strand promoters P_H and P_L, respectively, and the heavy strand origin of replication O_H. Also shown is the light strand origin of replication O_L and the location of the A3243G MELAS (mitochondrial encephalomyopathy, lactic acidosis, and strokelike episodes) mutation within the transfer RNA[Leu] gene. Cyt, cytochrome.

Table 8–1. Nuclear and Mitochondrial DNA-Encoded Subunits of the OXPHOS Complexes

Respiratory Complex	Nuclear DNA	Mitochondrial DNA
I	39	7
II	4	0
III	10	1
IV	10	3
V	14	2

matrilinear inheritance. A typical pedigree of a family with MELAS is shown in Figure 8-6. Note the strict maternal inheritance. Only offspring of affected mothers are themselves affected; none of the affected males pass on their mitochondrial disease.

Maternal inheritance is one of several interesting features of mitochondrial genetics. There are three other aspects of mitochondrial inheritance that are important. The first is replicative segregation leading to heteroplasmy (the presence of both mutant and wild-type mtDNA molecules within a cell or tissue). During cell division, mitochondria distribute to daughter cells according to their position in the cell during cytokinesis. Thus, if mutant mitochondria are concentrated in a particular area of the cytoplasm, then these mutant mitochondria may locate as a group in one of the daughter cells. Thus, a parental cell containing only 10% mutant mitochondria may give rise to a daughter cell with 20% mutant mitochondria after a single cell division. In this way, the mutant load in a muscle or brain cell may steadily increase during the natural aging process.

The second is the threshold effect describing the different degrees of dependency of various tissues on OXPHOS. For example, the brain and CNS have the highest demand of all the cells in the body for OXPHOS to provide ATP for normal function. Cardiac and skeletal muscle have the next highest need for OXPHOS, while the endocrine system and skin have lesser requirements for OXPHOS. Thus, as mitochondrial function fails due to deleterious mutations in mtDNA, often the earliest manifestations of such mitochondrial distress is seen in neurological and muscular abnormalities.

The third aspect is the high error rate and lack of efficient DNA repair systems, leading to a high mutation rate for mtDNA. It is estimated that mtDNA is 7–17 times more prone to mutation than somatic DNA. These aspects of mitochondrial biogenesis lead to the production of mutant mtDNA, contributing to the overall degree of heteroplasmy in human tissues.

MELAS is a mitochondrial genetic disease. At least 10 different causative point mutations have been described in mtDNA, 5 of which are located in the same gene, the tRNA$^{Leu\ (UUR)}$ gene. The most common mutation, initially reported in 1990 by Goto and coworkers (Goto et al., 1990) and found in 80% of individuals with MELAS, is an A → G transition at nucleotide pair (np) 3243 (A3243G) in the dihydrouridine arm of the tRNA$^{Leu\ (UUR)}$ gene. An additional 7.5% have a heteroplasmic T → C point mutation at np 3271 (T3271C) in the terminal nucleotide pair of the anticodon stem of the tRNA$^{Leu\ (UUR)}$ gene. Other mutations in this gene known to be associated with MELAS are A3252G, C3256T, and T3291C. In addition, there are several other mutations in this gene that are linked to other mitochondrial diseases having characteristics different from the group defining the MELAS syndrome.

Since both normal and abnormal mitochondria may be present in tissues (heteroplasmy),

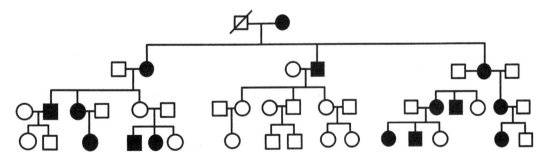

Figure 8-6. Four generations of a family with the mitochondrial disorder MELAS (mitochondrial encephalomyopathy, lactic acidosis, and strokelike episodes). Note that only female affected members will pass on the mutation to their offspring.

the clinical presentation of MELAS can be heterogeneous. Measurements of respiratory enzyme activities in intact mitochondria have revealed that more than one half of the patients with MELAS may have Complex I or Complex I + IV deficiency. The occurrence of strokelike episodes, sensorineural hearing loss, pigmentary retinal degeneration, heart involvement, and recurrent vomiting or abdominal pain can vary significantly among individual cases.

In the United States, as in the worldwide population, the frequency of the A3243G MELAS mutation is 16.3 per 100,000. Males and females are equally affected. This high prevalence suggests that mitochondrial disorders may constitute one of the largest diagnostic categories of neurogenetic diseases among adults.

The presence of this most abundant MELAS-associated mutation, the A3243G mutation, can be quickly determined using a combined PCR amplification of mtDNA followed by treatment of the PCR product with the restriction enzyme Apa I. As seen in Figure 8-7, a 372-base pair (bp) PCR product would be generated from this region of the mtDNA molecule. The cleavage of this 372-bp product by Apa I (which recognizes and cleaves at the sequence 5'-GGGCCC-3') into 263- and 109-bp fragments would indicate the presence of the A3243G mutation. The intensity of the DNA bands can be quantitated and related to the proportionate amounts of wild-type and mutant mtDNA present in the sample. This assay, therefore, not only detects the presence of the mutation but also measures the degree of heteroplasmy. This is very useful because often the level of heteroplasmy will correlate with the severity of the symptoms observed and can be predictive of the effective response to treatment protocols. All of the family members tested in Figure 8-7 possessed the A3243G mutation. The sample from the proband had the highest proportion of mutant mtDNA, 71%.

Mutations in tRNA$^{Leu (UUR)}$ may be expected to have an important effect on protein synthesis in mitochondria. The MELAS-associated human mitochondrial tRNA$^{Leu (UUR)}$ mutation causes aminoacylation deficiency and a concomitant defect in translation initiation (Borner et al., 2000). The expected result would be a deficit in general mitochondrial protein synthesis with resulting deficiencies of multiple OXPHOS components. Patients with MELAS disorder have been found to have a marked decrease in the activity of respiratory Complex I with a secondary reduction in the activity of Complex IV.

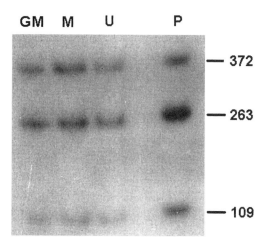

Figure 8-7. MELAS (mitochondrial encephalomyopathy, lactic acidosis, and strokelike episodes) assay using restriction enzyme Apa I to detect the presence of mutant mtDNA in skeletal muscle biopsies. GM, grandmother; M, mother; P, proband; U, maternal uncle. The uncut PCR product is 372 bp. The presence of the MELAS mutation results in cleavage into 263- and 109-bp fragments.

It is interesting to note the high number of mutations in this region of the mtDNA. There is a further interesting aspect of this particular region of the mtDNA that might explain the extraordinary number of pathologic mutations concentrated in this length of DNA sequence. In addition to encoding the tRNA$^{Leu(UUR)}$ gene, this region of mtDNA codes for a signal responsible for terminating transcription through the two rRNA genes. As seen in Figure 8-8, the tRNA$^{Leu(UUR)}$ gene follows immediately after the 16S large rRNA gene.

Although transcription of the heavy strand of mtDNA initiates from the heavy strand promoter (P$_H$) and proceeds completely around the circular mtDNA molecule, this full-length transcript is only made about 10% of the time. The other 90% of the time a truncated transcript from the heavy strand promoter terminates after the 16S rRNA gene. How does this happen? The nucleotides marked with an asterisk in Figure 8-8 form a transcription termination signal that, when bound by a mitochondrial termination factor, causes the mitochondrial RNA polymerase to dissociate from the mtDNA and cease transcription. It is proposed that alterations in the DNA sequence of this tRNA gene therefore not only may affect the role of the tRNA in protein synthesis but

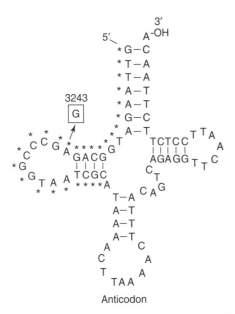

Figure 8-8. The mitcochondrial tRNA^{Leu(UUR)} gene. The diagram shows the position of the A3243G mutation. The nucleotides marked with an asterisk are involved in termination of transcription.

also may interfere with proper metabolism of mitochondrial RNA.

THERAPY

Although there is no cure for MELAS or any of the mitochondrial diseases, palliative treatments are available while others are being developed to alleviate symptoms and to slow the progression of the disease (Shoffner and Wallace, 1994). In general, the responses to treatment seem to be better for those patients with less-severe disease. Modifying the diet, adding vitamins and other supplements, and minimizing or avoiding external stresses are important approaches to managing the patient with MELAS. Although the long-term effects of dietary manipulations are unknown, it is important for the MELAS patient to maintain a good nutritional status, to remain properly hydrated, and to avoid fasting. Treatment must be tailored to each patient as the effectiveness of these treatments varies on an individual basis.

The goal of the metabolic therapies is to increase the production of ATP and interrupt

the progression of this mitochondrial disorder. Metabolic therapies used for the management of MELAS include: CoQ_{10}, idebenone, dichloroacetate (DCA), carnitine, menadione, phylloquinone, ascorbate, riboflavin, nicotinamide, succinate, and creatine monohydrate. A lack of long-term follow-up has hampered evaluation of these drug therapies.

The raison d'être for each of these metabolic therapies varies. CoQ_{10} is a naturally occurring substance that stabilizes respiratory complexes located in the mitochondrial inner membrane. It also scavenges free radicals and acts as a potent antioxidant. Treatment with CoQ_{10} has been reported to reduce serum lactate levels and to improve muscle weakness in some patients with MELAS. Idebenone (an analogue of coenzyme Q_{10} capable of crossing the blood-brain barrier) may stimulate OXPHOS function in the mitochondria of brain cells as well as increase cerebral metabolism. It also stimulates mitochondrial respiratory activity by protecting mitochondrial membranes from lipid peroxidation. However, CoQ_{10} has been shown to mediate mitochondrial uncoupling through the production of superoxide free radicals, so prolonged exposure to elevated concentrations of CoQ_{10} or idebenone may in fact lead to increased free-radical damage and compromised mitochondrial function.

DCA is an inhibitor of pyruvate dehydrogenase kinase, the enzyme that regulates pyruvate dehydrogenase (PDH) activity by phosphorylation of the E_1 subunit, leading to a decrease in PDH activity (see Chapter 7). DCA has been used to lower lactate levels in some patients with MELAS. Stimulation of PDH activity reduces the release of lactate from peripheral tissues and enhances its metabolism by the liver. Since prolonged use of DCA may lead to sensory neuropathy, treatment must be closely monitored.

Supplementing the diet with carnitine may stimulate the uptake of long-chain fatty acids into affected cells. Fatty acid oxidation within the mitochondrion will generate acetyl-CoA, which when oxidized in the TCA cycle will produce NADH and $FADH_2$ to feed into the ETC. Carnitine also shuttles potentially toxic fatty acid catabolic by-products out of the mitochondrial matrix to the kidney for excretion in the urine.

Succinate is an intermediate formed during the metabolism of acetyl-CoA that has entered the TCA cycle. This intermediate can donate electrons directly to RC II (succinate dehydrogenase). Succinate treatment has been used for a patient with MELAS, who showed significant improvement, suffering fewer strokelike episodes when treated with 6 g/day sodium succinate. Creatine monohydrate also has been used in some patients, and an increase in muscle strength in high-intensity anaerobic and aerobic activities has been reported. This effect may be related to increased intracellular creatine/phosphocreatine content, which may be involved in maintaining cellular ATP and in stabilizing the mitochondrial permeability transition pore, with subsequent reduction of neuronal death due to apoptosis.

Menadione (vitamin K_3), phylloquinone (vitamin K_1), and ascorbate (vitamin C) have been used to donate electrons to cytochrome c. For example, ascorbate is oxidized to dehydroascorbate as it uses its electrons to reduce cytochrome c directly. The dehydroascorbate is quickly reduced to ascorbate in the mitochondrion by NADH or $FADH_2$. Menadione appears to improve cellular phosphate metabolism and to enhance electron transfer after a respiratory Complex I block.

Riboflavin (vitamin B_2) has been reported to improve the exercise capacity of a patient with Complex I deficiency. After conversion to flavin monophosphate and FAD, riboflavin functions as a cofactor for electron transport in Complex I, Complex II, and electron transfer flavoprotein. Nicotinamide has been used because Complex I accepts electrons from NADH and ultimately transfers electrons to Q_{10}.

Medications such as β-blockers, calcium channel blockers, digoxin, and amiodarone can be used to control cardiac conduction abnormalities (arrhythmias), and a pacemaker may be inserted to combat heart failure. The general supportive care measures used in acute stroke syndromes also should be followed. Death in patients with MELAS is usually the result of cardiac failure, pulmonary embolus, or renal failure.

Status epilepticus can occasionally be fatal; therefore, seizures should be treated aggressively. Seizures can be managed with antiepileptic medications such as carbamazepine. The common antiepileptic drug valproic acid is contraindicated because it depletes the body of carnitine, which may in fact exacerbate symptoms. The potential risk of stroke may be reduced using appropriate medication. The complications

of diabetes can often be managed through dietary and nutritional modification and by appropriate medications.

In patients with MELAS and other mitochondrial disorders, moderate treadmill training may result in improvement of aerobic capacity and a drop in resting and postexercise lactate levels. Concentric exercise training (by which muscle cells shorten to exert force on an object, as in lifting a weight) also may play an important role since after a short concentric exercise training, a remarkable increase reportedly occurs in the ratio of wild-type to mutant mtDNAs and in the proportion of muscle fibers with normal respiratory chain activity (Taivassalo et al., 1999). If conditions such as cardiomyopathy (a structural or functional disease of heart muscle marked especially by hypertrophy of cardiac muscle) are present, then exercise should be restricted. A mild degree of aerobic activity may lead to an improvement of aerobic capacity; however, strenuous exercise may lead to rhabdomyolysis (the destruction of skeletal muscle tissue accompanied by the release of muscle cell contents into the bloodstream).

QUESTIONS

1. How can you explain the observation that, even within the same family, patients with the A3243G mutation may manifest very different severity of symptoms?

2. Why would a physician recommend avoiding fasting or to eat multiple smaller meals during the day rather than the traditional three meals?

3. Some pediatric patients with MELAS react badly when they are immunized against common childhood diseases. Can you suggest a reason why vaccination may exacerbate MELAS symptoms?

4. Which of the respiratory complexes would you expect to be least affected by mutations in mtDNA?

5. Although many mitochondrial diseases, such as MELAS, will involve multiple organs, neurological or neuromuscular abnormalities are often the earliest signs of disease. Why?

6. Why does the A3243G mutation associated with MELAS lead to reduced activity of respiratory complexes I and IV, while

the point mutation at 11778 (within the ND4 gene) associated with Leber's hereditary optic neuropathy affects only respiratory complex I?

7. Vitamin C (ascorbate) enhances the absorption of iron from the intestines. For this reason, it is recommended that vitamin C not be administered to a patient with MELAS immediately prior to or subsequent to a meal of red meat or other foods rich in iron. What is the biochemical basis for the concern about increased iron availability to a patient with MELAS?

BIBLIOGRAPHY

Borner GV, Zeviani M, Tiranti V, et al.: Decreased aminoacylation of mutant tRNAs in MELAS but not in MERRF patients. *Hum Mol Genet* **9**:467–475, 2000.

Goto Y, Nonaka I, Horai S: A mutation in the tRNA(Leu)(UUR) gene associated with the MELAS subgroup of mitochondrial encephalomyopathies. *Nature* **348**:651–653, 1990.

Howell N: Human mitochondrial diseases: answering questions and questioning answers. *Int Rev Cytol* **186**:49–116, 1999.

Lestienne P, Ponsot G: Kearns-Sayre syndrome with muscle mitochondrial DNA deletion. *Lancet* **1**:885, 1988.

Luft R, Ikkos D, Palmieri G, et al.: A case of severe hypermetabolism of nonthyroid origin with a defect in the maintenance of mitochondrial respiratory control: a correlated clinical, biochemical, and morphological study. *J Clin Invest* **41**:1776–1804, 1962.

Shoffner JM, Wallace DC: Oxidative phosphorylation diseases and mitochondrial DNA mutations: diagnosis and treatment. *Annu Rev Nutr* **14**:535–568, 1994.

Taivassalo T, Fu K, Johns T, et al.: Gene shifting: a novel therapy for mitochondrial myopathy. *Hum Mol Genet* **8**:1047–1052, 1999.

Wallace DC, Singh G, Lott MT, et al.: DNA mutation associated with Leber's hereditary optic neuropathy. *Science* **242**:1427–1430, 1988.

9

Systemic Carnitine Deficiency:
A Treatable Disorder

ERIC P. BRASS, HARBHAJAN S. PAUL, and GAIL SEKAS

CASE REPORT

A 3.5-year-old boy presented to the emergency room with hypoglycemia. The patient's history was remarkable for multiple episodes of altered consciousness resulting in hospital admissions since age 3 months. These episodes were characterized by depressed mental status or coma and hypoglycemia (blood glucose typically 15 mg/dL, normal 75–105 mg/dL). Seizure activity was noted on several admissions. On evaluation, the patient was consistently noted to have proximal muscle weakness, hepatomegaly, congestive heart failure, elevations of serum transaminases (aspartate aminotransferase [AST], and alanine aminotransferase [ALT]) to greater than 2000 IU/L (normal values 10–30 IU/L and 10–40 IU/L for AST and ALT, respectively) and elevated serum creatine phosphokinase to greater than 1500 IU/L (normal <175 IU/L).

The patient was born to nonconsanguineous parents from Chihuahua, Mexico, after an uncomplicated pregnancy and delivery. A brother had died at 3 months of age of a "liver problem" after an unexplained coma. The parents and three other siblings were well.

Developmental history was remarkable for delayed milestones and growth retardation (weight and height below the third percentile).

Previous diagnostic evaluation had included an electroencephalogram, brain scan, and chromosomal studies, which were unremarkable. Also normal were the plasma levels of electrolytes, calcium, phosphorus, magnesium, bilirubin, thyroxine, thyroid-stimulating hormone, and growth hormone. Results of total serum protein determination, serum electrophoresis, cerebrospinal fluid studies, and studies of immune function were normal. Between acute episodes, blood sugar, ammonia, ALT, AST, and creatine phosphokinase were all normal. A urinary organic acid profile was nondiagnostic. A muscle biopsy had been recently performed and microscopic examination revealed large amounts of neutral lipids. A liver biopsy also showed severe but nonspecific fatty changes.

As part of the evaluation during the current hospital admission, a 32-hour fasting study was performed. During the fasting period, the patient had no nausea or cramps. At the start of the fast, his blood glucose was 91 mg/dL, but by 24 hours it had fallen to 66 mg/dL and at 32 hours had fallen to 35 mg/dL. The fast was terminated at this point, and the patient was given glucose. During the fast, plasma triglyceride levels rose from 66 to 126 mg/dL, and free fatty acids increased from 0.1 to 2.0 mEq/L. Serum ALT rose from 36 to 1450 IU/L, with no increase in serum creatine phosphokinase or aldolase activities. Remarkably, acetoacetate and β-hydroxybutyrate concentrations did not increase during the fast. The patient's prefast serum carnitine concentration was markedly reduced (4.8 μmol/L vs. control range 30–45 μmol/L). Carnitine measurements were performed on the previously obtained liver and muscle biopsies and also showed low carnitine content (Table 9-1).

The patient was placed on a high-carbohydrate, low-fat diet and was treated with oral L-carnitine (2.0 g/day). After 3 months of

Table 9-1. Patient Carnitine Levels in Muscle, Liver, Serum, and Urine*

Analysis	Control Values	Patient Before Therapy	Patient After Therapy
Muscle total carnitine (mmol/kg wet weight)	2.5	0.02	0.2
Liver total carnitine (mmol/kg wet weight)	0.9	0.04	0.5
Serum carnitine (μmol/L)	33	4.8	18.5
Urine carnitine (μmol/24 hours)	100	40	1500

*Values are not from a single case but represent a composite from varied case reports.

treatment, the patient was symptomatically improved. While receiving carnitine therapy, laboratory studies showed an increase in the serum carnitine concentration to 18.5 μmol/L and a dramatic increase in urinary carnitine excretion (Table 9-1).

DIAGNOSIS

The patient's history strongly suggested a systemic disease based on the multisystem involvement (liver, heart, and skeletal muscle). The unknown disease in the patient's brother suggested the possibility of an inherited disease.The recurrent episodes of hypoglycemia suggested a metabolic basis for the clinical manifestations.

The fasting study that was performed provided a functional evaluation of the patient's integrative metabolic regulation. The development of hypoglycemia without increases in acetoacetate or β-hydroxybutyrate concentrations, pointed to a defect in hepatic fatty acid oxidation. Although, as discussed in the next section, there are many potential etiologies for impaired hepatic fatty acid oxidation, the extremely low serum, liver, and muscle carnitine concentrations strongly suggested carnitine deficiency as the primary etiology.

Carnitine is present in biological systems as both carnitine and acylcarnitines generated in tissues (see next section). Carnitine deficiency may be a primary defect due to a genetic defect in carnitine transport systems or may be secondary to other metabolic derangements. Normal carnitine homeostasis requires reabsorption of carnitine in the renal tubule via a specific transport protein. This same transport protein is responsible for the accumulation of carnitine in heart and skeletal muscle. If this transport system is not functional, then carnitine cannot reach tissues, and primary carnitine

deficiency results. Secondary carnitine deficiency results from the abnormal accumulation of acylcarnitines due to the accretion of metabolic intermediates associated with an underlying metabolic defect (for example, propionyl-CoA accumulation in propionic acidemia). Thus, in secondary carnitine deficiency, the low carnitine concentration is associated with a relative increase in acylcarnitines. Also, urinary organic acid analysis will typically result in diagnosis of the primary underlying metabolic disease.

The approach to diagnosis of a patient with suspected carnitine deficiency should be systematic and include

1. Case history: Frequency of illness, provocative factors, spectrum of symptomatology
2. Family history: Complete four-generation pedigree with all diseases noted
3. Physical examination: Cardiac, neurological, muscle strength, liver
4. Laboratory studies: Serum transaminases, blood glucose, plasma and urine carnitine and acylcarnitines, urinary organic acids
5. Metabolic studies: Response to fasting (glucose, free fatty acids, acetoacetate, β-hydroxybutyrate), response to medium-chain triglycerides
6. Tissue biopsy: Light and electron microscopy, tissue carnitine content, other metabolic enzymes as indicated
7. Genetic studies: Culture of fibroblasts for potential genetic and function studies, genetic testing for specific mutations

In obtaining the clinical history, particular attention should be paid to situations that may provoke episodic symptoms. Skipping meals, mild viral illnesses, and exercise are examples of metabolic stressors that may result in symptomatic decompensation. Importantly, results of each step of the evaluation should guide the specifics of subsequent steps to ensure efficient and definitive evaluation.

BIOCHEMICAL PERSPECTIVES

Fatty acid oxidation is a multistep process requiring orchestration of reactions in the cytoplasm and mitochondria (Fig. 9-1). Free fatty acids enter the cell and are activated to their coenzyme A (CoA) thioesters in the reaction catalyzed by fatty acyl-CoA synthetase:

$$\text{Fatty acid + ATP + CoASH}$$
$$\rightarrow \text{Fatty acyl-CoA + AMP + PPi}$$

The mitochondrial inner membrane is impermeable to fatty acyl-CoA. To be transported into mitochondria, the acyl moiety must first be esterified to L-carnitine (hereafter referred to simply as carnitine) to form the corresponding fatty acylcarnitine. This reaction is catalyzed by carnitine palmitoyltransferase I (CPT I) localized

on the outer surface of the mitochondrial inner membrane (Fig. 9-2):

$$\text{Fatty acyl-CoA + Carnitine}$$
$$\rightleftharpoons \text{Fatty acylcarnitine + CoASH}$$

A specific transport protein, the carnitine-acylcarnitine translocase, moves the fatty acyl-carnitine into the mitochondrial matrix while returning carnitine from the matrix to the cytoplasm. Once inside the mitochondria, another enzyme, carnitine palmitoyltransferase II (CPT II), located on the matrix side of the mitochondrial inner membrane, catalyzes the reconversion of fatty acylcarnitine to fatty acyl-CoA. Intramitochondrial fatty acyl-CoA then undergoes β-oxidation to generate acetyl-CoA. Acetyl-CoA can enter the Kreb's cycle for complete oxidation or, in the liver, be used for the synthesis of acetoacetate and β-hydroxybutyrate (ketone bodies).

Dysfunction of any of the steps in Figure 9-1, or in the enzymes of β-oxidation, can result in impaired fatty acid oxidation and clinical

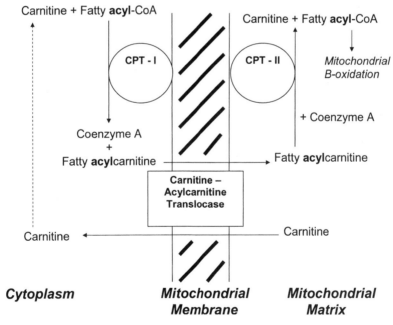

Figure 9-1. Role of carnitine in fatty acid oxidation. Long-chain fatty acids are activated as the thioester of CoA on the cytoplasmic side of the mitochondrial membrane. The fatty acyl group is then transferred to form the corresponding carnitine ester in a reaction catalyzed by carnitine palmitoyltransferase I (CPT I). The acylcarnitine then enters the mitochondrial matrix in exchange for carnitine via the carnitine-acylcarnitine translocase. The acyl group is transferred back to CoA in the matrix by carnitine palmitoyltransferase II (CPT II). The intramitochondrial acyl-CoA can then undergo β-oxidation.

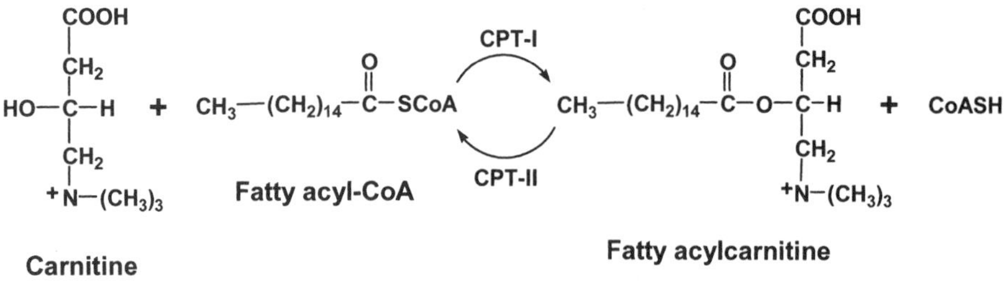

Figure 9-2. Carnitine palmitoyltransferase reaction. Palmitoyl-CoA is shown as a prototypic substrate. Carnitine palmitoyltransferase I (CPT I) and carnitine palmitoyltransferase II (CPT II) are shown illustrating the direction of the reaction catalyzed by each enzyme during physiological fatty acid oxidation.

disease. Interestingly, the transmitochondrial transport system depicted in Figure 9-1 is only required for the complete oxidation of long-chain fatty acids (12 carbon atoms or longer). Shorter-chain fatty acids are transported into mitochondria, can be directly activated to the acyl-CoA within the mitochondrial matrix, and then can undergo β-oxidation. Thus, the ability to differentially oxidize long-chain versus shorter fatty acids can be used *in vitro* or as a diagnostic test clinically to identify defects in the carnitine-dependent reactions of fatty acid oxidation.

It is clear from this discussion that carnitine is required in humans for the oxidation of long-chain fatty acids. In humans, carnitine is derived from both dietary sources and endogenous biosynthesis. Meat products, particularly red meats, and dairy products are important dietary sources of carnitine. Since biosynthesis can meet all physiological requirements, carnitine is not an essential nutrient. Premature infants are an exception to this rule as they lack a mature biosynthetic system and have limited tissue carnitine stores. As many infant formulas, particularly those based on soy protein, are low in carnitine, premature infants receiving a significant part of their nutrition from such formulas may be susceptible to carnitine deficiency.

Carnitine biosynthesis utilizes the essential amino acid lysine, with terminal methyl groups donated by S-adenosylmethionine. Only lysine incorporated into proteins is a substrate for the methylation reaction. In humans, the final reaction in the biosynthetic pathway, catalyzed by a cytosolic hydroxylase, occurs in liver and kidney but not in cardiac or skeletal muscle. The carnitine requirement of these tissues is met by carnitine transported to them via the plasma

from sites of biosynthesis or after intestinal absorption of dietary carnitine. Carnitine is accumulated in muscle against a concentration gradient with normal carnitine concentrations in skeletal muscle approximately 100-fold those in plasma. To prevent renal losses of carnitine during this trans-tissue transportation, 95% of the carnitine filtered by the kidney is reabsorbed into the plasma by the renal tubule. The membrane transport of carnitine into both muscle and the renal tubule is mediated by a sodium-dependent transport protein, organic cation transporter 2 (OCTN-2). OCTN-2 is essential for normal carnitine homeostasis. If OCTN-2 is defective, then the kidney will be unable to reabsorb the carnitine delivered to it. Thus, the bulk of any carnitine synthesized or obtained from dietary sources will simply be lost in the urine, resulting in systemic carnitine deficiency. Any residual carnitine in the plasma will be ineffectively taken up by critical tissues such as the heart and skeletal muscle. Mutations in OCTN-2 are responsible for clinical syndromes of primary carnitine deficiency such as the case presented in this chapter.

The clinical sequelae of OCTN-2 dysfunction and carnitine deficiency are readily predicted based on the biochemistry discussed here. Fatty acids are a major source of ATP in cardiac and skeletal muscle. Thus, carnitine deficiency will result in cardiac impairment (cardiomyopathy) and generalized skeletal muscle weakness. Under conditions of stress, skeletal muscle integrity may be compromised, resulting in significant muscle injury (rhabdomyolysis). Between meals, fatty acids are also a major source of energy for the liver. Under these conditions, fatty acid oxidation is required to support the critical functions of the liver, including gluconeogenesis and ureagenesis.

During starvation, the liver also uses acetyl-CoA generated from fatty acid oxidation to synthesize ketone bodies as a fuel source for the central nervous system. Thus, hypoglycemia may be a prominent clinical sign as peripheral tissues use glucose in the absence of the ability to burn fat, and the liver is unable to synthesize new glucose to meet the demand. The systemic dependence on fatty acid oxidation is greatest during periods of caloric deprivation, and delayed feedings are often a cause of episodic symptoms in patients with carnitine deficiency. CNS symptoms, including coma or seizures, may result from the hypoglycemia, absence of ketone bodies, and hyperammonemia (resulting from impaired ureagenesis). These manifestations of systemic carnitine deficiency are usually expressed early in life. As fatty acids delivered to tissues cannot be oxidized, they are esterified to form triglycerides, which accumulate in tissues and are evident on light microscopy of biopsied tissue. The case presented in this chapter demonstrates many of these clinical features, including an abnormal response to a controlled diagnostic trial of fasting.

THERAPY

Understanding the biochemical bases for carnitine deficiency and the resulting clinical syndrome forms the foundation for the two major approaches to therapy: avoidance of biochemical stressors and carnitine supplementation.

Biochemical stress can be minimized by using frequent feedings to minimize dependence on fatty acid oxidation, particularly for the liver. Meals should have a high-carbohydrate, low-fat content. Medium-chain triglycerides (synthetic or derived from coconut or palm kernel oils) can be used as these lipids can be oxidized independent of carnitine. These steps are particularly important when any external metabolic stress, such as a viral illness, is present.

Carnitine supplementation is also critical in these patients. In acute severe metabolic crises, carnitine can be administered intravenously. Oral carnitine supplementation can be used for chronic maintenance therapy. Note that as the primary transport defect will still be present, carnitine supplementation cannot normalize the patient's carnitine homeostasis.

In the present case, as soon as the diagnosis of carnitine deficiency was considered, the patient was given a high-carbohydrate, low-fat diet containing 20% of the calories as protein. In addition, the patient was given a total of 2.0 g of carnitine per day, which was administered in three equal doses. Carnitine therapy resulted in dramatic clinical and biochemical changes.

After 3 months of therapy (Table 9-1), serum levels of carnitine, though still lower than the controls, had increased markedly from the pretherapy levels. Muscle carnitine levels also increased but remained well below normal. Despite this, clinical muscle strength and tone were remarkably improved. Carnitine levels in the liver (where carnitine transport is not dependent on OCTN-2) increased more dramatically than those in muscle. Despite the low serum carnitine concentration, urinary carnitine losses were dramatically increased in the patient while on therapy as compared with controls. This reflects the continued dysfunction of the renal OCTN-2 and thus the continued urinary wasting of carnitine.

In addition to the biochemical changes, the patient experienced dramatic clinical improvements. Hepatomegaly was no longer evident after 2 weeks of carnitine therapy, and his transaminase levels returned to normal. Neurological disturbances, including hyperreflexia of the lower extremities, bilateral Babinski responses, and walking disability due to weakness and ataxia disappeared after 2 weeks of therapy. His muscle strength increased from 2/5 to 4/5 and he could run for the first time in his life. Sensory nerve conduction in the left peroneal nerve, virtually unmeasurable before therapy, was normal. Somatosensory evoked potentials, strikingly abnormal before therapy, showed marked improvement after 3 months of treatment. The cardiomyopathy was largely resolved.

After establishing the diagnosis and instituting carnitine therapy, the prognosis in such cases is generally quite favorable. Cases of carnitine deficiency have been reported since the mid-1980s, and limited long-term follow up of these patients is encouraging.

QUESTIONS

1. What are the reasons for lipid accumulation in the liver of this patient?
2. Why was the patient unable to produce ketone bodies after 24 hours of fasting prior to carnitine therapy?
3. What is the cause of hypoglycemia observed in this patient?

4. Why did skeletal muscle carnitine content remain below normal despite high-dose carnitine therapy in this patient?

5. What is the biochemical basis for the differential handling of medium-chain versus long-chain fatty acids in liver?

BIBLIOGRAPHY

Bremer J: Carnitine—metabolism and function. *Physiol Rev* **63**:1420–1480, 1983.

Cederbaum SD, Koo-McCoy S, Tein I, et al.: Carnitine membrane transport deficiency: a long-term follow up and OCTN2 mutation in the first documented case of primary carnitine deficiency. *Mol Gen Metab* **77**:195–201, 2002.

Kerner J, Hoppel C: Genetic disorders of carnitine metabolism and their nutritional management. *Annu Rev Nutr* **18**:179–206, 1998.

Rebouche CJ, Seim H: Carnitine metabolism and its regulation in microorganisms and mammals. *Annu Rev Nutr* **18**: 39–61, 1998.

Stanley CA, Treem WR, Hale D, et al.: A genetic defect in carnitine transport causing primary carnitine deficiency. *Prog Clin Biol Res* **321**: 457–464, 1990.

Tang NLS, Ganapathy V, Wu X, et al.: Mutations of OCTN2, an organic cation/carnitine transporter, lead to deficient cellular carnitine uptake in primary carnitine deficiency. *Hum Mol Genet* **8**:655–660, 1999.

Treem WR, Stanley CA, Finegold DN, et al.: Primary carnitine deficiency due to a failure of carnitine transport in kidney, muscle and fibroblasts. *N Engl J Med* **319**:1331–1336, 1988.

Wang Y, Ye J, Ganapathy V, et al.: Mutations in the organic cation/carnitine transporter OCTN2 in primary carnitine deficiency. *Proc Natl Acad Sci U.S.A.* **96**:2356–2360, 1999.

10

Neonatal Hypoglycemia and the Importance of Gluconeogenesis

IAN R. HOLZMAN and J. ROSS MILLEY

CASE REPORT

Female infant L. weighed 3.98 kg at birth to a 29-year-old mother after a 35-week pregnancy. Mrs. L. was an insulin-requiring diabetic who had had type 1 diabetes since she was 15 years old and had not yet shown signs of vascular disease. Her pregnancy had been complicated by multiple episodes of hyperglycemia (excess sugar in the blood) and glycosuria (presence of abnormal amounts of sugar in the urine). Her prenatal care was only episodic because her husband had been part of a layoff at work, and the family was without health insurance.

On the day of delivery, Mrs. L. had a routine nonstress test (a test that records changes in fetal heart rate with fetal movement and is used to assess whether the fetus is suffering from a lack of oxygen or blood flow to the brain) because she noticed that her fetus had decreased movement over the preceding 2 days. The nonstress test showed a flat baseline heart rate without any variation, a finding suggesting that the fetus was at risk for asphyxia (lack of oxygen leading to an accumulation of lactic acid and carbon dioxide in the blood). Following the rupture of membranes, a blood sample taken from the fetal scalp revealed an acidotic pH of 6.9 (normal > 7.3). Because these findings were clear evidence of fetal distress, an immediate cesarean section was performed.

The infant's Apgar scores (scale 0–10, with 10 being best) of 2 at 1 minute and 6 at 5 minutes suggested depression of neurological and cardiopulmonary function. The physicians resuscitated the infant, who was then taken to the neonatal intensive care unit. She had a normal pulse, respiratory rate, and rectal temperature. The infant's head circumference and length were both normal for her gestational age; however, she was clearly macrosomic (large body and organs) and plethoric (ruddy with an increased RBC mass) and had a protuberant, firm abdomen and a disproportionate amount of adipose tissue around the upper body. The liver edge was 4 to 5 cm below the right costal margin; the kidneys were large bilaterally but of normal shape and position, and the initial cardiac examination revealed no abnormalities. The pulses were symmetric but difficult to feel in all extremities. There were no other congenital anomalies.

When the infant was aged 30 minutes, the hematocrit was 0.63 (normal is 0.45–0.62), and the serum glucose was 2.5 mmol/L (normal is 2.8–3.3 mmol/L). An intravenous line was established. The initial intravenous fluid was 10% dextrose in water and was administered at a rate of 10 mL/hour or a total of 60 mL/kg/day (4 mg/kg/minute of glucose). Several minutes later, the infant's blood glucose concentration was 1.2 mmol/L, and 10 mL of 25% dextrose in water was given via intravenously over a 5-minute period (125 mg/kg/minute).

The first arterial blood gas determination at 45 minutes of life revealed a pH of 7.18 (normal is 7.30–7.35), a PO_2 of 6.3 kPa (normal is 6.7–9.3 kPa), a PCO_2 of 6.1 kPa (normal is 4.7–6.0 kPa), and a bicarbonate concentration of 17 mmol/L (normal is 18–21 mmol/L), with a base excess (anion gap; see chapter 7), of (−11 mmol/L. A chest radiographic film showed that the lungs were clear, and the heart was large. One hour and 10 minutes after birth, the infant's blood sugar was 21.0 mmol/L (after infusion of 10 mL of 25% dextrose noted above).

About 45 minutes later, the blood sugar was 1.8 mmol/L, and 8 mL of 10% dextrose was given intravenously over 5 minutes (40 mg/kg/minute). The intravenous infusion was changed to 12.5% dextrose in water at a rate of 13 mL/h (78 mL/kg/day or 6.8 mg/kg/min of glucose). Within 10 to 15 minutes, the serum glucose level had fallen to between 0 and 1.4 mmol/L, and an additional 4 mL of 12.5% dextrose was given intravenously. A catheter was then inserted into the umbilical vein to lie in the lower part of the right atrium, and an infusion of 15% dextrose was begun.

By 5 hours of age, this infant was receiving glucose at a rate of 13.5 mg/kg/min. The blood glucose concentration continued to be less than 1.1 mmol/L, and the infant was given 15 mg of hydrocortisone every 6 hours. Echocardiography showed decreased left ventricular contractility and hypertrophy of the ventricular septum but no other structural abnormalities. These findings were consistent with the cardiomyopathy often seen in infants of diabetic mothers.

By 12 hours of age, the infant had seizure activity that included rhythmic movement of both upper extremities, hiccupping, and repetitive chewing movements. An electroencephalogram was grossly abnormal, showing paroxysmal bursts of activity (seizures) and periods of suppression. Phenobarbital was given to alleviate the seizure activity.

Eventually, the infant's need for hydrocortisone began to decrease so that by the ninth day of life she no longer required steroids, and she maintained serum glucose concentrations above 2.8 mmol/L with a glucose infusion of less than 7 mg/kg per minute. Subsequently, glucose control was no longer difficult, and no further medications were given for this problem.

Sonar examination of this infant's head at 1 week of age showed an infarction of the right parieto-occipital area and hemorrhage within the right ventricle. This brain damage was manifested clinically: Infant L. had great difficulty with sucking and swallowing. She was also diffusely hypotonic (decreased muscle tone), with fewer movements of the lower extremities than of the upper extremities. Hearing tests revealed severe bilateral central hearing loss. At age 1 month, the infant was discharged to a transitional care center, where she could receive developmental stimulation, and the parents could be educated regarding how to feed her.

DIAGNOSIS

This case exemplifies many of the problems classically associated with infants born to diabetic mothers (Cowett, 1998). Inadequate maternal glucose control during pregnancy generates potential metabolic difficulties in the infant (see Biochemical Perspectives). Meticulous attention to diabetic control during pregnancy has markedly improved the outlook for these infants in terms of both morbidity and mortality. Indeed, in many high-risk centers, the outlook for a diabetes-associated pregnancy is indistinguishable from that of a normal pregnancy.

The size of this infant at birth (nearly 4 kg in a preterm infant), however, categorizes her as large for gestational age, a finding characteristic of affected infants of diabetic mothers. This infant is therefore likely to have the other manifestations associated with this pathophysiology. Indeed, many characteristics of this infant are typical for a child born to a mother with inadequately treated diabetes mellitus. Specifically, the macrosomia (large organs), round facies, plethora, and overall weight, length, and head circumference are all consistent with poorly controlled maternal diabetes mellitus that has significantly affected fetal growth and metabolism.

As the end of gestation approaches, the fetus of a diabetic mother is more likely to be poorly oxygenated *in utero*. The markedly decreased scalp pH and low Apgar scores are convincing evidence that this infant's supply of oxygen was insufficient to meet her need. The etiology of the hypoxemia is not always apparent at the time of birth. Any mechanical disruption of the fetal-placental circulation (e.g., abruption or separation, placenta previa or placenta located over the cervical os, or cord accidents) could compromise fetal oxygen supply, as could a fetal infection. In the present case, however, there was no evidence of such problems. Consequently, it seems more likely that the fetus exhibited the chronic oxygen deficit that occurs in infants of diabetic mothers and becomes more severe as the pregnancy progresses.

Hypoglycemia beginning soon after birth is typical for infants of diabetic mothers. Indeed, the physicians caring for this child should have expected this problem because the infant was so conspicuously affected by her mother's diabetes. Fortunately, the severity of the present case, including the need for glucocorticoids, has become rare since the advent of more sophisticated maternal care during pregnancy. Seizures are an unfortunate and serious complication of hypoglycemia, but it is not possible to determine whether the lack of oxygen during prenatal life, the hypoglycemia, or a combination of both is responsible for the infant's brain damage.

BIOCHEMICAL PRESPECTIVES

To understand the etiology of hypoglycemia in the newborn, it is first necessary to know the principles of fetal metabolism that form the basis for newborn physiology and pathology. A unique characteristic of the fetus is the need for the continual provision of substrates across the maternal and placental circulations for growth and energy. A second unique characteristic of the fetus is its biochemical development so that it no longer needs this constant substrate supply (i.e., is capable of independent existence) at birth.

The primary metabolic substrates the fetus receives from the mother are glucose, lactate, amino acids, essential fats, free fatty acids (primarily stored and not oxidized), and oxygen. Each of these is required for three ongoing processes: energy metabolism, growth, and preparation for extrauterine life. The provision of glucose is especially important because of its central role in fetal brain metabolism; cerebral glucose utilization proceeds under most conditions at a rate of about 5 mg/min/0.1 kg of tissue. The brain of the term human fetus weighs approximately 0.4 kg and thus would require approximately 20 mg/kg per minute of glucose for brain use alone.

Most of this glucose is needed for cerebral oxidative metabolism, but there is a further requirement for the synthesis of macromolecules. Other fetal tissues are less dependent on glucose as an oxidative fuel but still require glucose for growth. In addition, tissues such as liver, lung, heart, and skeletal muscle use glucose to form glycogen, and adipocytes distributed throughout the fetus convert glucose into lipid (triglycerides). To provide glucose for all these purposes, the fetus must receive glucose at a rate of 6 to 8 mg/kg per minute.

What system is in place to ensure that the fetus receives this constant supply of glucose? The transport of glucose from the maternal to the fetal circulation occurs by facilitated diffusion across the placental syncytiotrophoblast layer from maternal blood to the fetal capillaries. The carrier-mediated transport occurs via a glucose transporter named GLUT1 (one of a large family of GLUT proteins that are responsible for glucose transport into and out of mammalian cells). GLUT1 is present in the majority of fetal cells, and because it has a very high glucose affinity, it ensures maximal glucose transport to the rapidly growing fetal cells. A second glucose transporter, GLUT3, is also present in placental villi, and its concentration decreases as term approaches. It is primarily found in vascular endothelium and may also play a role in glucose transport from mother to fetus (Simmons, 2004).

This system of membrane transport equilibrates glucose concentrations across cell membranes but will not move sugar against a concentration gradient; therefore, the amount of glucose received by the fetus depends on the concentration gradient between the fetus and mother. Consequently, under circumstances of increased maternal glucose concentration, the fetomaternal glucose concentration gradient will increase, and more glucose will be delivered to the fetus. Conversely, if the maternal glucose concentration falls, then the fetomaternal glucose concentration gradient will decrease, and the fetus will receive less glucose. In pregnancies complicated by maternal diabetes, the larger placentas have an increase in GLUT1 protein, consistent with the increase in glucose transport to the fetus (Simmons, 2004).

The maternal glucose concentration is extremely critical in determining fetal glucose supply, and a normal fetal endocrine environment is important in modulating the way the fetus uses this supply of glucose. The endocrine milieu of the fetus provides an anabolic environment within which the fetus can produce complex macromolecules from simpler precursors. Although the placenta is essentially impermeable to maternal insulin, the fetal pancreas releases insulin in response to increases in fetal blood glucose concentration.

The pattern of insulin effects on the fetus makes sense if one knows which tissues have receptors to insulin and realizes that the effects of activation of these receptors differ in various tissues. Insulin is the major anabolic hormone that affects fetal growth. Because the fetus in late gestation begins to develop insulin-sensitive glucose transporters (GLUT4) in both fat and muscle, one of the major effects of fetal insulin is to regulate the use of glucose by these two tissues. Thus, in muscles, both skeletal and cardiac, higher insulin concentrations promote increased glucose uptake and oxidation as well as the storage of glucose in the form of glycogen. In adipose tissue, insulin promotes lipogenesis.

In addition, there are numerous effects of insulin, generally anabolic, not mediated through its well-known effects on glucose transport. For example, in muscle, insulin decreases glycogenolysis and proteolysis. Lipolysis is inhibited by insulin in adipocytes. The effect of insulin on hepatic tissue is to promote increased glycogen production and protein synthesis and to inhibit glycogenolysis, proteolysis, lipolysis, and gluconeogenesis (Fig. 10-1).

Other hormones, notably glucagon and epinephrine, are important counterregulators of the action of insulin in postnatal life; however, both fetal glucagon and epinephrine concentrations are normally quite low through fetal life and are even lower in infants of diabetic mothers. Thus, as the action of insulin is predominant, the endocrine milieu of fetal life is uniquely anabolic. A number of other growth factors are also believed to play a role in the excessive growth of infants of diabetic mothers. These include a family of insulin-like growth factors and their binding proteins as well as leptin, all of which are elevated in these infants.

The most obvious perinatal event is the loss of the constant supply of nutrients to the infant. At birth, the serum glucose concentration of a normal infant is approximately 4.2 mmol/L (the majority of glucose in the blood is located outside the red blood cells and thus is in serum), and the serum volume 45 mL/kg. Therefore, the total amount of available circulating glucose is 0.19 mmol/kg. At a utilization rate of 0.03 mmol/kg/min, the fetus receives enough glucose to support 7 minutes of normal metabolism. Obviously, continued existence depends on the ability of the infant to produce glucose or alternative fuels from endogenous sources. This is especially crucial for human brain cells, which have been shown to require some glucose constantly as a source of energy. Glucose transport into human brain cells is not regulated by insulin (although insulin may play a role in the expression of some glucose receptors in the brain); rather, it occurs by facilitated transport. Therefore, unlike muscle and fat cells, in which high insulin concentrations can continue to maintain glucose entry in the face of hypoglycemia, in brain cells the lower the serum concentration of glucose, the less glucose the brain cells receive. Consequently, prolonged periods without glucose may produce irrevocable brain damage.

The consequences of severe hypoglycemia to the newly born infant are significant; therefore, late fetal and early neonatal metabolism is specifically adapted to alleviate these effects. Initially, there is a precipitous decline of blood glucose in the newborn infant (Fig. 10-2). When the blood glucose pool is abruptly depleted, the initial source for replacement is from hepatic glycogen. The liver of the newborn infant contains about 0.012 kg of glycogen, representing sufficient glucose for about 12 hours of normal glucose use. Mobilization of these stores is dependent on a rapid change in the neonatal hormonal environment (Cowett, 2004). Over the first hours, there is a marked decline in the fetal insulin concentration and a striking rise in fetal glucagon concentration (Fig. 10-3).

Other counterregulatory hormones are also affected by birth. Plasma epinephrine and norepinephrine concentrations increase markedly, as does the concentration of cortisol. These rapid changes in hormone levels set in motion a cascade of enzymatic reactions that generate active phosphorylase, which in turn catalyzes the degradation of glycogen to glucose 6-phosphate. These same hormonal changes are likely also responsible for the remarkable postnatal induction of glucose 6-phosphatase, the enzyme responsible for the further metabolism of glucose 6-phosphate to glucose.

Because infants normally do not receive an adequate supply of exogenous glucose (from feeding) for the first days of life, however, hepatic glycogen stores are soon exhausted, and the glucose pool must be replenished from other endogenous sources (e.g., gluconeogenesis).

The only other endogenous source for glucose production is the generation of glucose from gluconeogenic amino acids. By late fetal life, all the enzymes needed for gluconeogenesis are present; however, because there is an easily obtainable source of glucose (i.e., across the placenta) and the fetal endocrine environment is not suitable for gluconeogenesis, the pathways

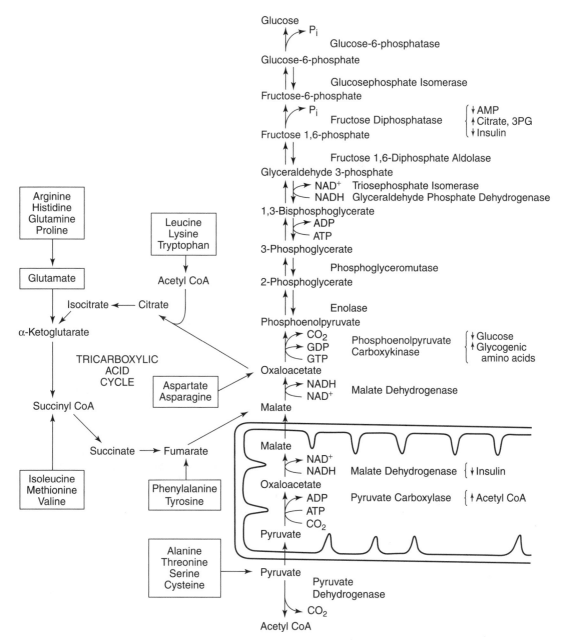

Figure 10-1. Enzymatic pathways for glucose synthesis from amino acids or pyruvate in mammalian liver. Enclosed in the boxes are the glucogenic amino acids with arrows indicating the points where carbon skeletons from these amino acids enter the pathways of gluconeogenesis or the tricarboxylic acid cycle. Bracketed next to the rate-controlling enzymes for gluconeogenesis are some of the substances that increase (↑) or decrease (↓) the activity of these enzymes. 3PG, 3-phosphoglycerate.

for the production of newly formed glucose are not used. Shortly after birth, the fall of the blood glucose concentration and the rise in concentrations of glucagon, catecholamines, and possibly the corticosteroid hormones serve as strong stimulants for the initiation of gluconeogenesis. These factors increase the synthesis and activity of cytosolic phosphoenolpyruvate carboxykinase, an enzyme that is directly related to hepatic gluconeogenic capacity. This activity of

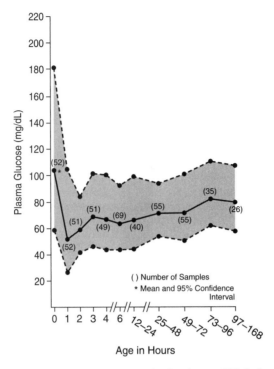

Figure 10-2. Decline in plasma glucose over the first hour of life in healthy term infants and its rapid increase by 3 hours without any intervention. Reproduced with permission from Srinivasan et al. (1986).

this enzyme, which is minimal in the near-term fetus, rises remarkably postnatally (Fig. 10-4). Amino acids derived from protein breakdown in skeletal muscle provide the most important source of gluconeogenic precursors. This source of glucose allows the newborn to maintain normal blood glucose concentrations during the period before the onset of adequate feeding (and adequate exogenous carbohydrates).

In addition, hepatic fatty acid oxidation is also required to sustain gluconeogenesis. These fatty acids may be obtained from exogenous feeding or metabolism of fatty acids released from endogenous lipid stores. β-Oxidation of fatty acids provides the acetyl-CoA needed to activate mitochondrial pyruvate carboxylase and the NADH used as the substrate in the reaction catalyzed by glyceraldehyde 3-phosphate dehydrogenase in the direction of gluconeogenesis (see Fig. 10-1).

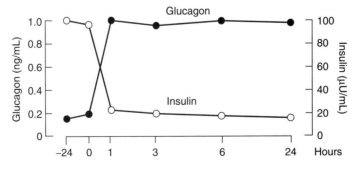

Figure 10-3. Postnatal changes in newborn rat plasma insulin and glucagon concentrations. Reprinted with permission from Girard et al. (1992).

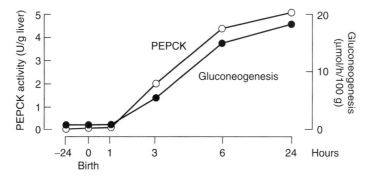

Figure 10-4. Postnatal changes in newborn rat liver cytosolic phosphoenolopyruvate carboxykinase (PEPCK) activity and gluconeogenic rate *in vivo* from [^{14}C-lactate]. Reprinted with permission from Girard et al. (1992).

Although glycogenolysis and gluconeogenesis represent the only pathways that the newborn can call on to produce glucose from endogenous sources, glucose usage could be minimized, and thus the blood glucose level maintained, if other substrates were to supply the metabolic needs of tissues. The newborn has a potential source of energy in the lipid stores present primarily in white adipose tissue (Girard et al., 1992). Indeed, among species, the human is unique in having a body fat content of about 16% of body weight. These stores are present almost entirely in the form of triacylglycerols, which contain significant amounts of palmitic and oleic acid. Mobilization of these stores in adipose tissue is controlled by a lipase that is regulated by the hormonal environment.

Insulin is probably the most important inhibitor of lipolysis. In contrast to adults, in whom catecholamines represent the most important stimulators of lipolysis, thyrotropin (TSH) is the most important stimulator of lipolysis in the newborn. Plasma free fatty acid concentrations rise markedly in the first hours after birth in response to a marked increase in the TSH concentration and a fall in the insulin concentration. The fatty acids released from lipid stores are oxidized by some extrahepatic tissues (e.g., heart and skeletal muscle, kidney, intestine, and lung). Because the respiratory quotient (the ratio of carbon dioxide production to oxygen use) falls from a value of 1.0 (showing that carbohydrate oxidation is the primary source of energy) to a value of 0.8 to 0.9 (showing increasing oxidation of protein or fatty acids) at 2 to 12 hours of age, at a time when protein catabolism is usually insignificant, fatty acid oxidation must represent a significant energy source in the early postnatal period.

Fatty acids are metabolized differently in the liver than they are in other tissues (Fig. 10-5). Only a small portion of the fatty acids is oxidized totally to the level of CO_2 and water in liver. Hepatic tissues convert most of the fatty acids they oxidize to ketone bodies, which are released into the bloodstream and carried to peripheral tissues, most notably the brain, where they are used as metabolic fuels. Because glucagon stimulates ketogenesis and insulin inhibits ketogenesis, the hormonal changes that occur at birth would be expected to promote ketone body formation; however, blood ketone bodies remain quite low during the first hours after birth, reaching a maximal value only after 1 to 2 days. The reason for this delay in ketone body formation may be the low concentrations of carnitine in the human newborn liver. Carnitine is needed to transfer long-chain fatty acids into the mitochondria, where β-oxidation occurs (Fig. 10-5). Because newborn infants have a limited capacity for carnitine synthesis, exogenous carnitine must be supplied through the diet before ketogenesis can proceed optimally. Thus, although cerebral oxidation of ketone bodies occurs shortly after birth and spares some of the cerebral glucose requirement, there still is a major need for glucose as an energy source in the brain.

With the above discussion in mind, it is possible to predict at least some of the consequences to the fetus and newborn of an elevated maternal blood glucose concentration, such as occurs in diabetes mellitus (Cowett, 1998). As the maternal blood glucose level increases, the gradient between fetal and maternal blood glucose

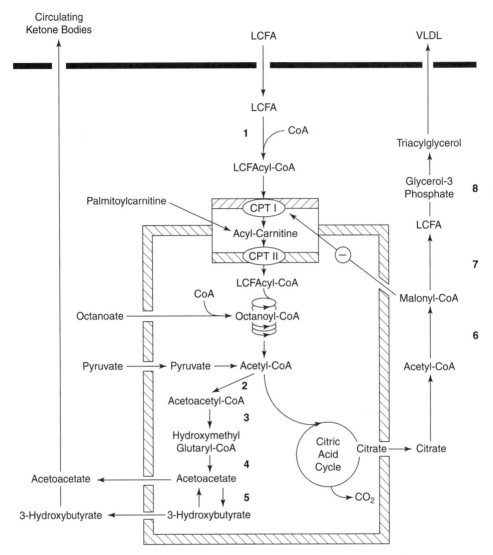

Figure 10-5. Intrahepatic metabolism of free fatty acids (FFA). CPT I, CPT II, carnitine palmitoyltransferase I, II, respectively; LCFA, long-chain fatty acid; VLDL, very low-density lipoprotein. 1, Long-chain acyl-CoA synthase; 2, acetoacetyl-CoA thiolase; 3, hydroxymethylglutaryl-CoA synthase; 4, hydroxymethylglutaryl-CoA lyase; 5, 3-hydroxybutyrate dehydrogenase; 6, acetyl-CoA carboxylase; 7, fatty acid synthase; 8, glycerolphosphate acyltransferase; Reprinted with permission from Girard et al. (1992).

concentrations increases, causing more glucose to be transported to the fetus. With the consequent rise in the fetal blood glucose concentration, the fetal pancreas releases more insulin (fetal hyperinsulinism). Fetal skeletal and cardiac muscles now become exposed to higher blood concentrations of both glucose and insulin. In response to the consequent increase in the rate of glucose transport, muscles metabolize more glucose and store more of it as glyco-

gen. The fetal liver also has a higher than usual glycogen content. In addition, the activities of the key gluconeogenic enzymes (see Fig. 10-1), phosphoenolpyruvate carboxykinase in particular, are depressed. The hyperinsulinemia stimulates fat cells throughout the body, including subcutaneous adipocytes to deposit lipid at a maximal rate, causing the fetus to weigh more than would be expected based on its length or head circumference.

In addition, the metabolic effects of insulin ultimately increase fetal oxygen consumption. The circulation of the fetus is unique; specifically, because blood in the fetal descending aorta contains a portion of venous return after tissue perfusion, the increased rate of consumption of oxygen by fetal tissues decreases the arterial oxygen concentration of the fetus. The fetal tissues supplied by this circulation (which include most of the mass of the fetus) are then at risk for inadequate tissue oxygenation.

There are two consequences of such tissue hypoxia. First, as renal oxygenation becomes inadequate, the fetal kidney produces erythropoietin, which in turn stimulates the production of new erythrocytes. This response leads to an increased hematocrit and an increase in the oxygen-carrying capacity of the blood of the fetus. Second, normal fetal metabolism may be altered if the supply of oxygen to the fetus becomes marginal. Generally, the normal fetus receives about twice as much oxygen across the placenta as needed for normal metabolism. For any fetus, labor increases the likelihood of decreased oxygen supply as uterine contractions interfere with blood flow to the intervillous space of the placenta. The fetus of the diabetic mother, even if it receives a normal oxygen supply, has, as noted, an accelerated rate of oxidative metabolism. The fetus of the diabetic mother is therefore at greater risk for hypoxic damage, as illustrated by the present case.

When the fetus lacks an adequate oxygen supply, it must satisfy its energy needs through anaerobic pathways (e.g., glycolysis); however, the glycolytic pathway of glucose utilization, while generating ATP, produces lactic acid (by reducing pyruvate). A fall in the blood pH is indicative of anaerobic metabolism. The use of glycolysis for energy production is an inefficient process that yields only 2 molecules of ATP per molecule of glucose metabolized, compared with the approximately 30 ATP molecules produced by the combined action of glycolysis, the citric acid cycle, and oxidative phosphorylation. Indeed, anaerobic glycolysis is too inefficient to provide the energy the fetus needs to survive for more than a few hours or days. The finding of a pH of 6.9 in the infant described in the present case report was evidence of significant anaerobic metabolism and impending fetal death. It was imperative that the physicians caring for this patient remove the fetus from the hostile intrauterine environment so that effective oxygenation and aerobic metabolism could proceed.

Once one understands the normal metabolic adaptation to extrauterine life, it is easy to see why the infant whose mother has diabetes is also likely to have problems maintaining neonatal glucose homeostasis. Before birth, infants of diabetic mothers whose placentas have functioned normally will receive a constant oversupply of glucose, which will induce high insulin levels and low concentrations of the principal counterregulatory hormones: glucagon and the catecholamines. Glucose utilization can be increased to rates as high as 10 mg/kg per minute in some infants of diabetic mothers. Even with the fetal blood glucose concentration (because of the maternal diabetes) as high as 8.3 mmol/L (representing a glucose pool of 0.45 mmol/L at birth), this source of glucose will be exhausted within 8 minutes. Therefore, the infant of a diabetic mother, like a normal infant, must generate endogenous glucose to maintain the metabolism of tissues, such as brain, that are constantly dependent on this metabolic substrate. Such infants have, as mentioned, abundant liver glycogen stores.

Over the first hours of life, however, such infants persist in having higher than normal insulin concentrations and lower than normal glycogen concentrations (Fig. 10-6). In addition, the concentrations of other counterregulatory hormones, such as catecholamines, remain low. This particular hormonal milieu will seriously inhibit glycogenolysis, thereby decreasing the rate of glucose release from the liver.

Unfortunately, the endocrine environment of the infant whose mother is diabetic also suppresses the production of glucose from its only other major potential source: amino acids. High insulin levels in both fetal and neonatal life inhibit protein breakdown, thereby decreasing the availability of amino acids from endogenous sources for potential use as gluconeogenic substrates. In addition, the marked increase that normally occurs in the activities of two important rate-controlling gluconeogenic enzymes, cytosolic phosphoenolpyruvate carboxykinase and glucose 6-phosphatase, is suppressed owing to the higher insulin and lower counterregulatory hormone concentrations of infants born to diabetic mothers. The combined effect of the decreased capacity for glycogenolysis and gluconeogenesis in infants of diabetic mothers is a marked decrease in the ability of the newborn to release glucose from the liver into the blood.

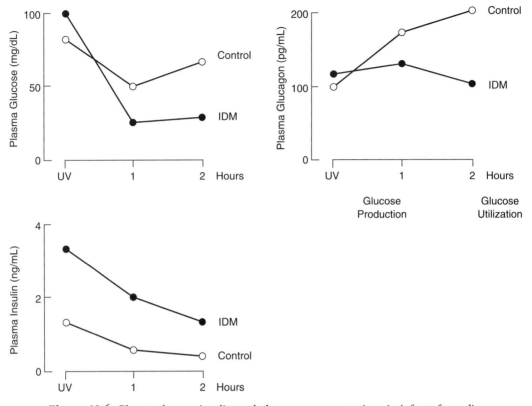

Figure 10-6. Plasma glucose, insulin, and glucagon concentrations in infants from diabetic mothers. UV, umbilical vein. Reprinted with permission from Girard et al. (1992).

Such a decrease in glucose production would have less impact if other metabolic fuels could be mobilized and used. As noted, the fetus whose mother has diabetes has greatly increased fat stores. In these infants, the amount of fat present is theoretically sufficient to supply adequate metabolic substrate for weeks, but the high insulin concentrations markedly inhibit lipolysis. As a consequence, tissues like heart and skeletal muscle, which are otherwise capable of using fatty acids to satisfy metabolic needs, are compelled to continue oxidizing glucose. The infant of a diabetic mother, therefore, in the face of impaired glucose production, has a higher than normal rate of glucose consumption. This circumstance precipitates a marked fall in the blood glucose concentration of the neonate.

The cerebral requirement for oxidative substrate can be met by only two substrates: glucose and ketone bodies. Unfortunately, the endocrine milieu of the infant of the diabetic mother inhibits both lipolysis (i.e., the mobilization of fatty acid stores) and hepatic ketogene-

sis (formation of ketone bodies). Consequently, the brain is left with no alternative to glucose as a metabolic substrate, and the use of glucose to support normal metabolism becomes obligatory. Unless steps are taken to supply exogenous glucose or to alter the endocrine environment so endogenous stores can be mobilized, the infant of a diabetic mother will be at great risk for brain injury.

The present case presentation and discussion of the consequences of maternal hyperglycemia presume that placental function is sufficiently preserved to allow maternal hyperglycemia to be reflected in fetal hyperglycemia. By contrast, some diabetic mothers whose disease is sufficiently long-standing or advanced to cause renal or retinal vascular disease will also have vascular disease that adversely affects the placenta and compromises its ability to transport substrates to the fetus. In such cases, the infants are affected by a chronic undersupply of both oxygen and other critical metabolic substrates, including glucose. Because the infants have received subnormal quantities of glucose, they have low insulin levels and higher than normal concentrations of counterregulatory hormones. Consequently, both their glycogen and lipid stores are minimal. Such an undersupply of fuel reserves results in an infant that is notably smaller than would be expected for its gestational age.

Despite the small size of the infant at birth, an obligate need for glucose (~4 mg/kg/min) still exists. Thus, an infant born with a subnormal serum glucose concentration of 3.3 mmol/L will have used up the entire circulating glucose pool within about 8 minutes. With such a rapid depletion of serum glucose, the infant must rely on glycogenolysis to replenish blood glucose. Although the endocrine environment of such infants, specifically one in which there are low insulin levels and higher than normal concentrations of counterregulatory hormones, favors glycogenolysis, complete depletion of glycogen reserves will occur in about 4 hours, which is much faster than normal. These infants must then resort to another source of endogenous glucose production, namely, gluconeogenesis. The endocrine environment of such infants is conducive to both mobilization of amino acids from protein breakdown and induction of the hepatic enzymes needed for gluconeogenesis. Nonetheless, gluconeogenesis remains deficient as a result of the lack of free fatty acid from lipolysis, which diminishes intramitochondrial acetyl-CoA and compromises hepatic gluconeogenesis. The free fatty acids are not available to provide metabolic substrate because lipolysis, although favored by the endocrine milieu, is limited by a lack of adipose triglyceride. Therefore, infants born to diabetic mothers, in whom placental function has been compromised, lack the endogenous sources of glucose and are also at risk for hypoglycemia; however, the etiology is one of decreased substrate stores rather than an inappropriate endocrine environment.

THERAPY

Because all the myriad consequences to the infant of a diabetic mother arise from maternal hyperglycemia, the therapy of hyperglycemia for the infant should begin before birth. Careful management of the maternal diabetes to prevent both hypoglycemia and hyperglycemia will lessen the likelihood to fetal death or neonatal hypoglycemia. In the present case, economic hardship (the husband's layoff and loss of health insurance) prevented Mrs. L. from obtaining adequate prenatal care. The resultant neonatal complications can be traced directly to this problem.

There are circumstances that preclude the preventive measures outlined above. In such cases, there are two main methods of relieving the hypoglycemia: provision of exogenous substrate or alteration of the infant's endocrine status. After delivery, assuming the infant is otherwise healthy, the early provision of calories by milk feedings can provide adequate exogenous sources of glucose to prevent hypoglycemia. In some infants, however, either because of other illnesses or because of the severity of the hypoglycemia (Cornblath and Ichord, 2000), it is necessary to provide intravenous glucose. Although this was done in the present case, the provision of glucose at only 4 mg/kg/min was inadequate to ensure a sufficient quantity of glucose for use by the brain. The initial intravenous therapy should provide at least 6 mg/kg/min.

When hypoglycemia does occur, it is imperative for the physician to respond rapidly and appropriately. Exogenous glucose delivered directly into a vein is the treatment of choice, but caution must be exercised because the rapid injection of quantities of glucose far in excess of requirements will lead to a sudden increase of blood glucose to hyperglycemic levels. For infants of diabetic mothers, this further stimulates insulin release, which then rapidly produces rebound hypoglycemia, as in the present case. The use of 10 mL of 25% dextrose produced a blood glucose concentration of nearly 22.2 mmol/L, followed by a rapid decrease. It is more prudent and efficacious to administer 1 to 2 mL/kg of 10% dextrose over approximately 5 minutes and then begin a continuous intravenous infusion calculated to supply 6 to 8 mL/kg of glucose per minute.

In an emergency, when an intravenous site cannot be rapidly obtained, the endocrine environment of the infant can be made more conducive to glucose release by use of intramuscular or subcutaneous injection of glucagon (0.3 mg/kg per dose) to produce a short-lived (<30 min) increase in blood glucose while an intravenous catheter is inserted. Glucagon acts not only by increasing glycogenolysis but also by stimulating phosphoenolpyruvate carboxykinase, which will increase gluconeogenesis. Glucagon may also increase the capacity for fatty acid oxidation, which is also essential for gluconeogenesis. Infants whose glycogen is depleted (i.e., growth-retarded neonates) cannot be expected to respond as effectively to glucagon as infants of diabetic mothers. If possible, milk feeding should also be instituted to stimulate the secretion of many glucoregulatory gut hormones and to supply an additional source of glucose and gluconeogenic precursors.

In a few infants, massive quantities of intravenous glucose fail to prevent repeated episodes of hypoglycemia, and manipulation of the neonatal endocrine status is required to minimize glucose use and maximize glucose production. The use of a brief course of glucocorticoids, one of the counterregulatory hormones, as in the present case, can effectively treat the hypoglycemia. The mechanisms of action are threefold: (1) glucocorticoids counteract the effect of insulin on peripheral muscle glucose uptake, thereby "sparing" glucose for brain use and raising the blood glucose concentration; (2) glucocorticoids stimulate hepatic glycogenesis and gluconeogenesis; and (3) glucocorticoids increase proteolysis in peripheral tissues, thereby increasing the availability of gluconeogenic substrates. The effectiveness of this therapy was clearly shown in the present case.

It is not surprising that infant L. suffered diffuse encephalopathy (brain disorder), a cerebral infarction, and seizures during the neonatal period (Yager, 2002). Both asphyxia and hypoglycemia are injurious to the brain. The treatment for seizures consists of providing normal metabolic substrates (e.g., glucose) and appropriate anticonvulsant therapy (phenobarbital), as was done in the present case. The long-term treatment for the child's developmental disabilities is complex and involves the skills of many members of the health care team.

The prognosis of infant L. is uncertain. Asymptomatic hypoglycemia in an infant of a diabetic mother is usually less injurious than those episodes associated with central nervous symptoms. Obviously, in the present case, although the child had symptoms of seizures and an abnormal neurological examination, it is not possible to differentiate these symptoms from those that might have resulted from the chronic inadequacy of cerebral oxygenation *in utero*. Nevertheless, the prognosis for an asphyxiated child with an abnormal electroencephalogram, a cerebral infarction, and persistent abnormalities on neurological examination is guarded at best. The bilateral hearing loss and the inability to swallow and feed adequately at the time of discharge are strong evidence of some degree of neurological disability in the future. Predictions about specific motor and mental potentials are impossible to make in the early neonatal period.

Generally, the prognosis for infants born to diabetic mothers is good; however, severe symptomatic hypoglycemia can lead to lifelong problems. Infants whose hypoglycemia reflects a long-term lack of adequate nutrition and oxygenation *in utero* (such as severe growth-retarded infants) are at even greater risk for developmental disabilities. In both cases, the additional burden of birth asphyxia will increase the likelihood of long-term problems. Obviously, the severity of illness in the infant described here and the ominous signs of cerebral disturbance at the time of discharge bode poorly for the child's future development.

QUESTIONS

1. Compare the hormonal changes that occur at birth and their effects on carbohydrate homeostasis with those that occur in adults during starvation.
2. What was the primary medical cause of infant L.'s problems? Why was appropriate therapy not initiated in the present case?
3. What substance is an important circulating oxidative substrate in fetal life but uncommon postnatally? What common metabolic substrate of postneonatal life is relatively less important during fetal life?
4. Can free fatty acids serve as a direct source of glucose (i.e., can fatty acids be converted into glucose)? Why or why not?
5. Would glucagon or glucocorticoids be as effective a therapy for hypoglycemia in the growth-retarded infant of a diabetic mother as in newborns who are large for gestational age?

BIBLIOGRAPHY

Cornblath M, Ichord R: Hypoglycemia in the neonate. *Semin Perinatol* 24:136–149, 2000.

Cowett RM: The infant of the diabetic mother, *in* Cowett RM (ed): *Principles of Perinatal-Neonatal Metabolism.* Springer-Verlag, New York, 1998, pp. 1105–1129.

Cowett RM: Role of glucoregulatory hormones in hepatic glucose metabolism during the perinatal period, *in* Polin RA, Fox WW, Abman SH (eds): *Fetal and Neonatal Physiology.* Saunders, Philadelphia, 2004, pp. 478–486.

Cowett RM, Farrag HM: Neonatal glucose metabolism, *in* Cowett RM (ed): *Principles of Perinatal-Neonatal Metabolism.* Springer-Verlag, New York, 1998, pp. 683–722.

Girard J, Ferre P, Pegorier J-P, et al.: Adaptations of glucose and fatty acid metabolism during the perinatal period and suckling-weaning transition. *Physiol Rev* **72:**507–562, 1992.

Simmons RA: Cell glucose transport and glucose handling during fetal and neonatal development, *in* Polin RA, Fox WW, Abman SH (eds): *Fetal and Neonatal Physiology.* Saunders, Philadelphia, 2004, pp. 487–493.

Srinivasan G, Pildes RS, Cattamanchi G, et al: Plasma glucose values in normal neonates: a new look. *J Pediatr* **109:**114–117, 1986.

Yager JY: Hypoglycemic injury to the immature brain. *Clin Perinatol* **29:**651–674, 2002.

Part III

Intermediary Metabolism

11

Glucose 6-Phosphate Dehydrogenase Deficiency and Oxidative Hemolysis

CATHERINE BURTON and RICHARD KACZMARSKI

CASE REPORTS

Case 1

A 50-year-old female presented passing black urine after having been unwell for 3 days with fever and headache. There was no previous history of blood disorders, anemia, or similar symptoms. Past medical history included a diagnosis of multiple sclerosis. Treatment included steroids and high-dose vitamins and minerals. These had been given on five separate occasions over the preceding 2 weeks and included 200 mg vitamin B_1, 25 mg B_2, 250 mg B_5, 100 mg B_6, 15 mg B_{12}, 50 g C, 2.5 mg folic acid, 15 mg zinc, 11 mg magnesium, 10 μg molybdenum, 100 μg selenium, and 50 μg chromium. In her social history, she was of Arabic descent from East Africa, currently living in Kuwait. Her nephew was reported to suffer from favism (an acute hemolytic condition occurring after ingestion of a certain species of bean [*Vicia faba*] in individuals with glucose 6-phosphate dehydrogenase [G6PD] deficiency). There was no recent history of travel or malaria exposure.

Laboratory tests showed that hemoglobin was 7.5 g/dL (normal range is 12–15 g/dL), and the reticulocyte count was 262×10^9/L (normal range is $50–100 \times 10^9$/L). The tests also indicated neutrophilia, a white cell count of 34×10^9/L (normal range is $4–11 \times 10^9$/L), and a platelet count of 328×10^9/L (normal range is $150–400 \times 10^9$/L). Renal function was normal. Malarial parasite screen and direct Coombs test were negative. Blood film showed nucleated red blood cells and anisocytosis with "bite cells"

and irregularly contracted cells consistent with acute oxidant drug-induced hemolysis (Fig. 11-1). G6PD deficiency screen was positive. On quantitative assay, G6PD measured 2.27 enzyme units (normal range 5.34–11.34), compatible with a diagnosis of severe G6PD deficiency. Management included blood transfusion, intravenous fluids, folic acid, and iron supplementation. All current medications were stopped.

Over the following days, her hemoglobin continued to drop but stabilized after a further transfusion. Her hemoglobinuria (dark rust-colored urine) gradually improved and the patient made a full recovery. No further hemolytic episodes have occurred. Family members have been screened (two brothers, two sons). The high dose of vitamin C administered to this patient was thought to be the precipitating factor (see Table 11-1), but it is possible that the high doses of the other vitamins may have contributed to the hemolysis.

Case 2

A 2-day-old baby boy was noted to be jaundiced (yellowing of skin and eyes). His initial bilirubin was 25 mg/dL (normal range is 2–10 mg/dL). By the following day, he was clinically more jaundiced. Phototherapy was initiated. Preparation was made for exchange transfusion, but by day 5 of age, bilirubin levels began falling and continued to fall over the subsequent few days. There was an associated fall in hemoglobin to a minimum of 12 g/dL (normal range is 15–21 g/dL), and the reticulocyte count was raised at 20% (normal range 2%–5%). On direct questioning of

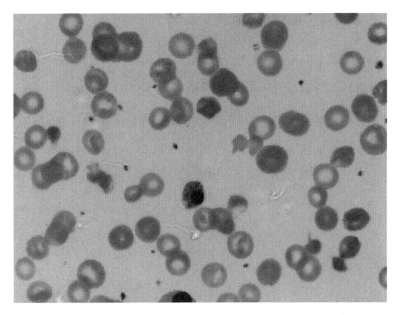

Figure 11-1. Peripheral blood features of oxidative hemolysis showing bite cells, irregularly contracted red cells, and nucleated erythrocytes.

his family history, he had an older brother who had also suffered with neonatal jaundice, which had resolved spontaneously. There was also history of a maternal uncle having had intermittent jaundice and one episode of dark urine when he had a respiratory tract infection as a child. A G6PD assay was performed and confirmed erythrocytic G6PD deficiency.

His parents have been counseled regarding the significance of G6PD deficiency. They have been advised to avoid certain drugs and to seek medical attention on development of dark urine. His older brother has been screened and has been confirmed to be G6PD deficient. Any future sons born to this mother should also be screened.

DIAGNOSIS

G6PD deficiency is the most common enzymatic disorder of red blood cells and should be considered in the differential diagnosis of any case of hemolytic anemia. It affects 400 million people worldwide with a wide variation in prevalence. It is very rare in the indigenous populations of northern Europe but increases to frequencies of 20% in parts of southern Europe, Africa, and Asia and up to 40% in certain areas of Southeast Asia and the Middle East.

G6PD deficiency is expressed clinically by a spectrum of hemolytic syndromes. Clinical variation in presentation from asymptomatic to episodic anemia to chronic hemolysis is due to genetic heterogeneity. The majority of patients are asymptomatic and initially present with anemia due to a precipitating cause, for example, an infectious illness, exposure to certain drugs, or metabolic disturbance.

The diagnosis should be considered in the clinical setting of a patient from an appropriate geographic or ethnic origin who presents with evidence of hemolytic anemia. Clinically, acute intravascular hemolysis is characterized by hemoglobinuria, jaundice, and symptoms and signs of anemia. Less-acute presentations may present in the course of investigation of jaundice. Chronic hemolysis may lead to gallstone formation, which may become symptomatic with abdominal pain.

The complete blood count will show a varying degree of anemia and a raised reticulocyte count. The mean cell volume may be raised due to the reticulocytosis or concurrent folate deficiency. As the oxidative denaturation of hemoglobin occurs, hemoglobin collects at one side of the cell with an adjacent membrane-bound clear zone. This gives the characteristic bite cell appearance on blood smears (Fig. 11-1). Other blood film appearances include red cell fragments, irregularly contracted erythrocytes, and Heinz bodies (seen on supravital stains; represent precipitated denatured hemoglobin). The

Table 11-1. Drugs and Chemicals to Be Avoided in Patients with Glucose 6-phosphate Dehydrogenase (G6PD) Deficiency

Sulfonamides/Sulfones	Cytotoxic/Antibacterial
Dapsone	Chloramphenicol
Sulfacetamide	Cotrimoxazole
Sulfanilamide	Nalidixic acid
Sulfapyridine	Furazolidone
Sulfasalazine	Furmethonol
Salazopyrin	Nitrofurantoin
Septrin	Nitrofurazone
Sulfamethoxypyrimidine	P-Aminosalicylic acid
Sulfisoxazole	
Antimalarials	*Cardiovascular Drugs*
Chloroquine	Procainamide
Hydroxychloroquine	Quinidine
Mepacrine (quinacrine)	α-Methyldopa
Pamaquine	Ascorbic acid
Pentaquine	Dimercaprol
Primaquine	Mestranol
Quinine	Hydralazine
Quinocid	
Analgesics/Antipyretics	*Miscellaneous*
Probenicid	Vitamin K (water-soluble) analogues
Acetanilid	Naphthalene
Amidopyrine (Aminopyrine)	Methylene blue
Antipyrine	Toluidine blue
Pyramidone	

biochemical profile will show elevated serum bilirubin levels, mainly unconjugated (indirect) bilirubin, consistent with intravascular hemolysis. Serum levels of red cell enzymes such as lactate dehydrogenase (LDH) will also be raised due to the hemolysis. Renal function may be abnormal, and some patients develop renal failure, particularly adults who may have previously unrecognized renal damage. This is the result of the hemoglobinuria but may be exacerbated by the intercurrent infection or drugs. Occasionally, this will require hemodialysis.

The diagnosis of G6PD deficiency is made by quantitative or semiquantitative assay. The methods used are based on the normal function of the G6PD enzyme in catalyzing the initial step in the pentose phosphate pathway (PPP). Screening tests depend on the inability of cells from deficient subjects to convert an oxidized substrate to a reduced state. The substrates

used may be the natural one of the enzyme, namely, NADP+, or other substrates linked by secondary reactions. The resultant reaction can be demonstrated by fluorescence, color change, or dye deposition methods. There are a number of screening tests available, using brilliant cresyl blue decolorization, methemoglobin reduction, or an ultraviolet spot test.

A simple method for diagnosis of G6PD deficiency is the fluorescent spot test. By adding a measured amount of hemolysate to glucose 6-phosphate (substrate) and NADP+ (substrate), the rate of NADPH production can be measured spectrophotometrically by measuring light absorbance of NADPH at 340 nm. Other screening tests include the estimation of NADPH generation indirectly by measuring transfer of hydrogen ions from NADPH to an acceptor. In the methemoglobin (metHb) reduction test, methylene blue is used to transfer hydrogen from NADPH to metHb, thereby promoting its reduction. This technique can detect relative G6PD sufficiency in individual red cells, detecting the carrier state with 75% accuracy. These tests will detect a threshold G6PD activity of about 30% of normal and will identify hemizygous deficient males and homozygous deficient females. An abnormal screening test should be followed by a quantitation of G6PD activity by spectrophotometric assay to confirm the diagnosis.

Although in most instances a screening test is adequate to make a diagnosis of G6PD deficiency, false-negative results and difficulties in diagnosis are a fairly common problem. False-negative results occur if the most severely deficient red cells have been destroyed by hemolysis. Therefore, the remaining cells analyzed have sufficient G6PD activity for the diagnosis to be missed, especially during the reticulocytosis that follows acute hemolysis. This is not usually a problem for male hemizygotes or female homozygotes but can result in a missed diagnosis in female heterozygotes and for both sexes in milder variants. Females have varying proportions of G6PD-deficient and normal red cells, and the reticulocytes of milder variants often have normal or near normal levels of G6PD activity. To investigate these cases further, family members should be studied especially in neonatal and pediatric cases. Alternatively, reevaluation can be repeated a few weeks after the hemolytic episode since red cells of all ages will be present. If a prompt diagnosis is required, then the oldest remaining cells can be isolated by differential centrifugation and demonstrated to have low G6PD activity. This technique can also be used if the patient has been transfused.

A conclusive diagnosis of G6PD deficiency can be made by DNA analysis. This is of particular use when the most likely variants in a population are known since polymerase chain reaction amplification of the appropriate region of the G6PD gene can be performed and the mutation identified.

BIOCHEMICAL PERSPECTIVES

Biology

G6PD deficiency was first reported in 1956 (Alving et al., 1956). The importance of G6PD for red cell integrity was recognized after African American soldiers taking the antimalarial drug primaquine developed acute hemolytic anemia with hemoglobinuria. This led to the discovery that one of the enzymes required to maintain adequate intracellular reduced glutathione levels was deficient in affected red blood cells.

The majority of glucose 6-phosphate produced by the phosphorylation of glucose by ATP is metabolized to lactate and pyruvate in the glycolytic or Embden-Myerhof pathway. The direct nonmitochondrial oxidation of glucose 6-phosphate occurs by the pentose phosphate pathway (PPP), and the G6PD enzyme is the initial enzyme in this alternative route of glucose metabolism (Fig. 11-2).

The PPP occurs in the cytosol of the cell. It comprises two irreversible oxidative reactions followed by a series of reversible sugar-phosphate interconversions. Unlike glycolysis or the citric acid cycle, in which the direction

of reactions is well defined, the interconversions reactions of the PPP can occur in different directions, with the rate and direction of the reactions determined by the supply and demand of intermediates in the cycle. The pathway provides a major portion of the cell's NADPH, which functions as a biochemical reductant.

The oxidative portion of the PPP consists of three reactions that lead to the formation of ribulose 5-phosphate, CO_2, and two molecules of NADPH for each molecule of glucose 6-phosphate oxidized. The G6PD enzyme catalyzes an irreversible oxidation of glucose 6-phosphate to 6-phosphogluconolactone. This reaction is specific for $NADP^+$ as coenzyme. The PPP is regulated primarily at this level with NADPH as the potent competitive inhibitor of the enzyme. Under most metabolic conditions, the ratio of NADPH to $NADP^+$ is sufficiently high to inhibit enzyme activity substantially (Fig. 11-3). Increased demand for NADPH decreases the ratio of NADPH/$NADP^+$, and increases G6PD activity. Subsequently, 6-phosphogluconolactone is hydrolyzed by 6-phosphogluconolactone hydrolase (Fig. 11-4). This reaction is irreversible and not rate limiting. The 6-phosphogluconate produced undergoes oxidative decarboxylation catalyzed by 6-phosphogluconate dehydrogenase. This irreversible reaction produces a pentose sugar-phosphate (ribulose 5-phosphate), CO_2, and a second molecule of NADPH (Fig. 11-5).

G6PD is responsible for maintaining adequate levels of NADPH inside the cell. NADPH is a required cofactor in many biosynthetic reactions and also provides electrons to reduce oxidized glutathione (GSSG) to reduced glutathione (GSH) catalyzed by glutathione reductase (Fig. 11-6).

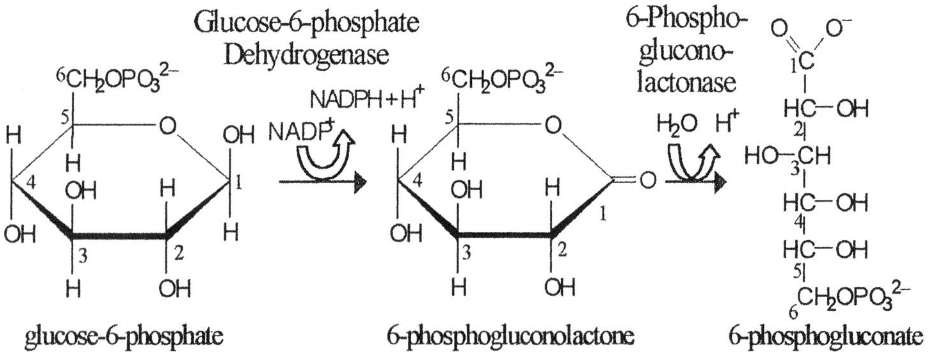

Figure 11-2. Initial oxidative reactions of the pentose phosphate pathway.

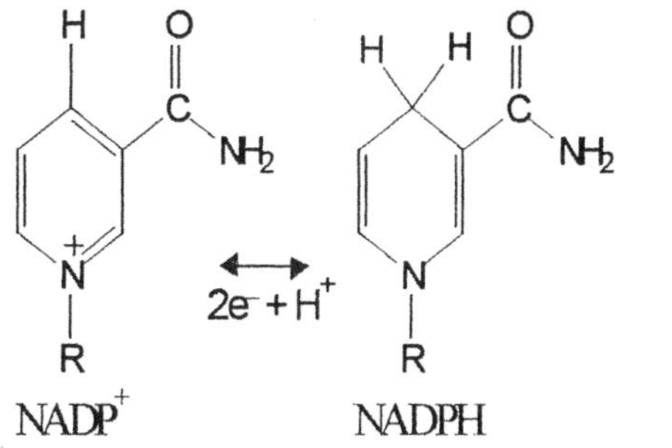

Figure 11-3. Reversible conversion of NADP⁺ to NADPH.

Reduced glutathione acts as a scavenger for dangerous oxidative metabolites in the cell; in particular, it converts harmful hydrogen peroxide to water with the help of the enzyme glutathione peroxidase (Yoshida and Beutler, 1986).

The malic enzyme also serves to generate NADPH in many cells including hepatocytes. A supply of NADPH is critical for the liver microsomal cytochrome P-450 mono-oxygenase system. This is the major pathway for the hydroxylation of steroids, alcohols, and many drugs. These oxidations also detoxify drugs and foreign compounds by converting them into soluble forms more readily excreted through the kidney. NADPH is also used as a source of electrons for the biosynthesis of fatty acids. The situation is unusual in red blood cells as this other NADPH-producing enzyme is lacking (Scriver et al., 1995). This has a profound effect on the stability of red blood cells since they are especially sensitive to oxidative stresses as well as having only one NADPH-producing enzyme to remove these harmful oxidants (Fig. 11-7).

The accumulation of hydrogen peroxidase affects many intracellular processes and results in hemolysis. These include the cross-linking of membrane proteins; hemoglobin denaturation (manifest as Heinz body formation), which in turn affects the physical properties of the erythrocyte; and lipid peroxidation, which may affect the cell membrane to cause direct hemolysis (Fig. 11-8). The resultant damage leads to a mixture of intravascular hemolysis and extravascular hemolysis (by which hemolysis occurs in the reticuloendothelial system). In acute hemolytic episodes, the clinical picture is of predominantly intravascular hemolysis, while predominantly extravascular hemolysis is seen in patients with chronic hemolysis.

The G6PD gene consists of 13 exons, which are the regions of the DNA that code for the enzyme, and 12 introns, which are intervening sequences serving no apparent functional purpose (Scriver et al., 1995). The enzyme's function is determined by the sequence and size of the G6PD gene and the mRNA encoded by the gene, which are 18,500 and 2,269 base pairs in length, respectively. The entire genomic sequence of the G6PD gene is described in the original research article by Chen and coworkers (1991). However, the complete three-dimensional structure of the enzyme, which determines the active enzyme's functional properties, has not yet been determined. G6PD, in its active enzyme form, is made up of either two or four identical subunits, each subunit having a molecular mass of about 59 kd (Scriver et al., 1995).

G6PD deficiency is known to have over 400 variant alleles or different forms of the same gene (Beutler et al., 1990). The biochemical characteristics of the particular G6PD variant determine the extent of enzyme deficiency,

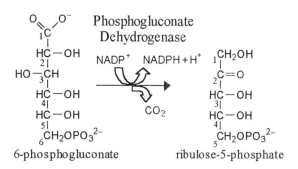

Figure 11-4. Subsequent oxidative reactions of the pentose phosphate pathway.

Glucose-6-phosphate + H_2O + $NADP^+$

⬇ **glucose-6-phosphate dehydrogenase**

6-phosphogluconate + NADPH + H^+

⬇

ribulose 5-phosphate + NADPH + H^+ + CO_2

Figure 11-5. Overview of oxidative reactions of the pentose phosphate pathway.

which subsequently affects the severity of hemolysis. Mutations can be in the form of point mutations or deletions that can range from one to several base pairs as well as replacements in the DNA (Scriver et al., 1995). Different populations have different types of mutations, but within a specific population, common mutations are usually shared (e.g., the "Mediterranean" variant in Egypt, the "Japan" variant in Japan) (Scriver et al., 1995). The World Health Organization has classified G6PD-deficient variants into five classes depending on the level of enzyme activity (Table 11-2). G6PD A⁻ is the most prevalent variant, mostly found in Africans and African Americans. G6PD Mediterranean is the second most common variant.

On a molecular level, most individuals with G6PD deficiency have a qualitative abnormality in the structure of the G6PD enzyme (Scriver et al., 1995). Various models have been proposed suggesting possible reasons why an abnormal enzyme is not fully active. As discussed in Scriver et al. (1995), it was suggested by Sharff that the decreased stability of a mutated enzyme results either from a change in the conformation of the G6PD molecule or from an increase in its susceptibility to proteolytic enzymes, resulting in accelerated decay of the

enzyme during the aging of the erythrocyte. Molecular analysis has demonstrated that each variant is associated with a particular biochemical and clinical phenotype, and that mutations can be found in every exon and are scattered throughout the G6PD gene.

Genetics

The gene for the G6PD enzyme is located at the q28 locus on the X chromosome (Pai et al., 1980; Scriver et al., 1995), so the expression of G6PD deficiency varies between males (XY) and females (XX). All X-linked genetic conditions, such as G6PD deficiency, are more likely to affect males than females. G6PD deficiency is expressed in males carrying a defective variant gene that produces sufficient enzyme deficiency to lead to symptoms. In heterozygous females, the mean erythrocyte enzyme activity can be normal, moderately reduced, or severely deficient. This is dependent on the degree of lyonization and the extent of expression of the abnormal G6PD variant.

Lyonization is the random inactivation by methylation of one of the two X chromosomes in each cell in females, so that the descendent of each cell inherits only one active X chromosome. This is a random event, and therefore normally a heterozygous female with inactivation of one X chromosome in each cell via lyonization has 50% normal G6PD activity (due to 50% normal erythrocytes) and 50% G6PD-deficient erythrocytes. Provided there is one good copy of the G6PD gene in a female, some normal enzyme will be produced, and this normal enzyme can then take over the function that the defective enzyme lacks. Excessive lyonization can occur when inactivation of a large proportion of the same X chromosome occurs. If this results in the majority of remaining red cells being G6PD

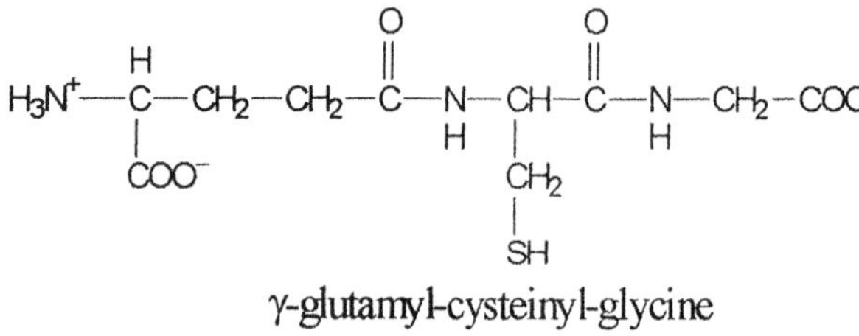

γ-glutamyl-cysteinyl-glycine

Glutathione

Figure 11-6. Chemical structure of glutathione.

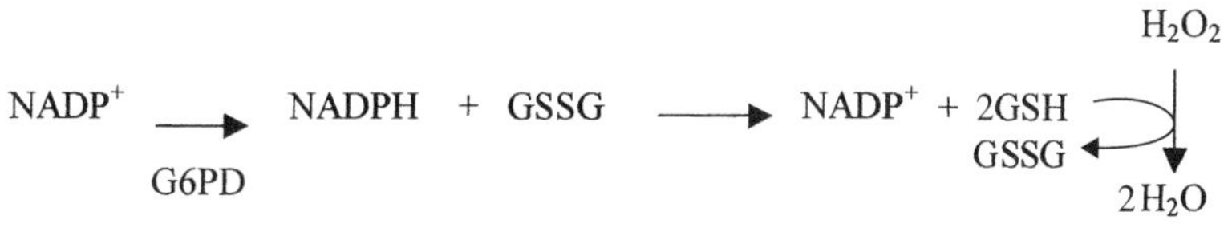

$$\text{NADP}^+ \xrightarrow{\text{G6PD}} \text{NADPH} + \text{GSSG} \longrightarrow \text{NADP}^+ + 2\text{GSH} \underset{\text{GSSG}}{\overset{\text{H}_2\text{O}_2}{\rightleftharpoons}} 2\,\text{H}_2\text{O}$$

Figure 11-7. Consequences of glucose 6-phosphate dehydrogenase (G6PD) deficiency. GSH, reduced glutathione; GSSG, oxidized glutathione.

deficient, then the phenotype is comparable to males and homozygous females. Compound heterozygosity can also result in G6PD deficiency manifestation in females when there are two defective copies of the gene in the genome.

CLINICAL PRESENTATION

Generally, all of the G6PD variants that occur with high frequency in various populations (e.g., G6PD A$^-$ and G6PD Mediterranean) are asymptomatic and are clinically important only because of the risk of acute hemolytic anemia. In contrast, symptomatic G6PD variants tend to be rare in any population. There are four clinical presentations of G6PD deficiency: acute hemolytic anemia, neonatal hyperbilirubinemia, congenital nonspherocytic hemolytic anemia, and favism.

Acute Hemolytic Anemia

As illustrated in case 1, acute hemolytic anemia occurs when there is destruction of the G6PD-deficient red cells. The fact that the most

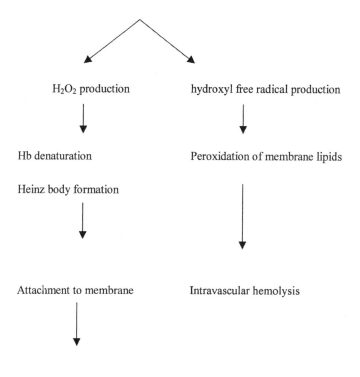

Figure 11-8. Mechanism of hemolysis in glucose 6-phosphate dehydrogenase deficiency.

Table 11-2. The World Health Organization Classification of Glucose 6-phosphate Dehydrogenase Activity Variants

Class	Level of Enzyme Deficiency	Clinical Presentation
I	Severe, < 10%	Chronic hemolytic anemia
II (e.g., G6PD Mediterranean)	Severe, < 10%	Intermittent hemolysis
III (e.g., G6PD A⁻)	Moderate, 10%–60%	Intermittent hemolysis, usually precipitated
IV	None	Normal
V	Increased activity	Normal

prevalent G6PD variants are normally asymptomatic in the steady state means that a level of enzyme activity of 20% (some studies suggest 3%) of normal is probably sufficient for normal red cell function under ordinary conditions. It can be demonstrated by isotopic techniques that there is slight shortening of the red cell survival, but generally there is no evidence of anemia, and blood film morphology is normal.

Destruction of the G6PD-deficient red cells is triggered by high redox potential drugs (as in case 1), certain infections, and metabolic disturbances such as acidosis or hyperglycemia. Typically, 2–4 days after drug ingestion there is a sudden onset of jaundice, pallor, dark urine, and often back or abdominal pain. This is associated with a rapid fall in hemoglobin. Morphological abnormalities such as red cell fragmentation, microspherocytes, and bite cells are present in the blood film. Both hepatic and splenic sequestration (pooling of red blood cells, which no longer contribute to the circulating volume, in these organs) can occur.

An appropriate stimulation of erythropoiesis is induced by the anemia. A reticulocytosis is apparent within 5 days and is maximal at 7 to 10 days after the onset of hemolysis. Even if there is continued drug exposure, the acute hemolysis usually resolves after 1 week. This spontaneous recovery reflects replacement of the older, enzyme-deficient erythrocytes by younger red cells with sufficient G6PD activity to withstand oxidative injury. Provided there is normally functioning bone marrow, the continued loss of aging red cells is compensated by the erythropoietic marrow response.

Neonatal Hyperbilirubinemia

As in case 2, some patients with G6PD variants experience hyperbilirubinemia in the neonatal period. Neonates with the rare class I variant are particularly at risk, but more common variants account for the majority of cases. The cause of neonatal hyperbilirubinemia is unclear because it does not occur in 50% or more of G6PD-deficient individuals. It is probably due to a combination of increased bilirubin production secondary to accelerated red cell breakdown and the immaturity of the neonatal liver, with the latter factor probably the most significant.

Congenital Nonspherocytic Hemolytic Anemia

Class I G6PD variants have such severe G6PD deficiency that lifelong hemolysis occurs in the absence of infection or drug exposure. Most have DNA mutations grouped around exon 10 of the gene which code for amino acids affecting the glucose 6-phosphate or NADP⁺/NADPH binding domains. These sites are central to the function of G6PD, and it is thought that the functional defect is so severe in patients in class I that the red cells are unable to withstand normal stresses within the circulation. Detection of anemia and jaundice normally occurs in the neonatal period. The degree of hyperbilirubinemia in these neonates is frequently severe enough to require exchange transfusion to prevent kernicterus. Most individuals have chronic hemolysis with mild-to-moderate anemia (hemoglobin of 8–10 g/dL) and a persistent reticulocytosis. Acute hemolysis can be aggravated by exposure to precipitants such as infection, fava beans, or drugs and chemicals with oxidant potential, as described above, resulting in acute hyperhemolysis. Drugs with mild oxidant potential that can be safely given to individuals with class II or III variants can increase hemolysis in class I variants.

Generally, these individuals only have mild anemia as increased erythropoiesis compensates for the chronic hemolysis. The anemia may worsen if there is reduced erythropoietic capacity for any reason, such as hematin deficiency, infection, or parvovirus-induced aplastic crises.

In patients who are severely G6PD deficient, on rare occasions an associated abnormality occurs in which there is neutrophil dysfunction secondary to G6PD deficiency. This defect leads to impaired neutrophil bactericidal activity, resulting in recurrent infections with catalase-positive organisms.

Favism

Favism usually results from the ingestion of fresh, uncooked fava beans, although it can occur with dried, cooked, canned, or frozen beans. It occurs most commonly in males between the ages of 1 and 5 years. Clinical symptoms and signs of acute intravascular hemolysis develop 5 to 24 hours after fava bean ingestion. Preceding symptoms of headache, nausea, back pain, chills, and fever are followed by hemoglobinuria and jaundice. The fall in hemoglobin is normally acute and severe and can be fatal if blood transfusion is not performed.

The glucoside divicine (or its aglycone isouramil) is the oxidant implicated in favism. It overwhelms the low GSH-generating capacity of the G6PD-deficient cells and directly compromises red cell function. The vast majority of individuals developing favism are G6PD deficient, although only a small percentage of G6PD-deficient individuals are sensitive to the fava bean. Also, the same individual's response can vary. It is unclear why fava bean ingestion is not always followed by hemolysis in G6PD-deficient individuals. There are probably a number of factors that are important in contributing to the phenotype. It is likely that hepatic metabolism of fava bean oxidants is important as well as the amount of divicine or isouramil in each fava bean and how the fava beans are consumed. The degree of hemolysis is known to correlate with the quantity of beans consumed and the intestinal surface area of the individual. Favism is most commonly associated with the G6PD Mediterranean variant and therefore most commonly occurs in Italy and Greece. Although Africans and African Americans with G6PD deficiency are less susceptible, favism nevertheless does occur with the G6PD A$^-$ variant.

Precipitants of Oxidative Hemolysis

Infection

Infection is probably the most common precipitating factor for hemolysis in G6PD-deficient individuals. The degree of hemolysis is normally mild, but severe intravascular hemolysis has occasionally been described. The mechanism of accelerated red cell destruction is not entirely clear. It is likely that phagocytosing macrophages generate oxidants while combating the infection, with resulting red cell damage. Commonly implicated infectious agents are *Salmonella*, *Escherichia coli*, β-hemolytic streptococci, rickettsiae, and viral hepatitis.

Drugs

Compounds known to induce hemolysis in G6PD-deficient individuals are listed in Table 11-1 (Avery, 1980; Koda-Kimble, 1978). All of these drugs interact with hemoglobin and oxygen, resulting in the intracellular formation of H_2O_2 and other oxidizing radicals (e.g., O_2^-, OH•). These oxidants accumulate in enzyme-deficient red cells with low GSH levels. This results in oxidation of hemoglobin and other proteins, leading to loss of function and cell death. Some drugs are dangerous for all G6PD-deficient individuals, whereas some can be given to individuals with less-severe deficiency as they only cause modest shortening of the lifespan of their red blood cells. Also, for drugs such as aspirin previously implicated in causing severe hemolysis, it is likely that the infection for which the drug was given was the true culprit.

THERAPY

The majority of patients with G6PD deficiency will be unaware of the problem and go through life clinically undiagnosed. For patients who are diagnosed with G6PD deficiency, their family members and offspring should be offered screening and counseling. Counseling should cover an explanation of the genetic background of the condition, ways it can affect health, and how to recognize symptoms and signs of hemolysis and should provide a list of drugs to avoid. Particular advice should be given regarding travel where malaria prophylaxis is required. The patient should be advised to carry a Medicalert tag and be sure to advise any health care professional with whom they are dealing (doctor, nurse, pharmacist) of their problem. Patients should be given this written information in an easily accessible form. The Internet also provides a number of useful and patient-friendly sites (e.g., http://rialto.com/g6pd/index.htm).

Treatment of a patient with G6PD deficiency is dependent on the clinical syndrome of the individual. All individuals known to be G6PD deficient should avoid exposure to known precipitants. This includes pregnant and lactating women who are heterozygous for G6PD deficiency as in some cases drugs can cross the placenta and be present in breast milk.

In acute hemolytic episodes, the use of the offending drug should be stopped and any infection treated. Supportive measures, including folic acid, are normally sufficient. Occasionally, iron supplements may be required since iron is lost in intravascular hemolysis. Transfusion is only rarely required if there is impaired erythropoiesis for some reason or if anemia causes cardiovascular compromise. The management of acute renal failure associated with hemoglobinuria does not differ from that of acute renal failure from any other cause. This will require appropriate management of fluid and electrolyte disturbance and addressing any cofactors, such as sepsis or drug toxicity. Hemodialysis sometimes may be required, but the prognosis for recovery is good.

The treatment of neonatal jaundice due to G6PD deficiency does not differ from that for other causes. Phototherapy and occasionally exchange transfusion may be required to prevent kernicterus (bilirubin neurotoxicity). Phototherapy results in photo-oxidation, configurational isomerization, and structural isomerization of bilirubin. The product of these reactions is lumirubin, a compound that can be efficiently excreted without hepatic conjugation. Exchange transfusion rapidly removes serum bilirubin, but the procedure may need to be repeated to remove the residual bilirubin subsequently released from the tissue-bound pool. With appropriate management, full recovery can be expected, but where good medical care is not available, severe neurological disability will occur. This therefore remains a major health issue in underdeveloped parts of the world where G6PD deficiency is prevalent.

Both vitamin E supplements and splenectomy have been suggested as potential therapeutic options, but neither has proven to be beneficial. Gene therapy is a potential future treatment under development but would only be clinically justified in the most severe cases affected by chronic hemolysis.

It is not common practice to screen routinely for this disorder as the milder variants are not clinically hazardous, and screening for the rarer variants is impractical. In high-prevalence populations (Africans, Mediterranean) however, there should be a high index of suspicion in patients presenting with appropriate clinical symptoms.

QUESTIONS

1. What are in the abnormalities in the chemical pathways that result in the clinical symptoms of G6PD deficiency?
2. What are the causes of false-negative assays for G6PD deficiency?
3. How might the clinical presentation of G6PD deficiency vary between individuals?
4. Why does the level of G6PD activity vary with the degree of maturity of the RBC?
5. By what mechanisms is G6PD deficiency clinically apparent in females?

BIBLIOGRAPHY

Alving A, Carson P, Flanagan C, et al.: Enzymatic deficiency in primaquine-sensitive erythrocytes. *Science* **124:**484–485, 1965.

Avery G: *Drug Treatment.* 2nd ed. ADIS Press, New York, 1980.

Beutler E: G6PD deficiency. *Blood* **84:**3613–3636, 1994.

Beutler E, Lisker R, Kuhl W: Molecular biology of G6PD variants. *Biomed Biochim Acta* **49:**S236–S241, 1990.

Chen E, Cheng A, Lee A, et al.: Sequence of human glucose-6-phosphate dehydrogenase cloned in plasmids and a yeast artificial chromosome. *Genomics* **10:**792–800, 1991.

Koda-Kimble M: *Applied Therapeutics for Clinical Pharmacists.* 2nd ed. Applied Therapeutics, San Francisco, 1978.

Luzzatto L, Gordon-Smith E: Inherited haemolytic anaemias, *in Postgraduate Haematology.* 4th ed. Hoffbrand, AV, Arnold, London, 2001, pp. 120–143.

Luzzatto L, Mehta A: Glucose-6-phosphate dehydrogenase deficiency, *in* Scriver C, Beaudet A, Sly W, Valle D (eds): *The Metabolic and Molecular Bases of Inherited Disease.* 7th ed. McGraw-Hill, New York, 1996, pp. 3367–3398.

Pai G, Sprenkle J, Do T, et al.: Localization of loci for hypoxanthine phophoriboxyltransferase and glucose-6-phosphate dehydrogenase and bio-chemical evidence of non-random X-chromo-some expression from studies of a human X-autosome translocation. *Proc Natl Acad Sci U.S.A.* **77:**2810–2813, 1980.

Scriver C, Beaudet A, Sly W, et al.: *The Metabolic and Molecular Bases of Inherited Disease.* 7th ed. McGraw- Hill, New York, 1995, pp. 3367–3398.

Yoshida A, Beutler E: *Glucose-6-phosphate Dehy-drogenase.* Academic Press, New York, 1986.

12

Biotinidase Deficiency:
A Biotin-Responsive Disorder

BARRY WOLF

CASE REPORT

A 6-month-old male was brought to the emergency department because the parents observed that he had "jerking" of his arms and legs. They said that the child had been sleeping for longer periods of time over the last few days and had episodes of vomiting that were not related to the time of feeding. He had been less responsive than usual, and they were concerned because his rate of breathing had markedly increased this morning. The parents had called their pediatrician, who recommended that they bring the child to see him. While preparing to bring the child to the physician's office, the child began jerking and "twitching." Instead of bringing their child to the pediatrician, the parents called the emergency medical service, which took him directly to the emergency department of the local hospital. By the time the emergency medical team arrived, the child had stopped seizing but was somnolent.

The child had had a normal and uneventful prenatal and birth history. He was born after a full-term gestation and weighed 3.3 kg. Until a few days prior to the incident, he had no medical problems. His weight, length, and head circumference had always followed the 40th percentile on growth charts. He had attained normal developmental milestones for age. There was no known consanguinity between the parents and no family history of similar problems, and there was a normal 3-year-old brother.

On physical examination, the child was afebrile with mild tachypnea and tachycardia.

He was lethargic and exhibited no overt seizure activity. He also had a fine eczemalike skin rash around his eyes, mouth, and genital areas and patchy loss of scalp hair (Fig. 12-1A). Neurologically, he was hypotonic (poor muscle tone) in both the upper and lower extremities with decreased deep tendon reflexes. His lung, cardiovascular, and abdominal examinations were unremarkable. The remainder of his physical examination was normal.

On further questioning, the parents stated that they thought the rash was just a diaper rash and had not noticed the redness around his eyes and mouth. They related that just a few days prior they had found hair on the child's bed but thought the hair loss was normal.

The major concern of the emergency department physicians was the lethargy, hypotonia, and seizure activity. Initial laboratory studies revealed that the child had a normal complete blood count and smear. Other blood tests revealed metabolic acidosis with a bicarbonate concentration of 11 mEq/L (normal is 20–25 mEq/L) and an anion gap of 22 mEq/L (normal is < 15 mEq/L). His serum glucose, calcium, and magnesium concentrations were normal. To exclude the diagnosis of meningitis, a spinal tap was performed. The cell counts and chemistries of the cerebrospinal fluid were normal. The physicians considered that the child might have sepsis and administered antibiotics and intravenous fluids. Prior to administration of antibiotics, blood, urine, and cerebrospinal fluid were sent for bacterial culture.

A urinalysis showed no signs of infection, but

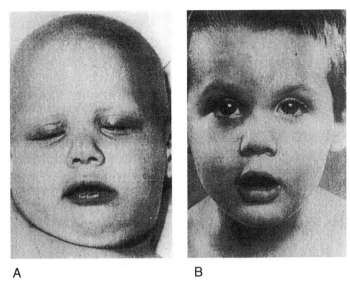

A   B

Figure 12-1. A child with biotinidase deficiency (*A*) prior to diagnosis and therapy and (*B*) after several months of biotin treatment.

there was marked ketonuria. Plasma ammonia concentration was mildly elevated. Based on the metabolic acidosis, increased base deficit, hyperammonemia in the presence of the lethargy, hypotonia, and decreased responsiveness, the possibility of an inherited metabolic disorder was considered. To screen for a variety of metabolic disorders, plasma amino acid concentrations were tested and found to be normal. Urinary organic acid analysis showed increased concentrations of lactate, β-hydroxisovalerate, β-methylcrotonylglycine, and methylcitrate. These findings were consistent with multiple carboxylase deficiency (Fig. 12-2). Based on these results, the child was given 10 mg of oral biotin (Fig. 12-3) and 10 mg per day thereafter.

To determine the type of multiple carboxylase deficiency, blood was obtained to determine the biotin holocarboxylase synthetase activity in leukocytes, and serum was sent to determine the biotinidase activity. The results of the serum biotinidase activity returned first and indicated less than 1% of mean normal serum activity, confirming that the child had profound biotinidase deficiency (less than 10% of mean normal serum biotinidase activity). Subsequently, biotin holocarboxylase synthetase activity was found to be normal. Although many states screen for biotinidase deficiency in the newborn period, this child was born in a state where newborn screening for biotinidase deficiency is not performed.

Over the next few days, the child became markedly more alert and exhibited no seizure activity. All the bacterial cultures were negative after 72 hours, and the antibiotics were discontinued. His skin rash disappeared in a week, and hair growth returned to the areas of alopecia (Fig. 12-1B). The child has had no further biochemical, neurological, or cutaneous abnormalities since the biotin was started.

Because ophthalmologic problems and hearing loss occur commonly in symptomatic children with profound biotinidase deficiency, extensive eye and auditory testing were performed. The child was found to have mild optic atrophy and moderate mid- and high-frequency hearing loss. To ensure normal language development, he was given hearing aids.

The parents and the sibling were shown to have about 50% of mean normal serum biotinidase activity, consistent with heterozygosity. Mutation analysis of DNA from the child revealed homozygosity for a common missense mutation.

DIAGNOSIS

Symptoms, such as vomiting, respiratory problems, hypotonia, and seizures, in young children often are characteristic of various serious infections, including meningitis and sepsis. Although these are usually accompanied by fever, neonates with sepsis may be hypothermic or euthermic (normal temperature). In the absence of seizures, gastrointestinal obstruction and cardiorespiratory problems are in the differential

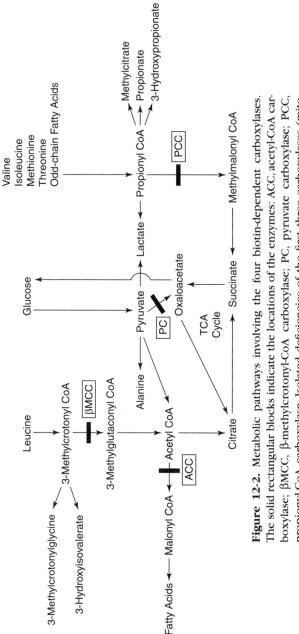

Figure 12-2. Metabolic pathways involving the four biotin-dependent carboxylases. The solid rectangular blocks indicate the locations of the enzymes: ACC, acetyl-CoA carboxylase; βMCC, β-methylcrotonyl-CoA carboxylase; PC, pyruvate carboxylase; PCC, propionyl-CoA carboxylase. Isolated deficiencies of the first three carboxylases (mitochondrial) have been established (isolated ACC deficiency has not been confirmed). At least the activities of the three mitochondrial carboxylases can be secondarily deficient in the untreated multiple carboxylase deficiencies, biotin holocarboxylase synthetase deficiency and biotinidase deficiency. Lowercase characters indicate metabolites that are frequently found at elevated concentrations in urine of children with both multiple carboxylase deficiencies. The isolated deficiencies have elevations of those metabolites directly related to their respective enzyme deficiency.

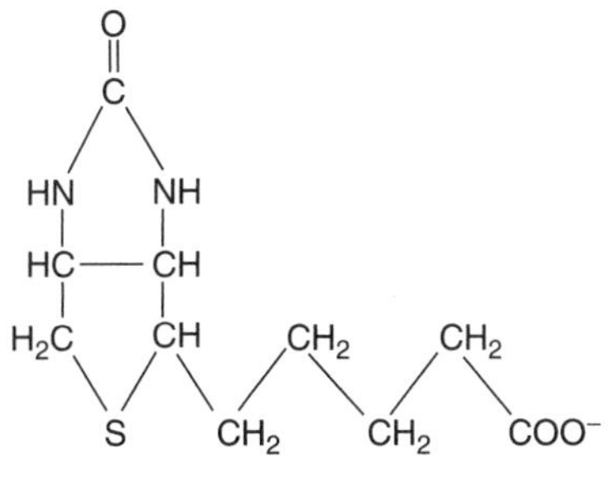

Figure 12-3. The structure of d-biotin and *N*-carboxybiotin covalently attached to an ε-amino group of a lysyl residue of a carboxylase. Biocytin is the biotin similarly attached to the ε-amino group of a lysine. The dotted line indicates the amide bond linkage.

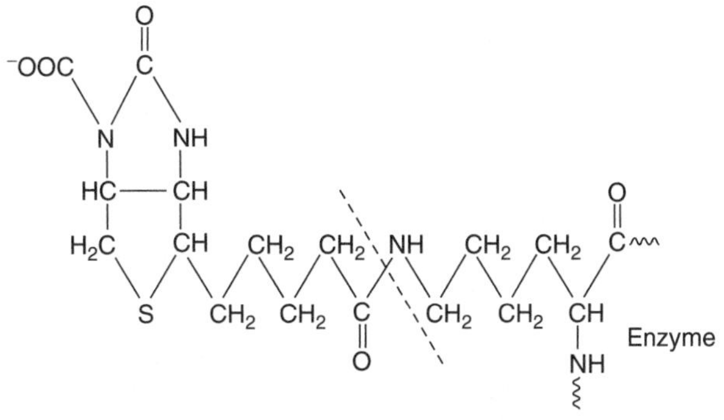

diagnosis. However, when these symptoms occur together with biochemical abnormalities, such as metabolic acidosis, ketonuria, or hyperammonemia, an inborn error of metabolism must be suspected. In addition, occasionally there are symptoms that are more specific for particular inherited metabolic disorders, such as skin rash and alopecia that lead the physician to the correct diagnosis. Plasma amino acid and urinary organic acid analyses are helpful screening tools to include or exclude disorders from the large group of possible inborn errors of metabolism.

Urinary organic acid analysis is useful for differentiating isolated carboxylase deficiencies from the biotin-responsive multiple carboxylase deficiencies. β-Hydroxyisovalerate is the most common urinary metabolite observed in isolated β-methylcrotonyl-CoA carboxylase deficiency, biotinidase deficiency, biotin holocarboxylase synthetase deficiency, and acquired biotin deficiency. In addition to β-hydroxyisovalerate, elevated concentrations of urinary lactate, methylcitrate, and β-hydroxypropionate are indicative of multiple carboxylase deficiency.

Children with any of the isolated carboxylase deficiencies do not improve with biotin supplementation, whereas those with multiple carboxylase deficiency do. A trial of biotin is often expedient and useful in discriminating between the isolated carboxylase deficiencies and the multiple carboxylase deficiencies. Isolated carboxylase deficiencies can be definitively confirmed by demonstrating deficient enzyme activity of one of three mitochondrial carboxylases in extracts of peripheral blood leukocytes (prior to biotin therapy) or cultured fibroblasts, whereas the activities of the other two carboxylases are normal.

The organic acid analysis in the urine of this child was consistent with biotin deficiency or multiple carboxylase deficiency. Biotin deficiency usually can be excluded unless there is a history of dietary indiscretion, such as consuming a diet containing raw eggs or few biotin-containing foods, or there is a history of prolonged parenteral hyperalimentation without biotin supplementation. Low serum biotin concentrations can be useful in differentiating biotin and biotinidase deficiencies from biotin holocarboxylase synthetase deficiency, but these determinations are laborious, only performed in a few laboratories, and depending on the methodology, can provide uninformative information. For example, only the methods that can distinguish biotin from biocytin or bound biotin provide useful information. Methods that measure total biotin and biotin plus biotin derivatives may not indicate biotin deficiency.

Children with both biotin holocarboxylase synthetase deficiency and biotinidase deficiency often exhibit similar nonspecific clinical features, such as feeding problems, vomiting, hypotonia, and lethargy. Other symptoms characteristic of biotin-responsive multiple carboxylase deficiencies, such as skin rash or alopecia, can lead more rapidly to the correct diagnosis, but also can be seen in children with zinc or essential fatty acid deficiencies. Frequent viral, bacterial, or fungal infections, due to immunological dysfunction, may occur in children with multiple carboxylase deficiency. On the other hand, an infection may be the stress than precipitates the symptoms of a metabolic disorder. Children with biotin holocarboxylase synthetase deficiency may have metabolic acidosis, a large anion gap, and elevated concentrations of lactate in the serum and urine. An amino acid analysis may reveal hyperglycinemia, which also can occur in other organic acidemias.

Biotinidase deficiency must be differentiated from biotin holocarboxylase synthetase deficiency. The majority of patients with biotinidase deficiency exhibit metabolic lactic acidosis, ketosis, and organic aciduria similar to that seen in biotin holocarboxylase synthetase deficiency. Patients with both disorders have elevated concentrations of urinary β-hydroxyisovalerate and β-methylcrotonylglycine. However, some symptomatic patients with biotinidase deficiency (about 20%) do not excrete the characteristic organic acids, even when they are seriously ill and metabolically compromised. Therefore, the presence of normal urinary organic acids, even when the child is symptomatic, does not exclude a diagnosis of biotinidase deficiency. Patients with both disorders may have mild hyperammonemia. When neurological or cutaneous symptoms are suggestive of multiple carboxylase deficiency, appropriate enzyme testing should be performed.

The age of onset of symptoms may be useful in discriminating between these two multiple carboxylase deficiencies. Although children with biotin holocarboxylase synthetase deficiency usually exhibit symptoms before 2 months of age and whereas those with biotinidase deficiency usually manifest symptoms after 3 months of age, there are, however, exceptions for both disorders.

Both multiple carboxylase deficiencies are characterized by deficient activities of the three mitochondrial carboxylases in peripheral blood leukocytes prior to biotin treatment. The carboxylase activities increase to near normal or normal after treatment with pharmacological doses of biotin. Patients with biotin holocarboxylase synthetase deficiency have deficient activities of the three mitochondrial carboxylases in fibroblasts incubated in medium with low biotin concentrations (containing only the biotin contributed by fetal calf serum added to the medium for cell growth), whereas patients with biotinidase deficiency have normal carboxylase activities under these conditions. The activities of the carboxylases in biotin holocarboxylase synthetase deficiency become near normal to normal when cultured in medium supplemented with high concentrations of biotin.

Biotinidase deficiency and biotin holocarboxylase synthetase deficiency can be definitively diagnosed by direct enzymatic assay. Biotinidase activity in plasma or serum is usually determined by using the artificial substrate, biotinyl-p-aminobenzoate. If biotinidase activity is present, then biotin is cleaved, releasing p-aminobenzoate. The p-aminobenzoate then is reacted with reagents that result in the development of purple color that can be quantitated colorimetrically. In the absence of biotinidase activity, p-aminobenzoate is not liberated. Biotinidase activity in patients with an isolated carboxylase deficiency or biotin holocarboxylase synthetase deficiency is normal.

Plasma biotin concentrations may be deficient in patients with biotinidase deficiency, but also can be normal prior to therapy. Again, it is important to be certain that the method used to determine the biotin concentration measures free biotin and does not also measure biotin derivatives, such as biocytin.

The age of onset of symptoms of children with profound biotinidase deficiency varies from several months to 10 years old, with a mean age of presentation between 3 and 6 months old. The most common neurological features of this disorder are seizures, hypotonia, and ataxia. Myoclonic seizures are the most common type of seizure, but some children have exhibited grand mal and focal types, and a few have been described as infantile seizures. Some children have exhibited breathing abnormalities, such as hyperventilation, laryngeal stridor, and apnea. One child who was initially diagnosed as having sudden infant death syndrome was retrospectively found to have biotinidase deficiency.

Older children with biotinidase deficiency often exhibit ataxia and developmental delay. Sensorineural hearing loss and eye problems, such as optic atrophy, have been described in many untreated children. A recent study has shown that 76% of symptomatic children with profound biotinidase deficiency have sensorineural hearing loss. Frequently, these children have cutaneous symptoms, including skin rash and alopecia. Several patients have had cellular abnormalities, manifested by fungal infection. These immunological aberrations are varied and may represent the effects of abnormal organic acid metabolites or biotin deficiency on normal immunological function. Biotin therapy rapidly corrects the immunological dysfunction. Some children with biotinidase deficiency only exhibit one or two of these features, whereas others have many of the neurological and cutaneous findings.

Children who are diagnosed and treated with biotin at birth, before developing symptoms, or who did not experience recurrent episodes of metabolic compromise will usually remain asymptomatic. Severe neurological problems most frequently occur in those children who have had recurrent symptoms and metabolic compromise. The irreversible symptoms include deafness, optic atrophy, and developmental delay.

BIOCHEMICAL PERSPECTIVES

Biotin, an essential water-soluble B-complex vitamin, is the coenzyme for four human carboxylases (Fig. 12-2): These include the three mitochondrial enzymes: pyruvate carboxylase, which converts pyruvate to oxaloacetate and is the initial step of gluconeogenesis; propionyl-CoA carboxylase, which catabolizes several branched-chain amino acids and odd-chain fatty acids; and β-methylcrotonyl-CoA carboxylase, which is involved in the catabolism of leucine; and the principally cytosolic enzyme, acetyl-CoA carboxylase, which is responsible for the

first, committed step in the synthesis of fatty acids (Fig. 12-2). Therefore, these enzymes are involved in carbohydrate, protein, and lipid metabolism.

Biotin is attached to the various apocarboxylases by the enzyme biotin holocarboxylase synthetase forming holocarboxylases through the two partial reactions shown below:

$$\text{A. Biotin} + \text{ATP} \leftrightarrows \text{Biotinyl-5'-AMP} + \text{PP}_i$$

$$\text{B. Biotinyl-5'-AMP} + \text{Apocarboxylase} \rightarrow \text{Holocarboxylase} + \text{AMP}$$

$$\text{Net: Biotin} + \text{ATP} + \text{Apocarboxylase} \rightarrow \text{Holocarboxylase} + \text{AMP} + \text{PP}_i$$

All four carboxylases bind a carbon dioxide moiety to a nitrogen atom in the heterocyclic portion of biotin and transfer the carbon dioxide to an acceptor molecule through the following two partial reactions:

$$\text{A. Enzyme-Biotin} + \text{ATP} + \text{HCO}_3^- \leftrightarrows \text{Enzyme-Biotin-CO}_2 + \text{ADP} + \text{P}_i$$

$$\text{B. Enzyme-Biotin-CO}_2 + \text{Acceptor} \leftrightarrows \text{Enzyme-Biotin} + \text{Acceptor-CO}_2$$

$$\text{Net: HCO}_3^- + \text{ATP} + \text{Acceptor} \leftrightarrows \text{Acceptor-CO}_2 + \text{ADP} + \text{P}_i$$

The carboxyl group of biotin is linked by an amide bond to an ε-amino group of a specific lysine residue of the apoenzymes (Fig. 12-3). After the holocarboxylases are degraded proteolytically to biocytin (biotinyl-ε-lysine) or small biotinyl peptides, biotinidase cleaves the amide bond, releasing lysine or lysyl peptides and free biotin, which can then be recycled (Fig. 12-4). Biotinidase also plays a role in the processing of protein-bound biotin, thereby making the vitamin available to the free biotin pool. Recent studies suggest that biotinidase also plays a role in the transfer of biotin from biocytin to specific proteins, such as histones.

Inherited isolated deficiencies of the three mitochondrial biotin-dependent carboxylases were described during the 1970s (Fig. 12-2). Children with each of the isolated deficiencies exhibit neurological symptoms during infancy or early childhood associated with metabolic compromise caused by the accumulation of abnormal metabolites resulting from the respective enzyme block. Each isolated deficiency is due to a structural abnormality in the respective mitochondrial enzyme, whereas the activities of

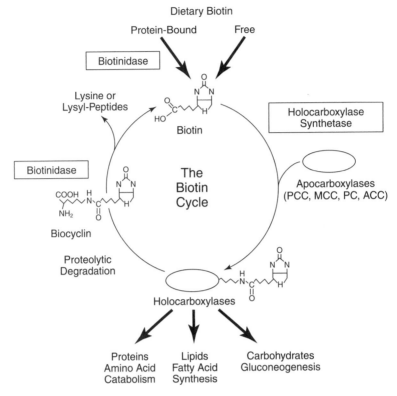

Figure 12-4. The biotin cycle shows the actions of biotin holocarboxylase synthetase in biotinylating carboxylases and of biotinidase in cleaving biocytin, thereby recycling biotin.

the other carboxylases are normal. Each disorder is treated by dietary restrictions, but all fail to improve following treatment with pharmacological doses of biotin.

In 1971, a child with biotin-responsive β-methylcrotonylglycinuria was reported. This individual had metabolic ketoacidosis and elevated concentrations of urinary β-methylcrotonic acid and β-methylcrotonylglycine. Several days after being given oral biotin, his symptoms resolved, and the urinary metabolites cleared. He subsequently was shown to have deficient activities of all three mitochondrial carboxylases in his peripheral blood leukocytes and skin fibroblasts. This was the first child to be diagnosed with what was called multiple carboxylase deficiency.

Additional children with multiple carboxylase deficiency were reported. Initially, these children were classified as having either the early-onset form (referred to as the neonatal or infantile form) or the late-onset form (referred to as the juvenile form) of multiple carboxylase deficiency, depending on the age of onset of

symptoms. Most of the children with the early-onset form ultimately were shown to have biotin holocarboxylase synthetase deficiency.

Two children with the late-onset form initially were reported as having a defect in intestinal transport of biotin. This conclusion was supported by finding low plasma biotin concentrations when these children were administered oral biotin compared to the concentrations of plasma biotin of unaffected control subject. In 1983, it was demonstrated that the primary biochemical defect in most patients with late-onset multiple carboxylase deficiency was a deficiency of serum biotinidase activity. The two children with a putative defect in intestinal biotin transport both were confirmed to have biotinidase deficiency. This disparity was reconciled by demonstrating that, in both cases, the children were biotin depleted at the time the biotin-loading studies were performed. Therefore, when the children initially were given biotin, although the vitamin was transported into the blood normally, it was rapidly taken up by the tissues, thereby resulting in low plasma biotin concentrations. When these children were replete in biotin, their plasma biotin concentrations increased normally in response to the biotin. These latter studies indicated that neither child had a defect in intestinal biotin transport.

Children with profound biotinidase activity have less than 10% of mean normal serum enzyme activity. Deficient biotinidase activity has also been demonstrated in extracts of leukocytes and fibroblasts. At least one patient was shown to have deficient biotinidase activity in his liver. More than 300 symptomatic individuals have been reported with biotinidase deficiency. The parents of these children usually have serum enzyme activities intermediate between those of the patients and those of normal individuals.

Biotinidase deficiency may present with varying degrees of metabolic acidosis, ketosis, and hyperammonemia. The metabolic acidosis is usually accompanied by an increased anion gap and lactate elevations. The ketosis is due to the accumulation of abnormal organic acid metabolites, such as propionate and lactate, in blood, and β-hydroxypropionate, methylcitrate, β-hydroxyisovaleric acid, β-methylcrotonylglycine, and β-hydroxybutyrate in urine. Hyperammonemia plays a major role in causing the lethargy, somnolence, and coma that can occur in the disorder. The hyperammonemia is due to the secondary inhibition of *N*-acetylglutamate synthetase, which produces *N*-acetylglutamate, the activator of carbamyl phosphate synthetase in the urea cycle.

Individuals with untreated biotinidase deficiency develop biotin deficiency because they cannot recycle endogenous biotin. The biotin deficiency subsequently results in the lack of substrate for biotin holocarboxylase synthetase. Without the availability of biotin to be added to the apocarboxylases, multiple carboxylase deficiency occurs, and the abnormal metabolites accumulate.

Serum biotinidase activity is not altered by biotin deficiency. This was demonstrated by finding normal serum biotinidase activity in several patients who became biotin deficient while being treated with parenteral hyperalimentation lacking biotin. Biotinidase appears to play an important role in the processing of protein-bound biotin, either by being secreted into the intestinal tract, where it can release biotin from

bound dietary sources that can subsequently be absorbed, or by cleaving biocytin or biotinyl peptides in the intestinal mucosa or in blood.

Most patients with biotinidase deficiency excrete large quantities of biocytin in their urine, but there has been no evidence of accumulation of this metabolite in tissues. It remains to be determined whether biotin therapy is harmful because it may increase the concentration of biocytin in these children.

Biotinidase activity in cerebrospinal fluid and the brain is very low. This suggests that the brain may not recycle biotin effectively and depends on biotin transported across the blood-brain barrier. Several symptomatic children who have failed to exhibit peripheral lactic acidosis or organic aciduria have had elevated lactate or organic acids in their cerebrospinal fluid. This compartmentalization of the biochemical abnormalities may explain why the neurological symptoms usually appear before other symptoms. Peripheral metabolic ketoacidosis and organic aciduria subsequently occur with prolonged metabolic compromise.

Most patients with biotinidase activity who have hearing loss had this problem before beginning biotin therapy. Hearing loss is usually irreversible, although several young affected children have shown some improvement in hearing with biotin therapy. Some researchers have speculated that the biocytin or biotinyl peptides accumulate and are toxic and even aggravate hearing deficits. This remains to be proven, however. Recently, biotinidase has been localized to discrete regions of the brain and cochlea, including the hair cells and spiral ganglion. Lack of biotinidase in these areas likely has a direct role in causing the hearing loss.

Electroencephalographic findings in individuals with untreated profound biotinidase deficiency have ranged from normal to markedly abnormal and are usually nonspecific. Demyelination and other cerebral abnormalities have been seen in some children with biotinidase deficiency. These findings sometimes improve following biotin treatment.

Human serum biotinidase has been purified to homogeneity and characterized. The cDNA that encodes for the enzyme and the genomic organization have been elucidated. The gene that encodes for the serum enzyme has been localized to chromosome 3p25. Over 100 different mutations that cause biotinidase deficiency have been identified.

THERAPY

A child with biotinidase deficiency should be adequately hydrated to facilitate the excretion of the abnormal organic acid metabolites (Fig. 12-2). Adequate nutrition is essential. In the acute stage of the disorder, protein may be restricted. It is imperative to supply sufficient calories in the form of parenteral glucose or oral polysaccharides, such as polycose. Severe acidosis may initially require bicarbonate supplementation.

The mainstay of therapy in biotinidase deficiency is biotin supplementation. To date, all symptomatic children with biotinidase deficiency have improved after treatment with 5 to 10 mg of biotin per day. Biotin appears to be required in the free form as opposed to the bound form. This is based on the findings of two children who were fed yeast as a form of therapy. Neither improved because essentially all of the biotin in yeast is protein bound, and these children could not recycle the biotin. These children, however, did improve when treated with free biotin. Treatment with biotin is essential and sufficient to prevent or resolve the symptoms. It is not necessary to treat children with biotinidase deficiency with protein-restricted diets as it is in some of the isolated carboxylase deficiencies because with biotin therapy all the carboxylase activities are normal. Symptoms of biotinidase deficiency are preventable if patients are diagnosed and treated at birth or before symptoms occur.

If the child with profound biotinidase deficiency is symptomatic, then the biochemical abnormalities and seizures resolve rapidly after biotin treatment. This is usually followed by improvement of the cutaneous abnormalities. Hair growth returns over a period of weeks to months in the children with alopecia. Optic atrophy and hearing loss are usually resistant to therapy, especially if several months have elapsed between the time of diagnosis and the initiation of treatment. Some treated children have rapidly regained lost developmental milestones, whereas others have continued to show deficits.

Biotinidase deficiency met most of the criteria for inclusion in a neonatal screening program, such as ease and efficacy of treatment, frequency of the disorder, and the relatively low cost of testing. Therefore, a simple colorimetric method to determine biotinidase activity using the same soaked filter-paper blood spots required for other neonatal screening tests was developed. Usually, this colorimetric enzymatic assay uses the same reagents described for confirmational testing. Currently, more than 25 countries and 25 states in the United States screen for biotinidase deficiency in the newborn period. The frequency of biotinidase deficiency is about 1 in 60,000 newborns.

Biotinidase activity can be measured in cultured amniotic fluid cells and in amniotic fluid. Therefore, prenatal diagnosis of biotinidase deficiency is possible. Prenatal diagnosis has been performed in two at-risk pregnancies in which amniocentesis was performed because of advanced maternal age. The fetuses were found to be unaffected, and this was confirmed after birth. In addition to enzyme determination in amniocytes, a fetus was correctly shown to be a heterozygote by molecular mutation analysis in an at-risk pregnancy. Because treatment is so effective in this disorder, some laboratories are now performing prenatal diagnosis.

Biotinidase deficiency represents a readily diagnosable inherited metabolic disorder for which the symptoms can be prevented or ameliorated with simple, direct therapy. If a child must have an inborn error of metabolism, then biotinidase deficiency is the disorder to have.

QUESTIONS

1. Although there have been reports of inherited isolated deficiencies of the three mitochondrial biotin-dependent carboxylases, there have not been any confirmed reports of inherited isolated acetyl-CoA carboxylase deficiency. What is a possible explanation for why isolated acetyl-CoA carboxylase deficiency has not been observed?

2. Some children with profound biotinidase deficiency exhibit symptoms, such as seizures, but do not have metabolic acidemia or elevations of the characteristic organic acids in their plasma or blood. What is a possible explanation for this observation?

3. Biotinidase activity in newborn screening and in confirmational testing is usually determined by using the artificial substrate biotinyl-p-aminobenzoate in the colorimetric assay. What are the ramifications of not using the natural substrate biocytin to

identify children with biotinidase deficiency?

4. Children with biotinidase deficiency cannot cleave biocytin. It has been suggested that biocytin may accumulate in tissues. Can you design an experiment to determine if biocytin is toxic or harmful?

5. Biotinidase activity in extracts of brain tissue is very low (when activity is expressed on a per-mg of-protein basis) relative to the activity in plasma, liver, or kidney. What might this finding suggest about the distribution of biotinidase in the brain?

6. Children with biotinidase deficiency are usually treated with 5–10 mg of oral biotin. We often use the same dose for infants as we do for older children. This obviously means that the dose of biotin per body weight is decreasing as the child gets older. How might one determine if the dose of biotin is adequate or if higher doses are necessary?

7. Yeast contains large concentrations of biotin or biotinyl derivatives. However, when yeast extracts are administered to symptomatic children with profound biotinidase deficiency, there has been no clinical improvement. What is a possible explanation for this observation?

8. A mouse can be made biotin deficient by feeding the animal food lacking biotin and supplemented with the egg white protein avidin, which strongly binds biotin, for 8 weeks. If the animal is then given radiola-beled biotin, as much as 50% of the biotin localizes to the nucleus of hepatocytes. What is a possible role of biotin in the nucleus?

BIBLIOGRAPHY

Cole H, Reynolds TR, Buck GB, et al.: Human serum biotinidase: cDNA cloning, sequence and characterization. *J Biol Chem* **269:**6566–6570, 1994.

Hymes J, Wolf B: Biotinidase and its roles in biotin metabolism. *Clin Chim Acta* **255:**1–11, 1996.

Wolf B: Disorders of biotin metabolism, *in* Scriver CR, Beaudet AL, Sly WS, Valle D (eds): The Metabolic Basis of Inherited Disease. McGraw-Hill, New York, 1992a, pp. 2083–2103.

Wolf B: Disorders of biotin metabolism: treatable neurological syndromes, *in* Rosenberg R, Prusiner SB, DiMauro S, Barchi RL, Kunkel LM (eds): *The Molecular and Genetic Basis of Neurological Disease*. Butterworth, Stoneham, MA, 1992b, pp. 569–81.

Wolf B: Biotinidase deficiency: new directions and practical concerns. *Curr Treat Options Neurol* **5:**321–328, 2003.

Wolf B, Feldman GL: The biotin-dependent carboxylase deficiencies. *Am J Hum Genet* **34:**699–716, 1982.

Wolf B, Grier RE, Allen RJ, et al.: Biotinidase deficiency: the enzymatic defect in late-onset multiple carboxylase deficiency. *Clin Chim Acta* **131:**273–281, 1983.

Wolf B, Heard GS, Weissbecker KA, et al.: Biotinidase deficiency: initial clinical features and rapid diagnosis. *Ann Neurol* **18:**614–617, 1985.

13

Adrenoleukodystrophy

MARGARET M. McGOVERN

CASE REPORT

An 11-year-old Caucasian male was referred for evaluation of deteriorating school performance and the recent onset of ataxic (i.e., wide-based and unsteady) gait. He had been previously diagnosed with attention deficit disorder and had been treated with Ritalin for the past 3 years. There was no history of trauma or infection. He came to attention after his fifth grade teacher noted that his handwriting skills had declined noticeably from the end of fourth grade, and that there was a general decline in his cognitive abilities, including difficulties with mathematical calculations. In addition, his mother reported that he was having difficulty reading, had become clumsy, and was displaying behavioral changes.

On physical examination, he had slightly slurred speech, was unable to follow complex commands, and had right-left disorientation. His gait was abnormal with circumduction (i.e., active circular movement of the leg) on the right and a steppage gait, right-sided weakness, and a positive Romberg sign (falling forward when eyes are closed, and feet are close together due to loss of position sensation). Further neurological assessment revealed dysgraphia (i.e., inability to write) and dyscalculia (i.e., inability to perform mathematical calculations). No other physical findings were present. Magnetic resonance imaging (MRI) of the brain revealed diffuse abnormal signal in the white matter of the posterior hemisphere extending anteriorly (Fig. 13-1).

Based on the clinical history and findings and the results of the brain MRI, the diagnosis of

X-linked adrenoleukodystrophy (X-ALD) was suspected. Plasma was obtained for the measurement of very long chain fatty acids (VLCFA), which revealed a C26:0 concentration of 1.32 μg/mL, a C24:0/C22:0 ratio of 1.88, and a C26:0/C22:0 ratio of 0.08 (normal is < 0.02), confirming the biochemical diagnosis of X-ALD. Subsequent formal neuropsychological testing was obtained and revealed a performance IQ of 70. Adrenal function was assessed by corticotropin (ACTH) stimulation test and revealed adrenal insufficiency that was treated with replacement therapy with hydrocortisone.

The family history was significant for a maternal uncle, who had died at the age of 18 years from sepsis and who was reported to have bronze skin, both of which presumably resulted from unrecognized adrenal insufficiency, and for another maternal uncle, who had been diagnosed with mental illness and was living in an adult residence. In addition, the 70-year-old maternal grandmother had been confined to a wheelchair for almost 15 years due to weakness, the cause of which had not been previously identified. Biochemical studies to determine VLCFA ratios confirmed the carrier status of the patient's mother and revealed that his only sibling, a 9-year-old brother, had the biochemical defect. Two of his three maternal aunts also were found to be carriers of X-ALD, one of whom was found to have an affected 1-year-old son.

After the diagnosis of X-ALD was established, the patient was placed on a regimen of 45 cc daily (qd) of Lorenzo's oil, 30 cc qd glycerol trioleate oil, and dietary restriction of VLCFA, which resulted in normalization of the plasma VLCFA. His family had decided to pursue bone

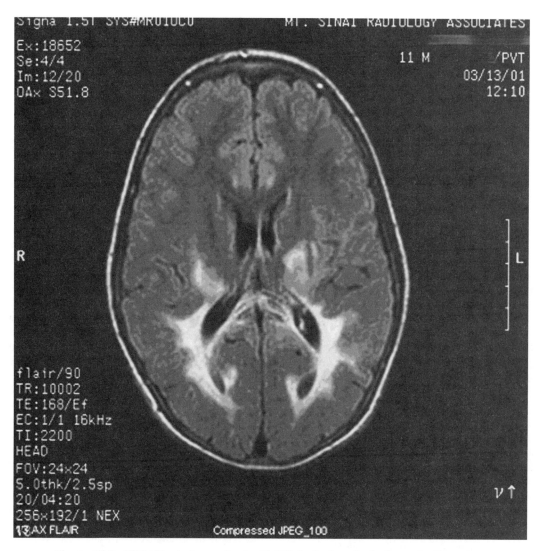

Figure 13-1. MRI of brain in a patient with X-linked adrenoleukodystrophy. Brain magnetic resonance image obtained shortly after diagnosis shows diffuse abnormal signal in the white matter of the posterior hemisphere extending anteriorly.

marrow transplantation (BMT) using marrow derived from his father, who was a histocompatible, antigen-identical match. In the post-transplant period, he continued to decline neurologically, lost all speech, and became progressively demented. Several months later he succumbed to an infection.

DIAGNOSIS

X-ALD is a clinically heterogeneous disorder that can result in progressive nervous system manifestations, adrenal insufficiency, and in-

volvement of the testis. The diagnosis should be considered in boys who present with behavioral disturbances, vision loss, deteriorating handwriting, incoordination, and other progressive neurological deficits. A concomitant history of attention deficit disorder is frequently present. A family history and pedigree should be obtained to look for a pattern of X-linked transmission of disease, although a high index of suspicion must be employed since the phenotype can vary markedly even among affected members of the same family. The diagnosis of X-ALD also should be considered in men who present with progressive gait disorders and abnormalities of sphincter control and sexual dysfunction, which characterize a later onset form of the disease called adrenomyeloneuropathy (AMN). In addition, specific biochemical testing should be obtained in males with primary adrenocortical insufficiency even if no neurological symptoms are present.

Clinical studies that contribute to the diagnosis include a thorough neurological examination and MRI of the brain in patients with neurological symptoms. Brain MRI is always abnormal in neurologically symptomatic males. The imaging findings usually include a characteristic pattern of symmetrical enhanced T-2 signal in the parieto-occipital region with contrast enhancement at the advancing margin.

Definitive diagnosis is achieved by the measurement of VLCFA in plasma. The results of this analysis are abnormal in nearly all males with X-ALD. The specific analyses that are included are the concentration of C26:0, the ratio of C24:0/C22:0, and the ratio of C26:0/C22:0, all of which are elevated in most cases. Increased concentration of VLCFA in plasma and/or cultured skin fibroblasts also is present in approximately 85% of female carriers, although identification of carriers is now available using molecular methods which are more reliable. Testing of at-risk family members is recommended and can identify affected males who may be candidates for therapy (see Therapy). In addition, it facilitates assessment of adrenocortical function in biochemically affected males, permitting treatment of those with adrenal insufficiency. This testing is accomplished by ACTH stimulation.

BIOCHEMICAL PERSPECTIVES

Historical Perspective and Clinical Phenotypes

X-ALD is a disorder of peroxisomal β-oxidation of VLCFA and is estimated to occur in approximately 1:20,000 males. The first description of an affected patient was in 1910. This patient was a previously healthy boy who developed visual disturbances at the age of 6 years, followed by deterioration of his schoolwork, and then spastic gait. His older brother had died of a similar illness in childhood. The brain pathology in this child revealed diffuse loss of myelin in the cerebral hemispheres. Involvement of the adrenal gland was subsequently reported in later-identified patients,

and the name adrenoleukodystrophy (ALD) was proposed in 1970.

Studies of the adrenal gland revealed the presence of lamellar inclusions and led to the recognition that X-ALD involved the abnormal storage of lipids. Identification of the stored material as cholesterol esterified with VLCFA led to the recognition that patients with X-ALD have impaired degradation of VLCFA. This discovery resulted in X-ALD being classified as a peroxisomal disorder. It was hypothesized that the defect was an enzymatic deficiency of VLCFA-CoA synthase, the first enzymatic step in the metabolism of VLCFA, although this theory was later disproven when the gene was identified in 1993 (see below). Nevertheless, the identification of the biochemical defect allowed the establishment of a diagnostic assay by quantitation of VLCFA in plasma.

The availability of a diagnostic assay led to the identification of patients with the biochemical defect who had varying phenotypic presentations that have now been delineated as several distinct X-ALD phenotypes (Table 13-1). These phenotypes range from a severe childhood cerebral form with progressive demyelination of the brain, to a milder adult form, adrenomyeloneuropathy (AMN), that is slowly progressive and limited to the spinal cord, and an even milder form characterized by Addison's disease only, with no neurodegeneration. The childhood form, which accounts for 35% of patients, usually presents between the ages of 4 and 8 years with behavioral or learning deficits, often diagnosed as attention deficit disorder or hyperactivity, followed by neurological symptoms suggestive of a more serious underlying disorder.

The neurological symptoms can include inattention, deterioration of handwriting skills, diminishing school performance, difficulty in understanding speech; reading difficulties, clumsiness; and visual disturbances. In some patients, behavioral disturbances predominate and can include aggression. The rate of disease progression is highly variable, with some patients progressing very rapidly and succumbing within several years, and others surviving for years, albeit with significant deficits. The cerebral phenotype is not only observed in childhood but may also present later in adolescence (adolescent cerebral ALD) or in adulthood (adult cerebral ALD).

AMN, which accounts for 45% of cases, usually presents in the second or third decade with progressive stiffness and weakness of the legs,

Table 13-1. Phenotypic Presentations of X-linked Adrenoleukodystrophy in Affected Males

Phenotype	Age of Onset	Clinical Features
Childhood cerebral	<10 years	Progressive neurological and behavioral deficits with total disability within 3 years
Adolescent cerebral	10–21 years	Progressive neurological and behavioral deficits with eventual total disability
Adrenomyeloneuropathy	Second or third decade	Progressive paraparesis, late cerebral involvement in 45%
Addison disease only	Any	Adrenocortical dysfunction with no neurological disease
Asymptomatic		Biochemical defect with no symptoms

abnormalities of sphincter control, and sexual dysfunction. A subset of these patients also have abnormal findings on MRI, and in a small number, the brain disease can be progressive, leading to cognitive and behavior abnormalities. The disorder also can manifest as Addison's disease only, which presents with unexplained vomiting and weakness or coma and increased skin pigmentation resulting from excessive ACTH secretion. A major pathophysiological difference between the cerebral and noncerebral forms of the disease is the presence of an inflammatory reaction in the cerebral white matter in the former, which resembles multiple sclerosis.

In addition to the manifestations in affected males, some carrier females also display disease symptoms. In particular, up to 40% of women have mild-to-moderate spastic paraparesis (i.e., weakness and stiffness of the legs) in middle age or later. Although adrenal insufficiency in females has been reported, it is rare, as is cerebral involvement.

Peroxisomal Function and Peroxisomal Diseases

X-ALD is a disorder of peroxisomal function. Normally, the peroxisome is the cellular site for β-oxidation of VLCFA and is also involved in the synthesis of bile acids, cholesterol, and plasmalogens. β-Oxidation of some long-chain fatty acids also occurs in the peroxisome, although most long-chain fatty acids are metabolized in the mitochondria. The peroxisome also plays a role in amino acid and purine metabolism. There are a number of genetic disorders associated with defects in the peroxisome. These include defects in genes that encode specific proteins, usually ones with enzymatic activity, and peroxisomal biogenesis defects that affect all of the metabolic pathways of the organelle. The former group includes hyperoxaluria type I

due to alanine:glyoxylate aminotransferase deficiency; Refsum's disease resulting from deficiency of phytanoyl-CoA hydroxylase; *X-ALD* due to deficiency of a membrane protein as described below; rhizomelic chondrodysplasia punctata types II and III due to dihydroxyacetone phosphate acyltransferase deficiency; and the β-oxidation disorders due to acyl-CoA oxidase, bifunctional protein, and thiolase deficiencies. The peroxisomal biogenesis disorders, which result from defects in the peroxisome biogenesis (PEX) genes, are severe disorders that include Zellweger syndrome, neonatal ALD, infantile Refsum disease, and rhizomelic chondrodysplasia punctata type I.

The Biochemical and Molecular Defect in X-linked Adrenoleukodystrophy

The biochemical abnormality in X-ALD is the accumulation of saturated VLCFA such as tetracosanoic (C24:0) and hexacosanoic acid (C26:0) in the brain, adrenal glands, testes, and plasma. Although the mitochondria are the primary site for the oxidation of ingested and stored fats, VLCFA are metabolized in the peroxisome. The metabolic pathway, which is shown in Figure 13-2, leads to the shortening of the carbon chain of the VLCFA by two carbons and the release of acetyl-CoA. This β-oxidation pathway involves consecutive reactions, including dehydrogenation, hydration of the double bond, dehydrogenation again, and thiolytic cleavage. Through this four-step mechanism a two-carbon unit is split from the fatty acid in the form of an acetyl-CoA unit, which can then be transported to the mitochondria and further oxidized in the citric acid Krebs cycle to produce CO_2, H_2O, and energy.

The source of the VLCFA substrates metabolized in the peroxisome is from both dietary

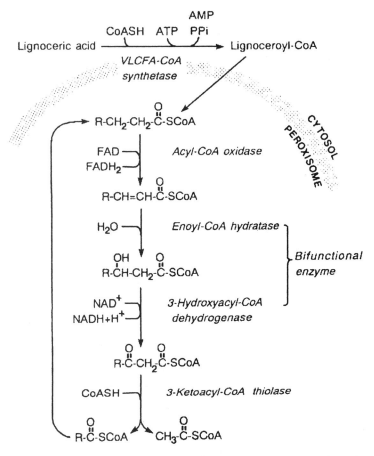

Figure 13-2. The metabolic pathway for the metabolism of very long chain fatty acids (VLCFA) in the peroxisome.

intake and endogenous synthesis. The latter occurs via the microsomal fatty acid elongation system. Both dietary and endogenously synthesized VLCFA have been implicated in the pathogenesis of X-ALD, which has led to the development and evaluation of a variety of therapeutic interventions that have attempted to decrease exposure to VLFCA from each of these sources.

The elevation of VLCFA can be detected in most body tissues and fluids and forms the basis for a diagnostic assay for the identification of affected individuals. The most frequently used test is the measurement of VLCFA in plasma which has been shown to be very sensitive. Although VLCFA are increased in some of the other peroxisomal disorders, including Zellweger syndrome, infantile Refsum disease, and neonatal ALD, the clinical presentations of these disorders are very different from X-ALD, and the discrimination of

these patients from those with X-ALD is usually apparent from the clinical findings. In female carriers of X-ALD, the measurement of VLCFA in the plasma also reveals elevations in about 85% of obligate carriers. Therefore, the test does have some false negatives in carriers, and more definitive diagnosis can be achieved using molecular methods as detailed below.

For many years, it was assumed that the inability of patients with X-ALD to degrade VLCFA was due to a primary deficiency of the first enzyme in this pathway, very long chain fatty acyl-CoA (VLCF-CoA) synthase. Indeed, studies in cultured skin fibroblasts from patients with X-ALD have revealed that this enzyme activity is decreased when compared to cells from normal controls. However, when the X-ALD gene was isolated in 1993, it was discovered that the underlying defect is the deficiency of a peroxisomal membrane protein, called ALD protein (ALDP). The gene maps to Xq28 and encodes a protein product that is a member of the adenosine triphosphate binding cassette (ABC) transporter superfamily. There are three other mammalian peroxisomal ABC transporters that are closely related to ALDP: ALDRP, PMP70, and PMP69.

The precise functions of the peroxisomal ABC transporters and the nature of their interaction with VLCFA-CoA synthase are not well understood, although their sequence similarities suggest that they may have related or overlapping functions in peroxisomal metabolism. Indeed, the fact that X-ALD cells, which lack ALDP, maintain residual activity of the synthase enzyme suggests that the presence of one or more of the other ABC transporters allows partial expression of the enzymatic function. However, to date the precise nature of the interaction beetwen ALDP and VLCFA-CoA synthase has not been completely elucidated, although recent studies have shown that peroxisomes from X-ALD cultured cells contain normal levels of VLCFA-CoA synthase protein. This finding suggests that ALDP is not required for the localization or stability of the VLCFA-CoA synthase but may play a role in its activation.

Since the identification of the genetic defect that results in X-ALD, the underlying molecular defects in affected patients have been extensively studied. Most families have been found to have private missense mutations, although nonsense and frameshift mutations, splice defects, and deletions also have been identified. As might be expected from the fact that different phenotypes can manifest in the same family, no genotype-phenotype relationships have been identified. Similarly, although 70% of patients have no demonstrable ALDP, no correlation between disease severity and the level of expressed protein has been established, and the VLFCA levels also do not correlate with phenotype. Therefore, it has been suggested that modifier genes play an important role in the expression of the phenotype.

Pathophysiology in X-linked Adrenoleukodystrophy

Studies of the pathophysiology of the disorder have focused on the metabolic and pathologic effects of high levels of VLCFA, although it is possible that future studies may identify other roles for ALDP that have yet to be recognized. To date, these investigations have revealed that VLCFA accumulation has an adverse effect on membrane structure and function. For example, in cultured adrenocortical cells, the addition of C26:0 to the media results in increased microviscosity of the cell membrane and decreased secretion of cortisol after ACTH stimulation. Although similar studies have not been carried out in nerve cells, the effect of VLCFA on neural cell membranes may also result in the neurological manifestations of patients with X-ALD.

In addition to the effect of increased VLCFA on membrane and possibly cellular function, the rapid cerebral form of X-ALD is characterized by an inflammatory response that is believed to contribute to the demyelination that characterizes this phenotype and which is similar to that seen in multiple sclerosis. These cerebral lesions are characterized by breakdown in myelin with sparing of the axons accompanied by the accumulation of cholesterol ester in the neurons. A perivascular inflammatory response with infiltration of T cells, B cells, and macrophages also is present. Therefore, it is believed that the rapid cerebral disease has an immunologically-mediated component. It has been suggested that the inflammatory response occurs in response to the elevated levels of VLCFA in lipids, which elicits an inflammatory cascade that may be mediated in part by cytokines. Once this cascade begins, it may be more difficult to intervene in the disease process, and in general therapeutic interventions studied to date have been most effective when initiated early. Therefore, prevention of the initiation of the immune response is important for improving outcome.

THERAPY

To date, no definitive therapeutic approach has been identified that is applicable to all patients with X-ALD, although a number of interventions have been evaluated as described in this section. The clinical evaluation of the efficacy of therapeutic approaches for this disorder is complicated by the wide spectrum of phenotypic severity, even within the same family, and the lack of a biochemical or genetic marker to predict phenotype. For example, it is not known when a particular patient enters a clinical trial what that patient's precise disease course will be. Therefore, it requires carefully planned clinical trials to determine whether the intervention is having a beneficial effect, taking into consideration that not all patients would go on to have the rapid cerebral form of the disease.

In addition to the attempts described below to interfere with the onset or progression of neurological disease, it is also important to carry out endocrine testing on all biochemically identified males to assess their adrenocortical axis. In particular, all patients who have adrenal insufficiency require adrenal hormone replacement to prevent life-threatening complications of insufficiency.

Dietary Therapy

The fact that VLCFA ingested in the diet has been implicated in the pathogenesis of the disorder led to the development of a diet that restricts intake of saturated VLCFA by limiting total fat intake to 20 to 30 g per day. However, the use of this low-fat diet alone does not reduce the plasma VLCFA concentrations and does not have an impact on clinical progression, most likely due to the fact that endogenous production of VLCFA continues to occur and contributes to the disease phenotype. Therefore, attempts have been made to disrupt the endogenous production of VLCFA by administration of a 4:1 mixture of glycerol trioleate oil and glyceryl trierucate oil, which is commonly refereed to as Lorenzo's oil, so named after a child affected with X-ALD whose parents actively participated in the development of this therapy. This mixture, which includes erucic acid, an unsaturated 22-carbon fatty acid, acts by competing with saturated fatty acids for the microsomal VLCFA elongation system.

Although Lorenzo's oil has been found to normalize VLCFA levels in the plasma of patients with X-ALD, this therapy has not been shown to improve outcomes in patients who already have neurological degeneration. Clinical trials have shown, however, that it may prevent neurological disease when provided to biochemically identified males who have not yet begun to manifest any neurological symptoms and who have a normal MRI. Therefore, it has been advocated by some that the administration of Lorenzo's oil to reduce endogenous production of VLCFA in combination with dietary therapy to reduce intake may be useful in asymptomatic boys, although careful follow-up and frequent clinical evaluation is needed to facilitate early identification of those patients who progress despite this intervention and who may become candidates for BMT.

Bone Marrow Transplantation

BMT has been attempted in a number of affected boys with X-ALD. The rationale for the use of BMT in this disorder is that bone marrow-derived cells are known to be capable of degrading VLCFA. Perhaps more important, it was expected that some bone marrow-derived cells would enter the brain since infiltration of the brain with perivascular lymphocytes and macrophages is known to occur. Experience with the procedure has shown that it can stabilize the disease course in a subset of patients, and several cases of reversal of neurological damage also have been reported in patients in the early stages of their disease.

Currently, BMT is not recommended for patients who already have advanced disease and who will most likely continue to deteriorate despite the intervention, presumably because the inflammatory cascade has already begun. Similarly, it is not recommended for boys with a biochemical diagnosis but with no symptoms or MRI changes as it is possible that they may never develop the rapid cerebral form. For these patients, exposing them to the high morbidity and mortality associated with BMT is not justified. However, careful neurological assessment, imaging studies, and neuropsychological testing are needed in asymptomatic patients in order to detect cerebral abnormalities early enough to permit the consideration of this intervention if evidence of disease progression is found. In general, BMT for this disease is now carried out primarily in patients with the biochemical defect who also have early evidence of cerebral involvement. It is not recommend in AMN.

Lovastatin

Lovastatin, commonly known as an inhibitor of cholesterol synthesis, is another agent that has been shown to reduce plasma levels of VLCFA and to increase the ability of X-ALD fibroblasts to metabolize VLCFA. The mechanism for this effect may involve upregulation of ABCD2, which encodes a protein (ALDR) that can substitute for the function of ALDP. However, clinical trials with this agent have demonstrated variable reactions, and no clear clinical benefit has been demonstrated.

QUESTIONS

1. What is the underlying genetic defect in X-ALD?
2. How does peroxisomal β-oxidation differ from mitochondrial β-oxidation?
3. How does the concept of genetic heterogeneity apply to the phenotypic expression of X-ALD?
4. How would you evaluate a patient suspected of having X-ALD?
5. What is the most reliable method for identifying carriers of X-linked ALD? Why?
6. Which patients with elevated levels of VLCFA are the most suitable candidates for BMT?

BIBLIOGRAPHY

Kemp S, Pujol A, Waterham HR, et al.: ABCD1 mutations and the X-linked adrenoleukodystrophy mutation database: role in diagnosis and clinical correlations. *Hum Mutat* **18:**499–515, 2001.

Moser AB, Kreiter N, Bezman L, et al.: Plasma very long chain fatty acids in 3,000 peroxisome disease patients and 29,000 controls. *Ann Neurol* **45:**100–110, 1999.

Moser HW.: Adrenoleukodystrophy: phenotype, genetics, pathogenesis and therapy. *Brain* **120:** 1485–1508, 1997.

Moser HW, Raymond GV, Koehler W, et al.: Evaluation of the preventive effect of glyceryl trioleate-trierucate ("Lorenzo's oil") therapy in X-linked adrenoleukodystrophy: results of two concurrent trials. *Adv Exp Med Biol.* **544:**369–387, 2003.

Moser HW, Smith KD, Watkins PA, et al.: X-linked adrenoleukodystrophy, *in* Scriver CR, Beaudet AL, Sly WS, Valle D (eds): *The Metabolic and Molecular Bases of Inherited Disease.* 8th ed. McGraw-Hill, New York, 2000, pp. 3257–3301.

Mosser J, Douar AM, Sarde CO, et al.: Putative X-linked adrenoleukodystrophy gene shares unexpected homology with ABC transporters. *Nature* **361:**726–730, 1993.

Paintlia AS, Gilg AG, Khan M, et al.: Correlation of very long chain fatty acids accumulation and inflammatory disease progression in childhood ALD: implications for potential therapies. *Neurobiol Dis* **14:**425–439, 2003.

Shapiro E, Krivit W, Lockman L, et al.: Long-term effect of bone-marrow transplantation for childhood-onset cerebral X-linked adrenoleukodystrophy. *Lancet* **356:**713–718, 2000.

van Geel BM, Bezman L, Loes DJ, et al.: Evolution of phenotypes in adult male patients with X-linked adrenoleukodystrophy. *Ann Neurol* **49:**186–194, 2001.

Whitcomb RW, Linehan WM, Knazek RA.: Effects of long-chain, saturated fatty acids on membrane microviscosity and adrenocorticotropin responsiveness of human adrenocortical cells *in vitro.* *J Clin Invest* **81:**185–188, 1988.

14

Low-Density Lipoprotein Receptors and Familial Hypercholesterolemia

MARINA CUCHEL and DANIEL J. RADER

CASE REPORT

A 10-year-old girl from China was evaluated at the University of Pennsylvania for homozygous familial hypercholesterolemia (FH) and possible participation in an experimental gene therapy protocol for her condition. Cutaneous xanthomas (lesions characterized by abnormal accumulation of lipids in macrophages) were first observed at 3 months of age. However, the origins were not fully investigated until the age of 3 years, when she was found to have a total cholesterol level of 1150 mg/dL (desirable levels are < 200 mg/dL) with normal triglyceride levels, and the diagnosis of homozygous FH was made. Both of her parents' total cholesterol levels were in the range of 300–400 mg/dL, consistent with the diagnosis of heterozygous FH. A positive family history for premature coronary artery disease was present on both sides.

The proband remained in apparent good health until she was 9 years old, when she developed progressive symptoms of exertional chest tightness and shortness of breath. Her physical examination at 10 years of age revealed numerous cutaneous and tendon xanthomas (overlying her elbows, wrists, knees, and buttocks and on the Achilles' tendons) as well as a systolic ejection murmur radiating to the neck and bilateral carotid bruits (abnormal sound heard during auscultation that suggests the presence of blockage). A carotid Doppler showed the presence of a stenosis (blockage) of approximately 50% in both common carotid arteries. She underwent a thallium exercise stress test that was negative; an exercise echocardiography that showed inferoseptal and inferobasal hypokinesis (decreased contractile function of the myocardium) during exercise that resolved at rest; and a cardiac catheterization that showed a 90–99% stenosis of the right coronary artery's ostium and a 40% stenosis of left anterior descending artery, in addition to mild aortic regurgitation.

Functional and genetic studies were performed to confirm the diagnosis of homozygous FH. Low-density lipoprotein (LDL) receptor activity, measured in an *in vitro* functional assay that used fibroblasts isolated from the patient's skin, was less than 2% of the normal value (functionally confirming the diagnosis of homozygous FH). LDL metabolism studies showed that she removed LDL from her blood at a markedly slower rate than normal, consistent with lack of LDL receptors. Finally, genetic analysis confirmed that she was homozygous for an LDL receptor gene mutation in exon 10 (W462X) that created a premature stop codon at amino acid 462; this mutant truncated LDL receptor has been shown to be nonfunctional.

She underwent coronary artery bypass grafting of the right coronary artery. Her exertional chest tightness and shortness of breath were noted to be entirely resolved following surgery. Two months after surgery, she was readmitted at the Hospital of the University of Pennsylvania for a research protocol of *ex vivo* liver-directed gene therapy. This was an experimental protocol designed to genetically correct liver cells taken from the patient with the normal LDL receptor gene and then readminister these liver cells to the patient (Raper et al., 1996). The first stage of the protocol consisted of the resection of the left lateral segment of the patient's liver and the isolation of hepatocytes (liver cells) to establish primary hepatocyte cultures. The cultures were then infected with a recombinant retrovirus that contained the human LDL receptor gene. One day later, the genetically modified hepatocytes were harvested and reinfused into the patient's liver via a portal venous catheter. The patient tolerated the procedure well and left the hospital several days later.

Three months later, her cholesterol levels were about 20% lower than prior to the gene therapy protocol. Repeat LDL metabolism studies showed that she cleared LDL from her blood significantly faster than prior to the gene therapy, consistent with some liver expression of the LDL receptor. A liver biopsy was done and demonstrated clusters of liver cells that were expressing the normal LDL receptor gene.

The patient was followed yearly. Because her cholesterol level remained very high, she was treated with a low-fat, low-cholesterol diet and the maximal dose of a statin (the most common drug class for treating high cholesterol) with modest effects. Although LDL apheresis (a physical method of purging the blood of cholesterol) is strongly recommended in patients with homozygous FH, it was not an available option where she lived. Her cardiovascular condition got progressively worse, and she experienced myocardial infarction at the age of 14 years. Her risk of developing recurrent atherosclerotic vascular disease remains high because of her very elevated cholesterol.

DIAGNOSIS

FH is a well-characterized genetic disorder caused by mutations in the gene encoding the LDL receptor, the receptor responsible for the uptake and subsequent removal of LDL from circulation. As a consequence, LDL levels in plasma are increased. FH is autosomal codominant: Heterozygotes have elevated LDL cholesterol levels (250–500 mg/dL), and homozygotes have even higher levels (500–1200 mg/dL). Its frequency is 1 in 500 subjects in the heterozygous state and 1 in 1 million in the homozygous state. In certain populations, such as Ashkenazi Jews, Afrikaners in South Africa, French Canadians, and Christian Lebanese, the frequency is substantially higher due to a "founder effect"

(i.e., to the fact that these population groups originated from a small number of individuals carrying LDL mutations at higher frequency than that of the general population).

Heterozygous FH patients have LDL cholesterol levels that are two- to threefold higher than normal subjects, tendon xanthomas (accumulation of cholesterol in tendons, causing them to be thickened and irregular, especially in the backs of the hands and the Achilles' tendons) in adulthood, and coronary atherosclerosis that becomes clinically manifest usually after age 30 years in men and 40 years in women. On the other hand, patients with homozygous FH have LDL levels that are more than three times the normal values; tendon, tuberous, and cutaneous xanthomas in childhood; and premature atherosclerosis with symptomatic coronary artery and other atherosclerotic vascular disease frequently before the age of 20 years. Interestingly, as in the case presented, the early atherosclerosis manifestation in homozygous FH is often due to the formation of atheroma along the aortic root, aortic valve, and coronary ostia, which result in the presence of systolic murmur as well as a pressure gradient across the aortic valve, narrowing of the root, and obstructive ostial coronary disease. This often requires surgical intervention that may include coronary bypass and/or valve replacement.

There is a substantial interindividual variation in LDL cholesterol levels among patients with FH. Generally, LDL cholesterol levels are inversely related to the residual LDL receptor activity, as measured in the *in vitro* assay that uses skin fibroblasts. Patients with homozygous FH are classically divided into two groups based on the fibroblast LDL receptor activity. Patients with less than 2% activity, as the patient described in the case report, are classified as receptor-negative. Patients with 2%–20% LDL receptor activity are classified as receptor-defective. The natural history of the disease is much more severe in receptor-negative patients, who, if left untreated, rarely survive beyond the second decade of life. Receptor-defective patients, in contrast, have less-severe hypercholesterolemia and a more delayed onset of coronary artery disease and mortality.

The diagnosis of FH is made on clinical grounds. The diagnosis of homozygous FH is usually made on the basis of markedly elevated LDL cholesterol levels, normal triglyceride level, presence of xanthomas, and family history of hypercholesterolemia and/or premature coronary artery disease. The differential diagnosis of heterozygous FH includes other less-frequent monogenic causes of hypercholesterolemia, such as familial defective apolipoprotein B-100 (apoB-100; due to mutations in apoB, the major protein in LDL and the ligand for binding to the LDL receptor), autosomal recessive hypercholesterolemia (due to mutations in the ARH gene encoding a novel adaptor protein important for the internalization of the LDL receptor), autosomal dominant hypercholesterolemia (due to mutations in PCSK9, a gene of unknown function), and sitosterolemia (due to mutations in ABCG5 or ABCG8 that are responsible for excretion of sterols from the body) (Rader et al., 2003).

BIOCHEMICAL PERSPECTIVES

The landmark studies by Brown and Goldstein (see Goldstein et al., 2001 for review) that led to the discovery of the genetic cause of FH and its metabolic and clinical consequences are fascinating and of historical importance because they were the first to elucidate the mechanisms of receptor-mediated endocytosis. Brown and Goldstein received the Noble Price in Medicine in 1985 for their work on the LDL receptor and molecular basis of FH.

Cells need cholesterol to survive. Cells can either synthesize cholesterol *de novo* or obtain it from exogenous sources, such as lipoproteins present in the circulation (see Table 14-1 and Rader and Hobbs, 2005, for review). All of the lipoprotein classes contain phospholipids, esterified and unesterified cholesterol, and triglycerides to varying degrees. LDL are the most abundant lipoproteins in humans. They are composed of a core of neutral lipids, mainly cholesteryl ester, surrounded by a shell of phospholipids and held together by a protein called apoB. Their precursors are very low density lipoproteins (VLDL), triglyceride-rich lipoproteins that are synthesized and secreted by the liver. Once in circulation, VLDL undergo lipolysis of the triglyceride by two enzymes called lipoprotein lipase and hepatic lipase and are converted to their remnants, intermediate-density lipoproteins (IDL), and finally to LDL.

The LDL receptor is a cell-surface glycoprotein able to bind both apoB, the sole protein of LDL, and apoE, an apolipoprotein that is present in multiple copies on other lipoproteins, including VLDL and IDL, but not LDL. ApoE has a twofold higher affinity than apoB for the receptor, and in general IDL are removed from the circulation more efficiently than LDL. In addition, while its precursors may be metabolized via other pathways, LDL removal from circulation depends heavily on functional LDL receptors.

LDL receptors are synthesized in the endoplasmic reticulum (ER), undergo glycosylation in the Golgi, and are then transported to the plasma membrane, where they localize in coated pits, specialized regions of the cell membrane capable of invaginating and forming coated vesicles (Fig. 14-1). Once at the cell surface, the LDL receptor can bind to the apoB on LDL, triggering invagination of the coated pit and internalization of the LDL receptor/LDL complex in a coated vesicle. Coated vesicles fuse with larger vesicles called endosomes. In the acidic environment of the endosomes, the LDL receptor undergoes conformational changes that cause the dissociation of bound LDL. The receptor is then recycled to the membrane surface, while the

Table 14-1. Major Lipoprotein Classes

	Density (g/mL)*	Size (nm)†	Electrophoretic Mobility‡	Apolipoproteins	
				Major	Other
Chylomicrons	<0.95	75–1200	Origin	B-48	A-I, A-IV, C-I, C-II, C-III
VLDL	<1.006	30–80	Pre-beta	B-100	E, A-I, A-II, A-V, C-I, C-II, C-III
IDL	1.006–1.019	25–35	Slow pre-beta	B-100	E, C-I, C-II, C-III
LDL	1.019–1.063	18–25	Beta	B-100	
HDL	1.063–1.21	5–12	Alpha	A-I	A-II, A-IV, E, C-I, C-II, C-III
Lp(a)	1.050–1.120	25	Pre-beta	B-100	Apo(a)

VLDL, very low density lipoprotein; IDL, intermediate-density lipoprotein; LDL, low-density lipoprotein; HDL, high-density lipoprotein; apo, apolipoprotein; C, cholesterol; TG, triglycerides; PL, phospholipids.

*The density of the particle is determined by ultracentrifugation.

†The size of the particle is measured using gel electrophoresis.

‡ The electrophoretic mobility of the particle on agarose gel electrophores reflects the size and surface charge of the particle, with beta the position of LDL and alpha the position of HDL.

dissociated LDL is transferred into lysosomes, where its lipid and protein components are hydrolyzed.

Numerous mutations (>1000) at the LDL receptor locus have been described as causing FH. Interindividual phenotypic variation among patients with either heterozygous or homozygous FH is at least partly dependent on the residual activity of the LDL receptor. This in turn depends on the site of mutation within the LDL receptor gene. The gene contains 18 exons and 17 introns and encodes a protein of 860 amino acids. The protein contains multiple domains (ligand-binding domain, EGF or epidermal growth factor homology domain, O-linked sugar domain, membrane-spanning domain, and cytoplasmic domain), all of which are important for its function. Numerous mutations have been reported in each of the exons.

LDL receptor mutations can be divided into five different functional classes as shown in Figure 14-1. Class 1 mutations (null alleles) do not produce immunoprecipable protein. Class 2 mutations produce proteins that are not (completely, 2A; partially, 2B) transported to the Golgi due primarily to defective folding of the protein, which is then targeted for degradation. Class 3 mutations produce proteins that are normally transported to the plasma membrane but do not bind to LDL normally. Class 4 mutations

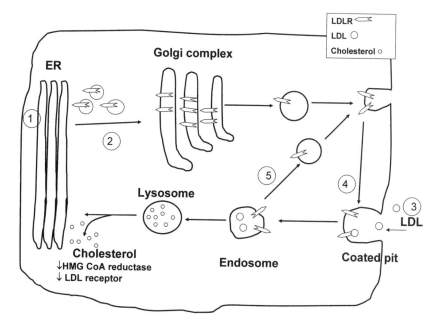

Figure 14-1. The biochemical role of the low-density lipoprotein (LDL) and the classes of mutations that affect its function. The LDL receptors are synthesized in the endoplasmic reticulum (ER), undergo glycosylation in the Golgi, and are transported to the plasma membrane, where they localize in coated pits. Once at the cell surface, the LDL receptors bind to the apolipoprotein B on low-density lipoprotein (LDL), triggering invagination of the coated pit and internalization of the LDL receptor/LDL complex in a coated vesicle. Coated vesicles fuse with larger vesicles called endosomes. In the endosomes, the LDL receptor undergoes conformational changes that cause the dissociation of bound LDL. The receptor is then recycled to the membrane surface, while the dissociated LDL is transferred into lysosomes, where its lipid and protein components are hydrolyzed. The free cholesterol obtained from the degradation of LDL diffuses into the cytoplasm and plays an important role in regulating intracellular cholesterol homeostasis through several mechanisms, including downregulation of hydroxymethylglutaryl-coenzyme A (HMG-CoA) reductase activity and LDL receptor expression. There are five classes of LDL receptor mutations, indicated by circled numbers in the figure: class 1 mutations are null alleles. Classes 2–5 affect different stages of processing, ligand binding, and internalization of the LDL receptor. See text for details.

produce proteins that are able to bind LDL but do not cluster on the coated pits and fail to internalize. Class 5 mutations produce proteins that are not able to release the LDL in the endosome and cannot be recycled. Class 1 and class 2A are usually associated with less than 2% LDL receptor activity in cultured fibroblasts, while other classes are associated with some degree of activity. As discussed earlier, subjects with homozygous FH who are receptor-negative (less than 2% activity) tend to have higher cholesterol levels and more severe clinical manifestation than patients who are receptor-defective.

The importance of functional LDL receptors for the removal of LDL from circulation in subjects with FH has been confirmed studying *in vivo* the clearance rate of radiolabeled LDL injected intravenously, as was done for the patient described in the case report before and after gene therapy. The removal time of LDL in subjects with heterozygous FH is approximately twice as long and in those with homozygous FH more than three times as long compared to that of normal controls.

Free cholesterol obtained from the degradation of LDL diffuses into the cytoplasm and plays an important role in the feedback mechanism that regulates intracellular cholesterol concentration through several mechanisms. Among these are the suppression of the activity of hydroxymethylglutaryl-coenzyme A (HMG-CoA) reductase (the rate-limiting enzyme in cholesterol synthesis) and the downregulation of LDL receptor synthesis to prevent excess cholesterol accumulation. In the absence of an exogenous source of cholesterol, both HMG-CoA reductase activity and LDL receptor synthesis are upregulated and hydrolysis of esterified cholesterol is increased, so that ultimately the needed amount of intracellular cholesterol is maintained.

Members of a family of nuclear transcription factors called sterol regulatory element-binding proteins (SREBP) are responsible for the regulation of these cholesterol feedback mechanisms. SREBP are able to activate a number of genes encoding for proteins involved in the homeostasis of cholesterol and other lipids, including the LDL receptor gene itself.

The promoter region of the LDL receptor gene contains several regulatory elements that control its expression. One in particular, sterol regulatory element 1, is the binding site for SREBP. Under baseline conditions, SREBP are inactive proteins bound to the endoplasmic

reticulum (ER). In the ER, SREBP bind to another protein called SREBP-cleavage activating protein (SCAP). SCAP is a sensor of sterols. When the cholesterol content in the cell is low, the SCAP-SREBP complex is able to move to the Golgi, where the SREBP are sequentially cleaved by two proteases, S1P and S2P, thus releasing the NH_2 terminal of the SREBP to the cytoplasm. Once in the cytoplasm, SREBP translocate to the nucleus, where they activate transcription by binding to the SRE-1 in the promoter regions of the LDL receptor gene, the HMG-CoA reductase gene, and other sterol-regulated genes, thus generating more cellular cholesterol in a homeostatic response.

Conversely, if intracellular sterols are in excess, then SCAP undergoes conformational changes, and the complex SCAP-SREBP can no longer migrate to the Golgi. The net resulting effect is that the NH_2 terminal of SREBP is not cleaved. Under these circumstances, the SREBP do not translocate to the nucleus and do not activate transcription of the target genes HMG-CoA reductase and the LDL receptor.

This finely regulated mechanism is physiologically very important as it is this mechanism that regulates the response to a high-fat diet as well as the response to therapeutic intervention with cholesterol-lowering drugs. A diet rich in saturated fat and cholesterol is associated with an increased flux of dietary cholesterol and fats from the intestine to the liver. This causes an increase in intracellular cholesterol concentration and the downregulation of LDL receptor gene expression in the liver, mediated by the SREBP-regulated feedback just described. The net effect is that LDL cholesterol is removed more slowly from circulation and accumulates in the plasma, causing an increase in its levels.

An opposite effect is at the basis of the upregulation of LDL receptors in response to treatments with bile acid sequestrants, intestinal cholesterol absorption inhibitors, and HMG-CoA reductase inhibitors. The first class of drugs inhibits the intestinal reabsorption of bile acids, thus promoting increased conversion of cholesterol to bile acids in the liver. The increased demand for cholesterol results in activation of the SREBP system and upregulation of LDL receptor synthesis (as well as cholesterol synthesis via upregulation of HMG-CoA reductase). Similarly, inhibition of intestinal cholesterol absorption with ezetimibe results in a reduction in the hepatic cholesterol pool and compensatory upregulation of the LDL receptor. Finally, upregulation of the LDL receptors is also obtained with HMG-CoA reductase inhibitors (statins) that decrease intracellular cholesterol synthesis by inhibiting the rate-limiting enzyme in the cholesterol synthesis pathway.

THERAPY

The primary goal of therapy is the control of the hypercholesterolemia and prevention of atherosclerotic cardiovascular disease. Patients with heterozygous FH can usually be successfully treated with medications to lower the LDL cholesterol to acceptable levels (Table 14-2). They are generally responsive to treatment with statins, alone or in combination with other drugs, such as bile acid sequestrants (such as cholestyramine) or cholesterol absorption inhibitors (such as ezetimibe) that act additively to upregulate the expression of the functioning LDL receptor as described in the "Biochemical Perspectives" section. In a few cases, a more aggressive treatment with LDL apheresis (discussed in this section) may have to be considered in order to reach acceptable LDL cholesterol levels.

In contrast, individuals with homozygous FH are largely unresponsive to conventional drug therapy and have limited treatment options. In particular, the response to statins is practically nil in receptor-negative patients, while it may be present to a small degree in receptor-defective patients. Surgical interventions, such as portacaval shunt and ileal bypass, have been used in the past in an attempt to decrease circulating cholesterol levels; however, they resulted in partial and transient LDL cholesterol lowering at best. The replacement of the patient liver with a healthy donor liver (orthotopic liver transplantation) has been demonstrated to substantially reduce LDL cholesterol levels in patients with homozygous FH, but it is not the treatment of choice due to the disadvantages and risks that are associated with this invasive approach and the lifelong need for immunosuppressive therapy.

Currently, the preferred treatment option for homozygous FH is LDL apheresis. This is a procedure in which apoB-containing lipoproteins (VLDL, IDL, and LDL) are selectively removed from the plasma when passed extracorporeally over a column designed to bind apoB. HDL and other plasma protein concentrations are not affected by this selective method. This procedure has been shown to result in regression of xanthomas and may reduce the rate of progression of atherosclerotic plaques. However, because rapid reaccumulation of LDL occurs, it has to be repeated frequently (every 1–2 weeks), and many patients with homozygous FH remain at high risk for atherosclerotic cardiovascular disease. Furthermore, this is a procedure that is available only in few specialized centers, and many patients with homozygous FH, like the one described in the case report, do not have access to it.

For these reasons, there is a great medical need for more effective treatments. Among future treatment options, liver-directed gene therapy is certainly a possibility. Gene therapy is an intervention with the goal of modifying the genetic material of a target organ's cells, and it is considered a theoretically attractive approach for the treatment of rare monogenic diseases such as homozygous FH. In the *ex vivo* approach, cells are genetically modified *ex vivo* and then returned to the patient. In the *in vivo* approach, cells are modified *in vivo* via the administration of vectors containing the gene that target the desired tissue. The young patient

Table 14–2. Low-Density Lipoprotein-Cholesterol Lowering Treatments Frequently Used in Patients with Familial Hypercholesterolemia

Treatment	Major Mechanism	Major Effect
Statins	↓ C synthesis	↑ LDLR activity
Bile acid sequestrants	↓ Bile acids reabsorption	↑ LDLR activity
Cholesterol absorption inhibitors	↓ Intestinal C absorption	↑ LDLR activity
Nicotinic acid	↓ VLDL production	↓ VLDL synthesis
Low-fat, low-C diet	↓ Dietary C and fats	↑ LDLR activity
LDL apheresis	Remove LDL	↓ LDL

C, cholesterol; LDL, low-density lipoprotein; LDLR, LDL receptor; VLDL, very low density lipoprotein.

described in the case report above was one of the five patients who participated in a pilot study to test the feasibility of *ex vivo* gene transfer for homozygous FH (Grossman et al., 1995). Current efforts focus on delivering the LDL receptor gene *in vivo* using viral vectors that have hepatic specificity.

Viral vectors are preferentially used in gene therapy because their higher efficiency in transducing cells *in vivo* as compared with other vectors such as liposomes or the administration of DNA only. In the lipoprotein research field, adenoviruses have been extensively used as vectors in animal studies because of their ability to efficiently infect the liver and to result in high levels of hepatic transgene expression. However, their administration is associated with cellular immune responses, which limits the duration of the gene expression. Recent efforts have been focused on the use of adeno-associated viruses (AAV). Adeno-associated viruses are parvoviruses that depend on other viruses (such as adenovirus) for replication. Importantly, they have not been associated with toxicity or inflammatory response, and stable long-term gene expression has been achieved in animal studies. Although homozygous FH remains an excellent candidate for the development of liver-directed gene therapy, more work must be done on the development of safe, liver-specific vectors that will provide long-term expression of the LDL receptor.

Alternative pharmacological approaches are also being explored. Preliminary results in animal models of FH using an inhibitor of the microsomal transfer protein, a key enzyme in the assembly and secretion of apoB-containing lipoproteins by the liver (see chapter 27 on abetalipoproteinemia for details) showed a significant decrease in LDL cholesterol levels and suggests that this may be a more realistic therapeutic approach in the near future.

QUESTIONS

1. What are the clinical characteristics of both heterozygous and homozygous FH?
2. What is the genetic cause of FH?
3. Once LDL is bound to the LDL receptor, what is the intracellular fate of this complex?
4. What is the effect of dietary cholesterol and saturated fats on the expression of the LDL receptor by the liver?
5. What is the mechanism of action of commonly used lipid-lowering drugs, such as statins and ezetimibe?
6. What are SREBP and SCAP? What role do they play in the regulation of cholesterol homeostasis?
7. What are the therapeutic options for the treatment of both heterozygous and homozygous forms of FH?

BIBLIOGRAPHY

Brown MS, Anderson RG, Goldstein JL: Recycling receptors: the round-trip itinerary of migrant membrane proteins. *Cell* **32**:663–667, 1983.

Brown MS, Goldstein JL: A receptor-mediated pathway for cholesterol homeostasis. *Science* **232**: 34–47, 1986.

Goldstein JL, Hobbs HH, Brown MS: Familial hypercholesterolaemia, *in* Scriver CR, Beaudet AL, Sly WS, Valle D (eds): *The Metabolic and Molecular Bases of Inherited Disease*. vol. 2. McGraw-Hill, New York, 2001, pp. 2863–2913.

Grossman M, Rader DJ, Muller DWM, et al: A pilot study of *ex vivo* gene therapy for homozygous familial hypercholesterolaemia. *Nat Med* **1**: 1148–1154, 1995.

Horton JD, Goldstein JL, Brown MS: SREBPs: activators of the complete program of cholesterol and fatty acid synthesis in the liver. *J Clin Invest* **10**:1125–31, 2002.

Naoumova RP, Thompson GR, Soutar AK: Current management of severe homozygous hypercholesterolaemias. *Curr Opin Lipidol* **15**:413–422, 2004.

Rader DJ, Cohen J, Hobbs HH: Monogenic hypercholesterolemia: new insights in pathogenesis and treatment. *J Clin Invest* **111**:1795–1803, 2003.

Rader DJ, Hobbs HH: Disorders of lipoprotein metabolism, in Braunwald E, Fauci AS, Kasper DL, Hauser SL, Longo DL, Jameson JL (eds): *Harrison's Principles of Internal Medicine*. 16th ed. McGraw-Hill, New York, 2005, pp. 2286–98.

Raper SE, Grossman M, Rader DJ, et al: Safety and feasibility of liver-directed *ex vivo* gene therapy for homozygous familial hypercholesterolemia. *Ann Surg* **223**:116–116, 1996.

15

Tangier Disease: A Disorder in the Reverse Cholesterol Transport Pathway

LIEN B. LAI, VIJAYAPRASAD GOPICHANDRAN, and VENKAT GOPALAN

CASE REPORTS

Case 1

T. L. was a 5-year-old patient who underwent a tonsillectomy in 1960. His enlarged tonsils were yellowish-gray, with many septa running through multiple abnormally lobulated regions. On pathological examination, many foam cells (macrophages with lipid deposits) were found in and among the lymph follicles. This histiocytic appearance of the foam cells led to a tentative diagnosis of either Hand-Schüller-Christian (a multifocal eosinophilic granuloma) or Niemann-Pick (a lysosomal lipid storage) disease. Thinking that the tonsillar honeycomblike appearance was unusual for either of these diseases, the attending physician, Dr. Thomas Edmonds, referred T. L. for further analyses to the NIH and thereby initiated a series of investigations that led to the discovery of Tangier disease by Dr. Donald S. Fredrickson and colleagues in 1961.

A physical examination found T. L. to be normal except for moderate hepatosplenomegaly (liver enlargement) and scattered enlarged lymph nodes. The diagnosis of Hand-Schüller-Christian disease was quickly eliminated when liver and lymph node biopsies lacked the histiocytic granuloma manifestation of the disease. A neurological examination of T. L. was unremarkable, a finding that is extremely rare in Niemann-Pick disease for a 5-year-old patient. Histochemical analysis to characterize the lipids in the biopsies was negative with the Smith-Dietrich stain, considered to be specific for the unsaturated phospholipids normally associated with Niemann-Pick tissues but was positive for the Schultz test, suggesting high levels of cholesterol or a related sterol. In addition, this lipid deposit was not membrane-bound. Subsequent chemical analysis of the lipid confirmed an extraordinarily high cholesterol ester content but normal levels of phospholipids, including sphingomyelin, thus definitively dismissing the possibility of Niemann-Pick disease. The investigators involved in the case suspected a novel lipid accumulation disorder and named it Tangier disease after the locality where T. L. resided.

Tangier Island is a geographically isolated island in the Chesapeake Bay of Virginia. It had in 1961 about 900 inhabitants, a large number of whom descended from a few original inhabitants who settled there in the late 1600s. Since such a genetically insulated locale provides an opportune setting for manifestation of a rare genetic disorder, a throat examination of more than a tenth of the island inhabitants was carried out after the diagnosis of T. L. All were normal except for E. L., the patient's sister. Although E. L. was healthy without signs of hepatosplenomegaly or lymphadenopathy (abnormal enlargement of lymph nodes), she, like T. L., had enormous lobulated tonsils (Fig. 15-1) and no neurological abnormalities.

When the lipid content of the tonsils from E. L. was compared to a nonsymptomatic control, the main difference was a 50-fold increase in cholesterol esters. This finding prompted the investigators to focus their research on cholesterol metabolism in the probands. As all results of tests

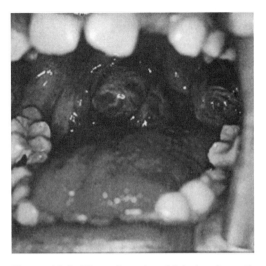

Figure 15-1. The enlarged and lobulated tonsils of E. L. Dr. Donald Fredrickson annotated his experience on encountering the sight: "When I saw those gigantic bright orange organs, I had the same feeling one gets at looking at a mountain that has never been climbed" (http://profiles. nlm.nih.gov/FF/B/B/L/G/_/ffbblg.txt). Photograph was reproduced from http://profiles.nlm.nih.gov.

for cholesterol synthesis were normal, plasma lipid profiling was subsequently explored. While the plasma triglyceride level was sixfold higher than that of controls, cholesterol and phospholipids levels were lower. Further analyses revealed that the high-density lipoproteins (HDL) were reduced to almost undetectable levels, but the low-density lipoproteins (LDL) appeared to be unaffected. The mother of T. L. and E. L. also had low levels of HDL. A partial pedigree of these children indicated consanguinity in their grandparents' (both maternal and paternal) and parents' generations.

Case 2

A 32-year-old man experienced weakness and burning pain in his hands for the 2 months. The weakness started insidiously and had been gradually progressing. As a professional pianist, he found that the mobility of his fingers was greatly limited since the onset of the problems. The burning pain started a few days after the weakness and was spontaneous with no specific aggravating or relieving factors.

His medical history was unremarkable except for a recurrent sore throat during child-hood that resulted in tonsillectomy at age 12 years. He was not diabetic or hypertensive and had no history of exposure to toxic metals.

Physical examination found him to be moderately built and nourished. Both hands showed diminished power of the flexors and the extensors to 2/5 on the right and 3/5 on the left. Wasting of the small muscles of the thenar eminence was also noted in both hands. Reflexes of the brachioradialis, biceps, and triceps were diminished to 1/4 in the right and 2/4 in the left arm. There was loss of pain and temperature sensation over the distribution of median and radial nerves. All other muscle groups and sensations were normal. Cranial nerves were normal. Abdominal palpation revealed hepatosplenomegaly, which was subsequently confirmed by ultrasound. Oral examination found yellowish plaques on the posterior pharyngeal wall. Eyes, ears, and nose were normal.

Differential diagnoses of peripheral neuropathy were entertained. Laboratory tests revealed that serum parameters for electrolytes and proteins were all within the normal range. Urine porphyrinogen and porphobilinogen levels were normal. Tests were negative for serum rheumatoid factor and antinuclear antibodies, the latter used in detection of connective tissue diseases such as systemic lupus erythematosus and polyarteritis nodosa that could present with features of peripheral neuropathy. Nerve conduction studies of the radial, ulnar, and median nerves revealed delayed conduction. Biopsies of the ulnar and radial nerves showed loss of nerve fibers and sudanophilic (indicating lipid) deposits in the Schwann cells of the neurons. Similarly, the yellowish plaques of the pharynx showed abundant macrophages filled with sudanophilic material. These deposits were not membrane-bound.

Subsequently, serum lipid and lipoprotein profiles were obtained: 70 mg/dL total cholesterol (normal is 130–200 mg/dL), 1 mg/dL HDL cholesterol (optimal is $\geq$ 60 mg/dL), 180 mg/dL triglycerides (normal is 100–150 mg/dL), and less than 5 mg/dL apolipoprotein A-I (apoA-I; normal is ~ 140 mg/dL). Cholesterol efflux from patient skin fibroblasts to apoA-I, the main protein component of HDL, was reduced to 30% of normal. These results indicated Tangier disease, the definitive diagnosis of which was made when the sequencing of the ATP-binding cassette transporter A1 (*ABCA1*) gene revealed a nonsense mutation within exon 12.

DIAGNOSIS

Tangier disease is an extremely rare genetic disorder with fewer than 100 cases reported since the index cases in 1961. Clinical signs and symptoms are variable and may depend on the age of the patients. For instance, signs of neuropathy were not observed in T. L. and E. L., in contrast to our 32-year-old patient. Assmann and colleagues (2001) have succinctly compiled the reported findings (Table 15-1), most of which are discussed here.

Of all the physical signs of Tangier disease (Table 15-1), perhaps the most remarkable feature is enlarged and lobulated tonsils with a distinctive yellow-orange color. Patients with tonsils removed are often found to have had a history of recurrent tonsillitis or oropharyngeal obstruction. Another physical diagnostic characteristic of the disease is the appearance of 1- to 2-mm discrete orange-brown speckles on the rectal mucosa. Similar speckles have also been reported in the colon, stomach, and intestine. These patients may be prone to frequent stools, intermittent diarrhea, and abdominal pain. In the eye, the most frequent finding is slight corneal opacification. Although about one third of Tangier patients have hepatomegaly, this sign might be transient as tests of liver function are often normal, and foam cells are found only occasionally. Many patients with splenomegaly (spleen enlargement) also have mild hemolytic anemia, stomatocytosis (erythrocytes with deep pitting on the cell membrane due to an altered membrane cholesterol:phospholipids ratio) and thrombocytopenia (low platelet count), with 30,000–120,000 platelets/mL (normal is 150,000–400,000/mL).

Lymphadenopathy is most often not clinically manifested; however, bright yellow plaques and a cholesterol ester content 100-fold higher than normal have been documented for both normal-size and enlarged lymph nodes in Tangier patients. Biopsies of bone marrow and the affected tissues have revealed many foam cells that are smaller than those observed in lipid storage diseases. In addition, these cells contain sudanophilic deposits which are not membrane-bound, as is the case for lysosomal storage diseases. Foam cells have also been found in otherwise normal skin, ureters, renal pelvises, tunica albuginea (white fibrous capsule) of testicles, mitral and tricuspid valves, and aorta, coronary, and pulmonary arteries.

About 30% of adult Tangier patients present with peripheral neuropathy, the onset of which usually takes place after 10 years of age. These neuropathic symptoms may be subtle or overt, transient or permanent, and include weakness, increased sweating, diplopia (double vision), ptosis (abnormally drooping eyelids), ocular muscle palsies, and diminished or absent deep-tendon reflexes. There are two prototypes of neuropathy found in Tangier dis-

Table 15-1. Frequencies of Clinical Symptoms and Findings in Tangier Disease

| | *Number of Cases* | | |
Symptoms	Present	Absent	Not Examined/Not Reported
Yellowish tonsils or pharyngeal plaques	44	6	18
Peripheral neuropathy	36	20	12
Splenomegaly	33	17	18
Abnormal rectal mucosa	28	4	36
Hepatomegaly	19	24	25
Corneal opacities	15	28	25
Coronary heart disease	15	33	20
Thrombocytopenia	14	1	44
Anemia or stomatocytes	9	6	53
Lymphadenopathy	6	26	36
Unexplained diarrhea	5	1	62

These data were obtained from the case reports of 66 Tangier patients whose ages ranged from 2 to 72 years (Assman et al., 2001). Reproduced with permission from McGraw-Hill Companies, Inc.©2001.

ease, a syringomyelialike syndrome and a multiple mononeuropathy. Of the two, the former is much more debilitating.

Syringomyelialike syndrome can appear early and be progressive, with loss of pain and temperature sensation, paresthesia (abnormal skin sensation with no physical cause), and muscle atrophy beginning in the face and distal parts of the upper limbs. Eventually, dysesthesia (impaired sensitivity to touch) may progress to the trunk and lower limbs. These symptoms are caused by axonal degeneration of small myelinated and unmyelinated fibers. Multiple mononeuropathy often presents with transient, relapsing, or no symptomatic complications. When manifested, impairments are either mononeuropathic or asymmetrically polyneuropathic and may involve cranial nerves. Morphologically, this type of neuropathy is characterized by de- and remyelination of peripheral nerves without axonal deficit. Atypical lipid accumulation in Schwann cells may be the underlying cause of these symptoms.

Profiling of plasma lipoproteins and serum lipids can often aid in the diagnosis of Tangier disease. There are four classes of lipoproteins: (1) chylomicrons, which transport dietary cholesterol and triglycerides from the intestines to the tissues; (2) very low-density lipoproteins (VLDL) and (3) low-density lipoproteins (LDL), both of which transport *de novo* synthesized cholesterol and triglyceride from the liver to the tissues; and (4) high-density lipoproteins (HDL), which mediate reverse cholesterol transport, a process in which excess cholesterol from peripheral tissues is transported to the liver.

In all Tangier patients, plasma HDL level is nearly undetectable (optimal is $\geq$60 mg/dL). Analysis of the major apolipoproteins on HDL by nephelometry (a technique that quantitates specific antigens by analyzing increases in turbidity caused by antigen-antibody complex formation) often reveals a marked decrease in apoA-I (1%–3% normal) and apoA-II (5%–10% normal). LDL levels are also reduced (~40% of normal) in Tangier patients. Analysis of serum lipids usually shows that the total cholesterol averages about 78 mg/dL (normal is 130–200 mg/dL). Triglyceride levels are usually higher than normal but vary significantly depending on diet.

Cultivated skin fibroblasts from Tangier patients fail to efflux cholesterol, phosphatidylcholine, or sphingomyelin to exogenous lipid-free apolipoproteins or artificial amphipathic polypeptides. Since 1999, definitive diagnosis of Tangier disease can be achieved by sequencing the *ABCA1* gene (Lapicka-Bodzioch et al., 2001), which encodes the ATP-binding cassette transporter responsible for the efflux of cholesterol and phospholipids from cells.

Several diseases have overlapping symptoms with Tangier disease, and differential diagnosis must be considered. First, very low plasma levels of HDL and apoA-I are also consistent with familial dyslipidemias, such as apoA-I and lecithin:cholesterol acyltransferase (LCAT) deficiencies and obstructive liver disease. Increased levels of proapoA-I (the precursor) relative to that of the mature apoA-I, a distinctive feature of Tangier disease, can be demonstrated by isoelectric focusing and be used to eliminate the possibility of a familial dyslipidemia. The hypercholesterolemic symptom found in obstructive liver disease distinguishes it from Tangier disease. Second, the presence of foam cells may indicate a lipid storage disorder (e.g., Niemann-Pick disease), but these disorders are not usually associated with the tonsillar abnormalities and low HDL levels. In addition, the absence of membrane surrounding the lipid deposits in foam cells is a clear indication of Tangier disease and not a storage disorder. Finally, low plasma cholesterol levels are also observed in abetalipoproteinemia, but patients with Tangier disease frequently also have elevated triglyceride and much lower HDL levels.

BIOCHEMICAL PERSPECTIVES

Almost four decades after the index cases of Tangier disease were reported, the gene responsible for the disease was identified as *ABCA1* by several groups (Bodzioch et al., 1999; Brooks-Wilson et al., 1999; Remaley et al., 1999; Rust et al., 1999). ABCA1 belongs to the ABC superfamily of ATP-binding cassette transporters, which are responsible for the translocation across cellular and intracellular membranes of various substances, including peptides, metabolites, drugs, and lipids. As one might expect from their ubiquitous presence and high degree of conservation, mutations in a number of these transporters have been incriminated in several human diseases, such as cystic fibrosis, macular degeneration, and immunodeficiency syndromes. We discuss next the role of ABCA1 in lipid metabolism and how mutations in this transporter result in Tangier disease.

Reverse Cholesterol Transport and ABCA1-Mediated HDL Formation

ABCA1 mediates the first step in the energy-dependent efflux of cholesterol from the cell to form HDL for reverse cholesterol transport (Fig. 15-2). While all tissues in the body can synthesize cholesterol, only the liver and steroidogenic tissues can metabolize it. Surplus cholesterol in cells of the peripheral tissues is transported to the liver for either redistribution to other cells or for excretion either as free cholesterol or as a bile salt after conversion in the liver. Therefore, this reverse cholesterol transport system plays a pivotal role in cholesterol homeostasis with HDL as one of the key players.

Due to dynamic remodeling within different HDL subfractions and between HDL and other lipoproteins, HDL is a heterogeneous class of lipoproteins that can be generalized by a high density (>1.063 g/mL) and a small size (5- to 17-nm diameter). Differences are characterized by shape, density, size, charge, and antigenicity, which are influenced by the lipid and apolipoprotein (e.g., A-I, A-II, C-II, E) content.

The formation of discoidal, nascent HDL particles commences with the two-step lipidation of apoA-I by ABCA1. These steps consist of the efflux of phospholipid followed by that of cholesterol and involve different mechanistic actions of ABCA1, the details of which are currently unknown. The function of ABCA1 was shown recently to include modification of late endocytic membranes to bring together pools of cellular cholesterol and those of endocytosed apoA-I (Neufeld et al., 2004). ABCA1 present on the cell surface stimulates apoA-I uptake into endosomes. These endosomes containing ABCA1 and apoA-I then travel to late endocytic compartments where ABCA1 appears to mediate the conversion of late endocytic pools of cholesterol to pools that associate with apoA-I. The lipidated apoA-I-harboring late endocytic vesicles may then move to the cell surface where their contents are released as nascent HDL particles. ABCA1-mediated lipidation of

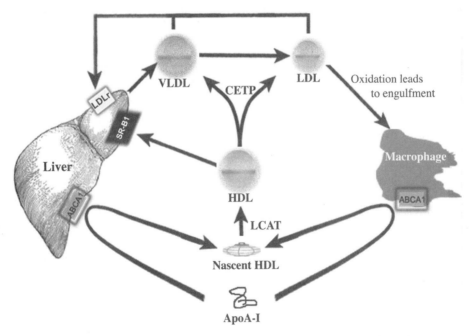

Figure 15-2. A simplified schematic of cholesterol transport. Cholesterol travels to non-hepatic cells, such as the macrophage, via VLDL and LDL particles, while excess cholesterol is shuttled to the liver via HDL particles. Note that *ABCA1* mediates nascent HDL formation by translocating cellular cholesterol and phospholipids to apolipoprotein A-I (apoA-I) in an active, energy-dependent reaction. CETP, cholesteryl ester transfer protein; LCAT, lecithin:cholesterol acyltransferase; LDLR, low-density lipoprotein receptor; SR-B1, scavenger receptor B1.

apoA-I could also take place at the plasma membrane and in early endocytic vesicles.

The nascent HDL particles change shape and composition as they acquire additional free cholesterol by passive cellular diffusion of free cholesterol from cell membranes or from other plasma lipoproteins. HDL surface-localized LCAT progressively converts the free cholesterol on the surface of the particles to cholesterol ester, which occupies the core of the lipoprotein particle. This process converts the shape of the HDL particles from discoidal to spherical. The lipid unloading of HDL in the liver follows at least two pathways. In the first route, the cholesterol ester transfer protein (CETP) mediates cholesterol ester transfer from HDL to VLDL and LDL in exchange for triglyceride; LDL in turn are taken up by the liver via the LDL receptor. In the second route, HDL binds to the scavenger receptor B1, and cholesterol esters are selectively taken into the liver cells without internalization of HDL proteins (Fig. 15-2).

In Tangier disease in which ABCA1 is defective, formation of nascent HDL particles is compromised, leading to the observed clinical findings. First, cellular levels of cholesterol are high in the absence of active reverse cholesterol transport. Second, lipophilic compounds such as vitamin E, retinyl esters (yellow), and carotenoids (orange) also accumulate inside the cell, perhaps due to their decreased efflux resulting from the ABCA1 mutation, thus accounting for the yellow-orange appearance of tissue plaques in Tangier disease. Third, failure to assemble functional HDL particles leads to rapid renal filtration and catabolism of apoA-I, thus accounting for the decreased level of HDL in plasma. Any residual HDL-like particles in Tangier plasma are small and lipid poor. Last, plasma triglyceride levels are often high (two- to threefold greater than normal) in adult patients. The elevated accumulation of triglyceride in VLDL and chylomicrons appears to result from the failure to activate lipoprotein lipase due to the absence of its activator apoC-II, which is normally transferred from HDL to VLDL.

ABCA1

The *ABCA1* gene has been localized to 9q31on the long arm of chromosome 9. It spans 149 kb and has 50 exons. The first intron has been shown to act as an alternative promoter. *ABCA1* is ubiquitously expressed, with notable expression in liver, brain, and steroidogenic tissues. Furthermore, it is expressed in confluent but not growing fibroblast cell culture, indicating the balance between cholesterol efflux and intracellular requirement. Consistent with this observation, overloading macrophages with cholesterol increased *ABCA1* transcription dramatically. This induction is mediated by the transcription activators liver X receptor (LXR) and retinoid X receptor (RXR), which act as obligate heterodimers in the presence of either oxysterols or retinoic acid (Costet et al., 2000). LXR/RXR binds to the DR4 elements in the *ABCA1* promoter and first intron. Hence, the accumulating cholesterol must be converted to an oxysterol to elicit *ABCA1* induction.

ABCA1 is a 2261-amino acid integral membrane protein consisting of two transmembrane domains, each with six transmembrane-spanning helices, connected by a regulatory domain rich in Ser and Thr residues. It also has two nucleotide-binding folds (NBFs) where ATP is bound and hydrolyzed, thus generating the energy needed for ABCA1 action. Each NBF, also known as an ATP-binding cassette, contains a signature motif (or C motif) inserted between two conserved regions, the Walker A and Walker B motifs. More than 50 mutations have been identified throughout the gene; these include various missense, nonsense, insertional, deletional, and even intronic mutations that can affect splicing (Singaraja et al., 2003). The genetic defect in the original Tangier disease kindred (case report 1) was determined to be a homozygous dinucleotide deletion (3283–3284TC) in exon 22, resulting in a frameshift at amino acid 1055 and a premature stop codon after amino acid 1084 (Remaley et al., 1999).

Although definitive answers are just forthcoming as to why these various mutations in ABCA1 cause a reduction in its ability to mediate cholesterol efflux, possibilities include mislocalization that causes a reduction in the fraction of ABCA1 that reaches the plasma membrane; altered NBFs that fail to bind and utilize ATP, thereby compromising active transport; and weaker interactions between ABCA1 and apoA-I that reduce lipidation of the latter. Establishing structure–function relationships in ABCA1 will be important in further elucidating the biochemical basis for Tangier disease.

ABCA1 Zygosity and Coronary Artery Disease

Tangier disease is inherited *clinically* as an autosomal recessive trait but *biochemically* as an autosomal codominant trait. This is because clinical phenotypes (e.g., hyperplastic tonsils) appear only in homozygotes, but biochemical phenotypes (e.g., reduced ABCA1 activity and cholesterol efflux) are also present in heterozygotes. This dichotomy can be appreciated by briefly examining the pathophysiology of the disease.

The main activity of tissue macrophages is to engulf apoptotic and necrotic cells. As the efflux of cholesterol extracted from the phagocytosed cell membranes is ABCA1-dependent, loss of function of both *ABCA1* alleles (in homozygotes) leads to tissue hyperplasia. As the heterozygotes do not have symptoms of lipid-loaded tissue macrophages characteristic of Tangier disease, one functional *ABCA1* allele may suffice to prevent cholesterol deposition in macrophages.

While the homozygotes display the various phenotypes typical for Tangier patients, the heterozygotes are associated with another disorder known as familial HDL deficiency, which is associated with an increased risk of coronary artery disease (CAD). Despite the well-documented inverse correlation between HDL levels and premature CAD, homozygotes with virtually no circulating HDL do not have a markedly increased risk of CAD compared to heterozygotes, who have half-normal levels of HDL. The underlying reason for this counterintuitive finding may be the low LDL levels (40% of normal) found in the homozygotes (Oram, 2000).

Why do low LDL levels confer antiatherogenic benefits? In arterial macrophages, most of the cholesterol comes from ingestion of oxidized LDL generated by reactive oxygen species in the bloodstream. To prevent endothelial injury, the oxidized LDL is engulfed by arterial macrophages. The combined assault of an impaired cholesterol efflux activity and low serum HDL levels (as in both homozygotes and heterozygotes) results in the transformation of these LDL-engorged arterial macrophages into foam cells due to their failure to egress their cellular stores of cholesterol. Under continued oxidative stress, these foam cells necrose and cause inflammation, stimulating further macrophage recruitment to the site and proliferation of smooth muscle and neointima, leading to atherosclerotic plaque formation (Frishman, 1998). Therefore, low serum LDL levels are considered to be atheroprotective.

This discussion highlights the interplay between pro- and antiatherogenic factors in dictating the overall risk of CAD in heterozygotes and homozygotes. However, why are LDL levels preferentially decreased in the Tangier homozygotes? Since a significant amount of cholesterol in LDL originates from HDL via the action of CETP, a decrease in HDL would be expected to lower LDL levels. Moreover, alterations in the HDL-mediated return of cholesterol to the liver might enhance LDL receptor activity and thereby facilitate a more rapid clearance of plasma LDL. The fact that Tangier patients do develop CAD despite their strikingly low LDL levels suggests that other proatherogenic abnormalities in lipid metabolism (such as the elevated levels of triglycerides, which can also cause arterial hardening) might partially offset the benefits of lower LDL levels. These observations shed light on why *ABCA1* mutations are associated with only a moderately increased risk of atherosclerosis, albeit not as high as that observed in other lipidemias, such as familial hypercholesterolemia.

THERAPY

Although there is no specific treatment for Tangier disease, symptom relief and alleviation of complications can improve the quality of life for the patients. Families with Tangier patients may also benefit from genetic counseling.

Surgical removal of tissues may be necessary in some cases to alleviate symptoms, such as oropharyngeal obstruction (tonsillectomy) and progressive anemia and thrombocytopenia (splenectomy).

Supplements frequently prescribed for patients with neuropathy, such as omega-3 fatty acids, antioxidants, and vitamin E, have not been effective in preventing the progression of neurological symptoms in patients with Tangier disease. Therefore, pain-relieving medications and physiotherapy are prescribed for these patients. Decompression surgery and nerve resection procedures may be used to alleviate intractable pain. The strength of the muscles can be improved by exercise, electrical stimulation, and physiotherapy.

Drugs used to increase HDL levels (fibrates, nicotinic acid, and statins) in otherwise normal people do not have the same effect in patients with Tangier disease. Therefore, it is necessary to identify and treat other risk factors associated with CAD. Exercise, weight reduction, dietary cholesterol and saturated fat reduction, and smoking cessation are the first line in management of low HDL cholesterol. Dietary management with low fat intake is beneficial in reducing the risk for CAD, as well as in preventing hepato- and splenomegaly. Although ineffective in increasing plasma HDL levels, fibrates have been useful in lowering triglyceride levels in patients with Tangier disease. In addition, drugs that lower HDL cholesterol, such as β-blockers, benzodiazepines, and androgens, should not be taken (if possible).

An exciting and intensively investigated area for therapeutic intervention in Tangier disease is the use of drugs to increase the expression of *ABCA1* at the transcriptional level. Even overexpression of a mutant version that possesses less than wild-type activity could confer some benefit. However, the success of such approaches will be predicated on the ability to elicit transcriptional activation of *ABCA1* specifically.

The prescient remarks of Fredrickson in 1961 that investigations into Tangier disease will shed light on poorly understood lipid and fat metabolic pathways have now been borne out. An unanticipated bonus has been the identification of a molecular target for pharmacological manipulation might help lower the risk of CAD in the normal population.

QUESTIONS

1. In general, do you expect biochemically dominant phenotypes for inherited recessive disorders? Using the reasoning for your answer, explain why patients with Tangier disease may have a lower risk of CAD than heterozygotes.

2. What would be the serum lipid and lipoprotein profile of a person homozygous or heterozygous for a mutation in the *ABCA1* gene?

3. Based on your understanding of the role of ABCA1 in the formation of HDL particles, how would you design a therapeutic modality to overcome a weakened interaction between ABCA1 and apoA-I that results from a mutation in *ABCA1* gene?

4. If an ABCA1 mutation does not completely eliminate the cholesterol efflux activity, then what approach would you take to enhance the level of expression of this mutant protein to alleviate the phenotypic consequences?

5. How would you modulate the reverse cholesterol transport pathway to increase cholesterol efflux from cells in normal individuals?

Acknowledgment: We thank Dr. Alan Remaley, NIH, for critical reading of the manuscript and providing valuable suggestions for improvement.

BIBLIOGRAPHY

Assmann G, von Eckardstein A, Brewer JB Jr.: Familial analphalipoproteinemia: Tangier disease, *in* Scriver CR, Beaudet AL, Sly WS, et al. (eds): *The Metabolic and Molecular Bases of Inherited Disease.* 8th ed. McGraw-Hill, New York, 2001, pp. 2937–2960.

Bodzioch M, Orsó E, Klucken J, et al.: The gene encoding ATP-binding cassette transporter 1 is mutated in Tangier disease. *Nat Genet* 22:347–351, 1999.

Brooks-Wilson A, Marcil M, Clee SM, et al.: Mutations in *ABC1* in Tangier disease and familial high-density lipoprotein deficiency. *Nat Genet* 22:336–345, 1999.

Costet P, Luo Y, Wang N, et al.: Sterol-dependent transactivation of the *ABC1* promoter by the liver X receptor/retinoid X receptor. *J Biol Chem* 275:28240–28245, 2000.

Fredrickson DS, Altrocchi PH, Avioli LV, et al.: Tangier disease—combined clinical staff conference at the National Institute of Health. *Ann Intern Med* 55:1016–1031, 1961.

Frishman, WH: Biologic markers as predictors of cardiovascular disease. *Am J Med* 104A:18S–27S, 1998.

Lapicka-Bodzioch K, Bodzioch M, Krull M, et al.: Homogeneous assay based on 52 primer sets to scan for mutations of the *ABCA1* gene and its application in genetic analysis of a new patient with familial high-density lipoprotein deficiency syndrome. *Biochim Biophys Acta* 1536:42–48, 2001.

Neufeld EB, Stonik JA, Demosky SJ, et al.: The ABCA1 transporter modulates late endocytic trafficking. *J Biol Chem* 279:15571–15578, 2004.

Oram JF: Tangier disease and ABCA1. *Biochim Biophys Acta* 1529:321–330, 2000.

Remaley AT, Rust S, Rosier M, et al.: Human ATP-binding cassette transporter 1 (ABCA1): genomic organization and identification of the genetic defect in the original Tangier disease kindred. *Proc Natl Acad Sci U.S.A.* 96: 12685–12690, 1999.

Rust S, Rosier M, Funke H, et al.: Tangier disease is caused by mutations in the gene encoding ATP-binding cassette transporter 1. *Nat Genet* 22:352–355, 1999.

Singaraja RR, Brunham LR, Visscher H, et al.: Efflux and atherosclerosis—the clinical and biochemical impact of variations in the *ABCA1* gene. *Arterioscler Thromb Vasc Biol* 23:1322–1332, 2003.

16

Gaucher Disease: A Sphingolipidosis

WILLIAM C. HINES and ROBERT H. GLEW

CASE REPORT

The patient was a 34-year-old woman of Ashkenazic Jewish ancestry. When she was four years old (September 1974), her parents noticed that she had frequent nosebleeds and bruised easily. In addition, she tired with little exertion and looked pale. They took her to the emergency department, and on admission to the hospital, a bone marrow biopsy revealed the presence of Gaucher cells as seen in Figure 16-1. She was diagnosed as having Gaucher disease, an inborn error of metabolism affecting β-glucosidase (also known as acid β-glucosidase or glucocerebrosidase). White blood cell (WBC) β-glucosidase assays were performed on the patient and her immediate family members. Her parents and only sibling had slightly reduced levels of WBC β-glucosidase, whereas the patient's β-glucosidase activity was only 9% of the control mean level, thus confirming the diagnosis of Gaucher disease on a biochemical-enzymatic basis. In addition, she was found to have an elevated level of serum acid phosphatase (ACP) activity, a characteristic of most patients with Gaucher disease.

At age 15 years, her spleen had greatly extended into the pelvis and right lower quadrant of the abdomen, and she subsequently underwent splenectomy to alleviate thrombocytopenia (low platelet count) aggravated by this splenomegaly. The pathologist reported that her spleen weighed 2070 g (normal range is 100–170 g), which is over 15 times normal size. Further microscopic examination of the spleen and of biopsies from the liver and adjacent lymph nodes confirmed the presence of Gaucher cells. Two months following the surgery, her hematological parameters were restored to normal levels: Her platelet count rose from 80×10^9 to 291×10^9/L (normal range is 140×10^9 to 440×10^9/L), and her hemoglobin had increased from 12.5 to 15.0 g/dL (normal range is 13.5–16.0 g/dL).

The patient felt well after her surgery until several months later, when she developed pain in her left hip. She began to limp to reduce her pain and resorted to the use of crutches to minimize the pressure placed on her left hip. Even with the use of crutches, however, she continued to have pain when walking. Prolonged sitting also caused her discomfort, particularly when rising. Radiological examination (Fig. 16-2) revealed the classical picture of Gaucher disease: osteonecrosis (death and degradation of bone tissue) of the left hip, with significant collapse of the head of the femur. In May 1990, she elected to undergo hip replacement surgery. The left femoral head was resected, and a total hip replacement device and acetabular implant were inserted.

Beginning in June 1991, the patient was administered a newly approved intravenous drug, Ceredase (the commercial name of a placental-derived glucocerebrosidase preparation). She was given a comprehensive evaluation at the beginning of the treatment and was monitored every 3 months thereafter. The initial assessment included a full blood analysis (hemoglobin, platelet count, biochemical markers) in addition to visceral, skeletal, and pulmonary evaluations. At her first evaluation after beginning therapy, her hematological parameters had

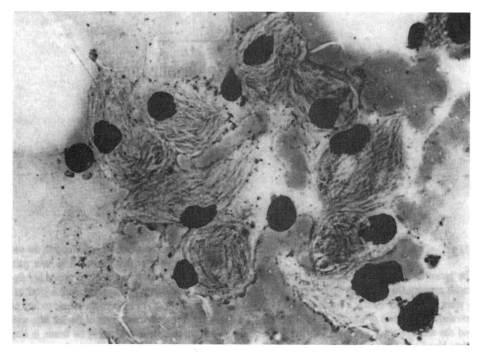

Figure 16-1. Wright-stained Gaucher cells obtained from bone marrow showing the typical wrinkled appearance of the cytoplasm (magnification 175×).

improved somewhat, but they had not normalized. Nevertheless, she reported increased stamina and a sense of well-being following Ceredase administration.

The patient experienced several bone crises (severe bone pain caused by ischemia from swelling and decreased blood supply) during the first year of treatment, but the duration and intensity were less severe than prior to enzyme replacement. Following the first year of treatment, a progressive reduction in generalized bone pain was noted. With subsequent attempts to titrate down the costly Ceredase dosage, the patient reported a gradual return of bone pain and lethargic feeling. These symptoms decreased after her dosage was returned to the higher levels. As shown in Table 16-1, over the course of 4 years of treatment, there was an improvement in the patient's hematological indices, including significant increases in platelet count and size. Furthermore, there was a notable reduction of liver volume. In 1995, a recombinant form of glucocerbrosidase, Cerezyme, was approved by the Food and Drug Administration. In 1996, the patient was switched to this less-expensive form and has been receiving it ever since. She remains stable to this day

and has not reported any additional complications.

DIAGNOSIS

Patients suffering from Gaucher disease are placed in one of three clinical subtypes (Table 16-2). The most common form, type I, originally described by Gaucher, is also termed chronic nonneuropathic or adult form Gaucher disease—even though the onset of symptoms in two thirds of patients occurs during childhood. This form of the disease usually follows a chronic progressive course characterized by hepatosplenomegaly, anemia, thrombocytopenia, and erosion of the long bones. The range of clinical severity is great; some patients suffer intensely before their third decade of life, whereas others remain undiagnosed into their sixth or seventh decade of life, hence the adult-onset designation.

The other, and much rarer, clinical subtypes, type II (acute neuropathic or, less commonly, malignant or infantile) and type III (chronic neuropathic or, less commonly, juvenile or subacute neuropathic), are distinguished from type I, as

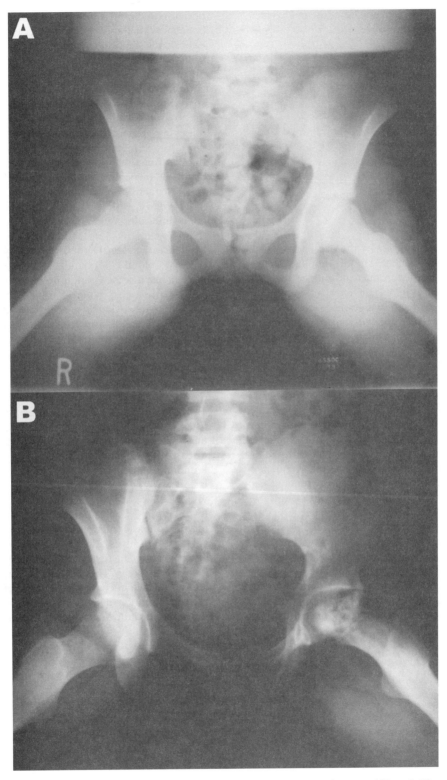

Figure 16-2. (*A*) X-ray of the patient's normal-appearing hip taken in 1982 and (*B*) a collapsed and necrotic left femoral head in 1986.

Table 16-1. Therapeutic Response to Enzyme Replacement Therapy

Therapeutic Response	December 1991	October 1995
Liver volume (cc)	3151	2271
RBC count ($10^6/mm^3$)	3.87	4.67
Hemoglobin (g/dL)	12.4	13.9
Hematocrit (%)	36.8	42.6
MCV (fL)	95	91
Platelet count ($10^3/mm^3$)	133	326
MPV (fL)	10.3	93.0

MCV, mean corpuscular volume; MPV, mean platelet volume; RBC, red blood all.

their names indicate, by the presence of neurological involvement. These neurological forms are distinguished from each other by their clinical severity. Type II Gaucher disease is the most drastic form, with symptoms occurring earlier and death usually following the third year of life, whereas type III Gaucher disease usually appears later in childhood and displays a slower course of progression.

Gaucher disease is the most common of the lysosomal storage diseases. It is an autosomal recessively inherited disorder that is prevalent within all populations; however, it is most prevalent in members of the Ashkenazic Jewish population, occurring at a rate of 1 in 450 individuals (the heterozygote "carrier" frequency is about 4%). In fact, it is the most frequent genetic disorder within this population. Consequently, descendants of this lineage account for the majority of cases within the United States, accounting for nearly two thirds of all Gaucher disease cases.

The suspicion of Gaucher disease often occurs when a relative of the patient suffers the disease; however, diagnosis is not always this straightforward. In the absence of any suspicions due to bloodlines, it may be difficult to identify patients with Gaucher disease because the disease shares signs and symptoms with other disorders. Therefore, physicians from several different specialties (pediatrics, hematology, pathology, radiology, orthopedics, neurology) should be prepared to suspect Gaucher disease on observing a patient with one or more of the following: reduced platelet count, abnormal x-ray, frequent nosebleeds, fatigue, bone pain, frequent fractures, enlarged abdomen, cognitive problems, myoclonic seizures, or disturbances in gait (characterized by a particular manner of moving the feet or walking—a common disturbance indicating neurological involvement).

Bone marrow biopsies are commonly performed to investigate the origin of cytopenias (reduced blood cell counts), and the diagnosis of Gaucher disease is often made or confirmed by a pathologist, who identifies the highly characteristic "Gaucher cells" within the stained aspirate of bone marrow. Gaucher cells, which are pathognomonic for Gaucher disease, are mononuclear cells of the macrophage-reticuloendothelial system (Figs. 16-1 and 16-3). They occur in abundance in sites of this system, namely, the spleen, liver, and bone marrow. They occur elsewhere in reduced numbers, usually in the lymph nodes and lungs. With patients having the neurological forms of Gaucher disease, these unique storage cells are also found in the brain, particularly in the perivascular areas. When cellular aspirates are treated with the Wright stain (a commonly used stain for blood and bone marrow that consists of a mixture of basic [methylene blue derivates] and acidic [eosin] dyes), Gaucher cells appear large with an abundant cytoplasm resembling wrinkled tissue paper. The nucleus is usually oval and positioned eccentrically. The wrinkled, striated appearance of the cytoplasm is due to the accumulation of the glucocerebroside-rich

Table 16-2. Clinical Features of the Gaucher Phenotypes

Clinical Features	Type I	Type II	Type III
Onset	Child/adult	Infancy	Juvenile
Hepatosplenomegaly	+	+	+
Hypersplenism	+	+	+
Bone crises/fractures	+	−	+
Neurodegenerative course	−	+++	++
Life expectancy	Variable	<2 years	Third to fourth decade
Ethnic predilection	Ashkenazic	Panethnic (Norrbottnian)	Swedish

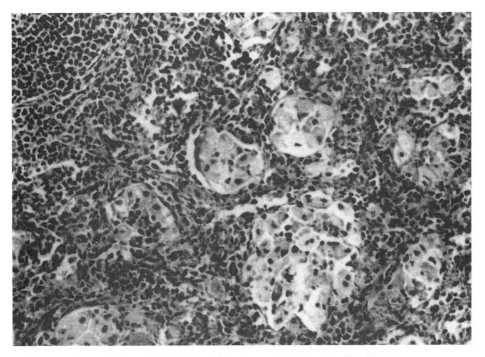

Figure 16-3. Splenic Gaucher cells, light micrograph.

storage material referred to as Gaucher deposits (Fig. 16-1). This finding, although indicative of Gaucher disease, can occur in other diseases, such as thalassemia or chronic granulocytic leukemia. Complicating the issue, the bone marrow aspiration procedure may not provide a sample (a "dry" tap) or contain enough Gaucher cells needed to make a diagnosis. Therefore, the β-glucosidase enzymatic assay, specific only to Gaucher disease, should always be performed to make a definitive diagnosis.

Although the β-glucosidase assay can be performed on any tissue, the tissues of choice are peripheral blood leukocytes or cultured fibroblasts grown from a punch biopsy of the skin. Antenatal diagnosis can be made using extracts of cultured amniotic cells obtained from amniocentesis. There are several different β-glucoside substrates that can be used in the assay: the natural substrate glucocerebroside or structurally similar, artificial substrates.

In the case of the glucocerebrosidase-dependent assay, the two products, glucose and ceramide, are separated based on their differing solubilities to assess the degree of enzymatic activity. It is convenient to use [³H]glucocerebroside labeled in the glucose moiety ([³H]glucose-ceramide) because it is soluble in chloroform and insoluble in water, whereas the radiolabeled product of the reaction, [³H]glucose, is water soluble:

$$[^3\text{H}]\text{Glucocerebroside} + \text{H}_2\text{O}$$
$$\rightarrow [^3\text{H}]\text{Glucose} + \text{Ceramide}$$

After incubating the substrate and tissue extract at 37°C in the appropriate buffer (0.2 M sodium acetate, pH 5.5) and in the presence of activator lipid (e.g., sodium taurocholate, 2% w/v), the reaction is terminated by extraction of the incubation medium with CHCl$_3$-methanol (2:1 v/v); the top layer (the water phase) containing [³H]glucose is counted in a liquid scintillation spectrometer to give a measure of the extent of reaction. Extracts from tissues from persons with Gaucher disease will usually generate less than 10% as much [³H]glucose as controls.

Since radiolabeled molecules are hazardous and difficult to dispose, most researchers and clinical laboratories prefer to use nonisotopic methods of labeling molecules. For this reason, investigators have established β-glucosidase assay conditions that allow the estimation of glucocerebrosidase content of human tissues when nonphysiological β-glucosides serve as the substrate. The artificial substrate of choice, and in widest use today, is 4-methylumbelliferyl-β-D-glucopyranoside (MUGlc). MUGlc is non-fluorescent, but one of the products of the reaction, 4-methylumbelliferone, is intensely fluorescent when the solution is brought to an alkaline pH (Fig. 16-4). Thus, the extent of the reaction may be determined by measuring the quantity of fluorescence generated by a particular tissue extract and comparing it to the fluorescence of standard solutions of 4-methylumbelliferone.

Complicating matters, however, is the presence of a second β-glucosidase in most human tissues, particularly leukocytes. This second β-glucosidase, which is not associated with Gaucher disease, does not cleave glucocerebroside and is not deficient in most cases of Gaucher disease; however, it does cleave the artificial substrate MUGlc, which can lead to misleading results when this artificial substrate is used in the diagnostic assay. Fortunately, it was found that the inclusion of bile salts, such as sodium taurodeoxycholate, in the assay media (used to keep the substrate soluble) inhibited the activity of the second β-glucosidase, while stimulating the activity of lysosomal glucocerebrosidase. Thus, one can use the nonphysiological β-glucoside (MUGlc) within the assay and remain confident that the activity is from the lysosomal, and Gaucher-specific, β-glucosidase

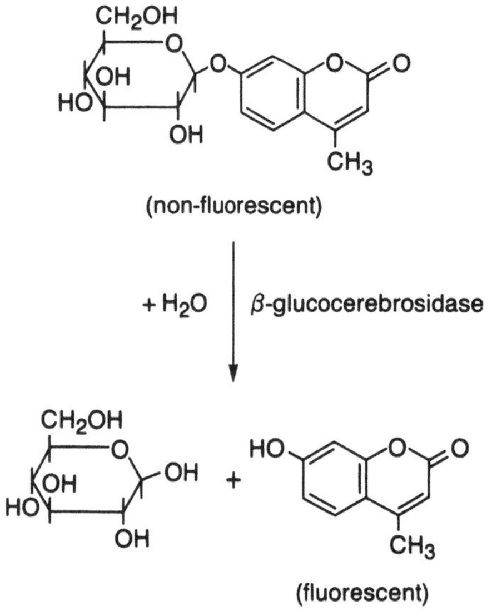

and not from the coexisting nonspecific isoenzyme.

Although not currently used for the diagnosis, there are other enzymes (serum acid phosphatase, chitinase) that are of significant clinical value due to their ability to signal abnormal physiological changes, and these are used to monitor the progression of Gaucher disease. These cell-specific enzymes, whose activities that are usually low in the serum, are commonly elevated in disorders that cause bone degradation or macrophage destruction. The first serological enzymatic marker identified as correlated with Gaucher disease was serum acid phosphatase (ACP). The elevation of ACP activity occurs in most, but not all, cases of Gaucher disease. Hence, there is the possibility that a patient may have a normal serum ACP level. Therefore, the diagnosis of Gaucher disease cannot be ruled out just because of normal serum ACP activity. Nevertheless, the finding of an elevated serum ACP value along with other clinical symptoms should heighten suspicion of Gaucher disease (95% of patients with Gaucher disease exhibit an elevated serum ACP value). One confounding problem regarding the diagnostic utility of the ACP test is its lack of specificity. The sera of patients with other lysosomal storage diseases, such as Niemann-Pick disease, may also exhibit elevations of ACP. This is why ACP is not used to make a diagnosis; however, once the diagnosis of Gaucher disease has been made, results of this enzymatic test are highly useful as they closely reflect the onset and progression of common symptoms and sequelae.

Another enzyme, chitotriosidase (also known as chitinase) has also been found to be elevated in the plasma of patients with Gaucher disease. This enzyme, which is synthesized in macrophages and Gaucher cells, is believed to be involved in the degradation of chitin walls of microorganisms. It is a stable protein and is readily analyzed; however, a drawback is the high frequency of a null allele within the general population that leads to the complete absence of activity in 3%–5% of individuals. Nevertheless, because plasma chitotriosidase activity is so closely associated with glucocerebroside storage and clinical manifestations, it has recently become an important clinical marker for Gaucher disease.

A new marker, a chemokine named CCL18/PARC, has recently been identified to be increased within the serum of patients with Gaucher disease, much like that of chitotriosi-

(non-fluorescent)

+ H₂O | β-glucocerebrosidase

(fluorescent)

Figure 16-4. The β-glucosidase reaction illustrating use of the artificial substrate MUGlc (4-methylumbelliferyl-β-D-glucopyranoside).

dase. However, unlike chitotriosidase, null alleles are not believed to exist in the general population; thus, this new marker may take the place of chitotriosidase or provide a mechanism to monitor the clinical manifestations within individuals who have chitotriosidase null alleles.

It should be emphasized that, although the enzymatic assays have proved 100% effective in diagnosing Gaucher disease, the β-glucosidase assay is not completely reliable in identifying Gaucher disease heterozygotes. Experience has shown that when using the β-glucosidase assay, about 1 of every 10 obligate heterozygotes will be incorrectly assigned to the control category. Thus, identification of heterozygotes must rely on other methods; in this case, molecular methods are the preferred and logical choice. Molecular diagnosis of Gaucher disease relies on the identification of the mutation(s) within the glucocerebrosidase gene. There are several different molecular strategies for identifying patients, and the most common methods include complete gene sequencing, restriction site analysis, or detection based on polymerase chain reaction (PCR). These analyses are easily performed on DNA isolated from blood leukocytes or buccal (cheek) cells. Each method has its limitations, but when used in combination, they can correctly identify carriers of β-glucosidase mutations in nearly all cases.

BIOCHEMICAL PERSPECTIVES

Gaucher disease is the most common of the sphingolipidoses, a group of related genetic diseases that result from the impaired lysosomal enzyme function. Figure 16-5 shows the relationships among the lysosomal enzymes that constitute the pathway of sphingolipid catabolism. The substrates and products that comprise the pathway are linked by a series of irreversible reactions that remove a sugar moiety, a sulfate residue, or a fatty acid; all of these reactions are hydrolytic (use water for cleavage), and the product of one reaction becomes the substrate for the next enzyme in the sequence. In the case of sugar residues, the oligosaccharide domains are disassembled by removal of monosaccharides one at a time from the nonreducing end of the sugar chain (the reducing end of sugar describes the anomeric carbon containing the free carbonyl group; the nonreducing end does not have a carbonyl group, (e.g., carbon-4 of glucose)). All reaction sequences

converge on ceramide, which is degraded in turn by an amidase called ceramidase.

Interestingly, all of the enzymes that comprise the sphingolipid-catabolic pathway are glycoproteins and may be found in different places within the organelle. For example, glucocerebrosidase is firmly associated with the lysosomal membrane, whereas others, like hexoseaminidase A, exist largely in soluble form in the lysosomal matrix. A common property of the lysosomal hydrolases, however, is their expression of maximum activity at a relatively acidic pH (i.e., pH 4.0-5.5), hence the term *acid hydrolase*. This is not unexpected because ATP-driven proton pumps sustain an acidic milieu (pH 5.2) within the lysosome.

All tissues of the patient under discussion, like each patient with Gaucher disease, are markedly deficient in lysosomal glucocerebrosidase activity. Glucocerebrosidase catalyzes the reaction shown in Figure 16-6, and insufficient activity results in the accumulation of substrate within cells, such as macrophages, where glucocerebroside precursors are being catabolized. Most of the glucocerebroside stored in the liver, spleen, and bone marrow is derived from the catabolism of membranes of white blood cells (WBC) and red blood cells (RBC) by the macrophages of the reticuloendothelial system.

In Gaucher disease, as the oligosaccharide chains of the sphingolipids are catabolized, metabolism is aborted at the level of glucocerebroside. This lipid molecule self-associates to form bilayers when it accumulates and will subsequently stack to form membranous sheets that create the histological tissue paper appearance within cells. The insolubility of glucocerebroside in water or bodily fluids is problematic because the lipid cannot be readily excreted in the urine, and only a relatively low rate of excretion occurs by way of the hepatic-biliary route. Thus, glucocerebroside molecules aggregate and accumulate in the lysosomes of cells (Fig. 16-7) within spleen and liver, giving rise to splenomegaly and hepatomegaly. The enlarged spleen and liver in turn destroy RBC, WBC and platelets prematurely, thereby contributing to the anemia, leukopenia, and thrombocytopenia that are common in patients with Gaucher disease.

The storage cells in the bone marrow have a myelophthisic effect; that is, they crowd out the normal hematopoietic tissues. As a result of Gaucher cell accumulation in the bone marrow,

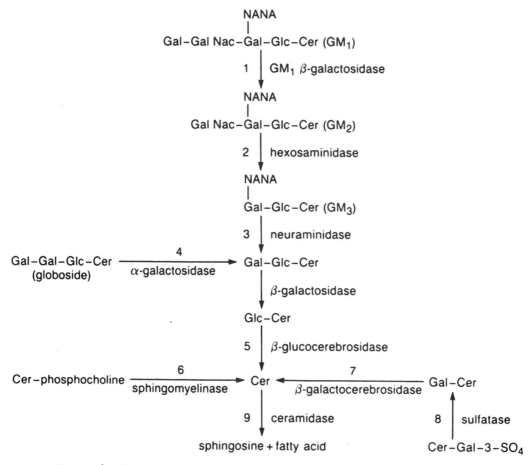

Figure 16-5. The pathway of sphingolipid catabolism. Diseases that result from specific enzyme deficiencies are as follows: (1) GM, gangliosidosis; (2) GM$_2$ gangliosidosis (Tay-Sachs disease); (3) sialidosis; (4) Fabry disease; (5) Gaucher disease; (6) Niemann-Pick disease; (7) Krabbe disease; (8) metachromatic leukodystrophy; (9) Farber disease. Cer, Ceramide; Glc, glucose; Gal, galactose; GalNAc, *N*-acetylgalactosamine; NANA, *N*-acetylneuraminic acid.

Gaucher patients often suffer from skeletal involvement; this includes frequent fractures and severe bone and joint pain, particularly in the femur, and is accompanied by swelling and tenderness of the surrounding tissue. These acute attacks, or "bone crises," are a major impairment for patients with Gaucher disease. Avascular necrosis and collapse of the femoral head occur in many patients and are often severe enough to require hip replacement surgery, as exemplified by the subject of the case report. Frequently seen in younger patients undergoing rapid bone growth is the "Erlenmeyer flask" deformity that arises from expansion of the cortex of the distal femur.

The patient described in the present report has the type I form of Gaucher disease and is spared central nervous system (CNS) involvement. However, in infants with the type II form of the disease, the brain contains Gaucher cells, and CNS involvement is extensive. This form is characterized by strabismus (lack of parallelism of the visual axes of the eyes), muscle hypertonicity (spasticity), retroflexion of the head, and failure to thrive. These infants usually die before the age of 2 years. Patients with type III Gaucher disease usually live longer than type II patients, but they also suffer from neurological involvement. Gaucher cells are also present in neuronal and nonneuronal tissues from type III patients, whose condition, although similar to that of type II patients, is usually less severe.

The accumulation of storage lipid within lysosome-rich cells of the reticuloendothelial

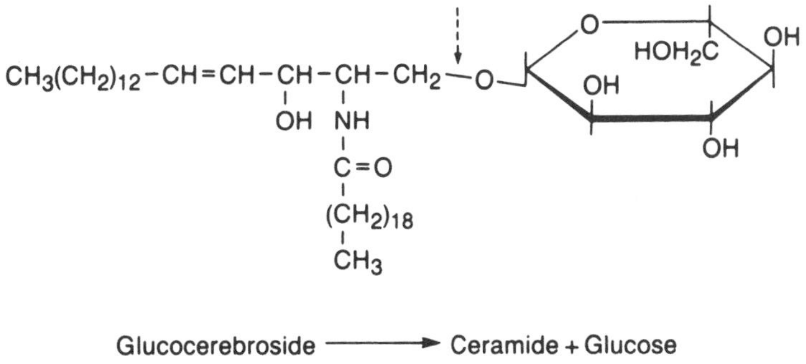

$$CH_3(CH_2)_{12}-CH=CH-CH-CH-CH_2-O$$
$$OH \quad NH$$
$$C=O$$
$$(CH_2)_{18}$$
$$CH_3$$

Glucocerebroside ⟶ Ceramide + Glucose

Figure 16-6. The reaction catalyzed by glucocerebrosidase.

system produces other effects, including the rupture of glucocerebroside-laden cells. After rupturing, the cellular contents of these cells enter the lymphatic system and eventually the bloodstream, causing elevated enzyme activities (ACP, chitinase) that are common in patients with Gaucher disease.

Glucocerebrosidase has a subunit molecular weight of about 67,000, and these inactive subunits have a tendency to aggregate into catalyt-ically active dimers, tetramers, and even larger forms. The enzyme is firmly embedded in the lysosomal membrane, and solubilization requires extraction with detergents such as Triton X-100 or bile salts (e.g., sodium cholate). Subsequent separation of enzyme protein and detergents using a butanol extraction step not only renders glucocerebrosidase soluble in aqueous media, but also removes endogenous, natural lipid activators that are found within

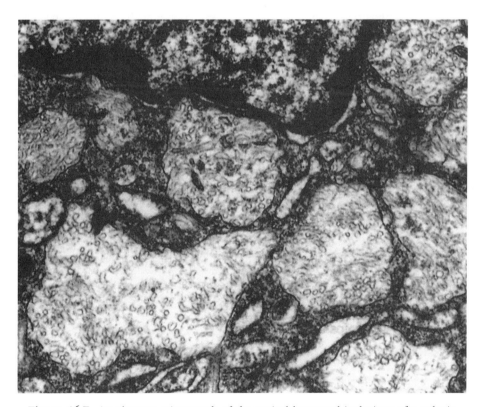

Figure 16-7. An electron micrograph of the typical lysosomal inclusions of a splenic Gaucher cell.

the lysosomal membrane. Thus, the *in vitro* demonstration of activity after such a procedure requires inclusion of some phospholipid or bile salt in the assay medium. The enzyme's pH optimum is in the range of 5.0–5.8, and the specific activity of the enzyme depends on the nature of the lipid activator used in the assay.

Glucocerebrosidase is particularly responsive to acidic lipids and an 11,000 molecular weight heat-stable glycoprotein, referred to historically as heat-stable factor (HSF), and more recently as sphingolipid activator protein (SAP). The acidic membrane lipids that are most effective in reconstituting glucocerebrosidase are phospholipids such as phosphatidylserine and phosphatidylinositol and gangliosides such as GM_1. These acidic lipids activate glucocerebrosidase by increasing the V_{max} and decreasing the K_m, and the activation, at least in dilute aqueous buffers, occurs with conversion of the enzyme from a low to a high molecular weight form. Regarding substrate specificity, glucocerebrosidase has a rather strict specificity for β-D-glucosides; it will cleave the glucose moiety from glucocerebroside as well as from non-physiological substrates like MUGlc and *p*-nitrophenyl-β-D-glucopyranoside but has little or no activity toward β-D-galactosides or β-D-xylosides.

In terms of molecular genetics, the human glucocerebrosidase gene is located within a gene-rich region within band q21 of the long arm of chromosome 1. It consists of 7,620 base pairs that reside within 11 exons separated by 10 introns (Fig. 16-8). A consensus sequence representing an inducible promoter occurs immediately upstream of two independent start codons. The 5.6-kb primary transcript is processed and translated into a polypeptide containing 497 amino acids which has an approximate molecular mass of 67,000 d. Within the primary structure of the enzyme, there are five consensus sequences for N-linked oligosaccharide chain glycosylation sites (Asn-X-Ser or Asn-X-Thr), four of which are occupied by complex-type oligosaccharide chains containing mannose, fucose, galactose, *N*-acetylglucosamine, and sialic acid (Fig. 16-9). The active site of glucocerebrosidase is localized to the carboxyl terminal region of the enzyme and is encoded by exons IX and X.

Notably, there exists a glucocerebrosidase pseudogene located 16 kb downstream from the functional gene (a pseudogene is a region of DNA that has sequence similarity to a known gene but is not functional). It shares a high exonic sequence homology (96%) to the active gene but does contain many sizable intronic and exonic deletions as well as several nonsense and missense point mutations. The pseudogene is actively transcribed from a weak promoter but is not translated or processed further. Several types of mutations have arisen from the homologous recombination between this pseudogene and the glucocerebrosidase gene.

To date, over 250 different mutations have been found within the glucocerebrosidase gene, comprising both private (unique) and public (common) mutations. Five mutations (N370S, L444P, R436C, 84insG, and IVS2+ 1G→A) are most commonly detected but have varying frequencies among differing populations. The first three mutations represent changes that have occurred in the coding region of the gene that cause a substitution of one amino acid for another. The 84insG mutation denotes a frameshift/nonsense mutation, a single base insertion of guanine at the 84th base pair within the coding region that creates a premature translational termination codon.

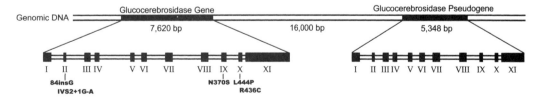

Figure 16-8. The glucocerebrosidase gene and sites of the most common mutations. The glucocerebrosidase pseudogene is located 16 kbp downstream. Over 250 different mutations have been identified. The most common mutations shown here are described in the text.

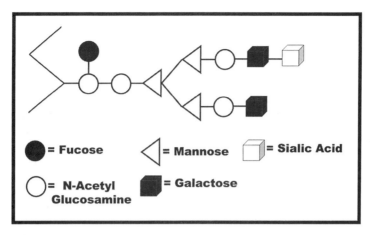

Figure 16-9. Schematic representation of the complex N-linked oligosaccharides contained in glucocerebrosidase.

The IVS2+1G→A mutation is a G-to-A change within the splice-donor site of intron 2, resulting in the deletion of the second exon from the mRNA.

The most commonly occurring mutation within most populations is N370S, whereas the others are found with variable frequencies among the different populations. For example, a recent study found that the 84insG mutation occurred only in Ashkenazi Jewish patients with Gaucher disease, whereas these same patients did not have any of the pseudogene-recombinant alleles that were found in members of the general population.

Gaucher disease is autosomal recessive, resulting from the inheritance of two copies of a mutated gene. *Homoallelic* disease is the result of inheriting precisely the same mutation from both parents. *Heteroallelic*, or *complex*, defects arise when an alteration in one allele coexists with a different mutation (or mutations) in the corresponding allele. Thus, numerous combinations of two of the 250+ mutations could possibly exist within a particular individual. Although the precise mutations can be identified within Gaucher patients, this knowledge cannot, with confidence, be used to predict the severity of the disease within a particular patient. However, some associations do exist; for example, the presence of at least a single copy of the N370S allele within a patient is largely associated with the nonneuropathic (type I) variant of the disease. Although some generalizations like this can be made, there is great clinical heterogeneity between patients

with Gaucher disease, even when they have identical mutations.

THERAPY

Successful implementation of enzyme replacement therapy was initiated in 1990, and has greatly improved the quality of life for many persons suffering from Gaucher disease. Before that time, the therapy, like that of the other sphingolipidoses, remained largely supportive, aimed at lessening the impact of the various manifestations of the disease process. As the splenomegaly associated with Gaucher disease often results in anemia and thrombocytopenia, the latter placing the individual at risk for bleeding diathesis, splenectomy was eventually performed on almost all patients. Although some physicians contend that postponing splenectomy as long as possible reduces the age of onset and rate of development of bone and liver involvement, there is little evidence to support this position. Surgical intervention—for example, the implantation of a hip prosthesis in the woman discussed in this chapter—usually results in decreased bone pain and increased mobility. Two years after her left hip was reconstructed, the patient's artificial hip was functioning well, and she was free of pain at the site.

In 1966, just a year or two after the enzymatic basis of Gaucher disease was identified, Brady and coworkers proposed a novel protocol for treating the disease, namely, the intravenous infusion of exogenous glucocerebrosidase (as discussed in Brady and Barranger, 1983). Eight years later, the earliest attempts at enzyme supplementation were undertaken using native glucocerebrosidase purified from human placenta. Despite the modest reductions in plasma and hepatic glucocerebroside levels that were achieved with a single infusion of glucocerebrosidase, the outcome of the initial treatment was disappointing because the infused enzyme did not effectively penetrate into the affected cells (i.e., macrophages) where the offending glycolipid is stored. The principal obstacle was the rapid clearance of the infused enzyme from the circulation via selective uptake by hepatocytes. Because glucocerebroside accumulates in the reticuloendothelial system of patients with Gaucher disease, a strategy was needed to target the placental enzyme specifically to macrophages. At about the same time, lectinlike receptors on the plasma membrane of macrophages were identified that selectively bind glycoproteins with oligosaccharide chains that terminate in α-linked mannose residues. It was subsequently shown that macrophages use a receptor-mediated endocytotic mechanism to internalize glycoproteins that contain exposed mannose residues at the nonreducing ends of their oligosaccharide chains. Hepatocytes, in contrast, express surface receptors that bind galactose-terminated glycoproteins.

Native placental glucocerebrosidase contains four oligosaccharide chains, all of which terminate with sialic acid (Fig. 16-9). To optimize glucocerebrosidase uptake by macrophages, the enzyme must be treated sequentially with neuraminidase, β-galactosidase, and β-N-acetylglucosaminidase, a process that results in the exposure of mannose residues.

In the early 1990s, macrophage-targeted glucocerebrosidase supplementation was proven to be a highly effective and safe therapy for most cases of Gaucher disease. Several accounts describe a gradual resolution of the clinical features of the disease, an overall decrease in lipid accumulation in organs and the circulation, and a dramatic improvement in the quality of life of the patients. No adverse effects following treatment were reported. As seen in Table 16-1, the patient in the present report experienced an improvement in hematological parameters and a significant reduction in liver volume after enzyme replacement therapy.

To treat more severe forms of the disease, a more aggressive regimen is advised. In most cases, therapy results in a significant decrease in splenic volume and in the level of circulating glucocerebroside. Generalized improvement in hematologic variables follows clearance of Gaucher cell infiltrates from the bone marrow. In a few subjects, there is slow and partial recovery from skeletal complications. Patients gain weight, grow taller, and experience increased vigor, satiety, decreased bone pain, and relief from chronic fatigue. Normalization of hematological parameters, including elevations in hemoglobin concentration and platelet count, an increase in the survival time of autologous labeled RBC, and decreased percentage of reticulocytes, occurs after 3–4 months of enzyme supplementation. Clearance of Gaucher infiltrates from the bone marrow and as much as a 60% reduction of splenic volume is thought to underlie the basis of such changes. Analysis of bone marrow aspirates of patients receiving enzyme supplementation therapy reveals qualitative changes in Gaucher cells, specifically a reduction in size and a decrease in lipid content. Amelioration of hematological variables is dose dependent; discontinuing therapy causes the hematological indices to revert to pretreatment values.

The cost of treating a single patient with glucocerebrosidase is several hundred thousand dollars per year, raising several concerns regarding compensation since insurance plans may refuse to authorize coverage. Such prohibitive cost often places a severe financial burden on patients in this country and makes enzyme replacement therapy in less-developed nations an impossibility.

One year of therapy for a patient infused with Ceredase, the placental-derived glucocerebrosidase drug, requires more than 22,000 placentas for production. To meet demand for therapy, Genzyme, the manufacturer of Ceredase, built a processing plant to extract glucocerebrosidase from donated placentas, and at one point, 35% of all unwanted placentas from the United States were passing through this French plant. Even with this large-scale processing, it was evident that not all patients with Gaucher disease would be able to receive enzymatic therapy. Fortunately, due to advancements in molecular biology, researchers were able to clone the glucocerebrosidase coding region and produce a recombinant form of the enzyme. This recombinant form could be altered for macrophage uptake, just as the placental-derived enzyme, and it demonstrated equivalent clinical efficacy. This recombinant form was approved by the Food and Drug Administration in 1995 and is produced by Genzyme under the name Cerezyme.

A formidable challenge remains in targeting glucocerebrosidase to the involved cells in the CNS of those afflicted with type 2 disease. Intraventricular infusion or temporary alteration of the blood-brain barrier have been suggested; at this time, no effective delivery strategy has yet been formulated for the neuronopathic Gaucher phenotype.

QUESTIONS

1. What are some of the ethical questions that would arise if (a) one attempted to implement a screening program to detect carriers of Gaucher disease that employed a biochemical test with a diagnostic specificity of 0.95? (b) a woman was encouraged to undergo amniocentesis to determine if the fetus was affected?
2. How would you go about determining the nature of the phospholipid in the lysosomal membrane that is the true *in vivo* activator of glucocerebrosidase?
3. What is the cause of elevation in serum acid phosphatase (ACP) activity in Gaucher disease?
4. What is the major source of the accumulated glucocerebroside in Gaucher disease? In what form is the accumulated lipid stored in the lysosome?
5. How would you assess whether glucocerebrosidase replacement therapy was effective in a teenager with Gaucher disease?
6. What consequences of immunoglobulin production against glucocerebrosidase might occur in a patient receiving placental enzyme replacement therapy?
7. What is the cause of the pancytopenia associated with Gaucher disease?
8. Assume you have discovered a new mutation at base position 276 in the glucocerebrosidase gene. How would you use this information to design an assay based on polymerase chain reaction for the presence of this mutation in the parents and siblings of the index case?

BIBLIOGRAPHY

Baldellou A, Andria G, Campbell PE, et al.: Paediatric non-neuronopathic Gaucher disease: recommendations for treatment and monitoring. *Eur J Pediatr* **163**:67-75, 2004.

Barton NW, Brady RO, Dambrosia JM, et al.: Replacement therapy for inherited enzyme deficiency—macrophage-targeted glucocerebrosidase for Gaucher's disease. *N Engl J Med* **324**:1464-1470, 1991.

Basu A, Glew RH: Characterization of the phospholipid requirement of a rat liver β-glucosidase. *Biochem J* **224**:515-524, 1984.

Basu A, Glew RH, Daniels LB, et al.: Activators of spleen glucocerebroside from controls and patients with various forms of Gaucher's disease. *J Biol Chem* **259**:1714-1719, 1984.

Beutler E.: Gaucher disease as a paradigm of current issues regarding single gene mutations of humans. Proc Natl Acad Sci U.S.A. **90**:5384-5390, 1993.

Boot RG, Verhoek M, de Fost M, et al.: Marked elevation of the chemokine CCL18/PARC in Gaucher disease: a novel surrogate marker for assessing therapeutic intervention. *Blood* **103**:33-39, 2004.

Brady RO, Barranger JA: Glucosylceramide lipidosis: Gaucher's disease, *in* Stanbury JB, Wyngaarden JB, Frederickson DS, et al. (eds): *The Metabolic Basis of Inherited Disease.* McGraw-Hill, New York, 1983, pp. 842-56

Brady RO, Barton NW, Grabowski GA: The role of neurogenetics in Gaucher disease. *Arch Neurol* **50**:1212-1242, 1993.

Brady RO, Furbish FS: Enzyme replacement therapy: specific targeting of exogenous enzymes to storage cells, *in* Martonosi AN (ed): *Membranes and Transport.* Vol. 2. Plenum Press, New York, 1982, pp. 587-92

Brady RO, Murray GJ, Oliver KL, et al.: Management of neutralizing antibody to Ceredase in a patient with type 3 Gaucher disease. *Pediatrics* **100**: E11, 1997.

Cox TM.: Future perspectives for glycolipid research in medicine. *Philos Trans R Soc Lond B Biol Sci* **358**:967-973, 2003.

Daniels LB, Glew RH: β-Glucosidase assays in the diagnosis of Gaucher's disease. *Clin Chem* **28**:569-577, 1982.

Elstein D, Abrahamov A, Hadas-Halpern I, et al.: Recommendations for diagnosis, evaluation, and monitoring of patients with Gaucher disease. *Arch Intern Med* **159**:1254-1255, 1999.

Furbish FS, Steer CJ, et al.: Uptake and distribution of placental glucocerebrosidase in rat hepatic cells and effects of sequential deglycosylation. *Biochim Biophys Acta* **673:**425-434, 1981.

Gauchers Association Web site. Available at: http://www.gaucher.org.uk. Accessed 03/12/06.

Genezyme Web site. Available at: http://www.genzyme.com. Accessed 03/12/06.

Glew RH, Basu A, Prence EM, et al.: Biology of disease—lysosomal storage diseases. *Lab Invest* **53:**250-269, 1985.

Glew RH, Daniels LB, Clark LS, et al.: Enzymic differentiation of neurologic and nonneurologic forms of Gaucher's disease. *J Neuropathol Exp Neurol* **41:**630-641, 1982.

Grabowski GA: Gaucher disease: gene frequencies and genotype/phenotype correlations. *Genet Test* **1:**5-12, 1997.

Grabowski GA, Andria G, Baldellou A, et al.: Pediatric non-neuronopathic Gaucher disease: presentation, diagnosis and assessment. Consensus statements. *Eur J Pediatr* **163:**58-66, 2004.

Grabowski GA, Barton NW, et al.: Enzyme therapy in type 1 Gaucher disease: comparative efficacy of mannose-terminated glucocerebrosidase from natural and recombinant sources. *Ann Intern Med* **122:**33-39, 1995.

Hill SC, Parker CC, et al.: MRI of multiple platyspondyly in Gaucher disease. *Arch Neurol* **50:**1212-1224, 1993.

National Gaucher Foundation Web site. Available at: http://www.gaucherdisease.org. Accessed 03/12/06.

Parker RI, Barton NW, et al.: Hematologic improvement in a patient with Gaucher disease on long term-enzyme replacement therapy: evidence for decreased splenic sequestration and improved red blood cell survival. *Am J Hematol* **38:** 130-137.

Sidransky E, Bottler A, Stubblefield B, et al.: DNA mutational analysis of type 1 and type 3 Gaucher patients: how well do mutations predict phenotype? *Hum Mutat* **3:**25-28, 1994.

Zhao H, Grabowski GA: Gaucher disease: perspectives on a prototype lysosomal disease. *Cell Mol Life Sci* **59:**694-707, 2002.

17

I-Cell Disease (Mucolipidosis II)

JAMES CHAMBERS

CASE HISTORY

The patient (Fig. 17-1) was a 38-week-gestation product of a 22-year-old $G, P_1 Ab_o$ (gravida 1, first pregnancy; paradelivery, first delivery; abortion, 0) woman and her 31-year-old first-cousin partner. Pregnancy was complicated by oligohydramnios (deficiency in the amount of amniotic fluid); an amniocentesis revealed a normal male karyotype. The infant was delivered by cesarean section because of maternal preeclampsia (development of hypertension due to pregnancy). Apgar scores were 8/9, weight was 2200 g, and length was 18.5 inches. On newborn examination, microcephaly (a broad nasal bridge with anteverted nostrils), micrognathia (smallness of the jaws, especially the underjaw), hypospadias (a defect in the wall of the urethra), and undescended testes were seen. A tentative diagnosis of Smith-Lemli-Opitz syndrome was postulated.

By 9 months of age, marked developmental delay was noted. Repeat evaluation revealed bilateral inguinal hernias, dysmorphic features with synophrys (growing together of the eyebrows), and thick upper lip with gum hypertrophy; limitation of motion at the knees, hips, elbows, and wrists; camptodactyly (bending of fingers); rib flaring; hepatosplenomegaly; corneal clouding; and hypotonia in addition to those findings reported at birth. A lysosomal enzyme screen indicated elevated levels of a number of lysosomal enzymes in plasma and urine and sialyloligosaccharides in the urine. These findings and the physical examination are consistent with a diagnosis of I-cell disease.

DIAGNOSIS

Postnatal

I-cell disease (mucolipidosis II, ML-II) is a rare autosomal recessive lysosomal storage disorder first described in 1966 by DeMars and Leroy while studying a group of suspected Hurler patient biopsies. The histopathologic hallmark of I-cell disease is the presence of characteristic phase-dense, cytoplasmic, spherical (approximately $0.5-1.0$ µm in diameter) vesicles (i.e., inclusions) (Fig. 17-2) surrounding the nucleus and juxtanuclear Golgi apparatus within the mesenchyme-derived tissues throughout the body. These cells were so distinctive compared with cells cultured from other patients with similar clinical symptoms that the appellation I cell was coined. Ultrastructurally, the inclusions are bound by a single membrane and contain fibrogranular and membranous lamellar material. Subsequently, I-cell disease was classified as a mucolipidosis (designated ML-II by Spranger and Wiedemann in 1970), characterized by intracellular (i.e., lysosomal) accumulation of acid mucopolysaccharides, sphingolipids, or glycolipids in visceral and mesenchymal cells.

I-cell disease is suspected clinically by the phenotype and is confirmed biochemically (cf. "Biochemical Perspectives" section). The infant with I-cell disease is usually small for gestational age and is clinically differentiated from having Hurler's syndrome by earlier onset of signs and symptoms, the absence of excessive mucopolysacchariduria, short stature, and the rapidly progressive course, leading to death usually by age 4 years.

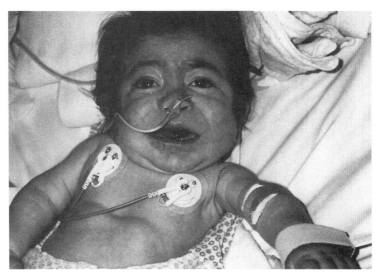

Figure 17-1. A 9-month-old Hispanic male infant with I-cell disease. From the Division of Medical Genetics, Children's Hospital, Los Angeles.

The disease progresses with the child developing coarse facial features with puffy eyelids, prominent epicanthal folds, flat nasal bridge, anteverted nostrils, macroglossia (enlargement of the tongue), and severe skeletal abnormalities. Craniofacial abnormalities (i.e., microencephaly and metopic craniosynostosis), restricted joint movement with generalized hypotonia, congenital hip dislocation, hernias, and bilateral talipes equinovarus (clubfoot) may be observed in the neonatal period. Gingival hypertrophy is more striking than in Hurler syndrome. Hard, firm subcutaneous nodules may represent accumulation of storage material. In addition, severe gingival hyperplasia is also observed in some presentations.

By 6 months of age, psychomotor retardation is usually obvious. Joint immobility progresses with development of claw-hand deformities and kyphoscoliosis. Hepatomegaly is prominent, but splenomegaly is minimal. Corneal haziness may be present but is subtle, and corneal opacities due to the accumulation of storage material are not as striking as in Hurler syndrome. Examination of peripheral blood smears reveals the presence of abnormal inclusions in cells such as lymphocytes, and increased lysosomal enzyme activity in whole blood as well as cultured fibroblasts is confirmatory of I-cell disease.

Radiographically, I-cell disease is manifested in two successive stages of infancy, one observed in the neonatal period and the other at about 1 year of age. When detected at birth, peculiar radiographic changes of the bones reflect a more severe disturbance in bone development and growth, and strongly resemble rickets or osteomalacia (softening and bending of the bones) as evidenced by the presence of rachiticlike (related to rickets) lesions and changes similar to those observed in hyperparathyroidism. The radiographic abnormalities found in older children appear to be more nonspecific and are typical of Hurler-like signs of dysostosis multiplex (roentgenographic abnormalities indicating bone changes at multiple sites).

Biochemically, I-cell disease is characterized by excessive secretion of newly synthesized lysosomal enzymes into body fluids and concomitant loss of respective intracellular activities in fibroblasts. Shown in Table 17-1 are representative lysosomal enzyme activity levels in serum from patients with I-cell disease and those with the closely related disorder pseudo-Hurler polydystrophy, indicating significantly increased levels of lysosomal enzyme activity. Germane to the biochemical diagnosis is the characteristic pattern of lysosomal enzyme deficiency in cultured fibroblasts, that is, an increase in the ratio of extracellular to intracellular enzyme activity (Table 17-2). It is interesting to note that not all lysosomal (i.e. intracellular)

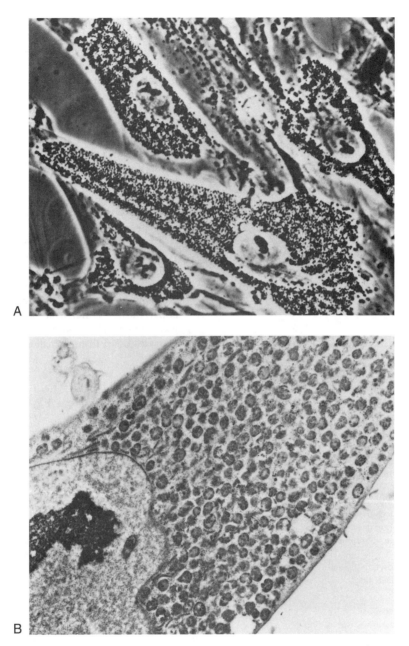

Figure 17-2. Microscopic examination of cultured I-cell skin fibroblasts. (*A*) Phase contrast microscopy. (*B*) Electron microscopy showing the inclusions. Photographs courtesy of Dr. Robert DeMars.

enzyme activities are decreased in I-cell fibroblasts, suggesting alternative lysosomal routing; acid phosphatase and β-glucosidase are the exceptions. Major increases in glycosylasparaginase activity in I-cell patient serum and urine and the markedly reduced activity in cultured fibroblasts can also be used as a diagnostic aid for detecting I-cell disease (Ylikangas and Mononen, 1998). It is important to note that increased levels of lysosome enzymes in serum cannot distinguish between ML-II and ML-III (pseudo-Hurler polydystrophy), which usually

Table 17-1. Lysosomal Enzyme Activities in Serum from Patients with I-Cell Disease and Pseudo-Hurler Polydystrophy

Enzyme	Controls	I-Cell	Pseudo-Hurler
β-Galactosidase*	16.3	30.6	ND
α-Galactosidase*	4.6	14.5	ND
α-Mannosidase*	31.4	1116	3976
β-Glucuronidase*	14.2	163	740
α-Fucosidase*	235	5184	4389
Arylsulphatase A*	14.2	1664	ND
α-Glucosaminidase*	15.8	1531	76
β-Glucosaminidase*	621	5040	4194
Glycosylasparaginase†	13.4	142	ND
β-Galactosidase†	58.9	926.5	ND

ND, nondetermined.

*Data from Poenaru et al. (1988). Specific activity is expressed as nmol/h/ml serum.

†Data from Ylikangas and Mononen (1998). Specific activity is expressed as mU/L.

must be differentiated on the basis of clinical events.

Degradation of most lysosomal substrates occurs by the stepwise activity of a series of hydrolases, with each step requiring the action of the previous hydrolase to modify the substrate, so that the substrate can be further degraded by the next enzyme in the pathway. If one step in the process fails, then further degradation ceases, and the partially degraded substrate accumulates. Thus, lysosomal accumulation of partially degraded substrate in many cases give rise to a metabolic "traffic jam" affecting the architecture and function of cells, tissues, and organs.

Analysis of I-cell patient glycosphingolipids reveals elevations in trihexosylceramide (GL-3) and the ganglioside GM_3 (Fig. 17-3) but not the massive accumulation associated with the glycosphingolipidoses. In the spleen, the only apparent lipid abnormality is an increase in the level of GM_3. The brain has normal levels of gangliosides, apart from a small increase in GM_3 and

Table 17-2. Intra- and Extracellular Levels of Various Lysosomal Enzymes of Cultivated I-Cell Disease Fibroblasts

Enzyme	Control	I-Cell Disease
Intracellular activity		
α-Fucosidase*	72	2.2
β-Galactosidase*	584	6.7
α-Mannosidase*	98	9.3
Neuraminidase*	39	0.5
Acid Phosphatase*	2,954	2,620
β-Glucosidase*	162	148
Phospholipase†	2.8	0.45
Palmitoyl-protein thioesterase‡	Detected, immunoblot	Undetected, immunoblot
Glycosylasparaginase§	70	6.0
β-Galactosidase§	21,800	890
Extracellular activity		
α-Fucosidase*	0.8	2.7
β-Glucuronidase*	41	345
Hexosaminidase A*	97	878
α-Mannosidase*	2.3	24
β-Glucosidase*	0.2	0.2
Phospholipase†	0.0	0.58
Palmitoyl-protein thioesterase‡	Undetected, immunoblot	Detected, immunoblot

*Data from Ben-Yoseph et al. (1986). Specific activity of intracellular enzymes is expressed as nmol/h/mg protein. Activities detected in the medium (extracellular) were those secreted by 1 mg cell protein in 24 hours.

†Data from Jansen et al. (1999). Intracellular and extracellular specific activities are expressed as nmol/h/mg fibroblast protein and nmol/h/ml medium, respectively.

‡Data from Verkruyse et al. (1997). Intracellular palmitoyl-protein thioesterase (PPT) was determined using whole cell lysates and anti-PPT antibody. PPT protein in the medium (extracellular) was detected following partial purification to enrich for PPT prior to immunoblotting with anti-PPT antibody.

§Data from Ylikangas and Monenen (1998). Specific activity is expressed as pmol/min/mg protein.

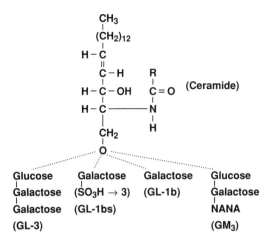

Glucose   Galactose   Galactose   Glucose
|
Galactose   (SO$_3$H → 3)   (GL-1b)   Galactose
|
Galactose   (GL-1bs)   NANA

(GL-3)   (GM$_3$)

Figure 17-3. Important glycolipids affected in I-cell disease. The dotted lines represent the respective β-linked glycosides. Ceramide, 2-*N*-acylsphingosine; NANA, *N*-acetylneuraminic acid. GL-1bs is shown sulfated in the 3 position of galactose (SO$_3$H → 3).

lower than normal concentrations of sulfatide GL-1bS and cerebroside GL-lb (Fig. 17-3).

Due to the extensive mesenchymal tissue involvement in I-cell disease, the observation of large amounts of unsulfated chondroitin in the cartilage matrix and compensatory decrease of chondroitin 4-sulfate has been viewed as suggesting possible abnormalities in the posttranslational assembly and subsequent modification of glycosaminoglycans. However, I-cell fibroblasts have been shown to (1) internalize cell-surface proteoglycans; (2) remove glycosaminoglycan chains from the proteoglycan core protein; and (3) partially degrade heparan sulfate glycosaminoglycan chains in identical fashion as that observed for normal fibroblasts (Brauker and Wang, 1987). Also suspect is the degradation of collagen (type I) in I-cell disease fibroblasts as a result of the greatly reduced levels of cathepsin B, which possesses potent collagenolytic activity; however, the rate of intracellular degradation of proline analogues by I-cell disease fibroblasts is comparable to rates of degradation observed for normal fibroblasts.

Many tissues from patients with I-cell disease exhibit normal levels of "intracellular" lysosomal enzymatic activities (e.g., brain, liver, kidney, and spleen). In the liver, lysosomal enzyme levels are normal except for diminished β-galactosidase and elevated β-hexosaminidase, β-xylosidase, and α-galactosidase. This fairly spe-

cific decrease in liver activity of β-galactosidase contrasts with the diminution of almost all lysosomal enzymes in cultured fibroblasts.

Prenatal

Prenatal diagnosis of I-cell disease has been based on greatly reduced phosphotransferase activity (cf. "Biochemical Perspectives" section) and abnormal intracellular-extracellular distribution of lysosomal enzymes in cultured amniotic fluid cells (Table 17-3). As indicated in Table 17-3, amniotic fluid cells secrete large amounts of lysosomal enzymes into the extracellular medium. Decreased levels of lysosomal enzymes in chorionic villi obtained by biopsy have also been observed in I-cell disease; however, the characteristic secondary effect (i.e., increased levels of lysosomal enzymes in the extracellular compartment) is only partially expressed or not expressed at all in chorionic villi, suggesting an alternative mechanism for the transport of lysosomal proteins. Although

Table 17-3. Prenatal Diagnosis: Levels of GlcNac-PO$_4$ Transferase and Various Lysosomal Enzymes in Amniotic Fluid and Cultivated Amniotic Fluid Cells

Enzyme	Control	I-Cell Disease
Amniotic fluid cells		
GlcNac-PO$_4$ Transferase	0.68	0.05
Intracellular activity		
α-Fucosidase	478	22.3
β-Galactosidase	745	27.3
β-Glucosidase	136	278
β-Glucuronidase	244	17.4
Hexosaminidase A	1345	119
α-Mannosidase	190	14.7
β-Mannosidase	462	31.1
Extracellular activity		
α-Fucosidase	53.4	285
β-Galactosidase	14.6	69.0
Hexosaminidase A	242	1843
α-Mannosidase	5.6	44.4
Amniotic fluid		
Hexosaminidase	155	1620
β-Glucuronidase	15.6	135
α-Fucosidase	18.0	140
α-Mannosidase	7.2	76
α-Galactosidase	0.78	2.4

Data from Parvathy et al. (1989) and Besley et al. (1990). Intracellular activities are expressed as nmol substrate cleaved/h/mg cell protein. Extracellular activities are expressed as the activity secreted into the medium/24 h/mg cell protein. Activities in amniotic fluid are expressed as nmol/h/mg protein.

the diagnosis is made more reliably using cells obtained by amniocentesis, direct examination of the phosphotransferase activity of chorionic villi has been effectively used to diagnose I-cell disease prenatally. This approach affords a more rapid diagnosis than the 2 to 4 weeks required for diagnosis by amniocentesis. In addition, electron microscopic examination of chorionic villus tissue has been used for rapid prenatal diagnosis of I-cell disease (Carey et al., 1999). Although not the focus of this discussion, prenatal diagnosis of the closely related disorder exhibiting the same primary biochemical defect as I-cell disease (i.e., pseudo-Hurler polydystrophy) was accomplished using molecular tools targeting the γ-subunit of the phosphotransferase enzyme (Falik-Zaccae et al., 2003).

BIOCHEMICAL PERSPECTIVES

Initial Observations

Historically, the important observation made by Hickman and Neufeld (1972) that I-cell fibroblasts are capable of endocytosing (the process by which cells take up macromolecules) lysosomal enzymes secreted by normal cells but that normal cells are incapable of internalizing the enzymes secreted by I-cell fibroblasts suggested that some kind of recognition marker for internalization of lysosomal enzymes was absent in I-cell fibroblasts. This recognition marker has subsequently been identified as mannose 6-phosphate.

It is widely believed that I-cell disease (ML-II) and pseudo-Hurler polydystrophy (ML-III) are variants of the same disorder because fibroblasts from both these disorders are deficient in phosphotransferase activity. At the molecular level, the primary and most significant difference is that in I-cell disease the deficiency is essentially total, whereas in pseudo-Hurler polydystrophy there appears to be significant residual activity (approximately 10% of control values). The molecular basis for these two diseases may, however, be distinct, as evidenced by genetic complementation studies demonstrating complementation of ML-II by some ML-III fibroblasts (Mueller et al., 1983). Although two clinical presentations of I-cell disease have been described (i.e., the neonate and 6- to 12-month-old patient), correlation of the degree of deficiency of phosphotransferase activity with clinical severity in the two I-cell disease presentations remains controversial.

Molecular Theme

The Marking Event

The I-cell patient has proved invaluable for elucidation of the complex nature of intracellular packaging and sorting of lysosomal enzymes. The physiological importance of this signal-mediated pathway is evident in that fibroblasts from patients with I-cell disease and pseudo-Hurler polydystrophy *secrete* rather than target most of their lysosomal enzymes. Thus, the molecular theme of I-cell disease is that of "faulty" lysosomal targeting, the inability to transport (i.e., sort) lysosomal enzymes from their site of synthesis to the lysosome.

The biosynthetic pathways responsible for both membrane and secretory glycoproteins have been localized to specific lumenal regions of the Golgi and endoplasmic reticulum (for an excellent review see Kornfeld and Kornfeld, 1985). As shown in Figure 17-4, the "core" oligosaccharide (three glucose, nine mannose, and two N-acetylglucosamine residues) is preassembled in an "activated" form and is transferred en bloc from a lipid-linked (dolichyl-pyrophosphate) carrier to distinct asparagine residues of the nascent polypeptide while the protein is being synthesized on membrane-bound polysomes. This transfer usually takes place before the folding of the polypeptide chain. Once glycosylation of the protein has occurred, processing of the oligosaccharide is initiated by trimming reactions that remove three glucose residues and one mannose unit. The proteins then move by vesicular transport to the Golgi, where they undergo a variety of additional posttranslational modifications and are sorted for targeting to the proper destination, that is, to the lysosome, secretory granules, or plasma membrane.

The trafficking of lysosomal hydrolases to the lysosome in higher eukaryotes depends on the specific modification of asparagine-linked oligosaccharides to contain a mannose 6-phosphate recognition marker. This man-6-P-dependent sorting system requires the concerted action of two key enzymes (Fig. 17-5). The initial and determining step in the generation of the mannose 6-phosphate recognition marker is catalyzed by the enzyme UDP-N-acetylglucosamine:lysosomal-enzyme N-acetylglucosaminyl-1-phosphotransferase (EC 2.7.8.17), commonly referred to as phosphotransferase.

The primary biochemical defect in I-cell dis-

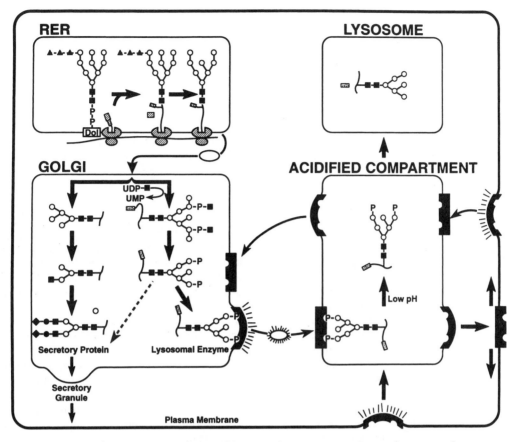

Figure 17-4. Schematic pathway of lysosomal enzyme targeting to lysosomes. Lysosomal enzymes and secretory proteins are synthesized in the rough ER (RER) and glycosylated by the transfer of a preformed oligosaccharide from dolichol-P-P-oligosaccharide (Dol). In the RER, the signal peptides (▨) are excised. The proteins are translocated to the Golgi, where the oligosaccharides of secretory proteins are processed to complex-type units, and the oligosaccharides of lysosomal enzymes are phosphorylated. Most of the lysosomal enzymes bind to mannose 6-phosphate receptors (MPRs) (▭) and are translocated to an acidified prelysosomal compartment, where the ligand dissociates. The receptors recycle back to the Golgi or to the cell surface, and the enzymes are packaged into lysosomes, where cleavage of their propieces is completed (▨). The Pi may also be cleaved from the mannose residues. A small number of the lysosomal enzymes fail to bind to the receptors and are secreted along with secretory proteins. These enzymes may bind to surface MPRs in coated pits (⏝) and be internalized into the prelysosomal compartment. (■), N-Acetylglucosamine; (○), mannose; (▲) glucose; (●), galactose; (◆) sialic acid. Reprinted with permission from Kornfeld (1987). Copyright 1987, *FASEB J.*

ease, as well as in pseudo-Hurler polydystrophy, is in the phosphotransferase enzyme. This metabolic error creates a secondary deficiency of most lysosomal enzymes, as described in this section. The reaction catalyzed by the phosphotransferase enzyme (cf. reaction 1, Fig. 17-5) results in formation of the phosphodiester N-acetylglucosamine-l-phosphate-6-mannose intermediate. A second "uncovering" enzyme (i.e., N-acetylglucosamine-l-phosphodiester-α-N-acetyl-glucosaminidase or EC 3.1.4.45) cleaves the terminal α-N-acetylglucosamine residue to uncover the mannose 6-phosphate group that serves as the required "recognition marker" component

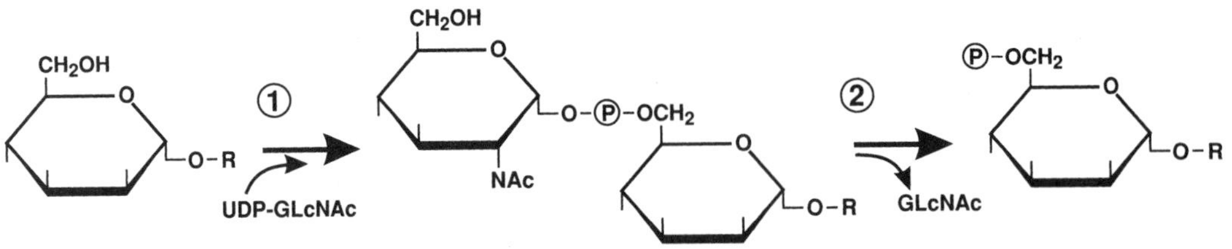

Figure 17-5. Synthesis of the mannose 6-phosphate recognition marker. R represents the high-mannose oligosaccharide of newly synthesized lysosomal enzymes. Reaction 1 is catalyzed by UDP-*N*-acetylglucosamine:lysosomal enzyme *N*-acetylglucosaminyl-1-phosphotransferase. Reaction 2 is catalyzed by *N*-acetylglucosamine-1-phosphodiester-*N*-acetylglucosaminidase.

responsible for high-affinity binding to mannose 6-phosphate receptors (MPRs) in the Golgi.

The MPRs and their bound ligands (i.e., lysosomal enzymes) are packaged into clathrin-coated vesicles that bud from the *trans*-Golgi network (TGN) and subsequently fuse with an acidic endosomal compartment, where the low pH promotes dissociation of receptor and ligand. Thus, these receptors mediate delivery of the "targeted" enzymes to endosomal compartments, where they are discharged and subsequently packaged into lysosomes (for reviews, see Kornfeld, 1986, 1992; von Figura and Hasilik, 1986). In I-cell disease, lysosomal enzymes are not modified by addition of mannose 6-phosphate. Thus, they are not segregated by the MPRs into the appropriate transport vesicles in the TGN and instead are carried to the cell surface and secreted.

The Enzyme

Bao and coworkers (1996) have purified bovine phosphotransferase as a 54-kd complex composed of three different subunits (α_2, β_2, and γ_2). Bovine phosphotransferase is the product of two genes, one encoding the α- and β-subunits, the second coding the γ-subunit. The multisubunit nature of the enzyme gives much insight into the relationship between subunits, ML-II complementation groups, and the mucolipidoses (ML-II and ML-III). The gene coding for the human γ-subunit has been localized to chromosome 16p. Examination of human γ-subunit in ML-III patients indicated a single nucleotide insertion difference in the phosphotransferase subunit.

Although both I-cell disease and pseudo-Hurler polydystrophy patients are deficient in phosphotransferase activity, they exhibit different patterns of intracellular and extracellular

lysosomal enzyme activities in cultured skin fibroblasts with respect to electrophoretic mobility, lectin-binding properties, and responsiveness to sucrose loading. Complementation studies of fibroblasts from I-cell disease and pseudo-Hurler polydystrophy indicate three genetic groups (A, B, and C) exhibiting altered phosphotransferase activity. In these studies, fibroblasts from individual patients are fused with cells from other patients. Variants have been categorized on the basis of phosphotransferase activity toward α-methylmannoside as acceptor in the phosphotransferase assay as well as decreased secretion of lysosomal enzymes into the extracellular compartment.

Complementation group A is the largest and includes all I-cell disease and many pseudo-Hurler polydystrophy patients. The defects in patients from group A are thought to be alleles at the same locus and are characterized by a change in the catalytic portion of the phosphotransferase that renders it unable to use the artificial acceptor substrate (α-methymannoside). In patients of complementation group A, the phosphotransferase enzyme appears to be smaller than normal, suggesting the absence of a catalytically important enzyme component.

Groups B and C consist entirely of the less-common pseudo-Hurler polydystrophy (ML-III) variants. Group B is comprised of patients with defective phosphotransferase catalytic function. The enzyme from patients with complementation group B phosphotransferase deficiency appears to be larger than normal, suggesting abnormal aggregation of the enzyme. Group C includes patients exhibiting a phosphotransferase with normal catalytic function toward α-methylmannoside but one that fails to recognize endogenous lysosomal enzymes as acceptor substrate. The mutation in group C is thought to affect a gene coding a noncatalytic phosphotransferase site or a component that is involved in the recognition of, or specific binding to, lysosomal enzyme precursors. Work by Raas-Rothschild and coworkers (2004) strongly suggests that, despite the existence of the three complementation groups, the γ-subunit of the phosphotransferase gene plays a major role in ML-III.

The Phosphotransferase Assay

As shown in Figure 17-5, the phosphotransferase transfers N-acetylglucosamine-l-phosphate residues *en bloc* to the C-6 oxygen of particular mannose residues in "high-mannose" oligosaccharide units of lysosomal enzymes. This reaction occurs in two stages: transfer of N-acetylglucosamine-l–phosphate to a mannose residue on the *a*-1,6 branch of a high-mannose oligosaccharide and addition of a second N-acetylglucosamine-l–phosphate to the *a*-1,3 branch. The two stages are thought to occur in a pre-Golgi compartment and the *cis* Golgi, respectively. A number of assay procedures have been described for the phosphotransferase using ^{32}P-, ^{3}H-, and ^{14}C-labeled UDP-GlcNAc (radioactivity is located in the GlcNAc moiety) as the N-acetylglucosamine-1-phosphate donor and a variety of acceptor substrates (e.g., β-hexosaminidase, glycopeptides, and α-methylmannoside).

Generally, phosphotransferase is assayed using α-methylmannoside as acceptor. After incubation, the reaction is terminated, and the phosphodiester product of the transfer reaction, (i.e., [^{14}C or ^{3}H]GlcNac-α-l-phospho-6-mannose-α-l-methyl) is chromatographically separated from the reaction components, and the radioactivity is determined. The general reaction scheme is

$$\text{UDP-}[^{3}\text{H}/^{14}\text{C}]\text{GlcNAc} + \alpha\text{-CH}_3\text{-Man} \leftrightarrow \text{UMP} + \alpha\text{-CH}_3\text{-Man-(6}\leftarrow\text{P)-GlcNAc}[^{3}\text{H}/^{14}\text{C}]$$

In vivo, the CH_3 group in the reaction scheme is representative of the rest of the high-mannose oligosaccharide intermediate.

Phosphotransferase Protein Target Recognition

Efficient targeting of enzymes to lysosomes requires the phosphotransferase to recognize and bind with high affinity to a protein determinant that is common to lysosomal enzymes but absent from nonlysosomal glycoproteins. Because lysosomal enzymes do not share linear amino acid sequences, the phosphotransferase must specifically interact with a conformation-dependent protein determinant that is expressed in 40 to 50 different lysosomal hydrolases while displaying low affinity for hundreds of other glycoproteins that contain identical high-mannose-type oligosaccharides.

The high-affinity interaction required for efficient phosphorylation *in vivo* and *in vitro* appears to be mediated primarily through protein–protein structural interactions (Lang et al., 1984). This is based on the fact that isolated high-mannose-type oligosaccharide and glycopeptides are extremely poor phosphotransferase acceptor substrates. Furthermore, the phosphorylation of intact lysosomal enzymes is markedly inhibited by the inclusion of deglycosylated lysosomal enzymes in reaction mixtures, supporting the hypothesis that the phosphotransferase recognizes a protein domain that is common to all lysosomal enzymes but absent in nonlysosomal glycoproteins.

Much insight into this problem has been derived from studies of cathepsin D, a bilobed lysosomal aspartylprotease that contains one asparagine-linked oligosaccharide per lobe. Using chimeric proteins containing either amino or carboxyl lobe sequences of cathepsin D substituted into a glycosylated form of the homologous secretory protein pepsinogen, the minimal elements of a recognition domain required for phosphorylation involving two specific lysine residues have been identified that are thought to be shared among lysosomal enzymes and recognized by the phosphotransferase.

Mutation of these two residues results in 70% inhibition of mannose phosphorylation (Sandholzer et al., 2000). A phosphotransferase recognition domain located on either lobe of the cathepsin/glycopepsinogen chimeric molecule is sufficient to allow phosphorylation of oligosaccharides on both lobes. Interestingly, the carboxyl lobe oligosaccharides of cathepsin D acquire two phosphates, whereas the amino lobe oligosaccharides acquire only one phosphate. Molecular modeling of the cathepsin D sequences inclusive of the lysosomal enzyme recognition domain indicates that these residues come together in three-dimensional space to form a surface patch on the carboxyl lobe of the molecule.

Although much of the focus of I-cell disease centers around lysosomal enzyme carbohydrate processing, it is important to remember that lysosomal enzymes are synthesized as pre-proenzymes with amino terminal extensions that require further proteolytic processing. In addition to removal of the signal peptide in the ER, the newly synthesized protein may be subject to additional limited proteolysis during transport (Fig. 17-4). This proteolytic processing appears to be initiated in the prelysosomal compartments and is completed after the enzymes arrive in the lysosomes. In some cases, there are further internal cleavages of the peptide as well as carboxyl-terminal processing. The biological significance of this processing is not well understood but may play an early role in the sorting process (e.g., maintenance of the correct folding and conformation of the nascent protein that subsequently becomes a substrate for the phosphotransferase).

Mannose 6-Phosphate Receptor: An Intracellular Lysosomal Enzyme Receptor

Newly synthesized lysosomal enzymes containing mannose 6-P residues are recognized by two distinct mannose 6-phosphate receptors (MPRs) with molecular masses of 46,000 and 300,000 d. Both mediate the transport of newly synthesized soluble lysosomal enzymes from the trans-Golgi network (TGN) to a prelysosomal compartment that is part of the endocytic route. There the receptor-ligand complexes are dissociated, and hydrolases are subsequently packaged into lysosomes. The smaller receptor requires divalent cations for its binding activity and is referred to as cation dependent (i.e., CD-MPR). In contrast, the larger MPR is cation independent (i.e., CI-MPR). Both MPR are type I trans-membrane glycoproteins. The two receptors recycle regardless of whether they are loaded with ligands or not between the TGN, the endosomal compartment, and the cell surface. MPR are never detected in the lysosomes. Through increasingly better-understood pathways (reviewed by Eskelinen et al., 2003), respective lysosomal substrates and the enzymes responsible for their breakdown are brought together in the endosomal compartment.

In humans and in many other species, the larger receptor is identical to the receptor for the insulinlike growth factor II (IGF-II) and thus is referred to as the mannose-6-P/insulin growth

factor II (man-6-P/IGF-II) receptor. The MPRs are distributed over several cellular compartments. A single pool of MPRs cycles constitutively between the Golgi, endosomes, and the plasma membrane. At the plasma membrane, the man-6-P/IGF-II receptor binds and mediates endocytosis of extracellular ligands, whereas the CD-MPR appears not to function in endocytosis under physiological conditions despite rapid internalization from the cell surface. The distribution of MPRs in fibroblasts from some I-cell patients is abnormal, with the receptors found almost exclusively in Golgi cisternae and in coated vesicles located near the cisternae. Thus, defective receptors, as well as functional receptors wrongly distributed, represent possibly yet additional mechanisms that can result in the I-cell phenotype.

Whereas both types of MPRs bind mannose 6-P with the same affinity ($7-8 \times 10^{-6}$ M), the man-6-P/IGF-II receptor binds diphosphorylated oligosaccharides with a significantly higher affinity than does the CD-MPR (2×10^{-9} M vs. 2×10^{-7} M, respectively). Because oligosaccharides with two phosphomonoesters bind to the MPRs with an affinity similar to that observed for lysosomal enzymes, the high-affinity binding of lysosomal enzymes can be explained by a two-site model in which two phosphomannosyl residues on the lysosomal enzyme interact with the receptor. Individual phosphomannosyl residues located on different oligosaccharides appear to interact with the receptor with higher affinity than do two phosphomannosyl residues present on the same oligosaccharide.

How Does Sorting Occur?

The signal for the rapid internalization of MPR 300 at the plasma membrane has been localized to the pentapeptide KYSKV (residues 24–29 in its 163-residue cytoplasmic tail). MPR 46 appears to contain in its cytoplasmic tail of 67 residues several distinct signals for rapid internalization and binding to clathrin adaptors. Both receptors have a leucine-based sorting signal close to their C terminus, which is critical for their ability to sort lysosomal enzymes (Denzer et al., 1997).

The question of why two MPR are present in mammalian cells remains unanswered. Analysis of cell lines made deficient in MPR by targeted disruption of the respective MPR gene from mice as well as from tumors has shown that each of the two MPRs contributes to the targeting of newly synthesized lysosomal enzymes and that the complement of lysosomal enzymes transported by either receptor is distinct but largely overlapping. However, neither type of MPR appears to be sufficient for targeting of lysosomal enzymes to lysosomes. This has been demonstrated by expression of either MPR 46 or MPR 300 in cells that lack endogenous MPRs (Kasper et al., 1996).

Does defective lysosomal catabolism in I-cell disease somehow feed back to affect the expression of lysosomal proteins and their receptors? Compared with control fibroblasts, twofold increases in man-6-P/IGF-II receptors have been observed for fibroblasts from patients with I-cell disease. This increase in receptor concentration stems from an increased rate of synthesis, not from differences of receptor stability. Interestingly, when they are exposed to insulinlike growth factors I and II or tumor-promoting phorbol esters, I-cell fibroblasts respond differently from control fibroblasts. These observations indicate multiple regulatory sites in the man-6-P/IGF-II receptor pathway.

Lysosomes have more complex functions than simply being the end point of a degradative pathway. It is now emerging that the limiting membranes around these organelles and their associated proteins (LAMP-1, LAMP-2, and lysosomal integral membrane protein 2/lysosomal membrane glycoprotein 85) exhibit very interesting functions. A multidomain family of proteins implicated in protein trafficking of mannose 6-phosphate receptors and associated cargo from the TGN to endosomes (the GGA or Golgi localizing, γ-adaptin ear homology domain, ARF binding) have now been shown to participate in lysosomal enzyme sorting via the CD-MPR (Doray et al., 2002), and specific GGA interact with an adaptor protein (AP-1) to package MPR cooperatively into coated vesicles at the TGN (Bai et al., 2004). Thus, these interactions may be physiologically important in ensuring proper transfer of the MPR into coated vesicles at the TGN.

The discovery that MPR 300 binds and internalizes IGF-II, which does not contain mannose 6-phosphate residues, raised the fascinating possibility that this receptor may function in two diverse biological processes: protein trafficking and transmembrane signaling. The results of several studies have shown that IGF-II mediates transmembrane signaling through an independent receptor. These responses include stimulation of glycogen synthesis, amino acid

uptake, cell proliferation, Na^+/H^+ exchange, inositol triphosphate production, and Ca^{2+} influx.

In light of the increased number of man-6-P/IGF-II receptors in I-cell fibroblasts, the above interactions of IGF could have far-reaching effects. For example, I-cell disease has not been typically associated with abnormalities in phosphorous/calcium metabolism. The extensive skeletal deformities could involve impairment of mechanisms of orderly calcium deposition. Rather than resulting from a primary disorder of calcium metabolism, it is possible that the bone lesions in I-cell disease are secondary to altered lysosomal processing events in the kidney or liver.

Terman and coworkers (2002) recently reported that although I cells can undergo apoptosis, their response to different proapoptotic agonists is substantially delayed, likely due to functional inefficiency of multiple lysosomal hydrolases resulting from their nonlysosomal compartmentalization. This finding supports the emerging notion that lysosomal enzymes are important inducers/mediators of apoptosis and suggests that I cells may be a suitable model for exploring this process.

THERAPY

The notion that lysosomal storage diseases could be treated by replacing the defective enzyme with its normal counterpart was first suggested by de Duve 40 years ago. Only recently has this approach become available for treatment of three human lysosomal storage diseases: Gaucher disease, Fabry disease, and mucopolysaccharidosis (MPS) type I (Barton et al., 1991; Desnick, 2001; Kakkis et al., 2001). Although promising, this approach has yet to be tried with I-cell disease, and except for symptomatic therapies, I-cell disease remains untreatable. Thus, the clinical course of I-cell disease is chronic, progressive, and fatal.

Because lysosomal hydrolases are synthesized in the rough ER and cotranslationally modified in the rough ER lumen, a major consideration in I-cell disease enzyme replacement therapy is one involving correct insertion of viable phosphotransferase enzyme in the Golgi. Alternatively, therapy could provide multiple normal enzymes to the lysosomes of abnormal cells.

One case of I-cell disease has been reported to exhibit biochemical and clinical improvement following bone marrow transplantation (Yamaguchi et al., 1989). The precise mechanism for this improvement remains obscure because lysosomal storage diseases are not specific to blood cells. However, macrophages are important therapeutic targets for many lysosomal storage diseases. These phagocytic cells have a complicated endocytosis mechanism involving several different receptors (mannose, mannose 6-phosphate, asialoglycoprotein, and various scavenger receptors) for internalization of specific lysosomal enzymes. One plausible explanation is that cells derived from hematopoietic progenitors of the donor (i.e., circulating leukocytes and tissue macrophages) can donate lysosomal enzymes to the deficient cells in all tissues of the host either through secretion or direct cell–cell interactions.

Considerable progress in gene replacement therapy has been made using retroviral vectors carrying lysosomal enzyme-encoding cDNAs since the initial work of Wolfe and coworkers (1990) correcting deficient human and canine fibroblasts. Several new animal models have recently been characterized (Ellinwood et al., 2004). A viral vector gaining increased interest for use in lysosomal storage is the adeno-associated viral vector, which exhibits low toxicity and supports long-term transgene expression in mice as well as large animals. Importantly, most of the cDNAs that encode lysosomal enzymes are relatively small.

A clever alternative to the above enzyme-replacement approach is that of LeBowitz and coworkers (2004) entailing the use of a peptide-based targeting system for delivery of enzymes to lysosomes in a murine MPS type VII model. This strategy depends on the interaction of a fragment of IGF-II with the IGF-II binding site on the bifunctional, IGF-II cation-independent mannose 6-phosphate receptor. A chimeric protein containing a portion of mature human IGF-II fused to the C terminus of human β-glucuronidase containing the catalytic site was taken up by MPS VII fibroblasts in a mannose 6-phosphate-independent manner, and its uptake was inhibited by the addition of IGF-II. The tagged enzyme was delivered effectively to clinically significant tissues in the MPS type VII mouse model and was effective in reversing the storage pathology. Although both mannose-6-phosphate receptors are involved in lysosomal targeting, this approach is ideal for I-cell disease, with the major consideration the generation of a family of chimeric proteins rather than just one to replace only one deficient enzymic activity.

QUESTIONS

1. In certain cell types (e.g., fibroblasts) from patients with I-cell disease, lysosomal enzymes are secreted into the extracellular milieu rather than targeted to lysosomes. In contrast, other cells (such as hepatocytes, Kupffer cells, and leukocytes) contain nearly normal levels of lysosomal enzymes, even though these cells are also deficient in phosphotransferase activity. What do these observations suggest about the targeting of lysosomal enzymes in these different kinds of cells?

2. You are interested in devising a method for prenatal diagnosis of I-cell disease. Using the enzymes listed in Table 17-3, which of these enzyme activities would be most useful in this endeavor and why?

3. Acid sphingomyelinase is a lysosomal enzyme that catalyzes the breakdown of sphingomyelin to ceramide and phosphorylcholine. A deficiency of this enzyme leads to lysosomal accumulation of sphingomyelin in patients with Niemann-Pick disease. Recent data indicate that correct intracellular targeting of acid sphingomyelinase to lysosomes is dependent on the mannose 6-phosphate-mediated pathway. Does this imply that the I-cell patient will present with Niemann-Pick symptoms? Can I-cell disease be viewed as a constellation of many lysosomal storage diseases?

4. In this chapter, we indicate that the metabolic error (i.e., deficiency of phosphotransferase activity in I-cell disease) gives rise to a secondary phenotype of generalized diminished lysosomal enzyme activity. What other metabolic defects in the mannose 6-phosphate-mediated uptake system could result in such a phenotype, and how would you confirm the defect?

Acknowledgments: I thank Dr. Robert DeMars for providing the original photographs first describing the I cell and Dr. Robert H. Glew for his helpful comments and suggestions.

BIBLIOGRAPHY

Bai H, Doray B, Kornfeld S: GGA1 interacts with the adaptor protein AP-1 through a WNSF sequence in its hinge region. *J Biol Chem* **279:**17411–17417, 2004.

Bao M, Elmendorf BJ, Booth JL, et al.: Bovine UDP-*N*-acetylglucosamine:lysosomal-enzyme *N*-acetyl-glucosamine-1-*N*-phosphotransferase.*J Biol Chem* **271**:31446-31451, 1996.

Barton NW, Brady RO, Dambrosia JM, et al.: Replacement therapy for inherited enzyme deficiency—macrophage-targeted glucocerebrosidase for Gaucher's disease. *N Engl J Med* **324**:1464-1470, 1991.

Ben-Yoseph Y, Pack BA, Mitchell DA, et al.: Characterization of the mutant *N*-acetylglucosaminyl-phosphotransferase in I-cell disease and pseudo-Hurler polydystrophy: complementation analysis and kinetic studies. *Enzyme* **35**:106-116, 1986.

Besley GTN, Broadhead DM, Nevin NC, et al.: Prenatal diagnosis of mucolipidosis II by early amniocentesis. *Lancet* **335**:1164-1165, 1990.

Brauker JH, Wang JL: Nonlysosomal processing of cell-surface heparan sulfate proteoglycans. *J Biol Chem* **262**:13093-13101, 1987.

Carey WF, Jaunzems A, Richardson M, et al.: Prenatal diagnosis of mucolipidosis II-electron microscopy and biochemical evaluation. *Prenat Diagn* **19**:252-256, 1999.

Demars R, Leroy JG: The remarkable cells cultured from a human with Hurler's syndrome: an approach to visual selection for *in vitro* genetic studies. *In Vitro* **2**:107-118, 1966.

Denzer K, Weber B, Hille-Rehfeld A, et al.: Identification of three internalization sequences in the cytoplasmic tail of the 46 kd mannose 6-phosphate receptor. *Biochem J* **326**:497-505, 1997.

Desnick RJ: Enzyme replacement and beyond.*J Inherit Metab Dis* **24**:251-265, 2001.

Doray B, Bruns K, Ghosh P, et al.: Interaction of the cation-dependent mannose 6-phosphate receptor with GGA A proteins. *J Biol Chem* **277**:18477-18482, 2002.

Ellinwood NM, Vite CH, Haskins ME: Gene therapy for lysosomal storage diseases: the lessons and promise of animal models. *J Gene Med* **6**:481-506, 2004.

Eskelinen EL, Tanaka Y, Saftig P: At the acidic edge: emerging functions for lysosomal membrane proteins. *Trends Cell Biol* **13**:137-145, 2003.

Falik-Zaccai TC, Zeigler M, Bargal R, et al.: Mucolipidosis III type C: first-trimester biochemical and molecular prenatal diagnosis. *Prenat Diagn* **23**:211-214, 2003.

Hickman S, Neufeld EF: A hypothesis for I-cell disease: defective hydrolases that do not enter lysosomes. *Biochem Biophys Res Commun* **49**:992-999, 1972.

Jansen SM, Groener JEM, Poorthuis VJHM: Lysosomal phospholipase activity is decreased in mucolipidosis II and III fibroblasts. *Biochim Biophys Acta* **1436**:363-369, 1999.

Kakkis ED, Muenzer J, Tiller GE, et al.: Enzyme-replacement therapy in mucopolysaccharidosis I. *N Engl J Med* **18**:182-188, 2001.

Kasper D, Dittmer F, von Figura K, et al.: Neither type of mannose 6-phosphate receptor is sufficient for targeting of lysosomal enzymes along intracellular routes. *J Cell Biol* **134**:615-623, 1996.

Kornfeld S: Trafficking of lysosomal enzymes in normal and disease states.*J Clin Invest* **77**:1-6, 1986.

Kornfeld S: Trafficking of lysosomal enzymes. *FASEB J* **1**:462-468, 1987.

Kornfeld S: Structure and function of the mannose 6-phosphate/insulin-like growth factor II receptor. *Annu Rev. Biochem.* 61: 307-330, 1992.

Kornfeld R, Kornfeld S: Assembly of asparagine-linked oligosaccharides. *Annu Rev Biochem* **54**:631-664, 1985.

Lang L, Reitman M, Tang J, et al.: Lysosomal enzyme phosphorylation. Recognition of a protein-dependent determinant allows specific phosphorylation of oligosaccharides present on lysosomal enzymes.*J Biol Chem* **259**:14663-14671, 1984.

LeBowitz JH, Grubb JH, Maga JA, et al.: Glycosylation-independent targeting enhances enzyme delivery to lysosomes and decreases storage in mucopolysaccharidosis type VII mice.*Proc Natl Acad Sci U.S.A.* **101**:3083-3088, 2004.

Leroy JG, Ho MW, MacBrinn MC, et al.: I-cell disease: biochemical studies. *Pediatr Res* **6**:752-757, 1972.

Mononen IT, Kaartinen VM, Williams JC: A fluorometric assay for glycosylasparaginase activity and detection of aspartylglycosaminuria. *Anal Biochem* **208**:372-374, 1993.

Mueller OT, Honey NK, Little LE: Mucolipidosis II and III. The genetic relationships between two disorders of lysosomal enzyme biosynthesis. *J Clin Invest* **72**:1016-1023, 1983.

Parvathy MR, Mitchell DA, Ben-Yoseph Y: Prenatal diagnosis of I-cell disease in the first and second trimesters.*Am J Med Sci* **297**:361-364, 1989.

Poenaru L, Castelnau L, Tome F, et al.: A variant of mucolipidosis II. Clinical, biochemical and pathological investigations. *Eur J Pediatr* **147**:321-327, 1988.

Raas-Rothschild A, Bargal R, Goldman O, et al.: Genomic organization of the UDP-*N*-acetyl-glucosamine-1-phosphotransferase γ subunit (GNPTAG) and its mutations in mucolipidosis III. *J Med Genet* **41**:e52, 2004.

Sandholzer U, von Figura K, Pohlmann R: Function and properties of chimeric MPR 46-MPR 300 mannose-6-phosphate receptors. *J Biol Chem* **275**:14132-14138, 2000.

Spranger JW, Wiedemann HR: The genetic mucolipidoses. Diagnosis and differential diagnosis. *Humangenetik* **9**:113-139, 1970.

Terman A, Neuzil J, Kagedal K, et al.: Decreased apoptotic response of inclusion-cell disease fibroblasts: a consequence of lysosomal enzyme missorting? *Exp Cell Res* **274:**9–15, 2002.

Verkruyse LA, Natowicz MR, Hofmann SL: Palmitoyl-protein thioesterase deficiency in fibroblasts of individuals with infantile neuronal ceroid lipofuscinosis and I-cell disease. *Biochim Biophys Acta* **1361:**1–5, 1997.

von Figura K, Hasilik A: Lysosomal enzymes mind their receptors. *Annu Rev Biochem* **55:**167–193, 1986.

Wolfe JH, Schuchman EH, Stramm LE, et al.: Restoration of normal lysosomal function in mucopolysaccharidosis type VII by retroviral vector-mediated gene transfer. *Proc Natl Acad Sci U.S.A.* **87:**2877–2881, 1990.

Yamaguchi K, Hayasaka S, Hara S, et al.: Improvement of tear lysosomal enzyme levels after treatment with bone marrow transplantation in a patient with I-cell disease. *Ophthal Res* **21:**226–229, 1989.

Ylikangas PK, Mononen IT: Glycosylasparaginase as a marker enzyme in the detection of I-cell disease. *Clin Chem* **44:**2543–2544, 1998.

18

Inborn Errors of Urea Synthesis

PRANESH CHAKRABORTY and MICHAEL T. GERAGHTY

CASE REPORT

A male infant was born at term following an uncomplicated pregnancy to a healthy woman pregnant for the first time. The delivery was uncomplicated, and growth was appropriate for gestational age. Initially, he was breastfed every 3 h. On the second day of life, he developed mild respiratory distress and fed poorly. Antibiotics were started, but no evidence for an infection was found. On day 3, he became increasingly unresponsive. Arterial blood gases revealed a normal Po_2 with a respiratory alkalosis (pH 7.56, Pco_2 17, HCO_3^- 15 µmol/L (normal 21–28 µmol/L)). Blood glucose and electrolytes were normal. He became comatose and required artificial ventilation. Repeat tests showed persistent respiratory alkalosis, and the plasma ammonium was 1250 µmol/L (normal 5–30). Serum electrolytes, plasma glucose, and lactate and a toxicology screen were normal. Plasma was obtained for quantitative amino acid analysis and quantitative carnitine and for an acylcarnitine profile; urine was obtained for orotic acid measurement and organic acid profiling.

All enteral feeds were stopped. The baby was given intravenous glucose, L-arginine, sodium benzoate, and sodium phenylacetate. Hemodialysis was initiated. At this time, there were no spontaneous respirations, there was no response to painful stimuli, and brainstem reflexes were absent. The plasma amino acid results revealed a glutamine level of 1500 µmol/L (normal 254–823), and citrulline was undetectable (normal 10–34 µmol/L). Quantitative carnitine, plasma acylcarnitine, and urine organic acid profiles were normal. The urine orotic acid concen-

tration was normal at 2 µmol/L. Over the next 12 h, the ammonium concentration decreased to 100 µmol/L; however, the baby remained comatose until the fifth day of life, when he began to regain brainstem reflexes, spontaneous respirations, and response to stimuli. He was treated with a low-protein diet and oral medications.

Blood leukocyte DNA was used for mutation analysis of the carbamoyl phosphate synthetase I (CPSI) gene, and he was found to carry two separate, previously described, disease-causing mutations. Subsequently, the boy suffered global developmental delay, reduced head growth, and a seizure disorder. He had several hospital admissions for episodic hyperammonemia associated with intercurrent viral illnesses. In a subsequent pregnancy, the parents had prenatal diagnosis by molecular analysis of chorionic villus. The fetus was not affected, and a healthy baby was born.

DIAGNOSIS

The clinical syndrome of acute neonatal hyperammonemic encephalopathy described in the case report represents the classical presentation of a patient with a urea cycle disorder (UCD). It is important to note that this neonatal course represents only the most common and severe presentation of a UCD. This holds true for all the diseases listed in Table 18-1, with the exceptions of arginase (ARG-1) deficiency, which results in progressive spasticity of the lower limbs, and of the mitochondrial membrane transporters citrin and ornithine transporter 1 (ORNT-1). Deficiency of citrin results in adult-onset encephalopathy; deficiency of

Table 18-1. Enzymes, Transporters, and Biochemical Features of Inborn Errors of Urea Synthesis

	Disease	Gene	Chromosome	Tissue	Plasma	Urine
Enzymes						
N-Acetylglutamate synthetase (NAGS)	NAGS deficiency	NAGS	17q21.31	Liver	Citrulline ↓ Arginine ↓	Orotic acid ↓
Carbamoyl Phosphate synthase 1 (CPS)	CPS-1 deficiency	CPS1	2q35	Liver	Citrulline ↓ Arginine ↓	Orotic acid ↓
Ornithine transcarbamoylase (OTC)	OTC deficiency	OTC	Xp21.1	Liver	Citrulline ↓ Arginine ↓	Orotic acid ↑↑
Arginino succinate synthetase (AS)	Citrullinemia type 1	AS	9q34	Liver Skin	Citrulline ↑↑ Arginine ↓	Orotic acid ↑ Homocitrulline ↑
Arginino succinate lyase (AL)	aciduria	AL	7cen-q11.2	Liver, skin, RBC	Citrulline ↑ Arinine ↓ ASA, arginino succinic acid ↑↑	Orotic acid ↑
Arginase	Argininemia	ARG1	6q23	Liver, RBC	Citrulline ↑ Arginine ↑↑ ASA, arginino succinic acid ↑	Orotic acid ↑
Transporters						
Ornithine transporter	HHH disease	ORNT1	13q14	Liver, skin	Citrulline ↑ Ornithine ↑	Orotic acid ↑ Homocitrulline ↑↑
Aspartate-glutamate transporter	Citrullinemia type 2	CITRIN	7q21.3	Liver	Citrulline ↑ Arginine normal-↑ ASA ↑	Orotic acid ↑

HHH, hyperornithinemia, hyperammonemia, homocitrullinuria; RBC, red blood cells.

ORNT-1 presents with recurrent hyperammonemia and protein aversion in infancy and childhood. For the remainder, variant clinical syndromes presenting at almost any age have been described.

Several classes of inborn errors of metabolism in addition to inborn errors of urea synthesis can cause neonatal hyperammonemia. These include organic acidurias, fatty acid oxidation defects, amino acidopathies, and mitochondrial respiratory chain disorders. All of these disorders have a number of features in common. Labor and delivery tend to be normal, and there are no predisposing risk factors. Clinical features present after 24 h of life and are progressive. They are inherited, and thus a family history of previously affected children or neonatal deaths may be present. While most are inherited in an autosomally recessive manner, ornithine transcarbamoylase (OTC) deficiency is X linked, and a family history of affected males in the maternal pedigree is not uncommon.

In the majority of cases, a UCD can be distinguished from other inborn errors of metabolism by routinely available clinical chemistry tests such as blood gases, acid/base balance, plasma glucose, ammonium, or lactate. Urea production, and hence serum urea nitrogen, is decreased in UCDs. Respiratory alkalosis has few causes and is an important diagnostic clue of hyperammonemia that should trigger measurement of plasma ammonium.

Alkalosis is a consequence of hyperventilation caused by increased intracerebral ammonium or glutamine accumulation. Hyperammonemia associated with an increased anion gap metabolic acidosis strongly suggests an organic acidemia (e.g., propionic or methylmalonic acidemia), while concomitant hypoketotic hypoglycemia is suggestive of a defect in fatty acid oxidation (e.g., very long chain acyl-CoA dehydrogenase deficiency). Analysis of urine organic acids, plasma carnitine levels, and a plasma acylcarnitine profile will distinguish these groups of disorders and often establishes a definitive diagnosis. As ammonium incorporation into urea occurs primarily in the liver, acute or chronic liver failure may result in hyperammonemia.

Several preanalytical factors can cause a false elevation of the measured plasma ammonium concentration. These include prolonged tourniquet application, hemolysis, specimen transportation at room temperature, delay in plasma separation, and even ambient ammonium from cleaning agents or cigarette smoke. These factors seldom cause measured ammonium concentrations exceeding 100 μmol/L.

Plasma Amino Acids

Quantitation of plasma amino acids, especially of citrulline, is the first step in determining the precise enzyme or transport protein defect in patients with a UCD. If the defect involves *N*-acetyglutamate synthetase (NAGS), CPSI, or OTC, then plasma citrulline concentration will be low. Marked hypercitrullinemia (>2000 μmol/L) is seen in argininosuccinate synthetase (AS) deficiency, while moderate increases (>200 μmol/L, normal undetectable) are found in argininosuccinate lyase (AL) and citrin deficiencies. In AL deficiency, the presence of argininosuccinic acid and its anhydrides further distinguishes this disorder.

Consideration of other plasma amino acids also informs the diagnosis of inborn errors of urea synthesis. The plasma concentrations of glutamine and alanine are often elevated in parallel with or prior to the ammonium concentration as they act as a nitrogen buffer. Plasma arginine concentrations are low since the only synthetic route for arginine in humans is via the urea cycle. In contrast, the arginine concentration is elevated in ARG-1 deficiency. Hyperornithinemia and homocitrullinuria are the characteristic features of the hyperammonemia, hyperornithinemia, and homocitrullinuria (HHH) syndrome caused by a defect in the ornithine transporter (ORNT-1).

Urine Orotic Acid

Orotic acid is an intermediate in pyrimidine synthesis. It is synthesized from the transcarbamylation of aspartic acid and subsequent intramolecular condensation. Any defect in ureagenesis causing accumulation of intracellular carbamoyl phosphate provides substrate for orotic acid synthesis. Therefore, a defect of OTC, or any defect distal to this step, can cause orotic aciduria. The detection of elevated orotic acid in the urine is most useful in differentiating between patients with OTC deficiency and either CPSI- or NAGS-deficient patients in whom orotic aciduria is not present.

Enzymology

Definitive diagnosis of a UCD can be made by specific enzyme assays. A deficiency of OTC,

CPSI, or NAGS is established by liver biopsy as these enzymes are expressed only in liver. Due to random X inactivation, women with OTC deficiency may have normal enzyme activity. The diagnosis in these women must be established by interpretation of the analytes described above or by mutation analysis. AS is assayed in skin fibroblasts as well as liver; AL is assayed in a number of additional tissues, including red and white blood cells. ARG-1 activity is measured in liver or red blood cells.

Mutation Analysis

The genes for the six enzymes and two transporters involved in the urea cycle have been identified, and disease-causing mutations have been reported in each. Most mutations are private, with no common mutation accounting for a large proportion of affected individuals. Mutation testing is therefore complicated by the need to screen for mutations in the entire coding region and, in some cases, for larger gene rearrangements or mutations in regulatory regions.

BIOCHEMICAL PERSPECTIVES

In contrast to the storage of glucose in glycogen, and two-carbon skeleton storage in fatty acids, animals do not possess a mechanism to store nitrogen. Amino acids are primarily used for the synthesis of protein and other nitrogenous compounds such as purine nucleotides and heme. Excess amino acids are deaminated, and their carbon skeletons are used directly as an energy source or for gluconeogenesis or ketogenesis. All animals therefore require a mechanism to excrete excess nitrogen.

Several evolutionary solutions exist to accomplish this. From a teleological viewpoint, there are two main reasons for the development of nonammonium nitrogen-containing excretion products. First, ammonium is poorly soluble and is therefore associated with a large obligate water loss. Second, ammonium is highly toxic to vertebrate central nervous systems. Humans, like other mammals, excrete urea and are therefore called *ureotelic* organisms. This word derives from the Greek *ouron* meaning "urine" and *telos* meaning "end." In contrast, birds and reptiles are primarily *uricotelic* (excreting uric acid), and marine animals are primarily *ammoniatelic* (excreting ammonium).

Urea is synthesized via the urea cycle (Fig. 18-1). In 1932, Krebs and Henseleit published data demonstrating that ornithine stimulates the synthesis of urea without stoichiometric consumption of this intermediate. This apparent catalytic function was determined to be the result of the cyclic nature of the pathway. This was a revolutionary idea since metabolic pathways were conceptualized as purely linear prior to the publication of these observations. In the following sections, we discuss the biochemical processes involved in urea formation.

Nitrogen Sources for Urea

Nitrogen incorporated into urea in the liver originates from both intrahepatic and extrahepatic sources. Urea contains two nitrogen atoms; one is derived from ammonium, while the other is derived from aspartic acid. In liver hepatocytes, ammonium is generated by the oxidative deamination of glutamic acid, catalyzed by glutamate dehydrogenase,

$$\text{Glutamate} + \text{NAD}^+ \leftrightarrow \alpha\text{-Ketoglutarate} + \text{NH}_3 + \text{NADH} + \text{H}^+$$

as well as from deamination of a number of other amino acids. Alternatively, the α-nitrogen from glutamate or alanine may be incorporated into urea via aspartate following transamination of oxaloacetate.

The extrahepatic organs involved in urea synthesis are muscle, small bowel, and kidney. Muscle is an important source of alanine that feeds both the hepatic urea cycle as well as hepatic gluconeogenesis. Once in the hepatocyte, the α-nitrogen of alanine may be transferred to α-ketoglutarate to produce glutamate used for ammoniagenesis or formation of aspartate. The other product of alanine transamination is pyruvate, which is used in gluconeogenesis. Muscle is also a net producer of glutamine, which is used in the small intestine to produce ammonium, alanine, and citrulline. These urea cycle precursors are efficiently transported to the liver via the portal circulation, where ammonium and alanine are metabolized as described. While citrulline may be used in the hepatic urea cycle, a substantial amount is metabolized to arginine by the kidney prior to completion of the urea cycle in the liver. There is also a renal glutaminase activity, which may supply ammonium for the hepatic urea cycle.

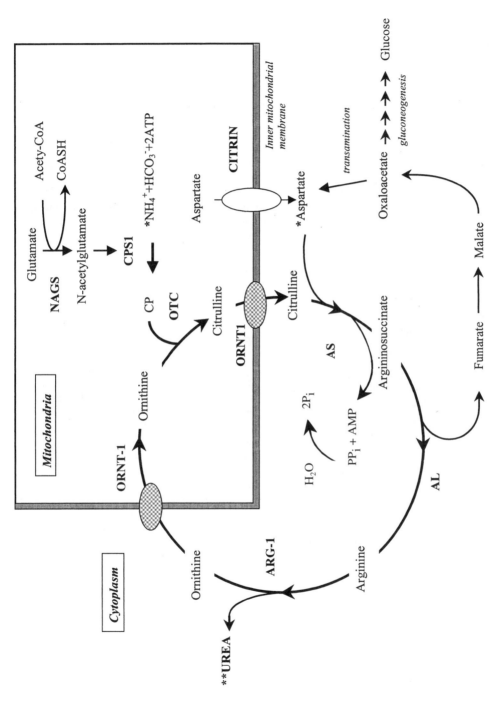

Figure 18-1. Urea synthesis in the liver. Enzymes and transporters are in bold. *N-Acetylglutamate* (NAG), an allosteric activator of carbamoyl phosphate synthetase (CPSI) is formed by NAG synthase (NAGS). Organic acids are competitive inhibitors of this reaction. CP, carbamoyl phosphate; OTC, ornithine transcarbamoylase; AS, argininosuccinate synthetase; AL, argininosuccinate lyase; ARG-1, arginase; ORNT-1, ornithine-citrulline antiporter. Nitrogen atoms are represented as *.

Carbamoyl Phosphate Synthetase I

CPSI catalyzes the formation of carbamoyl phosphate from bicarbonate, ammonium, and two adenosine triphosphate molecules (Fig. 18-1). This first step of the urea cycle occurs in the mitochondrial matrix and assimilates the first of the two nitrogen atoms that will eventually be found in urea. While two ATP molecules are hydrolyzed, there is formation of a lower energy bond in carbamoyl phosphate. CPSI is a homodimer that accounts for 15–30% of the total protein mass in liver mitochondria. N-Acetylglutamate (NAG) is an essential allosteric activator of CPSI activity, and magnesium ions are also required for its activity.

A second, cytosolic CPS activity (CPSII) occurs in mammals as part of the CAD trifunctional protein that catalyzes the first three steps of pyrimidine synthesis (CPSII, asparate transcarbamoylase, and dihydroorotase). The activities of these three enzymes—CPSII, aspartate transcarbamoylase, and dihydroorotase—result in the production of orotic acid from ammonium, bicarbonate, and ATP. CPSII has no role in ureagenesis, but orotic aciduria results from hepatocellular accumulation of carbamyl phosphate and helps distinguish CPSI deficiency from other UCDs. Defects in CPSI classically present with neonatal acute hyperammonemic encephalopathy. The plasma citrulline and urine orotic acid concentrations are both low. A definitive diagnosis can be established by enzyme assay of biopsied liver tissue or by mutation analysis.

N-Acetylglutamate Synthase

NAG is an essential allosteric activator of CPSI activity that is produced by intramitochondrial condensation of acetyl-CoA and glutamate catalyzed by NAGS. NAG plays an important role in the regulation of the urea cycle. Its production is upregulated by arginine; its transport into the cytosolic compartment for degradation is inhibited by glucagon. The clinical and laboratory presentation of NAGS deficiency is indistinguishable from CPSI deficiency. Diagnosis can be confirmed by NAGS mutation analysis.

Ornithine Transcarbamoylase

The second intramitochondrial step of the urea cycle is the reversible condensation of carbamoyl phosphate and ornithine, catalyzed by OTC. The high-energy phosphate bond in carbamoyl phosphate is cleaved during this reaction, and equilibrium favors the forward reaction to produce citrulline. OTC is a homotrimer of 35-kd polypeptides. It has a high specific activity and is found outside the liver in small intestine and to some extent in kidney.

OTC deficiency is the most common urea cycle defect. As it is X linked, affected boys typically have severe disease with neonatal presentation as described in this chapter. The disease in women who carry an OTC mutation on one X chromosome ranges from severe early-onset disease to complete absence of symptoms. Furthermore, affected women may decompensate in the context of a metabolic stress such as an infection or following parturition. OTC-deficient patients have low plasma citrulline and high urine orotic acid. Confirmation of the diagnosis requires mutation analysis or a liver biopsy for enzymology. The carrier status of women is most accurately determined by mutation analysis.

Ornithine-Citrulline Transporter

Citrulline is exchanged for ornithine across the inner mitochondrial membrane by ORNT-1. Ornithine is produced in the cytosol as the final step in the urea cycle and must be returned to the mitochondrial matrix for transcarbamoylation by OTC. A second ornithine-citrulline antiporter (ORNT-2) is also expressed in the liver mitochondria and may attenuate the severity of disease in patients with HHH (Hyperammonemia, Hyperornithinemia, Homocitrullinuria) disease due to ORNT-1 deficiency. This disorder typically manifests later in life with intermittent hyperammonemic encephalopathy and protein aversion. Intramitochondrial ornithine deficiency causes both hyperammonemia and hyperornithinemia due to a lack of substrate for OTC. Homocitrullinuria occurs due to the use of lysine by OTC as an alternate substrate. The diagnosis is confirmed by mutation analysis.

Argininosuccinate Synthetase

Once citrulline is in the cytosol, argininosuccinic acid is formed by condensation of citrulline with aspartate. This is where the second nitrogen atom enters the cycle. Argininosuccinate synthetase, a homotetramer of a 46-kd polypeptide catalyzes the reversible reaction accompanied by hydrolysis of ATP to AMP and pyrophosphate. The subsequent hydrolysis of pyrophosphate shifts the equilibrium to the right and results in the consumption of two high-energy phosphate bonds.

AS activity is found in liver, kidney, skin fibroblasts, and some areas of the brain. Patients with citrullinemia classically present with neonatal hyperammonemic encephalopathy. The disease is easily distinguishable by the very high concentration of citrulline in plasma. Urine orotic acid is usually elevated. The major source of circulating citrulline is extrahepatic. Observations of patients with OTC or AS deficiency who have undergone liver transplantation support this finding. Citrulline levels in such patients do not normalize; they remain low in the OTC-deficient patients and do not entirely normalize in AS-deficient patients.

Argininosuccinate Lyase

AL is found in a wide variety of tissues, including liver, kidney, skin fibroblasts, red blood cells, and parts of the brain. It cleaves argininosuccinic acid to form arginine and fumarate. The formation of arginine via the urea cycle is the reason that it is a nonessential dietary amino acid. The cytosolic fumarate hydratase and malate dehydrogenase activities act on fumarate to produce oxaloacetate. Oxaloacetate may be transaminated to form aspartate, which is then used again in the urea cycle or in cytosolic gluconeogenesis. Patients with AL deficiency or argininosuccinic aciduria usually develop early-onset hyperammonemic encephalopathy. Plasma citrulline is moderately elevated. Argininosuccinic acid and its two anhydrides are detected in the plasma amino acid profile. The anhydrides may coelute with the neutral amino acids isoleucine or leucine or with the dipeptide homocystine in many ion exchange chromatography methods used for amino acid quantitation. Patients often develop progressive liver dysfunction and developmental delays in spite of treatment.

Arginase

The final step of the urea cycle is the cleavage of arginine to release urea and regenerate ornithine. Ornithine then reenters the mitochondria via the ORNT-1 ornithine-citrulline antiporter. ARG-1 is a cytosolic homotrimeric enzyme of 35-kd monomers that is expressed in liver and red blood cells. A second mitochondrial arginase (ARG-2) most likely plays a role in nitric oxide synthesis and is most abundant in brain, kidney, and prostate. ARG-1 deficiency is unique among the urea cycle deficiencies as patients do not present with hyperammonemia and encephalopathy but rather develop progressive spasticity of the lower limbs. Biochem-

ically, the plasma arginine concentration is markedly elevated.

Aspartate-Glutamate Transporter (Citrin)

Citrin is an aspartate-glutamate antiporter that has a role both in the urea cycle and in the malate aspartate shuttle. It is necessary for the transport of aspartate produced in the mitochondria into the cytosol, where it is used by AS. Its role in the malate-aspartate shuttle is to transport cytosolic NADH reducing equivalents into the mitochondria, where they are used in oxidative phosphorylation. Defects in citrin cause citrullinemia type II. Patients manifest later-onset intermittent hyperammonemic encephalopathy as in HHH syndrome.

THERAPY

Treatment for patients with a UCD can be divided into two parts: acute management of hyperammonemic encephalopathy and long-term control to prevent further episodes of hyperammonemia while maintaining normal growth and development.

Acute Management of Hyperammonemic Encephalopathy

Ammonia is very toxic to the CNS, and elevated levels over a period of time result in irreversible brain damage and poor outcome. The treatment of choice for acute hyperammonemic coma is hemodialysis (or peritoneal dialysis if hemodialysis is not available). While awaiting hemodialysis, the following measures should be initiated immediately. Protein (exogenous nitrogen) intake must be stopped and adequate calories provided in the form of glucose and fat to prevent further catabolism (endogenous nitrogen).

Intravenous arginine should be provided since it becomes an essential amino acid in UCDs, and it promotes the formation of citrulline (in AS deficiency) or argininosuccinic acid (in AL deficiency), both of which are excreted in the urine, thus providing some waste nitrogen excretion. In addition, intravenous sodium benzoate and sodium phenylacetate can be given. These provide an alternate mechanism of waste nitrogen disposal (Fig. 18-2). Once the plasma ammonium has been normalized, these drugs can be continued while refeeding (intravenous or enteral) is reintroduced. Oral sodium benzoate and sodium phenylacetate (or alternatively sodium phenylbutyrate) is introduced, but careful matching of nitrogen intake versus waste disposal by these medications must be observed.

Long-Term Management of Patients with Urea Cycle Disorders

Long-term measures to reduce ammonium levels rely on dietary protein restriction. However, this approach alone is not sufficient. Two major advances in treatment have contributed to greater survival and improved outcome. First, the recognition that arginine is an essential amino acid in patients with a UCD, and that deficiency leads to endogenous protein breakdown and negative nitrogen balance. Second, it was recognized that one could provide an alternate pathway for waste nitrogen disposal by the use of sodium benzoate and sodium phenylacetate (Fig. 18-2). Sodium benzoate is conjugated with glycine (a non-essential amino acid containing a single nitrogen atom) to form hippuric acid. Sodium phenylacetate is conjugated with glutamine (a nonessential amino acid with two nitrogen atoms) to form phenylacetylglutamine. Both hippuric acid and phenylacetylglutamine are excreted in the urine.

The combination of protein reduction and alternate waste nitrogen establishes an alternate homeostasis. From the physician's point of view, it remains very difficult to balance the ongoing dynamic of nitrogen turnover using a static treatment of prescribed diet and fixed-dose medications. Changing growth rates, illness, and inadvertent protein intake all contribute to recurrent hyperammonemia. Constant surveillance of growth (e.g., height, weight, head circumference) and of adequate nutrition (blood concentrations of hemoglobin, prealbumin, vitamins, and trace elements) and monitoring of disease control (e.g., plasma concentrations of ammonium, glutamine, alanine, and other amino acids) are required throughout life.

Treatment of CPS, OTC, or NAGS deficiency generally requires daily restriction of dietary nitrogen to 0.7 g/kg/day milk protein and 0.7 g/kg/day essential amino acids. The latter contains roughly 12% nitrogen as opposed to approximately 16% in milk protein. Nitrogen requirements are normally increased in the very young, during accelerated growth phases (infancy and puberty), and after acute illness and surgery. Citrulline supplementation at 170 mg/kg/day is given. Citrulline has two ad-

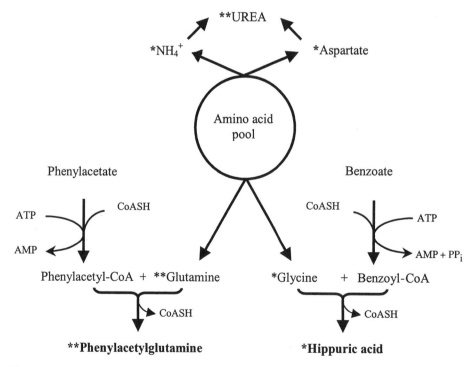

Figure 18-2. Nitrogen (*) incorporation into benzoate and phenylacetate as phenylacetylglutamine (PAG) and hippuric acid (HA) provide an alternate path to urea for waste nitrogen excretion.

vantages over arginine: It is deficient in both of these disorders, and it contains less nitrogen (3 atoms) than arginine (4 atoms), thus minimizing intake of nitrogen. Sodium benzoate (250 mg/kg/day) and sodium phenylactetate (250 mg/kg/day) are recommended. More recently, sodium phenylbutyrate (500 mg/kg/day or 12 g/m²/day), which has a less-offensive odor, has been used. Sodium phenylbutyrate requires one round of fatty acid oxidation to produce phenylacetyl-CoA, which is then conjugated with glutamine. A structural analog of NAG, carbamoylglutamate has been shown to bind and activate CPSI, and several patients with NAGS deficiency have been reported to respond to this compound.

Treatment of AS deficiency is similar to that for CPS and OTC deficiencies. Protein intake is restricted to 1.5–1.75 g/kg/day, and sodium benzoate and sodium phenylacetate (or sodium phenylbutyrate) are provided. Arginine supplementation is required not only for protein synthesis but also to stimulate waste nitrogen excretion in the form of citrulline. Unfortunately, citrulline formation allows incorporation of only a single ammonium nitrogen atom, and its renal clearance is only 25% that of the glomerular filtration rate. Nevertheless, citrulline does provide an alternative, albeit reduced, form of waste nitrogen excretion. Increasing attention is being paid to the long-term metabolic effects of chronic hypercitrullinemia and hyperargininemia as a result of therapy.

In AL deficiency, argininosuccinic acid is a much better waste nitrogen product than citrulline. It contains two waste nitrogen atoms (i.e., one from carbamoyl phosphate and one from aspartate), and its renal clearance is equal to that of the glomerular filtration rate. Thus, arginine supplementation alone allows sufficient waste nitrogen excretion to prevent hyperammonemia. Moderate protein restriction (1.5–1.75 g/kg/day) is also recommended. As in AS deficiency, the long-term metabolic effects of increased citrulline and argininosuccinic acid in this disorder are unclear. Despite adequate treatment (i.e., prevention of recurrent hyperammonemia), many patients have developmental delays and unexplained liver disease.

ARG-1 deficiency is treated by arginine restriction to about 300 mg/day. Patients thus require strict limitation of protein supplemented with essential amino acids. The effectiveness of such treatment is unclear. Patients with ORNT-1 or citrin deficiency are treated with low-protein diets. The use of sodium benzoate or sodium phenylbutyrate to provide an alternate waste nitrogen disposal pathway may be beneficial in these disorders.

QUESTIONS

1. List several metabolic fates of the amino acid arginine in the human. What is the difference between essential and nonessential amino acids? How is this relevant to the treatment of urea cycle defects?
2. Carbamoyl phosphate is a substrate for two separate enzymes. What are the enzymes involved and describe the metabolic fates of their respective products?
3. A patient with OTC deficiency has recurrent hyperammonemic events over a 3-month period despite reduced protein intake and increased doses of sodium benzoate and sodium phenylacetate. What are the factors that need to be considered as a cause of the hyperammonemia in this individual? (Consider the dynamic of nitrogen balance over this period.) What is the likely treatment?
4. Describe how recent advances in molecular genetics have contributed to our knowledge of the urea cycle. List some applications of these advances to medical practice.
5. How does the location of the gene that encodes OTC on the X chromosome contribute to greater clinical variation in patients with deficient enzyme activity? List reasons why the diagnosis of OTC deficiency is difficult in women.

BIBLIOGRAPHY

Brusilow SW: Treatment of urea cycle disorders, *in* Desnick RJ (ed): *Treatment of Genetic Diseases.* Churchill Livingstone, New York, 1991, pp. 79–94.

Brusilow SW, Horwich AL: Urea cycle enzymes, *in* Scriver C, Beaudet A, Sly W, et al. (eds): *The Metabolic and Molecular Bases of Inherited Disease.* 8th ed. McGraw-Hill, New York, 2001, pp. 1909–1963.

Brusilow SW, Maestri NE: Urea cycle disorders: diagnosis, pathophysiology and therapy. *Adv Pediatr* **43:**127–170, 1996.

McCabe RB, Bachmann C, Batshaw, et al (eds): New developments in urea cycle disorders. *Mol Genet Metab* **81**(suppl 1):S4–S91, 2004.

19

Phenylketonuria

WILLIAM L. ANDERSON and STEVEN M. MITCHELL

CASE REPORT

Penny Urick is a 22-year-old G1P0 (one pregnancy, no births) woman who was seen at the family practice clinic for routine prenatal care during her first pregnancy. Mrs. Urick described herself as "generally healthy." At the time of her visit, she stated that she took no medications and had no known medical allergies; however, her medical record revealed a history of phenylketonuria (PKU). When further questioned about her experience with PKU Mrs. Urick stated that:

> I had it as a child, but I am fine now. They put me on this diet, which I had to stay on until I was 18 years old, when I was told that I didn't need it anymore. I haven't had any problems at all since I stopped it.

On further questioning, it became clear that Mrs. Urick was concerned that her baby might inherit the disorder, and that if so, the baby would need to be on the PKU diet. Mrs. Urick described her experience with PKU management as follows:

> It [the diet] was terrible! You can't eat anything everyone else can. I couldn't eat meat or fish or cheese or eggs. While everyone else was eating these things, I had to eat potatoes and cereal. You get pretty sick of potatoes and cereal every day! I had to constantly watch everything I ate, exchanging one thing for another, depending on the amount of phenylalanine the various foods had. I also had to take a daily supplement which was not exactly tasty. I met with a dietician con-

stantly, which my parents said was pretty expensive. Plus, I had to get my blood tested all the time. That's why I stopped the diet when I turned 18. My doctor said he thought it would be fine if I tried stopping it. I haven't had any trouble being on regular food, and I don't want my child to have to go through all of that.

During the clinical interview Mrs. Urick expressed an interest in knowing more about changes in treatment should her baby have PKU. She was especially curious about tetrahydrobiopterin (BH_4) therapy, which she learned about while searching the Web, where she found several sites indicating that BH_4 therapy may be helpful in some patients with PKU.

DIAGNOSIS

The standard diagnostic test for PKU is the Guthrie bacterial inhibition assay. The test uses the growth of a strain of bacteria on a specially prepared agar plate as a sign for the presence of high levels of phenylalanine (PA), phenylpyruvate, or phenyllactate. The compound β-2-thienylalanine will inhibit the growth of the bacterium *Bacillus subtilis* (ATCC 6051) on minimal culture media. If PA, phenylpyruvate, or phenyllactate is added to the medium, then growth is restored. Such compounds will be present in excess in the blood or urine of patients with PKU. If a suitably prepared sample of blood or urine is applied to the seeded agar plate, then the growth of the bacteria in the test will be a positive indicator for PKU in the patient.

Despite the fact that widespread newborn screening for PKU has been in place since the 1960s, accurate data regarding the incidence and prevalence of PKU is sparse, and it becomes difficult to identify the best epidemiological evidence or clinical experience to use as the basis for a recommendation for Mrs. Urick or her baby. It is clear from existing data that Mrs. Urick's PA levels ought to be controlled as tightly as possible during her pregnancy. However, the questions of how closely dietary restriction should be controlled in nonpregnant adults and which other treatments are most effective and available are currently under debate. This chapter presents the basic science and current best clinical evidence regarding the most current potential care for Mrs. Urick and her baby.

EPIDEMIOLOGY

Some of the most convincing data regarding the epidemiology of PKU comes from the 1994 Newborn Screening Report of the Council of Regional Networks for Genetic Services. However, these data are limited, and there was a lack of uniformity of criteria used by individual states to screen for PKU and non-PKU hyperphenylalaninemia (HPA). In addition, there was considerable variability in the actual data reported. In the United States, the total incidence of phenylalanine hydroxylase (PAH) deficiency of varying degrees is about 1 in 10,000 births, and the prevalence of the heterozygous condition is roughly 2%. The incidence of frank PKU (serum PA levels >1 mM) is 1 in 13,500 to 19,000 births. There is wide variation regarding the reporting of the incidence of non-PKU HPA; however, current composite estimates suggest an incidence of 1 in 48,000 among newborns. HPA is less common in blacks, Asians, and Hispanics, with a higher incidence in white and Native Americans (NIH Consensus Statement, 2000).

CLINICAL MANIFESTATIONS

The clinical course of PKU is progressive and exhibits considerable variability among individuals. Mental retardation is the hallmark of the disease in untreated patients, but other neurological manifestations are often present (Table 19-1). Newborns initially appear normal but fail to attain early developmental milestones, including failure to roll by 4 months, failure to sit by 6

Table 19-1. Clinical Manifestations of Hyperphenylalanemia

Mental retardation
Cerebral and basal ganglion dysfunction
Rigidity, chorea, spasms, and hypotonia
Hyperactivity
Seizures
Gait abnormalities
Unstable temperature regulation
"Mousy" odor of skin, hair, and urine

months, failure to walk by 1 year, and delayed language development. These delays are usually noticeable by 6 months. All patients with untreated PKU will be mentally retarded, which cannot be accurately diagnosed until after age 6 years but can be strongly suspected based on poor language skills and late motor milestones. Mental dysfunction worsens during early childhood, with increasing dietary consumption of PA and continuing myelination during brain development. Commonly, patients eventually develop hyperactivity, abnormalities of gait, disturbances in posture and stance, seizures, and severe mental retardation, including autisticlike syndrome. Once brain maturation is complete, the condition is thought by some physicians to stabilize, while other investigators have documented neurological difficulties in adults who do not strictly adhere to a PA-restricted diet and recommend that all affected individuals remain on the diet for their lifetime (Koch, 2002; Longo, 1998; NIH Consensus Statement Online, 2000; Poustie, 2004).

The precise cause of brain damage in patients with PKU is unclear and likely multifactorial (Table 19-2) but most probably reflects the accumulation of aromatic metabolites of PA in neural tissues. Due to accumulation of phenylacetate, patients often have what is described as a "mousy" odor to their skin, hair, and urine. Hypopigmentation results from decreased availability of tyrosine and competitive inhibition of tyrosinase by an overabundance of PA (Longo, 2001; NIH Consensus Statement Online, 2000; Scriver, 2000).

BIOCHEMICAL PERSPECTIVES

The biochemical basis of Ms. Urick's problem is an inability to dispose of excess dietary PA. Mild forms of the condition lead to HPA, and in severe cases of PKU, mental retardation results from

Table 19-2. Potential Causes of Impaired Brain Development in PKU

Increased competitive inhibition of transport of other amino acids required for protein synthesis in the brain

Increased oxidative stress

Increased production of metabolites of phenylalanine that inhibit synthesis of a variety of substances required for normal brain growth

Inhibition of *N*-methyl-*D*-aspartate receptors, which are involved in memory and learning

Competitive inhibition of transport of other amino acids required for protein synthesis

Impaired polyribosome formation or stabilization

Reduced synthesis/increased degradation of myelin

Decreased formation of norepinephrine and serotonin

Altered myelin structure and function

accumulation of PA in the blood and tissues. Normal serum PA levels are less than 0.24 mM, and in an individual with PKU, this level increases above 0.9 mM. Normally, PA is not detected in the urine; however, an individual with PKU can excrete as much as 2 g of PA per day in the urine. Non-PKU HPA results from a partial deficiency of PAH, with serum PA levels in the range 0.24–0.9 mM. Both conditions are autosomal recessive disorders that are the result of different mutations to the PAH enzyme; consequently, severity and clinical presentation varies considerably between individuals.

As illustrated in Figure 19-1, there are two different competing pathways available for the catabolism of PA. One pathway involves transamination of PA to phenylpyruvate, followed by the phenylpyruvate dehydrogenase reaction to form phenylacetyl-CoA. The products of these reactions (phenylpyruvate, phenylacetyl-CoA) and the excretion products phenylacetate and phenyllactate cannot be further metabolized and consequently accumulate in the blood, urine, and tissues.

A second competitive pathway for the disposal of PA requires the initial conversion of PA into tyrosine. This reaction is catalyzed by the enzyme PAH (phenylalanine-4-monooxygenase; EC 1.14.16.1). The resulting tyrosine molecule can then be catabolized into fumarate and acetoacetate. Both products are nontoxic and can be further catabolized in the citric acid cycle. In Mrs. Urick and the majority of individuals suffering from HPA and PKU, there is a defect in the PAH enzyme system (NIH Consensus Statement Online, 2000). In the absence of an effective PAH, the alternate transaminase pathway is the only available route for the disposal of PA.

Phenylalanine Hydroxylase

A schematic representation of the phenylalanine hydroxylation reaction is shown in Figure 19-2. PAH reduces and cleaves molecular oxygen into two hydroxyl groups. One of the hydroxyl functional groups is found in the reaction product tyrosine, while the other oxygen atom is used to modify the reaction cofactor BH_4, creating the pterin 4α-carbinolamine.

PAH, a nonheme iron-containing enzyme, is a member of a larger BH_4-dependent amino acid hydroxylase family. In addition to PAH, the enzyme family includes tyrosine hydroxylase and tryptophan hydroxylase. The enzymes in this family participate in critical metabolic steps and are tissue specific. PAH catabolizes excess dietary PA and synthesizes tyrosine. In adrenal and nervous tissue, tyrosine hydroxylase catalyzes the initial steps in the synthesis of dihydroxyphenylalanine. In the brain, tryptophan is converted to 5-hydroxytryptophan as the first step of serotonin synthesis. Consequently, these enzymes are highly regulated not only by their expression in different tissues but also by reversible phosphorylation of a critical serine residue found in regulatory domains of the three enzymes. Since all three enzymes are phosphorylated and dephosphorylated by different kinases and phosphatases in response to the need for the different synthetic products, it is not unexpected that the exact regulatory signal for each member of the enzyme family is unique.

Although regulation is unique for each member of the aromatic amino acid hydroxylase family, the catalytic mechanism and cofactor requirements for members of the family are identical. During the reactions of all three enzymes, the dioxygen molecule is cleaved and incorporated as a hydroxyl group into both the aromatic amino acid and BH_4. Each enzyme in the family displays its own unique substrate specificity profile. Two interesting questions about this enzyme family relate to the actual hydroxylation mechanism and how enzyme activity is altered by changes in BH_4 levels. Problems in any one of these hydroxylation systems can arise from either an inadequate supply of the BH_4 cofactor or a defect in the enzyme or its expression.

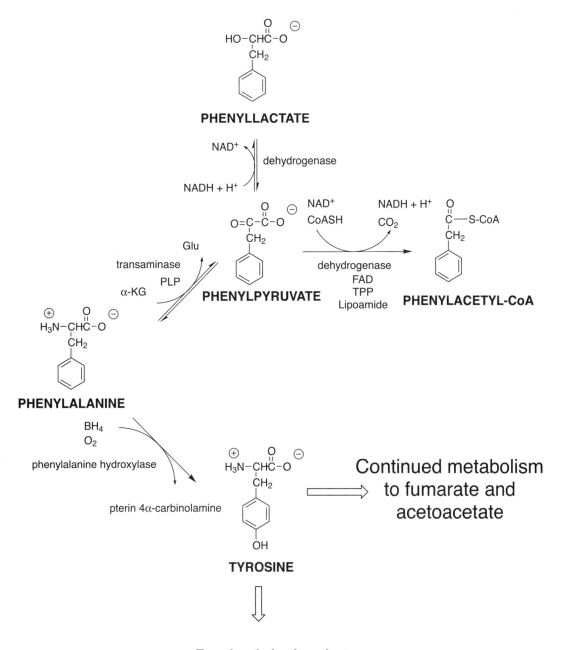

PHENYLLACTATE

PHENYLPYRUVATE

PHENYLACETYL-CoA

PHENYLALANINE

TYROSINE

Continued metabolism to fumarate and acetoacetate

Tyrosine derived products

Figure 19-1. Pathways for the metabolic disposal of phenylalanine. There are two competitive pathways for the disposal of phenylalanine. One pathway involves a transaminase enzyme phenylpyruvate, while the first step in the second pathway requires phenylalanine to be initially converted to tyrosine. Continued metabolism of the phenylpyruvate produced by the first pathway leads to products that cannot be further metabolized, while tyrosine can be converted into citric acid cycle intermediates. Glu, glutamate; αKG; CoASH, coenzyme A; BH_4, tetrahydrobiopterin; TPP, thiamine pyrophosphate.

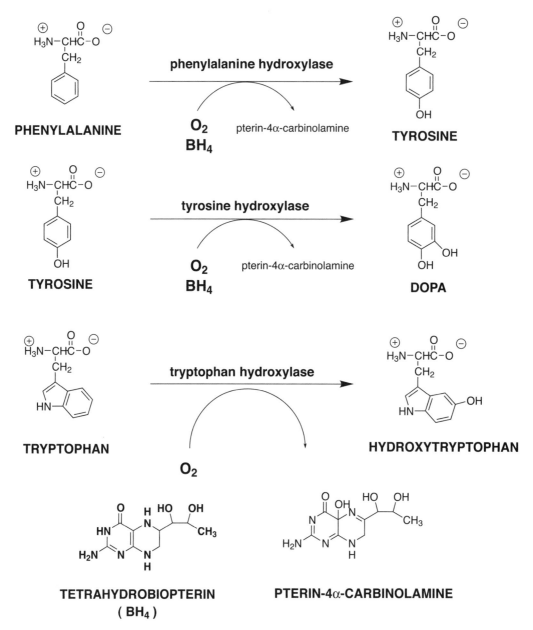

Figure 19-2. Aromatic amino acid hydroxylase reaction. Aromatic amino acids are hydroxylated by a common mechanism catalyzed by a family of hydroxylases. The enzyme family consists of phenylalanine hydroxylase, tyrosine hydroxylase, and tryptophan hydroxylase. In addition to substrate, all three enzymes require molecular oxygen and the cofactor tetrahydrobiopterin. Tetrahydrobiopterin is consumed in this reaction and converted into pterin 4α-carbinolamine. DOPA, dihydroxyphenylalanine.

Biopterin Synthesis and Recycling

Mrs. Urick's questions to her physician concerned the possible effectiveness of elevating BH_4 levels as a therapeutic intervention for this condition, which raises the possibility of BH_4 deficiency as a cause of her disease. As discussed, since BH_4 is consumed in the hydroxylation reaction, without adequate BH_4 it is possible that a BH_4 deficiency could be a causative factor in this disease. BH_4 can be either synthesized *de novo* from GTP or salvaged from the pterin-4α-carbinolamine product of the hydroxylase reaction. Both synthetic and recycling pathways for BH_4 are illustrated in Figure 19-3. Considering that these metabolic pathways include a number of different steps, there are several possible sources for an error in BH_4 production, and patients with most of these possible errors have been identified.

The specific difficulty in answering Mrs. Urick's question is illustrated by Figure 19-4, which compares the frequency of PKU cases known to be caused by a BH_4-related problem with reports on effectiveness of BH_4 supplementation therapy. Although defects in biopterin synthesis and the BH_4 recycling system account for less than 2% of all PKU cases (NIH Consensus Statement Online, 2000), there is a growing body of data that suggests that a significantly higher percentage of PKU and HPA cases will respond favorably (decreased serum PA levels) to BH_4 therapy. In one study, 41% of 41 random patients had PAH mutations that responded to BH_4 therapy (Trefz and Blau, 2003), while in a retrospective study of 1919 patients with mild PKU and HPA, greater than 60% responded to BH_4 therapy (Bernegger and Blau, 2002).

Both of these observations have led to suggestions that, in all newly diagnosed cases of PKU and HPA, serum levels of PA should be monitored following a BH_4 challenge to determine if the serum PA levels decrease in response to the BH_4 challenge. It has been suggested that this BH_4 challenge test be a routine part of patient management (Trefz and Blau, 2003). If the defect in the PAH enzyme resides in the BH_4 binding site and results in a lower affinity for the cofactor, then one can easily justify a mechanistic rationale for the proposed BH_4 therapy in more than 2% of patients.

Enzyme Structure

The active PAH enzyme is a tetramer of identical polypeptides. Each polypeptide subunit is composed of three different domains: an amino terminal regulatory domain, the iron-containing catalytic domain, and a carboxyl terminal polymerization domain. To date, the crystal structure of the intact enzyme has yet to be elucidated; however, the protein database contains several high-resolution human and rat PAH structures that were first truncated by removal of either the regulatory or the polymerization domain,

thereby allowing the structure of the intact protein to be determined by combining different crystal structures. A schematic structure of the monomeric regulatory and catalytic domains of the rat enzyme is illustrated in Figure 19-5.

Fitzpatrick (2003) reported that when several different crystal structures are superimposed on a single PAH monomer, the different molecules demonstrate a remarkable conservation of three-dimensional shape in the catalytic domain for all members of the enzyme family. Moreover, the catalytic domains exhibit about 80% amino acid sequence homology. As would be expected by both their different tissue expression and their biological functions, structural differences between the regulatory domains are significantly greater.

Erlandsen and Stevens (1999) used these different overlapping structures to create a composite model of the intact enzyme. The ferric iron atom, located in a deep pit of the catalytic domain, is coordinated by interactions with histidine residues, glutamic acid, water molecules, and the BH_4 cofactor. Prior to catalysis, the ferric iron must be reduced to the ferrous state. It has been assumed that BH_4 is the physiological reducing agent; however, this has yet to be confirmed. Descriptions of the iron coordination are variable and consist of reports of octahedral coordination and distorted pentahedral coordination, depending on which crystal structure is analyzed, suggesting structural alterations are possible on crystallization. More important, this observation complicates attempts at using crystal structure to propose or test a catalytic mechanism for the enzyme because unique contact residues and bond angles vary between crystal structures. Moreover, until recently, crystal structures of enzyme-substrate complexes have not been available.

The location of the BH_4 binding site and the amino acid contact to BH_4 are very relevant to Mrs. Urick's questions about the effectiveness of dietary BH_4 supplementation as a therapeutic intervention. This site has been located in several different structures and provides a second possible explanation for the large number of putatively BH_4-responsive individuals. Presumably, if the cofactor binding site represents a mutational "hot spot," then mutations to residues in the BH_4 binding site could lower the affinity for the cofactor, thus requiring an increased concentration of the cofactor to saturate the binding site, resulting in a higher-than-expected frequency of BH_4-responsive

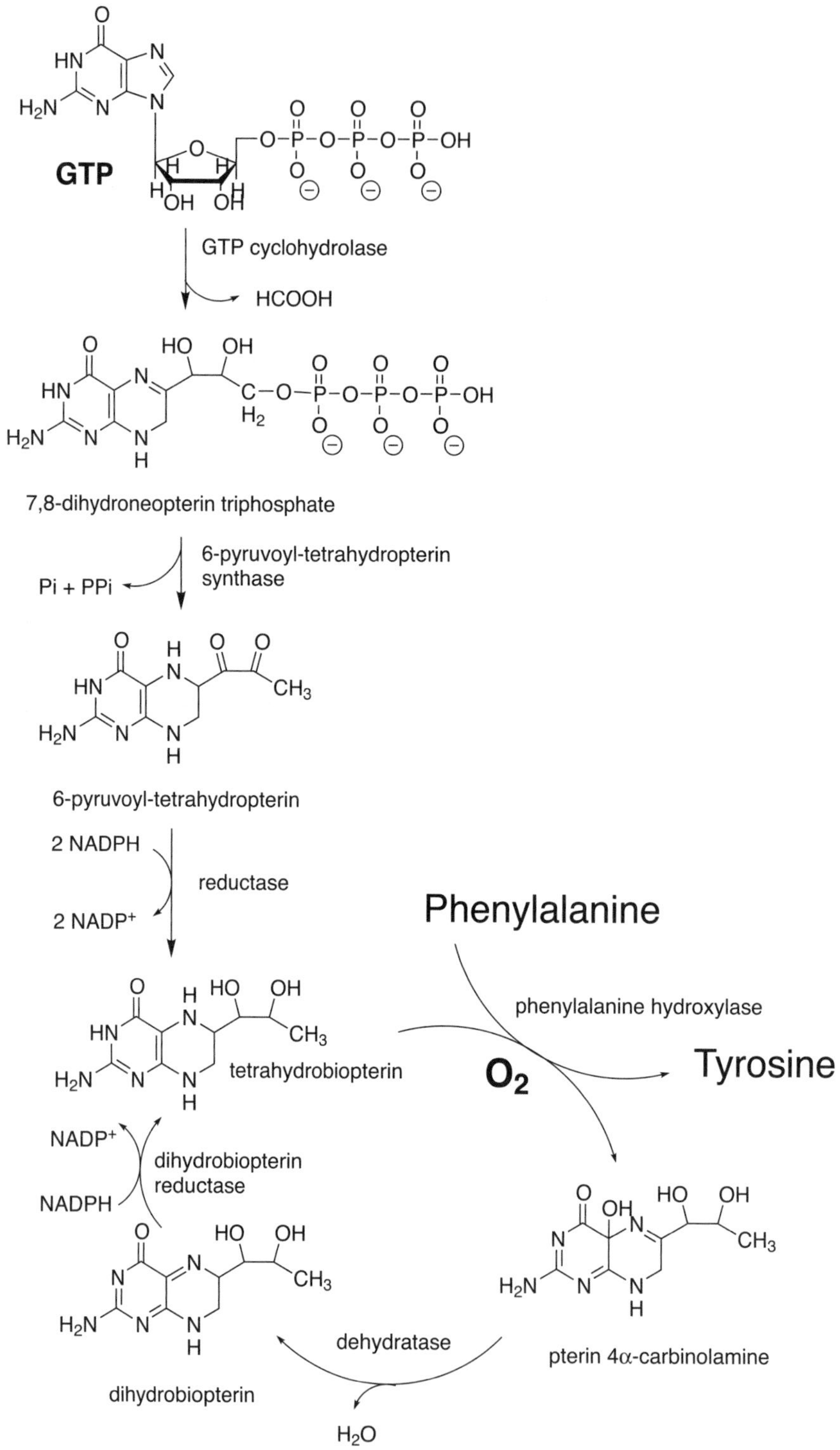

Figure 19-3. *De novo* biopterin synthesis and recycling. Tetrahydrobiopterin can be synthesized *de novo* from GTP or resynthesized from the pterin 4α-carbinolamine.

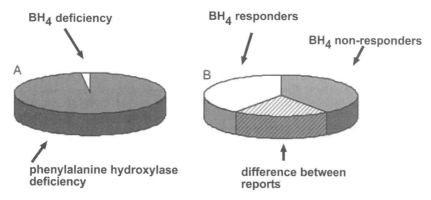

Figure 19-4. Differences between the frequency of phenylketonuria (PKU) and hyperphenylalaninemia (HPA) caused by problems in tetrahydrobiopterin (BH$_4$) metabolism and reports of positive therapeutic responses to BH$_4$ therapy. (*A*) Frequency of PKU and HPA cases documented to be caused by defects in BH$_4$ metabolism. □, Clinical cases documented to be caused by defects in BH$_4$; ■, clinical cases presumable due to a defect in the phenylalanine hydroxylase enzyme. (*B*) Frequency of PKU and HPA cases that have been reported to respond positively to BH$_4$ therapy. ■, Positive response to BH$_4$ therapy; ▨, no response to BH$_4$ therapy. Different reports in the literature varied with respect to the numbers of individuals responding to BH$_4$ therapy. The differences in reported numbers of BH$_4$ responders are indicated by the boxes with cross-hatching.

enzymes. Mutations of the PAH enzyme have been intensively studied, and currently 400 different mutations have been documented. By identifying single-nucleotide mutations and mapping the polymorphisms, the amino acid change involved in the mutation, and the location of the mutation, one should be able to predict whether a particular patient might be responsive to BH$_4$ therapy. The database on the mutations to PAH is extensive and rapidly growing. This database includes not only natural mutations to the enzyme but also the results of *in vitro* expression of laboratory manipulations to the PAH gene. An in-depth discussion of these modifications is beyond the scope of this chapter. Moreover, these data have been summarized (Pey et al., 2003; Teigen et al., 1999). One of the most up-to-date listings of PAH mutations can be obtained from the PAH Web site (http://www.pahdb.mcgill.ca).

The problem with a genetic approach to investigating BH$_4$ responsiveness is that (1) there is no evidence that the BH$_4$-binding site represents a mutational hot spot, and (2) mutations outside the known BH$_4$-binding site also have been shown to produce a BH$_4$-responsive PAH (Bernegger and Blau, 2002; Steinfeld et al., 2001). The dissociation between the location of the mutation in the x-ray crystal structure and

BH$_4$ responsiveness has led Dr. Blau to create a functional database for the PAH molecule in which individuals can contribute to the functional mapping of genetic mutations (http://www.bh4.org).

Catalytic Mechanism

The mechanism by which elevated BH$_4$ levels enhance the catalytic effectiveness of a mutated PAH, even when the mutation does not involve the BH$_4$-binding site, is unclear. The answer to this problem will likely be found in a fuller understanding of the enzyme mechanism itself. Understanding the catalytic mechanism of the PAH enzyme and how the dioxygen molecule is cleaved have proven to be difficult experimental challenges. Kinetic investigations indicated that a ternary complex of enzyme, biopterin, and oxygen must be formed prior to the binding of PA. In the active site of the enzyme, the oxygen molecule replaces one of the water molecules and is coordinated between the iron atom and the BH$_4$ cofactor. This complex, illustrated in Figure 19-6, effectively prevents substrate access to the oxygen molecule and suggests that a reactive oxygen molecule must be formed prior to substrate binding. Two different species have been suggested as the active oxygen molecule. One possibility is an

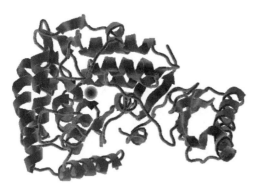

Catalytic domain   Regulatory domain

Figure 19-5. Phenylalanine hydroxylase structure. Ribbon structure of the catalytic and regulatory domain of the rat phenylalanine hydroxylase enzyme (PDB access number 1PHZ) (Kobe et al., 1999). The catalytic domain is on the left and a nonheme iron atom is present in the center of the domain. The regulatory domain is shown on the left.

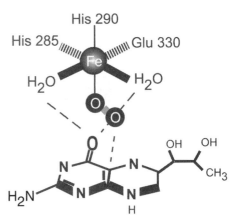

Figure 19-6. Hypothetical active site complex of phenylalanine hydroxylase. The nonheme iron atom of phenylalanine hydroxylase is coordinated with protein amino acid residues (top of the figure) and molecular oxygen. The BH_4 cofactor is also coordinated with molecular oxygen (bottom of the figure). It has been suggested that this complex decomposes to either an iron-oxygen complex or a biopterin-4 hydroperoxide complex prior to interaction with the amino acid substrate.

active Fe(IV)-oxygen complex (Bugg, 2001; Klinman, 2001; Solomon et al., 2000); the other suggestion requires the biopterin cofactor to be converted into a 4-hydroperoxide (Eberlein et al, 1984). Evidence supporting both hypotheses exist, but an in-depth evaluation of that evidence is beyond the scope of the present discussion. These data have been reviewed by several investigators (Bassan et al., 2003; Fitzpatrick, 2003), who concurred that that the Fe(IV)-oxygen intermediate is the most likely oxidizing species.

The difficulty in obtaining crystal structures from active substrate enzyme complexes has significantly hampered the ability to confirm the hypotheses about the mechanism of PAH action. This problem was solved by Andersen and coworkers (2002) using 3-(2-thienyl)-L-alanine as a substrate analogue. These authors reported that, during catalysis, the enzyme undergoes major structural changes as part of the activation of the dioxygen molecule. They also reported that a tyrosine residue (Tyr 138) thought to be exposed on the surface of the enzyme is moved to the interior and may play an important, but as-yet-unrecognized, role in the active enzyme-substrate complex.

These new findings also raise questions about the assignment of residues to roles in catalysis and suggest that the mutation databases should

be reevaluated in the light of these dramatic conformational changes. The possibility of a change in global enzyme conformation playing a role in the catalytic mechanism also provides an explanation for the observations related to the successful use of high levels of BH_4 in patient treatment (Erlandsen and Stevens, 2001). These investigators argued that a catalytic mechanism involving major structural changes could be dramatically influenced by cofactor levels. Mutations that cause slow or delayed folding of the enzyme would be cleared and degraded by the proteosome system. However, if high levels of BH_4 cofactor were present during the folding, then the interaction with enzyme might stabilize the enzyme or enhance proper folding, which might explain the observation that a BH_4 effect is found in more than just a few patients.

In the past two years the number of reported BH_4 responsive cases of HPA and classical PKU has increased dramatically, suggesting that the BH_4 response rate may be far greater than initially observed. Moreover, BH_4 responses have even been reported in classical PKU (Matalon et al., 2005). In response to this changing view about PKU, in addition to the holding the "First International Conference on the Role of BH_4 and Phenylketonuria Treatment" in 2005, the journal, Molecular Genetics and Metabolism, devoted an entire supplement to "New Developments in Phenylketonuria and Tetrahydrobiopterin Research" (Kock et al., 2005). Although the mechanism of the BH_4 effect remains elusive, evidence is accumulating that in addition to an elevated Km for BH_4 by the phenylalanine hydroxylase enzyme, BH_4: increases enzyme stability, protects against proteolytic degradation, has chaperon-like activity, alters regulation of BH_4 synthesis, induces PAH expression and the stability of its mRNA (Erlandsen et al., 2004; Blau and Erlandsen, 2004). The altered view about the potential role of BH_4 therapy in PHA and classic PKU has led to the suggestion that all cases of HPA and PKU be evaluated using the BH_4 loading test (Fiege et al., 2005). To date the only contraindication for BH_4 therapy appears to be the cost of the cofactor.

THERAPY

Testing

Unlike most other genetic diseases, PKU is unique in that, once diagnosed, it can be successfully treated. Moreover, while medical intervention is not inexpensive, it is far more cost-effective than treating the manifestations of the disease itself (NIH Consensus Statement, 2000). For these reasons, screening for HPA is public policy in the United States and many other countries. In patients with HPA, plasma PA levels are typically normal at birth but quickly rise after the initiation of protein feedings.

Screening must take place within 3 weeks after birth to prevent mental retardation. Blood PA levels are measured using the Guthrie bacterial inhibition assay. Elevated values are then confirmed using quantitative amino acid analysis. If screening reveals HPA (plasma levels persistently greater than 0.125 mM), then investigation of BH_4 homeostasis must be initiated to rule out dihydropteridine reductase deficiency. Deficiency of dihydropteridine reductase is confirmed by direct enzyme measurement in dried blood samples (Dhondt, 2002). Dihydrobiopteridine deficiency and subsequent block in BH_4 synthesis can also be detected *in utero* via assays on cultured amniocytes.

If BH_4 levels are normal, then HPA due to a problem with PAH becomes established by exclusion. About half of these patients will have PKU, with PA levels above 1 mM, and half will have non-PKU HPA, with PA levels between 0.125 and 1.0 mM. While not widespread as yet, DNA analysis is becoming more common and clinically relevant (NIH Consensus Statement Online, 2000; Scriver, 2000).

Treatment

As discussed in the preceding section, of all genetic diseases, screening for PKU is important because the manifestations of the disease can be prevented with proper medical intervention. Currently, the primary treatment of patients with HPA is dietary restriction of PA, which was first introduced by Bickel in 1953. Normal PA intake is more than 1000 mg per day, but in patients with PKU, only 250–500 mg/day PA can be tolerated. There are a variety of semisynthetic diets currently available that are devoid of or low in PA.

It is important to note that, while PA intake must be significantly reduced in affected individuals, PA is still an essential amino acid and cannot be completely eliminated from the diet. As such, growth rate and PA levels need to be monitored regularly. Unfortunately, as clearly identified by Mrs. Urick, these diets are often expensive and universally unpalatable. As such, compliance is frequently a clinical issue (Bodamer, 2003; Scriver, 2000). In this case, the physician is left with several questions: Was it appropriate for Mrs. Urick to discontinue her diet? What are the implications, if any, for her unborn baby? and Will she or her baby be a candidate for BH_4 therapy?

Unfortunately, few clinical studies have investigated the efficacy and timing of specific dietary intervention with patients who have PKU. In fact, there are no randomized clinical trials comparing treatment from diagnosis versus no treatment at all. On the other hand, evidence from nonrandomized studies overwhelmingly demonstrated that implementation of dietary restriction of PA early in life can significantly decrease the mental retardation and neurological impairments associated with PKU. While the need for intervention via a PA-restrictive diet is clear, some questions still remain regarding exactly how early to begin treatment, which dietary supplements should be added to PA restriction, what degree of metabolic control should be achieved, and when, if ever, the diet should be discontinued (Koch, 2002; NIH Consensus Online, 2000; Poustie and Rutherford, 2004).

Current evidence suggests dietary restriction should begin as soon as possible, preferably within the first week of life (NIH Consensus Statement Online, 2000), but certainly within the first 20 days after birth (Poustie and Rutherford, 2004). There is considerable evidence that earlier initiation of dietary restriction directly corresponds to higher IQ levels, and elevated PA levels even in the first 2 weeks of life may affect development of the visual system (NIH Consensus Statement Online, 2000).

Questions arise when discussing the necessary degree of control of plasma PA levels. While results from a variety of studies vary widely and there is no consensus what the optimal plasma PA level should be, current best evidence suggests that tighter metabolic control (low PA levels) correlates directly with improvements in IQ, motor skills, attention span, behavioral skills, and cognitive ability. In most of these areas, effects of lower PA levels have beneficial effects throughout the life of the patient (NIH Consensus Statement Online, 2000).

As discussed, PA restriction diets are poorly palatable, difficult to follow, and expensive, thus making compliance difficult. These diets also require regular support from specialists and may result in inappropriate eating behaviors. In addition, proper nutrition can be difficult to maintain. Adding to the problem, physicians have been giving patients inconsistent advice on the appropriate length of time the diet should be maintained (Poustie and Rutherford, 2004).

As such, and as illustrated by Mrs. Urick's experience, reduced compliance often begins in midchildhood. By late adolescence, a significant number of affected individuals have discontinued the diet. While screening and intervention for patients with PKU have been widely acceptable and established as public policy for over 40 years, there is considerable uncertainty about when, if ever, the diet should be discontinued and what other dietary supplements should be included. It seems clear that discontinuing the diet prior to 6 years of age has a negative effect on performance on IQ tests (NIH Consensus 2000; Poustie and Rutherford, 2004). However, it is less clear that discontinuation at later ages has adverse consequences and, if so, to what degree.

There are some data suggesting that continuing the diet as long as possible may be beneficial to long-term neurological health. First, upper motor neuron disturbances have been documented in older children and adults who have returned to a normal diet. In addition, elevated PA levels in these individuals can lead to white matter changes in the brain, as demonstrated by magnetic resonance imaging (Poustie and Rutherford, 2004). Adults who discontinue PA restriction do not usually exhibit poorer performance on IQ tests, but they do not do as well on measures of attention span or speed of processing. Surveys of physicians and evidence from several studies suggested that, if possible, the PA restrictive diet should be maintained throughout life for best neurological outcome in the individual. However, there is some evidence that metabolic control may be able to be relaxed later in life (NIH Consensus Statement Online, 2000).

Supplementation for patients who are restricting PA intake varies with the particular diet that patient is receiving. Many patients require vitamins and other supplements along with other essential amino acids that may be deficient in the restricted diets (Poustie and Rutherford, 2004). Several studies have investigated tyrosine supplementation. Given that individuals with PKU suffer from both an excess of PA and a deficiency of tyrosine, one would expect that tyrosine supplementation might be helpful in addressing the manifestations of this disease. However, there have yet to be shown any significant differences between patients taking tyrosine supplements and those who are not, other than an increase in plasma tyrosine. Due to the small number of individuals looked at in these studies, a definitive answer to tyrosine supplementation cannot be reached with certainty as yet, and a large multicenter randomized clinical trial would be necessary to do so.

EPILOGUE

Mrs. Urick immediately began following a restrictive diet and successfully maintained plasma PA levels below 0.9 mM. She reported that the diet was hard to follow, but it was well worth it to have a healthy child. She was also very interested in exploring BH$_4$ therapy. While she was unable to enroll in a clinical evaluation of BH$_4$ treatment during her pregnancy, she maintained good plasma PA levels throughout gestation, carried the baby to term, and delivered a healthy baby girl, who was screened for PKU and found not to have the disease. After the birth of her baby, Mrs. Urick decided to try to continue the restrictive diet "at least for a while." She also expressed interest in finding out more about BH_4 supplementation and other potential treatments.

QUESTIONS

1. How would you justify the observation that that two different patients possessing the same mutation in the PAH enzyme may exhibit very different phenotypes with respect to PA metabolism?
2. How can you explain the observation that in some individuals with a mutation to the PAH enzyme outside the BH_4-binding site show a decrease in serum PA levels when given dietary BH_4?
3. Although mutations to dihydrobiopterin reductase and PAH are equally likely to be found in the population, how can you account for the observation that mutations to dihydrobiopterin reductase accounts for only about 2% of patients with PKU and HPA?
4. What would you propose as the least-expensive and most rapid method to identify the existence of a defect in BH_4 metabolism as the cause of a patient's PKU or HPA?
5. Based on metabolic pathways, what phenotypic differences would you expect to observe between individuals suffering from either a defect in BH_4 metabolism or a defect in the PAH enzyme?
6. Mrs. Urick was initially counseled that as an adult she did not need to follow the strict PKU diet. How do you respond to this advice? Based on PA metabolism, how do you justify your response?
7. Based in biochemical and physiological mechanisms, how can you explain impaired brain development as a consequence of uncontrolled PKU?

BIBLIOGRAPHY

Andersen OA, Flatmark T, Hough E: Crystal structure of the ternary complex of the catalytic domain of human phenylalanine hydroxylase with tetrahydrobiopterin and 3-(2-thienyl)-L-alanine, and its implications for the mechanism of catal-

ysis and substrate activation. *J Mol Biol* **320:** 1095-1108, 2002.

Bassan A, Blomberg MRA, Siegbahn PEM: Mechanism of dioxygen cleavage in tetrahydrobiopterin-dependent amino acid hydroxylases. *Chem Eur J* **9:**106-115, 2003.

Bernegger C, Blau N: High frequency of tetrahydrobiopterin-responsiveness among hyperphenylalaninemias: a study of 1919 patients observed from 1988 to 2002. *Mol Genet Metab* **77:**304-313, 2002.

Bickel H, Gerrard J, Hickmans EM: Influence of phenylalanine intake on phenylketonuria. *Lancet* **265:**812-813, 1953.

Blau N, Erlandsen H: The metabolic and molecular bases of tetrahydrobiopterin-responsive phenylalanine hydroxylase deficiency. *Mol. Genet. Metab.* **82:**101-111, 2004.

Bugg TDH: Oxygenases: mechanisms and structural motifs for O_2 activation. *Curr Opin Chem Biol* **5:**550-555, 2001.

Dhondt JL: Screening of tetrahydrobiopterin deficiency among hyperphenylalanenic patients. *Ann Biol Clin Paris* **60:**165-71, 2002.

Eberlein GA, Bruice TC, Lazarus RA, et al.: The interconversion of the 5,6,7,8-tetrahydro-, 6,7,8-dihydro, and radical forms of 6,6,7,7-tetramethyldihydropterin. A model for the biopterin center of aromatic amino acid mixed function oxidases. *J Am Chem Soc* **106:**7916-7924, 1984.

Erlandsen H, Pey AL, Gámez A, et al.: Correction of kinetic and stability defects by tetrahydrobiopterin in phenylketonuria patients with certain phenylalanine hydroxylase mutations. *Proc. Natl. Acad. Sci. (USA)* **101:**16903-16908, 2004.

Erlandsen H, Stevens RC: The structural basis of phenylketonuria. *Mol Genet Metab* **68:**103-125, 1999.

Erlandsen H, Stevens RC: A structural hypothesis for BH_4 responsiveness in patients with mild forms of hyperphenylalaninaemia. *J Inherit Metab Dis* **24:**213-230, 2001.

Fiege B, Bonafé L, Ballhausen D, et al.: Extended tetrahydrobiopterin loading test in the diagnosis of cofactor-responsive phenylketonuria: A pilot study. *Mol Genet Metab* **86:**s91-s95, 2005.

Fitzpatrick PF: Mechanism of aromatic amino acid hydroxylation. *Biochemistry* **42:**14083-14091, 2003.

Klinman JP: Life as aerobes: are there simple rules for activation of dioxygen by enzymes? *J Biol Inorg Chem* **6:**1-13, 2001.

Kobe B, Jennings IG, House CM, et al.: Structural basis of autoregulation of phenylalanine hydroxylase. *Nat Struct Biol* **6:**442, 1999.

Koch R, Burton B, Hoganson B, et al.: Phenylketonuria in adulthood: a collaborative study. *J Inherit Metab Dis* **25:**333-346, 2002.

Kock R, Matalon R, Stevens RC (eds): New developments in phenylketonuria and tetrahydrobiopterin research. *Mol Genet Metab* **V86 (Supplement 1)**:1–156, 2005.

Longo N: "Inherited Disorders of Amino Acid Metabolism and Storage." *Harrison's Principles of Internal Medicine*. Eugene Braunwald (ed). 15th Edition. New York, NY. The McGraw-Hill Companies, Inc. 2001. Chap 352: 2301–2309.

Matalon R, Michals-Matalon K, Koch R, et al.: Response of patients with phenylketonuria in the U.S. to tetrahydrobiopterin. *Mol Genet Metab* **86**:s17–s21, 2005.

NIH Consensus Statement Online: Phenylketonuria: screening and management. October 16–18; **17**:1–27, 2000. http://consensus.nih.gov/2000/2000phenylketonuria113html.htm. Accessed 4/5/06.

Pey AL, Desviat LR, Gámez A, et al.: Phenylketonuria: genotype-phenotype correlations based on expression analysis of structural and functional mutations in PAH. *Hum Mutat* **21**:370–378, 2003.

Poustie VJ, Rutherford P: Dietary interventions for phenylketonuria, Cochrane Review, in: *The Cochrane Library, Issue 1*. Wiley, Chichester, UK, 2004. http://www.mrw.interscience.wiley.com/cochrane/clsysrev/articles/cd001304/frame.html. Accessed 4/5/06.

Scriver CR: "The Hyperphenylalaninemias and Alkoptonuria." *Cecil Textbook of Medicine*. Vol. 1. Ed. Lee Goldman and J. Claude Bennette. 21st edition. Philadelphia, PA, W.B. Saunders Company, 2000. Chap 209: 1108–1110.

Solomon EI, Brunold TC, Davis MI, et al.: Geometric and electronic structure/function correlations in non-heme iron enzymes. *Chem Rev* **100**:235–349, 2000.

Steinfeld R, Kohlschutter A, Zschocke J, et al.: Tetrahydrobiopterin-responsiveness associated with common phenylalanine hydroxylase mutations distant from the tetrahydrobiopterin binding site. *J Inherit Metab Dis* **24**:29, 2001.

Teigen K, Frøystein NÅ, Martínez A: The structural basis of the recognition of phenylalanine and pterin cofactors by phenylalanine hydroxylase: implications for the catalytic mechanism. *J Mol Biol* **294**:807–823, 1999.

Trefz FK, Blau N: Potential role of tetrahydrobiopterin in the treatment of maternal phenylketonuria. *Pediatrics* **112**:1566–1569, 2003.

20

HMG-CoA Lyase Deficiency

VIRGINIA K. PROUD and MIRIAM D. ROSENTHAL

CASE REPORT

D.E.C. was a normal female infant (weight 6 lb 4 oz, length 20 inches) born via spontaneous vaginal delivery to an 18-year-old primigravida (first pregnancy). The pregnancy was unplanned and complicated only by maternal use of antidepressants (Zoloft and Depakote) during the first months of gestation. When D.E.C. was 1 month of age, she appeared to have macrocephaly and mild hypotonia; a cranial sector scan was performed and was normal. She was initially breast-fed but was a poor feeder, had gastroesophageal reflux, and gained weight slowly (Fig. 20-1). She sweated profusely when sleeping, and at 4 months of age had hypotonia and poor head control.

She was initially hospitalized at 4 months of age during a family vacation. An initial viral illness with low-grade fever and vomiting led to lethargy within 12 h. When she developed generalized seizures, she was taken to the emergency room and admitted. She experienced respiratory decompensation, was intubated, and required ventilator support for 72 h. Laboratory studies demonstrated marked metabolic acidosis with hypoglycemia (45 mg/dL; normal >80 mg/dL) and hyperammonemia (plasma ammonium >1100 μmol/L; normal 50–200 μmol/L). Her liver enzymes were markedly elevated. Her urine contained a number of organic acids, including 3-hydroxyisovaleric acid, 3-methylglutaconic acid, and 3-hydroxy-3-methylglutaric acid, all by-products of leucine catabolism. Plasma amino acid values also suggested a problem in branched-chain amino acid metabolism. Studies with skin fibroblast cultures confirmed a defi-

ciency of 3-hydroxy-3-methylglutaryl (HMG)-CoA-lyase deficiency with zero enzyme activity.

Although leucine is an essential amino acid, it was necessary to restrict the diet of this patient to about half of the leucine intake of normal healthy infants. She was therefore placed on a low-leucine formula consisting of three components: Similac with iron (a common infant formula), I-Valex 1 (a medical food that is a leucine-free, carnitine-enriched formula), and Polycose powder (glucose polymers; Ross Laboratories) to provide additional carbohydrate calories. The initial formula was designed to provide her with age-appropriate infant nutrition of 150 mL/kg, 130 Kcal/kg, 2 g protein/kg while limiting leucine to 121 mg/kg, the minimum requirement to support normal growth. After a 10-day hospitalization, she was discharged taking the formula mixture, a multivitamin, and L-carnitine supplement. Due to poor oral intake, she required supplemental nasogastric tube feeding.

Physical exam at 5 months of age revealed a frail-appearing small girl with nasogastric tube in place (Fig. 20-2). Her weight was significantly below the fifth centile, and neurological exam revealed truncal hypotonia and focal increased deep tendon reflexes. The neurological findings suggested brain injury secondary to her initial metabolic insult. She laughed and smiled but had poor head control and could not lift her head from prone.

By 10 months of age, she had required several hospitalizations for viral illnesses with mild dehydration, hypoglycemia, and mild acidosis. She also had several brief episodes of right-sided focal seizures lasting as long as 10 s. As a

CDC Growth Charts: United States

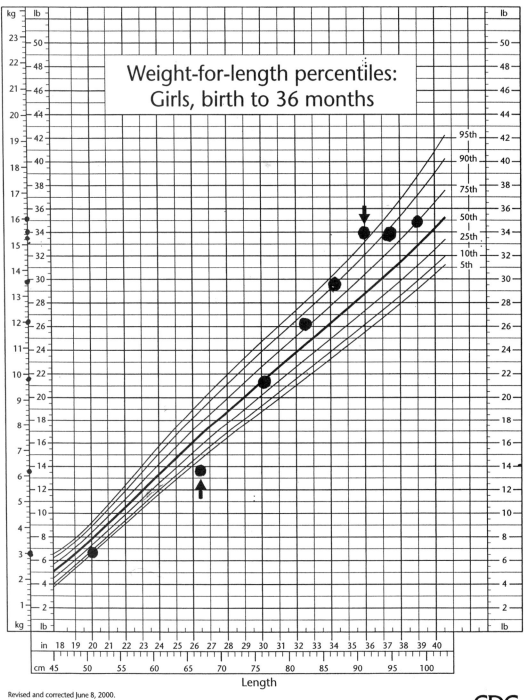

Weight-for-length percentiles:
Girls, birth to 36 months

Revised and corrected June 8, 2000.

SOURCE: Developed by the National Center for Health Statistics in collaboration with the
National Center for Chronic Disease Prevention and Health Promotion (2000).

Figure 20-1. Growth chart, weight for length, for D.E.C. Note poor weight for length at 5 months before placement of gastrostomy tube (first arrow) and increased weight for length by 2 years 6 months, when she was admitted for metabolic studies and feeding therapies.

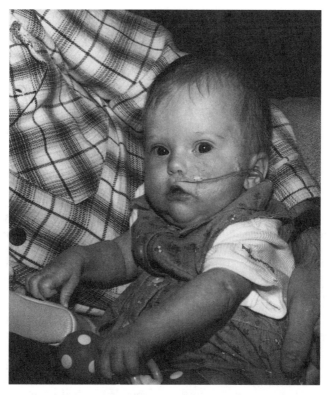

Figure 20-2. Photograph of D.E.C. at 5 months. Note nasogastric feeding tube and listless expression.

result of her chronic organic acidemia, reflux, frequent hospitalizations, hypotonia, and developmental delay, she developed oral aversion and poor feeding. There was constant concern about hypoglycemia, and at one clinic visit she had a blood sugar of 37 mg/dL (normal >80 mg/dL). A permanent gastrostomy tube (G-tube) was placed at 6 months of age, and a Nissen fundoplication was performed to treat gastroesophageal reflux. After the G-tube placement, metabolic balance was achieved more easily, with no further hospitalizations for dehydration, acidosis, or hypoglycemia.

By 2.5 years of age, her weight was greater than the 95th centile, but she was taking very little food by mouth (Fig. 20-1). Although it was necessary to decrease her caloric intake to allow her to lose weight and to stimulate her appetite, there was concern that she might develop hypoglycemia. She was therefore admitted to the special feeding unit at the Children's Hospital to monitor her metabolic status while her gastrostomy-tube intake was decreased and a team of feeding specialists, nutritionists, and occupational therapists worked

with her to improve her oral intake. During the 6-week hospitalization, a fasting study confirmed that she was stable for up to 14 h without hypoglycemia; this probably reflected improved availability and adequacy of glycogen stores with liver growth and maturation. With continued feeding therapy, all of her caloric intake was by mouth by 4 years of age, and by 6 years of age approximately 75% of her calories were from foods other than the medical formula. Her appetite remained poor, however, and mealtimes often extended over an hour.

At 7 years of age, she had a completely normal physical examination. Her weight was 22.1 kg (60th centile), height was 123.4 cm (60th centile), and head circumference was 51 cm (40th centile). The neurological exam was normal without focal findings. She did well in first grade and led a normal life in all areas with the exception of her diet. Although her eating was more mechanical than natural, her appetite had improved, and she was eating a variety of foods. She still could not eat meat, eggs, or other high-protein foods, and her family must still measure and weigh all foods to determine leucine content. Her mealtimes had decreased to only 30 min. She drank her medical food mixed with juice and must adhere to a consistent eating schedule to avoid fasting. The medical team continues to monitor her biochemical parameters by analyzing plasma amino acids and modifies her diet to optimize growth.

DIAGNOSIS

Organic acidurias comprise a unique group of disorders of amino acid and fatty acid metabolism characterized by a predisposition for metabolic decompensation. Several of these disorders, including methylmalonic aciduria, propionic aciduria, and isovaleric aciduria, can have similar clinical presentations. However, qualitative examination of urinary organic acids demonstrates a unique profile for each disease. In children with HMG-CoA lyase deficiency, the urine organic acids include 3-hydroxyisovaleric acid, 3-methylglutaric acid, and 3-hydroxy-3-methylglutaric acid. In addition, HMG-CoA lyase deficiency is unique among organic acidurias in that hypoglycemia is not associated with increased urinary levels of the so-called ketone bodies, acetoacetate and β-hydroxybutyrate.

The clinical presentation of HMG-CoA lyase deficiency depends on the amount of residual enzyme activity as well as the specific illness or metabolic stress that precipitates the clinical problems. There may be acute neonatal metabolic acidosis with hypoglycemia, hypotonia, and seizures, or there may be a more indolent course with several months of hypotonia, developmental delay, and failure to thrive. Older infants, between 6 months and 2 years, may present with profound metabolic acidosis, lactic acidosis, hypoglycemia, and hyperammonemia. The rapid-onset metabolic decompensation often results from an acute viral illness, especially if associated with fever, vomiting and diarrhea, and dehydration, but can also be precipitated by a fever secondary to routine immunizations. The clinical presentation often includes hepatomegaly and shock. If there is a change in neurological status, especially with lethargy, then diagnostic studies should include blood gas to determine degree of metabolic acidosis and compensatory respiratory alkalosis as well as plasma levels of glucose, lactic acid, ammonia, amino acids, carnitine (total and free), and urinary organic acids. In older children, MRI of the brain may also show changes in the white matter caused by poor myelinization, which with recurrent episodes of metabolic insult can progress to cortical atrophy, seizures, and neurological deterioration.

Many states have expanded newborn metabolic screening programs and are using tandem mass spectrometry to identify as many as 60 amino acid and fatty acid oxidation defects, including phenylketonuria, maple syrup urine disease, and homocystinuria, from the analysis of one small blood sample. An elevated plasma level of leucine is indicative of an inborn error in leucine catabolism. Further diagnostic tests are then required to characterize the specific enzyme deficiency. More widespread use of this technology will permit identification of many infants and children before acute metabolic decompensation occurs, thus preserving optimal neurological and cognitive function.

BIOCHEMICAL PERSPECTIVES

HMG-CoA lyase deficiency was first reported by Faull and co-workers (1976). The patient, a 7-month-old infant, presented with diarrhea, vomiting, dehydration, metabolic acidosis, hypoglycemia, and organic aciduria. Analysis of urinary metabolites by gas-liquid chromatography/mass spectrophotometry identified high concentrations of 3-hydroxylisovaleric, 3-methylglutaric, 3-methylglutaconic, and 3-hydroxyl-3-methylglutaric acids. This profile differed from that seen in previously described diseases related to leucine catabolism (including maple syrup urine disease) and suggested a deficiency in the cleavage of HMG-CoA to acetoacetate and acetyl-CoA.

HMG-CoA lyase is normally present in the mitochondrial matrix. To understand the complexity of the metabolic problems of a patient with HMG-CoA lyase deficiency, it is necessary to consider the role of this enzyme in two very distinct metabolic pathways: catabolism of leucine and ketogenesis.

Catabolism of Leucine

Leucine is a branched chain-amino acid that is essential or required in the diet. Mitochondrial catabolism of excess leucine occurs by the pathway shown in Figure 20-3. The initial transamination step (removal of the amino group) is followed by a decarboxylation reaction to produce isovaleric acid. It is this decarboxylation of the α-keto analogs of the three

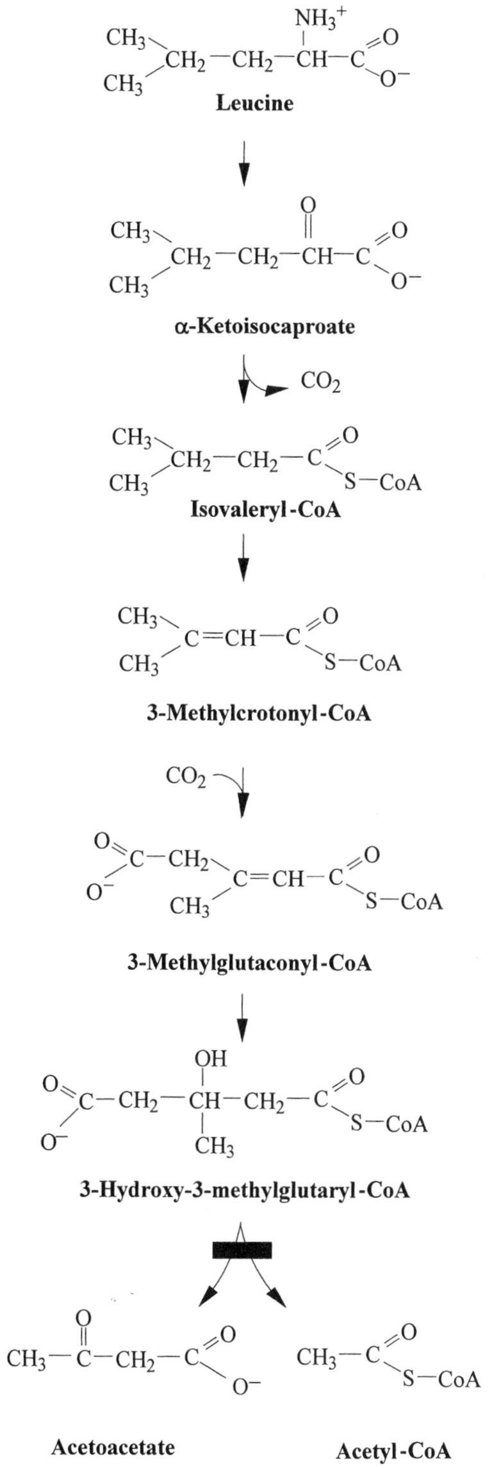

Figure 20-3. Pathway for the catabolism of leucine. The last step in the pathway is catalyzed by 3-hydroxy-3methyl-CoA lyase, which is deficient in 3-hydroxy-3-methylglutaryl-CoA lyase deficiency.

branched-chain amino acids leucine, isoleucine, and valine that is deficient in maple syrup urine disease. Catabolism of isovaleric acid ultimately produces HMG-CoA, which, as discussed, is cleaved by HMG-CoA lyase to produce acetoacetate and acetyl-CoA. Subsequent metabolism of acetoacetate involves an acetoacetyl-CoA intermediate that is cleaved to form two more molecules of acetyl-CoA.

Individuals who are deficient in HMG-CoA lyase are unable to complete the metabolism of leucine. The increased urinary excretion of 3-hydroxy-3-methylglutaric acids is the primary biochemical criterion that distinguishes this particular enzymatic defect from other defects in enzymes of leucine catabolism that also result in metabolic acidosis and abnormal organic aciduria. There is also substantial urinary excretion of intermediates of leucine catabolism, such as 3-methylglutaconic acid, and their metabolites, including 3-hydroxy-isovaleric acid produced from isovaleric acid.

Ketogenesis

Ketogenesis or "ketone body" formation occurs in the liver and, to some extent, renal cortex during the fasted state and is an obligatory pathway for energy metabolism during fasting. Under these conditions, the hormone glucagon stimulates hepatocytes to maintain blood sugar levels both by mobilizing glucose from liver glycogen stores and by gluconeogenesis. The major substrates for gluconeogenesis are amino acids such as alanine and glutamine. As shown in Figure 20-4, oxaloacetate is a key intermediate in gluconeogenesis. Oxaloacetate also plays a key role in the tricarboxylic acid (TCA) cycle, in which it is combined with the entering acetyl-CoA to form citrate. When gluconeogenesis occurs, diversion of oxaloacetate to glucose synthesis depletes the TCA cycle of this key intermediate, resulting in shutdown of the oxidation of acetyl-CoA to CO_2 and the ATP generation linked to reducing equivalents generated through the TCA cycle.

Utilization of amino acids for gluconeogenesis requires initial removal of their amino groups, usually by transamination linked to subsequent glutamate dehydrogenase activity. The resultant NH_4^+ is detoxified by urea synthesis.

Both gluconeogenesis and urea synthesis require net energy input as ATP. In the fasting

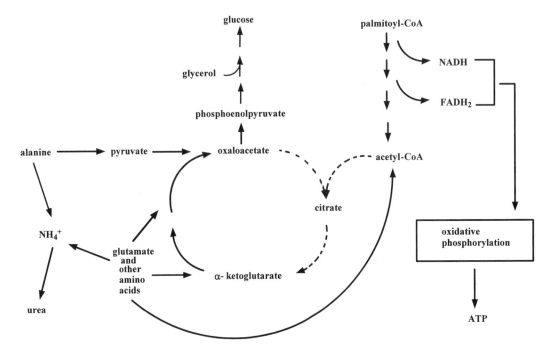

Figure 20-4. Biochemical pathways for gluconeogenesis in the liver. Alanine, a major gluconeogenic substrate, is used to synthesize oxaloacetate. The carbon skeletons of glutamine and other glucogenic amino acids feed into the TCA cycle as α-ketoglutarate, succinyl-CoA, fumarate, or oxaloacetate and thus also provide oxaloacetate. Conversion of oxaloacetate to phosphoenolpyruvate and ultimately to glucose limits the availability of oxaloacetate for citrate synthesis and thus greatly diminishes flux through the initial steps of the TCA cycle (dashed lines). Concurrent β-oxidation of fatty acids provides reducing equivalents (NADH and FADH$_2$) for oxidative phosphorylation but results in accumulation of acetyl-CoA.

state, the liver relies on β-oxidation of fatty acids for synthesis of ATP. The reducing equivalents (NADH and FADH$_2$) generated during each cycle of β-oxidation can flow directly into the electron transport chain, independent of the TCA cycle, and generate ATP via oxidative phosphorylation. There is, however, one problem: What do liver cells do with the acetyl-CoA generated by β-oxidation of fatty acids? The solution is the synthesis of so-called ketone bodies. This process (shown in Fig. 20-5) essentially converts two molecules of acetyl-CoA to one four-carbon acetoacetate, with release of the two molecules of reduced coenzyme A (CoA-SH). HMG-CoA, the six-carbon intermediate in this pathway, is formed by successive condensations of three acetyl-CoA molecules. HMG-CoA lyase then cleaves the HMG-CoA to release acetyl-CoA from acetoacetate.

Ketogenesis is thus an alternate pathway in which the partially oxidized intermediates of fatty acid oxidation are exported from the liver

as acetoacetate (and β-hydroxybutyrate). The acetoacetate can then be further oxidized by tissues such as muscle that are not gluconeogenic and that retain an active TCA cycle.

An individual who is deficient in HMG-CoA lyase cannot synthesize acetoacetate from HMG-CoA; in the absence of a pool of free CoA-SH molecules, β-oxidation of fatty acids cannot continue in the liver. This often causes *hepatomegaly* (liver enlargement) with diffuse accumulation of lipid droplets in swollen hepatocytes. Lack of sufficient ATP generation impairs urea synthesis and results in *hyperammonemia*. Most important, in the absence of ongoing ATP generation, gluconeogenesis cannot occur. Stores of liver glycogen, usually more limited in neonates and young children, are thus depleted more rapidly than normal. The resultant fasting *hypoglycemia* often precipitates a metabolic crisis.

For most patients with HMG-CoA lyase deficiency, strict dietary control can maintain

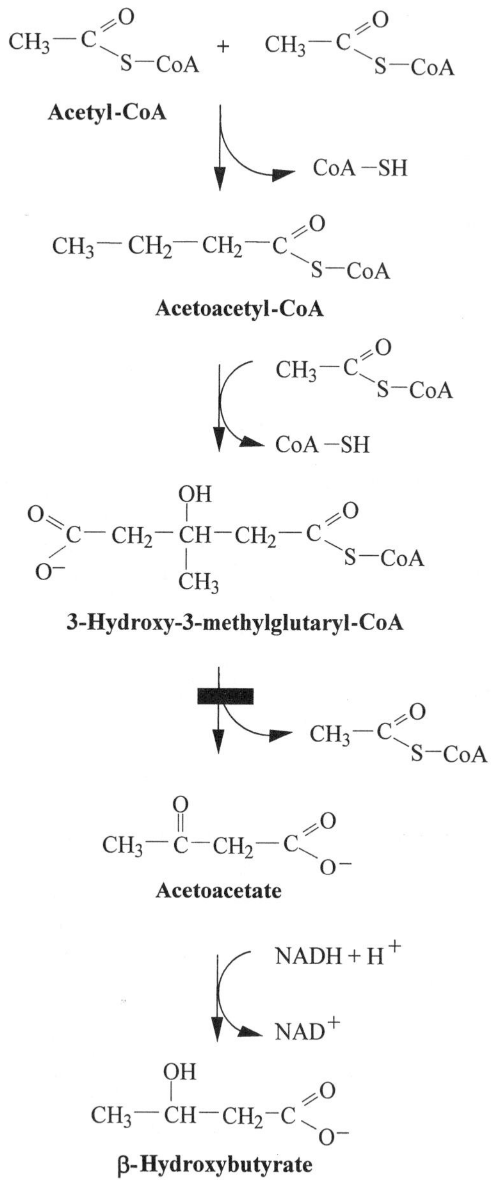

Figure 20-5. Biochemical pathway for ketogenesis. Condensation of three molecules of acetyl-CoA results in synthesis of 3-hydroxy-3-methyl-glutaryl (HMG)-CoA and release of free CoA-SH, which is then available for continued β-oxidation. Deficiency of HMG-CoA lyase results in the inability to cleave the HMG-CoA to form acetoacetate (the initial "ketone body") and its reduction product β-hydroxybutyrate.

homeostasis and prevent metabolic decompensation while providing adequate leucine intake for growth. A regimen of frequent feeding and sufficient carbohydrate intake is utilized to min-

imize the need for gluconeogenesis, particularly in neonates and young children, whose liver glycogen stores are often less adequate to meet long-term needs. As described, metabolic decompensation often occurs during illnesses, such as viral infections, when decreased dietary intake and fever result in dehydration and endogenous protein catabolism. In normal individuals, the endogenous protein catabolism provides amino acid substrates for synthesis of immunoglobulins and acute phase proteins as well as for gluconeogenesis to meet the increased needs of the stress response. However, individuals with HMG-CoA lyase deficiency cannot tolerate the increased mobilization of leucine from muscle proteins and will quickly decompensate and develop profound metabolic acidosis.

Leucine is a ketogenic amino acid with a carbon skeleton that cannot serve as a substrate for gluconeogenesis. Normally, much of the leucine (and other branched-chain amino acids) mobilized during fasting is actually not released from the muscle. Instead, the amino groups are removed by transamination and exported from the muscle as alanine or glutamine; the resultant branched α-keto acyl-CoA molecules are metabolized within the muscle for energy. In individuals who are deficient in HMG-CoA lyase, increased leucine mobilization during the catabolic state induced by illness results in increased accumulation of 3-hydroxy-3-methylglutaric acid and other organic acids.

Role of Carnitine

Carnitine deficiency complicates HMG-CoA lyase deficiency and other inborn errors of metabolism, which results in organic acidemia. L-Carnitine or β-hydroxy-γ-trimethylammonium butyrate is a carrier molecule that transports long-chain fatty acids across the inner mitochondrial membrane for subsequent β-oxidation. L-Carnitine also facilitates removal of toxic metabolic intermediates or xenobiotics via urinary excretion of their acyl carnitine derivatives. Indeed, individuals with HMG-CoA lyase deficiency have been shown to excrete 3-methylgluatarylcarnitine (Roe et al., 1986). In the absence of ketogenesis, the formation of the acyl carnitine derivative of 3-hydroxy-3-methylglutarate from HMG-CoA also serves to regenerate free CoA in the mitochondria and permits continued β-oxidation of fatty acids.

Individuals with HMG-CoA lyase deficiency are particularly susceptible to carnitine deficiency. With restriction of red meats and dairy products, dietary carnitine intake is quite low. Carnitine is also synthesized endogenously from the modified, methylated lysine resides of various proteins; free trimethyllysine is released when the protein is degraded. Since the therapy for patients with HMG-CoA lyase deficiency must minimize their endogenous protein catabolism, they also have limited availability of trimethyllysine for carnitine synthesis.

THERAPY

Nutritional therapy for HMG-CoA lyase deficiency has two major goals. First, the prescribed diet aims to provide enough total protein and calories to achieve normal growth and maintain metabolic balance in the context of a leucine-restricted diet. Equally important, the nutritional therapy focuses on preventing excess catabolism, acidosis, and hypoglycemia, especially during times of acute illness. For these patients, it is particularly important to avoid fasting at any time.

Monitoring plasma amino acids and growth on a regular basis in a metabolic clinic is necessary to ensure adequate leucine and total protein intake. Leucine tolerance varies widely from patient to patient. Furthermore, the leucine needs of each patient will change as a result of growth spurts, age, illness, and adequacy of total protein and energy intakes. Leucine deficiency can cause poor weight gain, hair loss, skin rash, loss of appetite, and irritability. Excess leucine intake, on the other hand, will lead to the accumulation of organic acids, metabolic acidosis, and potentially to acute decompensation. Plasma samples should be drawn 2–4 h postprandially (after a meal) and the diet adjusted to maintain leucine levels at the low end of normal (50–100 μmol/L). For the younger child, routine infant formula is used to supply the prescribed amount of leucine in the form of natural protein from milk. The medical food (I Valex 1) provides additional protein in the form of individual amino acids, but it is totally deficient in leucine. It also provides additional fluid, fat, carbohydrate, vitamins, and minerals. If consumed as prescribed, then the final formula, which is a combination of natural protein and medical food, will meet the nutritional needs of the growing child.

Manipulation of the intake from infancy, however, frequently results in oral aversion, a general refusal to engage in normal eating behavior. The child may exhibit poor oral-motor skills, decreased appetite, food refusal, and sensory problems, especially with textures. Causes of oral aversion include lack of eating experience, especially when a gastrostomy tube is necessary to facilitate feeding of special formula, anorexia secondary to organic acids in the blood, and loss of the normal hunger cycle in individuals whose diet is regulated to avoid fasting. Lack of adequate oral intake can result either in excessive dependence on continued gastrostomy tube feeding or in failure to thrive. Ultimately, failure to thrive leads to impaired brain growth and developmental delay or even metabolic encephalopathy with loss of motor and cognitive skills. Oral aversion is a very complex disorder and must be treated in a multidisciplinary way with parents, occupational and speech therapists, the nutritionist, and metabolic geneticist working together. Sometimes, medication is indicated to stimulate the child's appetite and optimize eating behavior. Often, months or years of feeding therapy and behavior modification are necessary to teach the child to eat normally.

Complications occur in spite of optimum nutritional therapy, especially if the child acquires a viral illness, ear infection, or gastroenteritis and cannot maintain the necessary formula intake. It is important that he or she be seen early to optimize hydration and maintain caloric and protein intake. Maintaining biochemical homeostasis requires a fine balance in these patients, especially during the infant and toddler years when their ability to maintain homeostasis during illness is much less than that of older children. Levels of plasma glucose, electrolytes, pH, and HCO_3^- together with the specific gravity of urine are important indicators of the extent of metabolic decompensation and the need for intravenous fluids with dextrose and HCO_3^-. Unlike children with other inborn errors of metabolism, individuals with HMG-CoA lyase deficiency will not accumulate either plasma or urinary ketones, and ketosis therefore cannot be used as an indicator of dehydration or catabolism. If the child is vomiting or cannot take food by mouth, then gastrostomy tube feeding or intravenous hyperalimentation must be started within 24–48 h to avoid further catabolism.

In summary, HMG-CoA lyase deficiency is a unique inborn error of metabolism with profound effects on both amino acid catabolism and metabolic homeostasis in the fasted state. Management of these patients is difficult and requires constant attention to daily nutrition and timely intervention during acute illness. Fortunately, nutritional therapy treatment that provides a diet adequate for growth but with limited intake of leucine and prevents fasting and hypoglycemia enables individuals with HMG-CoA lyase deficiency to live normal active lives.

QUESTIONS

1. Why does deficiency of HMG-CoA lyase result in the excretion of a large number of organic acids in the urine?
2. Why do individuals with HMG-CoA lyase deficiency have difficulty fasting?
3. Why might infection precipitate metabolic decompensation in an individual with HMG-CoA lyase deficiency?
4. What is the rationale for providing supplemental carnitine to individuals with HMG-CoA lyase deficiency?
5. Would you expect an individual with HMG-CoA lyase deficiency to have continued reliance on medical foods as an adult? Why?

Acknowledgments: We wish to thank genetic counselor Heather Creswick, metabolic nutritionist Melody Persinger-Yeargin, and administrative assistants Christina McCalla and Trina Moore for their contributions to this chapter and preparation of the manuscript.

BIBLIOGRAPHY

Acosta PB, Yannicelli S: Disorders of leucine catabolism, *in* Acosta PB, Yannicelli S (eds): *Nutrition Support Protocols; the Ross Metabolic Formula System.* 4th ed. Abbott Laboratories, Columbus, OH, 2001, pp. 103–122.

Elsas LJ II, Acosta PB: Nutritional support in inherited metabolic disease, *in* Shils ME, Olson JA, Shike M, and Ross AC (eds): *Modern Nutrition in Health and Disease.* 9th ed. Lippincott Williams and Wilkins, Baltimore, MD, 1999, pp. 1003–1056.

Faull K, Bolton P, Halpern B, et al.: Patient with defect in leucine metabolism. *New Engl J Med* **294:**1013, 1976.

Mitchell GA, Fukao T: Inborn errors of ketone body metabolism, *in* Scriver CR, Sly WS, et al. (eds): *The Metabolic and Molecular Bases of Inherited Disease.* 8th ed. McGraw-Hill, New York, 2001, pp. 2327–2356.

Nyhan WL, Barshop BA, Ozand PT: 3-Hydroxy-3-methylglutaryl CoA lyase deficiency, in Nyhan WL, Barshop BA, Ozand PT (eds): *Atlas of Metabolic Diseases*, 2nd edition. Chapman and Hall Medical, 2005, pp. 253–258.

Roe CR, Millington DS, Maltby DA: Identification of 3-methylglutarylcarnitine: a new diagnostic metabolite of 3-hydroxy-3-methylglutaryl-coenzyme A lyase. *J Clin Invest* **77:**1391–1394, 1986.

21

Hyperhomocysteinemia

ANGELA M. DEVLIN and STEVEN R. LENTZ

CASE REPORT

A 35-year-old man presented to his family physician after he noted a 20-min episode of slurred speech and weakness of his left arm. He had had a similar episode, lasting 10 min, 3 days earlier. He had never smoked cigarettes, and he had no history of high blood pressure, high cholesterol, diabetes, stroke, or neurological problems. He did have a history of blood clots in his right leg (deep vein thrombosis) and lungs (pulmonary embolism) at age 15 years. From age 15 until age 20 he took the anticoagulant drug warfarin, which inhibits blood clotting by blocking the synthesis of vitamin K-dependent coagulation factors.

At age 26, he first noted pain and swelling of his right leg. These symptoms worsened progressively over the next 2 years, becoming so severe that he was no longer able to jog or play basketball. At age 28, ultrasonography of his right lower extremity revealed chronic occlusion (blockage) of his right femoral vein with accompanying venous insufficiency (leaky valves in the veins of his leg). He then underwent catheter-directed thrombolysis, a procedure in which the drug urokinase, which dissolves blood clots, is infused into the femoral vein. Following the thrombolysis procedure, a metal stent was placed in the femoral vein to help prevent its reocclusion. He again took warfarin along with clopidogrel, a drug that inhibits blood clotting by preventing aggregation of platelets. Except for some intermittent swelling of his right ankle after exercise, he did well for the next 7 years.

At the time he noticed the episodes of slurred speech and left-sided weakness, he was taking no medications except for warfarin and clopidogrel. His diet consisted mainly of meats and fried potatoes, with very few fruits and vegetables. He admitted to drinking up to a 12-pack of beer on the weekends. His family history was negative for stroke or blood clots, but his father had suffered a fatal myocardial infarction (heart attack) at age 44.

On physical examination, his neurological function was completely normal, and his speech was intact. Magnetic resonance imaging of his brain was normal, but ultrasonography of his neck revealed a 50% stenosis (narrowing) of the right internal carotid artery. Laboratory valuation indicated that the concentration of total homocysteine in his blood plasma was elevated to 38 μmol/L (the normal range is 5–12 μmol/L). The level of vitamin B_{12} in his serum was within the normal range (312 pmol/L), but the level of folate in his serum was slightly below normal (3.4 ng/L; normal level >4.1 ng/L). His serum creatinine, an indicator of kidney function, also was normal (0.8 mg/dL). Genetic testing revealed that he was homozygous for the C677→T polymorphism of the methylene tetrahydrofolate reductase (*MTHFR*) gene.

He was diagnosed with moderate hyperhomocysteinemia and treated with 2.0 mg folic acid daily. He continued to take warfarin and clopidogrel. After 1 month, his plasma total homocysteine level had decreased to 9 μmol/L. He had no further episodes of weakness or other neurological symptoms during the ensuing 12 months.

DIAGNOSIS

Hyperhomocysteinemia is defined as an elevated level of homocysteine in the blood. It is diagnosed by measuring the concentration of total homocysteine (tHcy) in a sample of plasma or serum. The laboratory measurement of tHcy quantifies the total amount of homocysteine and all of its disulfide derivatives. The normal reference range for plasma tHcy is defined as the 2.5th-to-97.5th percentile interval for presumed healthy individuals. This range is typically 5–10 μmol/L, but the upper limit may vary between 10 and 15 μmol/L depending on age, gender, ethnic group, and dietary intake of folate. Levels tend to increase with age and are higher in men than women.

Mild hyperhomocysteinemia is defined as a plasma tHcy concentration of 10–30 μmol/L; moderate hyperhomocysteinemia is classified as 30–100 μmol/L. A very severe form of hyperhomocysteinemia, which produces plasma tHcy concentrations greater than 100 μmol/L, can be caused by one of several inborn errors of methionine metabolism. Patients with these disorders also have high levels of tHcy in their urine, a condition known as *homocystinuria*.

Because hyperhomocysteinemia may be associated with a variety of different nutritional and genetic factors, additional laboratory testing is often useful in confirming the diagnosis and defining the cause of hyperhomocysteinemia. Adjunctive tests may include measurement of blood levels of folate (vitamin B_9), cobalamin (vitamin B_{12}), or methionine and genetic testing for mutations or polymorphisms in genes, such as *MTFHR*, that are involved in homocysteine metabolism.

BIOCHEMICAL PERSPECTIVES

Homocysteine, first described by Butz and Vincent du Vigneaud in 1932, is a sulfur-containing amino acid that is structurally and metabolically linked to the dietary amino acids methionine and cysteine (Fig. 21-1). Homocysteine is found in both prokaryotic and eukaryotic organisms and is a sensitive marker of vitamin deficiency and kidney function.

Homocysteine is formed in the cytoplasm during the intracellular metabolism of methionine. Within the methionine cycle (Fig. 21-2), methionine is converted to *S*-adenosylmethionine (SAM) by methionine adenosyltransferase. SAM serves as a methyl donor for a variety of methyl acceptors, including DNA, protein, neurotransmitters, and phospholipids. *S*-Adenosylhomocysteine (SAH) is produced following methyl donation by SAM, and homocysteine is formed through the liberation of adenosine from SAH by the enzyme SAH hydrolase. Unlike methionine and cysteine, homocysteine is not incorporated into polypeptide chains during protein synthesis. Instead, homocysteine has one of two metabolic fates: transsulfuration or remethylation to methionine.

The transsulfuration pathway involves conversion of homocysteine to cysteine by the sequential action of two pyridoxal phosphate (vitamin B_6)-dependent enzymes, cystathionine-β-synthase (CBS) and cystathionine γ-lyase (Fig. 21-2). Transsulfuration of homocysteine occurs predominantly in the liver, kidney, and gastrointestinal tract. Deficiency of CBS, first described by Carson and Neill in 1962, is inherited in an autosomal recessive pattern. It causes homocystinuria accompanied by severe elevations in blood homocysteine (>100 μM) and methionine (>60 μM). Homocystinuria due to deficiency of CBS occurs at a frequency of about 1 in 300,000 worldwide but is more common in some populations such as Ireland, where the frequency is 1 in 65,000. Clinical features include blood clots, heart disease, skeletal deformities, mental retardation, abnormalities of the ocular lens, and fatty infiltration of the liver. Several different genetic defects in the *CBS* gene have been found to account for loss of CBS activity.

Cysteine is considered a nonessential nutrient because it can be synthesized from methionine via the transsulfuration pathway (Figs. 21-1 and 21-2). Production of cysteine is metabolically important because it serves as a source of sulfur for incorporation into proteins and detoxification reactions. A lack of cysteine needed for incorporation into the structural protein collagen may be responsible for the musculoskeletal abnormalities seen in patients with CBS deficiency. A major metabolic use of cysteine is in the production of glutathione (γ-glutamylcysteinylglycine), an important antioxidant. Another important pathway for cysteine metabolism is its oxidation to cysteinesulfinate, which serves as a precursor for taurine, an amino acid that stabilizes cell membranes in the brain.

Remethylation of homocysteine to methionine

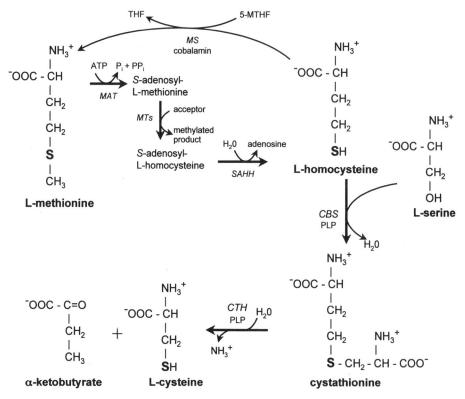

Figure 21-1. Structural and metabolic relationships between methionine, homocysteine, and cysteine. CBS, cystathionine b-synthase; CTH, cystathionine γ-lyase; MAT, methionine adenosyltransferase; MS, methionine synthase; 5-MTHF, 5-methyltetrahydrofolate; MTs, methyl transferases; PLP, pyridoxal phosphate; SAH, S-adenosylhomocysteine; SAHH, SAH hydrolase; THF, tetrahydrofolate.

is primarily accomplished by the cobalamin-dependent enzyme methionine synthase (MS), which uses 5-methyltetrahydrofolate (5-MTHF) as the methyl donor for the remethylation reaction. 5-MTHF is produced by the folate cycle enzyme methylenetetrahydrofolate reductase (MTHFR), which catalyzes the reduction of 5,10-methylenetetrahydrofolate to 5-MTHF. In addition to serving as the precursor to 5-MTHF, 5,10-methylenetetrahydrofolate also provides methyl groups for the synthesis of thymidylate, a pyrimidine required for the synthesis of DNA.

Deficiency of MTHFR can produce severe hyperhomocysteinemia and homocystinuria but is distinguishable from CBS deficiency in that blood levels of methionine are not elevated. The first case of homocystinuria caused by deficiency of MTHFR was described by Mudd et al. in 1972. The case was a patient who presented with homocystinuria without elevation of blood levels of methionine. Since then, several

genetic defects in the *MTHFR* gene resulting in severe deficiency of enzyme activity and homocystinuria have been described.

A common thermolabile variant of MTHFR, first described by Frosst et al. in 1995, results from a C→T substitution at nucleotide 677 of the *MTHFR* gene. Homozygosity for the C677→T variant produces deficient MTHFR activity and is associated with mild or moderate hyperhomocysteinemia. Individuals homozygous for the C677→T variant have an increased risk of cardiovascular disease, especially under conditions of low dietary folate intake (Klerk et al., 2002). The frequency of the 677TT genotype ranges from 10% to 20% in Caucasian populations in North America and Europe and has been shown to be slightly higher in Mexican American populations and lower in African American populations.

During the remethylation of homocysteine to methionine, the methyl group from 5-MTHF is transferred to cobalamin, which serves as an

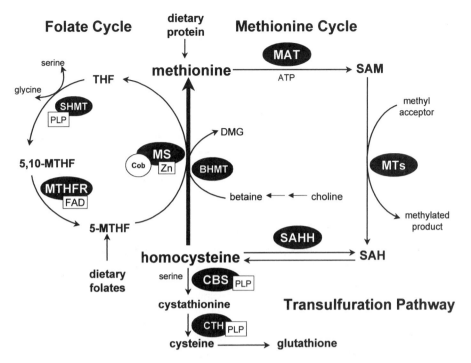

Figure 21-2. Metabolism of homocysteine. BHMT, betaine:homocysteine methyltransferase; CBS, cystathionine β-synthase; Cob, cobalamin; CTH, cystathionine γ-lyase; DHF, dihydrofolate; DMG, dimethylglycine; FAD, flavin adenine dinucleotide; MAT, methionine adenosyltransferase; 5-MTHF, 5-methyltetrahydrofolate; 5,10-MTHF, 5,10-methylenetetrahydrofolate; MTHFR, methylenetetrahydrofolate reductase; MS, methionine synthase; MTRR, methionine synthase reductase; MTs, methyl transferases; PLP, pyridoxal phosphate; SAH, *S*-adenosylhomocysteine; SAHH, SAH hydrolase; SAM, *S*-adenosylmethionine; SHMT, serine hydroxymethyltransferase; THF, tetrahydrofolate; Zn, zinc.

intermediate methyl carrier (Fig. 21-3). The methyl group is subsequently transferred to homocysteine, generating methionine. The other product of the reaction is tetrahydrofolate, which is then remethylated to 5,10-methylenetetrahydrofolate by the enzyme serine hydroxymethyltransferase, completing the folate cycle (Fig. 21-2). Over time, the catalytic activity of MS decays due to oxidation of its cofactor, cobalamin. Regeneration of active MS requires the reductive methylation of cobalamin via methionine synthase reductase (MTRR), which uses SAM as the methyl donor (Fig. 21-3).

Deficiency of MTRR can produce homocystinuria accompanied by megaloblastic anemia (a type of anemia characterized by the presence in the blood of large, immature red blood cells). This condition is also known as cobalamin-responsive homocystinuria and is classified as the cbl E complementation type of

cobalamin deficiency. Defects in the intestinal absorption, metabolism, or transport of cobalamin can also result in hyperhomocysteinemia with megaloblastic anemia (see Chapter 28 on Vitamin B$_{12}$ deficiency).

An alternative reaction for the remethylation of homocysteine to methionine can be accomplished by betaine homocysteine methyltransferase, which uses betaine instead of 5-MTHF as the methyl donor. Unlike the MS reaction, which is believed to be ubiquitously present in all tissues, the betaine homocysteine methyltransferase reaction occurs only in the liver and kidney. Betaine is not a required nutrient since the liver can synthesize betaine from choline. Betaine supplements, however, have been shown to lower plasma total homocysteine concentrations successfully in subjects with deficient homocysteine remethylation due to defects in MTHFR or MTRR and in those with deficient CBS activity.

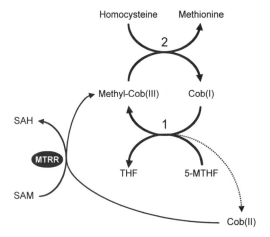

Figure 21-3. The methionine synthase reaction. Methionine synthase catalyzes the remethylation of homocysteine to methionine. In the first half reaction (1), a methyl group is transferred from 5-methyl tetrahydrofolate (5-MTHF) to the reduced form of cobalamin [Cob(I)], generating methyl-cobalamin [Methyl-Cob(III)] and tetrahydrofolate (THF). During the second half reaction (2), the methyl group is transferred from methylcobalamin to homocysteine, generating methionine. During the catalytic reaction, Cob(I) occasionally becomes oxidized, producing an inactive form of cobalamin, cob(II)alamin [Cob(II)]. The enzyme methionine synthase reductase (MTRR) then reactivates Cob(II) through reductive methylation, producing methyl-Cob(III). SAM, S-adenosylmethionine; SAH, S-adeno-sylhomocysteine.

Blood Homocysteine

The fraction of intracellular homocysteine that does not undergo transsulfuration or remethylation is secreted into the extracellular space and ultimately finds its way into the blood. One major source of blood homocysteine is the liver, but some homocysteine is secreted into the blood by endothelial cells, circulating blood cells, and other tissues. Only about 2% of homocysteine in blood remains in its reduced, thiol form. The remainder circulates as a variety of different oxidation adducts, which include the disulfide, homocystine, as well as homocysteine-cysteine mixed disulfide and several protein-bound disulfides. About 70% of total homocysteine in blood is bound to the protein albumin through a disulfide linkage. When blood homocysteine is measured in the clinical laboratory, a reducing agent is added to the sample

to convert all of the disulfide forms to homocysteine, which is then detected using either chromatographic or immunologic methods. The result is reported as tHcy.

Measurement of blood tHcy is usually performed for one of three reasons: (1) to screen for inborn errors of methionine metabolism; (2) as an adjunctive test for cobalamin deficiency; (3) to aid in the prediction of cardiovascular risk. Hyperhomocysteinemia, defined as an elevated level of tHcy in blood, can be caused by dietary factors such as a deficiency of B vitamins, genetic abnormalities of enzymes involved in homocysteine metabolism, or kidney disease. All of the major metabolic pathways involved in homocysteine metabolism (the methionine cycle, the transsulfuration pathway, and the folate cycle) are active in the kidney. It is not known, however, whether elevation of plasma tHcy in patients with kidney disease is caused by decreased elimination of homocysteine in the kidneys or by an effect of kidney disease on homocysteine metabolism in other tissues. Additional factors that also influence plasma levels of tHcy include diabetes, age, sex, lifestyle, and thyroid disease (Table 21-1).

Most cases of hyperhomocysteinemia are classified as mild (a plasma tHcy concentration of 10–30 μmol/L) or moderate (a plasma tHcy concentration of 30–100 μmol/L). Mild or moderate hyperhomocysteinemia can be caused by nutrient deficiencies (Table 21-2), genetic polymorphisms in genes encoding enzymes required for homocysteine or methionine metabolism, impaired kidney function, or excessive alcohol intake. Some drugs, such as nitrous oxide, antiepileptic drugs, and certain drugs used to treat asthma or high cholesterol, can produce mild hyperhomocysteinemia by altering the metabolism of homocysteine, folate, or cobalamin. The most severe form of hyperhomocysteinemia, which produces plasma tHcy concentrations greater than 100 μmol/L, is found in patients with homocystinuria caused by severe deficiency of CBS, MTHFR, or MTRR.

Hyperhomocysteinemia and Vascular Disease

It has been recognized for over 30 years that individuals with homocystinuria due to CBS deficiency have a very high incidence of cardiovascular disease. When untreated, affected patients have about a 50% chance of developing a myocardial infarction, stroke, or serious

Table 21-1. Factors Influencing Plasma Levels of Total Homocysteine

	Factor
Increase	Diabetes
	Increasing age
	Male sex
	Postmenopause
	Smoking
	Alcohol
	Coffee
	Hypothyroidism
	Renal disease
Decrease	Pregnancy
	Hyperthyroidism
	Exercise
	Vitamin intake (Table 21-2)

blood clot before the age of 30. Because the metabolic defect in CBS deficiency produces marked elevation of blood levels of both homocysteine and methionine, it was initially not known whether the high risk of vascular disease in these patients is related to elevation of homocysteine, methionine, or another factor.

In 1969, McCully made an important observation when he noticed severe vascular pathology caused by defects in homocysteine remethylation in children with homocystinuria (McCully, 1969). Like patients with CBS deficiency, these children had markedly elevated levels of tHcy in their blood and urine, but their blood levels of methionine were lower than

normal. It was McCully's observation that vascular disease is a characteristic feature of homocystinuria caused by either transsulfuration or remethylation defects; this led him to postulate that homocysteine itself may be a causative agent in cardiovascular disease.

Initial attempts to confirm McCully's hypothesis met with mixed results in the 1970s and 1980s. Progress in the field was hampered by a lack of reliable laboratory methods to measure circulating levels of plasma tHcy accurately. The introduction of newer, automated methods for determination of plasma tHcy levels in the 1990s led to an exponential increase in published research studies investigating the pathological effects of hyperhomocysteinemia. Elevations in plasma tHcy have now been proven to be associated with increased risk of developing coronary heart disease, stroke, and blood clots.

Like cholesterol, tHcy appears to be a graded risk factor, and even mild hyperhomocysteinemia confers an increased risk of cardiovascular events. A meta-analysis concluded that a 25% elevation in plasma tHcy (about 3 μmol/L) is predictive of about a 10% increased risk of myocardial infarction and a 20% increased risk of stroke (Homocysteine Studies Collaboration, 2002).

Despite a large amount of epidemiological evidence supporting the hypothesis that hyperhomocysteinemia is a risk factor for cardiovascular disease, the molecular mechanisms underlying the vascular pathogenic effects of homocysteine are still not fully understood. Homocysteine is a highly reactive amino acid that can undergo redox reactions, producing oxidants

Table 21-2. Nutrients Required for Homocysteine Metabolism

Nutrient	*Function*
Folate (vitamin B_9)	Methionine cycle: methyl donor in the remethylation of homocysteine to methionine via methionine synthase
Cobalamin (vitamin B_{12})	Methionine cycle: intermediate methyl carrier in the remethylation of homocysteine to methionine cofactor for methionine synthase
Pyridoxine (vitamin B_6)	Transsulfuration pathway: cofactor for cystathionine-β-synthase and cystathionine γ-lyase
	Folate cycle: methylation of tetrahydrofolate cofactor for serine hydroxymethyltransferase
Riboflavin (vitamin B_2)	Folate cycle: reduction of 5,10-methyltetrahydrofolate cofactor for methylenetetrahydrofolate reductase
Betaine*	Methionine cycle: methyl donor in the remethylation of homocysteine to methionine via betaine hydroxymethyltransferase
Choline*	Methionine cycle: required for the formation of betaine
Zinc	Methionine cycle: remethylation of homocysteine to methionine cofactor for methionine synthase

*Not considered to be essential nutrients in healthy adults.

such as hydrogen peroxide. Homocysteine also can participate in disulfide exchange and aminoacylation reactions, resulting in the chemical modification of proteins. Studies using mouse models of CBS deficiency and MTHFR deficiency have confirmed that mild hyperhomocysteinemia produces oxidative stress and vascular inflammation, resulting in dysfunction of the endothelium of blood vessels (Faraci and Lentz, 2004).

One major mechanism for endothelial dysfunction in hyperhomocysteinemic animals appears to be mediated by the oxidative inactivation of nitric oxide, a diffusible gas that relaxes blood vessels and prevents blood clotting. Impairment of NO-mediated dilation of blood vessels also has been observed in human subjects with chronic or acute hyperhomocysteinemia (Lentz, 2001).

Another mechanism contributing to the vascular pathogenic effects of homocysteine may be a diminished capacity for methylation reactions. Hyperhomocysteinemia is often accompanied by a decreased intracellular SAM/SAH ratio, which can inhibit the methylation of DNA and other methyl acceptors (Fig. 21-2). DNA hypomethylation, with resulting changes in gene expression, has been observed in white blood cells isolated from human subjects with hyperhomocysteinemia (Ingrosso et al., 2003).

Birth Defects and Pregnancy Complications

Hyperhomocysteinemia is associated with an increased risk of birth defects resulting from incomplete closure of the neural tube during early embryogenesis. The molecular mechanism responsible for this manifestation of hyperhomocysteinemia is not well understood, but the risk of a neural tube defect can be decreased by treatment with folic acid prior to and during pregnancy. Neural tube closure occurs very early in gestation, during a time when many women may be unaware of their pregnancy. To help prevent neural tube defects, therefore, the Food and Drug Administration mandated in 1998 that all grain products in the United States be fortified with folic acid. In addition, the American College of Obstetricians and Gynecologists recommends that all women of childbearing age take folic acid supplements for the prevention of neural tube defects.

Hyperhomocysteinemia also has been implicated as a risk factor for other complications of pregnancy, including intrauterine growth retardation, eclampsia, birth defects other than neural tube defects, and premature separation of the placenta from the wall of the uterus. It is not yet known, however, whether treatment with folic acid or other homocysteine-lowering therapies will protect pregnant women from these complications.

Neurological Disease

Regulation of homocysteine metabolism appears to be especially important in the central nervous system, presumably because of the critical role of methyl transfer reactions in the production of neurotransmitters and other methylated products. It has been known for decades that mental retardation is a feature of the genetic diseases, such as CBS deficiency, that cause severe hyperhomocysteinemia and homocystinuria. Impaired cognitive function is also seen in pernicious anemia, which causes hyperhomocysteinemia due to deficiency of cobalamin (see Chapter 28). Hyperhomocysteinemia also may be linked to depression, schizophrenia, multiple sclerosis, and Alzheimer's disease. The molecular mechanisms underlying these clinical associations have not yet been delineated.

THERAPY

Homocysteine-lowering therapy is lifesaving for patients with severe hyperhomocysteinemia due to CBS deficiency. Approximately 50% of patients respond to treatment with pharmacological doses (100 to 800 mg daily) of pyridoxine (a form of vitamin B_6). Adjunctive therapy may include betaine (2 to 6 g daily), folic acid (5 to 10 mg daily), or cobalamin (0.05 to 1.0 mg daily), or methionine restriction. Long-term homocysteine-lowering therapy substantially decreases cardiovascular risk in these patients.

Dietary supplementation with B vitamins is also highly effective in lowering homocysteine in most individuals with mild or moderate hyperhomocysteinemia. A meta-analysis of 12 randomized trials performed prior to folic acid fortification concluded that treatment with folic acid (0.5 to 5 mg daily) decreased homocysteine levels by 25%, and that the addition of cobalamin (0.5 mg daily) produced a further 7% decrease in homocysteine levels (Brattstrom et al., 1998). The addition of pyridoxine did not provide any additional lowering of homocysteine levels. In the current era of folic acid fortification, the degree of homocysteine lowering expected from treatment with folic acid may be attenuated. Nevertheless, it is still possible to achieve a normalization of plasma homocysteine in most individuals with mild or moderate hyperhomocysteinemia, although patients with renal failure may be resistant.

It is less clear, however, whether homocysteine-lowering treatment actually improves clinical outcomes in patients with mild or moderate hyperhomocysteinemia. Several randomized clinical trials of homocysteine-lowering therapy are now being conducted to address this question. These trials are designed to test the effectiveness of folic acid or cobalamin in preventing vascular events (such as myocardial infarction, stroke, or blood clots) in patients with known coronary heart disease or prior stroke. Until the results of these trials become available, homocysteine-lowering therapy will continue to be used mainly in selected patients (such as those with a history of premature cardiovascular disease, stroke, or blood clots or those felt to be at high risk due to the presence of other risk factors such as the *MTHFR* 677TT genotype).

When treatment is undertaken, the goal is to maintain plasma tHcy within the low-normal reference range for the laboratory performing the measurement. An American Heart Association science advisory statement has suggested that a homocysteine level of below 10 μmol/L is a reasonable target for subjects with high cardiovascular risk (Malinow et al., 1999).

QUESTIONS

1. How does a diet deficient in folate affect homocysteine and methionine metabolism?
2. What are the metabolic and clinical consequences of CBS deficiency?
3. What patient populations are at risk for hyperhomocysteinemia?
4. What is the predominant form of homocysteine in the blood, and what methods are employed to measure levels of blood homocysteine?
5. What potential mechanisms have been suggested to account for the vascular pathogenic effects of homocysteine?
6. Why is the U.S. food supply fortified with folic acid?

BIBLIOGRAPHY

Brattstrom L, Landgren F, Israelsson B, et al.: Lowering blood homocysteine with folic acid based supplements—meta-analysis of randomised trials. *BMJ* **316**:894–898, 1998.

Butz LW, du Vigneaud V.: The formation of a homologue of cystine by the decomposition of methionine with sulfuric acid. *J Biol Chem* **99**:135–142, 1932.

Carson NA, Neill DW.: Metabolic abnormalities detected in a survey of mentally backward individuals in Northern Ireland. *Arch Dis Child* **37**:505–513, 1962.

Faraci FM, Lentz SR.: Hyperhomocysteinemia, oxidative stress, and cerebral vascular dysfunction. *Stroke* **35**:345–347, 2004.

Frosst P, Blom HJ, Milos R, et al.: A candidate genetic risk factor for vascular disease: a common mutation in methylenetetrahydrofolate reductase. *Nat Genet* **10**:111–113, 1995.

Homocysteine Studies Collaboration: Homocysteine and risk of ischemic heart disease and stroke: a meta-analysis. *JAMA* **288**:2015–2022, 2002.

Ingrosso D, Cimmino A, Perna AF, et al.: Folate treatment and unbalanced methylation and changes of allelic expression induced by hyperhomocysteinaemia in patients with uraemia. *Lancet* **361**:1693–1699, 2003.

Klerk M, Verhoef P, Clarke R, et al.: MTHFR 677C→T polymorphism and risk of coronary heart disease: a meta-analysis. *JAMA* **288**:2023–2031, 2002.

Lentz SR: Homocysteine and cardiovascular physiology, *in* Carmel R, Jacobsen DW (eds), *Homocysteine in Health and Disease.* Cambridge University Press, Cambridge, UK, 2001, pp. 441–450.

Malinow MR, Bostom AG, Krauss RM: Homocyst(e)ine, diet, and cardiovascular diseases—a statement for healthcare professionals from the Nutrition Committee, American Heart Association. *Circulation* **99**:178–182, 1999.

McCully KS: Vascular pathology of homocysteinemia: implications for the pathogenesis of arteriosclerosis. *Am J Pathol* **56**:111–128, 1969.

Mudd SH, Uhlendorf BW, Freeman JM, et al.: Homocystinuria associated with decreased methylenetetrahydrofolate reductase activity. *Biochem Biophys Res Commun* **46**:905–912, 1972.

22

Neonatal Hyperbilirubinemia

JEFFREY C. FAHL and DAVID L. VANDERJAGT

CASE REPORT

A newborn male was the product of a 37-week gestation to a primagravida female whose blood type was O and Rh positive. During the pregnancy, the tests for syphilis and hepatitis B were negative. The pregnancy was uncomplicated, and the mother received excellent care. She denies alcohol consumption and does not smoke.

The labor was prolonged, but the delivery was spontaneous and vaginal. The child was vigorous, active, and breathing spontaneously. Prior to delivery, the mother decided to breastfeed and the child was allowed to suckle immediately following birth.

The initial physical exam revealed a birth weight of 2775 g, a birth length of 48 cm, and a head circumference of 33 cm, which are within normal limits for a near-term male child.

The child was vigorous and appropriate for gestational age. No bruises, skin rashes, or cyanosis were observed. The head, eyes, ears, nose, and throat were normal. He was normocephalic with appropriate molding of the cranial sutures from the delivery. The child had excellent sucking and swallowing coordination. The chest shape and movement were symmetrical with good air entry. No abnormal breath sounds were heard. The heart had a regular rate and rhythm. A slight holosystolic murmur was heard along the left sternal border and was thought to be normal. The abdomen was soft and nontender with no organomegally present. The umbilicus was clamped. Two arteries and one vein were visible. The genitourinary exam was normal, with a normal penis and bilaterally descended testes. His extremities demonstrated

a full range of motion. No deformities were found. Initial laboratory screening values were as follows: hematocrit 48%; blood sugar 55 mg/dL; total serum bilirubin 1.0 mg/dL (all within normal range). The child was given the standard eye care and vitamin K injection. He was allowed to room with the mother, and the mother was encouraged to allow the child to nurse at least every 2 h.

The following morning, nearly 24 h later, the change-of-shift nurse noted that the child appeared to be jaundiced, with the whites of the eyes appearing yellow and the skin yellow to the level of the chest. Following the nursery protocol, repeat laboratory screening values were obtained. These tests showed the following values: hematocrit 45%; total serum bilirubin 7 mg/dL; cord blood type A; and positive Coombs antibody test. The child's pediatrician was informed of the results.

DIAGNOSIS

Hyperbilirubinemia in newborn infants is very common and accounts for most of the laboratory testing done in the neonatal period. The greatest challenge to managing neonates with hyperbilirubinemia is the short hospital stay of mothers and infants. The length of stay is as little as 24 h in some cases, which does not allow adequate time for the normal bilirubin rise to occur. This requires the physician to make a diagnosis quickly and accurately but sometimes with only limited laboratory data.

Diagnosis of the cause of hyperbilirubinemia is made by (1) evaluating the total serum bilirubin

Table 22-1. Conditions That May Produce
Neonatal Jaundice

Prematurity

ABO incompatibilities

Rh-negative mothers with prior exposure to Rh-positive
    infants

Hemolysis

Infection

Dehydration

Breast-feeding

Hypothryoidism

Maternal drug use

Drugs given to infants

Familial nonhemolytic hyperbilirubinemia

and the hematocrit or the hemoglobin; (2) examining a blood smear for signs of hemolysis; (3) comparing the mother's and infant's blood type; and (4) obtaining a Coombs test. The differential diagnosis is broad but can be quickly refined based on simple laboratory tests done reliably by all hospital laboratories. This discussion focuses on the causes of unconjugated or indirect hyperbilirubinemia since conjugated hyperbilirubinemia, which should raise clinical alarms, has a very different differential diagnosis. The causes of neonatal jaundice are listed in Table 22-1.

The gestational age of the infant is a major factor in the development of neonatal hyperbilirubinemia. The more premature the infant is, the lower the level of expression of the enzymes necessary for synthesis of conjugated bilirubin (discussed in the section on Hepatic Metabolism of Bilirubin) and the more likely the child is to develop jaundice. Babies are not routinely screened for the cause of jaundice until the condition manifests itself. Testing would be instituted early if there were a sibling who had experienced prolonged jaundice, or if the mother is blood type O or is Rh negative. All mothers who have good prenatal care are tested for blood type and Rh antibodies. This alerts the physician to potential problems and allows the physician to anticipate the most common forms of jaundice, namely, ABO incompatibilities.

These incompatibilities occur because of small transfusions of maternal blood into the infant at the time of delivery. The naturally occurring antibodies that define blood groups then may initiate hemolysis. For example, a mother

with blood type O has antibodies to A and B blood types. If the child has either an A or B blood type, then the small maternal blood transfusion may lead to hemolysis of the child's blood. However, if the child is blood type O, then no reaction will occur. Even if the mother is blood type O, there is a low probability of jaundice developing. A higher risk occurs if the child is Coombs positive, which demonstrates antibody formation to the child's blood type. (The direct Coombs test detects antibodies on the erythrocytes using Coombs antiglobulin reagent. The indirect Coombs test detects antierythrocyte antibodies in serum).

Rh-negative mothers have an advantage now that RhoGAM, an antisera against Rh antibody formation, is available. RhoGAM is an immunoglobulin G globulin that, when given to an Rh-negative mother, prevents antibody formation to Rh-positive cells from the infant. This exposure occurs during pregnancy, particularly at the time of delivery. If given to the mother within 72 h of delivery, then RhoGAM effectively prevents the mother from developing antibodies to Rh-positive blood and prevents hydrops fetalis, which would often lead to major neonatal problems prior to 1965.

Although ABO incompatibility and Rh-antibody formation are the most common causes of hemolysis, other causes need to be considered, such as cephalohematoma formation during delivery with resultant increase in bilirubin production as the hematoma is resorbed; hereditary spherocytosis, which is a red cell membrane defect that results in premature breakdown of the red cells; and glucose 6-phosphate dehydrogenase deficiency, which is involved in maintaining adequate reduced glutathione levels in the red cell. Infection in the neonatal period is uncommon but still must be considered as a cause of jaundice. In particular, infections of the urinary tract lead frequently to jaundice as a preliminary symptom. The increase in infection associated with instrumentation in the premature infant is always a concern.

Infants are slow to begin nursing, often do not drink enough fluids during the first few days of life, and lose weight. Dehydration can occur, and it is a major effort to encourage mothers to feed or nurse their child during the neonatal time period. Dehydration concentrates the blood volume and increases the bilirubin concentration.

Breast-fed infants may have problems because

milk flow doesn't occur immediately after birth. Frequent suckling induces milk flow, but the presence of pregnandiol in the breast milk inhibits expression of bilirubin-UDP-glucuronyltransferase (discussed in the section on Hepatic Metabolism of Bilirubin), leading to the accumulation of indirect hyperbilirubinemia.

Hypothyroidism is sufficiently common that all infants are screened for this problem prior to discharge from the nursery. Most infants are asymptomatic because thyroxine diffuses across the placental membrane. When hypothyroidism does occur, it results in lethargy, slow movement, hoarse cry, macroglossia, umbilical hernia, large fontanels, hypotonia, dry skin, hypothermia, and prolonged unconjugated hyperbilirubinemia. These are late findings, so early detection and treatment will improve long-term outcome and avoid cretinism, which includes extremely poor developmental and physical growth.

One needs to keep in mind that the use of drugs by the mother will sometimes lead to impairment of the activity of bilirubin-UDP-glucuronyltransferase. Phenothiazines are an example of this kind of interaction. The use of drugs in the neonatal intensive care unit also can contribute to hyperbilirubinemia. Usually, the medications that compete for binding sites on albumin are the culprits in this case (see section on Bilburin Transport). An example of this type of interaction is the use of furosimide, which is a diuretic used to decrease fluid retention and improve cardiac function and renal output.

Finally, there are hereditary causes of non-conjugated, nonhemolytic hyperbilirubinemias. These are Crigler-Najjar types 1 and 2 and Gilbert's syndrome (discussed in the section on Genetic Diseases of Bilirubin Metabolism).

BIOCHEMICAL PERSPECTIVES

Bilirubin Metabolism

Heme Oxygenase

About 75% of bilirubin is derived from degradation of the heme obtained from hemoglobin that is ingested by phagocytic cells in the destruction of senescent erythrocytes, especially in spleen and liver. Most of the remaining bilirubin is derived from turnover of other heme-containing proteins, including myoglobin,

catalase, and cytochromes. Some hemoglobin is released into the circulation when senescent erythrocytes are destroyed. This hemoglobin is complexed as oxyhemoglobin dimers to haptoglobins, which are a family of α_2-globulins synthesized in the liver and secreted into the circulation. The haptoglobin-hemoglobin complexes are removed from the circulation by phagocytes, including Kupfer cells in the liver. Any free heme that might be released is complexed by the globulin hemopexin as well as by serum albumin and transported to the liver.

The heme that is dissociated from globin in the phagocytic process is Fe^{+3}-heme (ferriheme or ferriprotoporphyrin IX). This form of heme is the substrate for the microsomal heme oxygenases, which are mixed-function oxidases that utilize molecular oxygen and NADPH, similar to the family of cytochrome P450s (Fig. 22-1). The oxidation of heme, catalyzed by heme oxygenase, releases carbon monoxide, iron, and biliverdin IXα. The Fe^{+3} iron in heme is reduced by microsomal NADPH-dependent cytochrome P450 reductase in this process and is released as Fe^{+2}. The carbon monoxide is obtained from the α-methene carbon of the cyclic tetrapyrrole ring of heme.

Two genetically distinct heme oxygenases (HOs) have been characterized; HO-1 is an inducible form, whereas HO-2 is constitutive. HO-2 is abundant in selective tissues such as brain and the cardiovascular system. HO-1 is highly inducible in many tissues in response to a variety of stresses, including infection, exposure to xenobiotics, hypoxia, and proinflammatory cytokines. The recognition that heme oxygenase is expressed in many different tissues led to studies of the role of heme degradation apart from the pathway for formation and elimination of bilirubin derived from destruction of senescent erythrocytes.

Biology of Carbon Monoxide

It is well recognized that low levels of carbon monoxide (CO) derived from the heme oxygenase reaction in certain tissues play an important role in the physiological response to stress. CO participates in several signaling pathways in which CO exerts vasoregulatory, anti-inflammatory, antiapoptotic and antiproliferative effects. Evidence is accumulating that CO plays an especially important role in neural signaling. Thus, the pathway of heme degradation (Fig. 22-1) should be viewed in the context of both

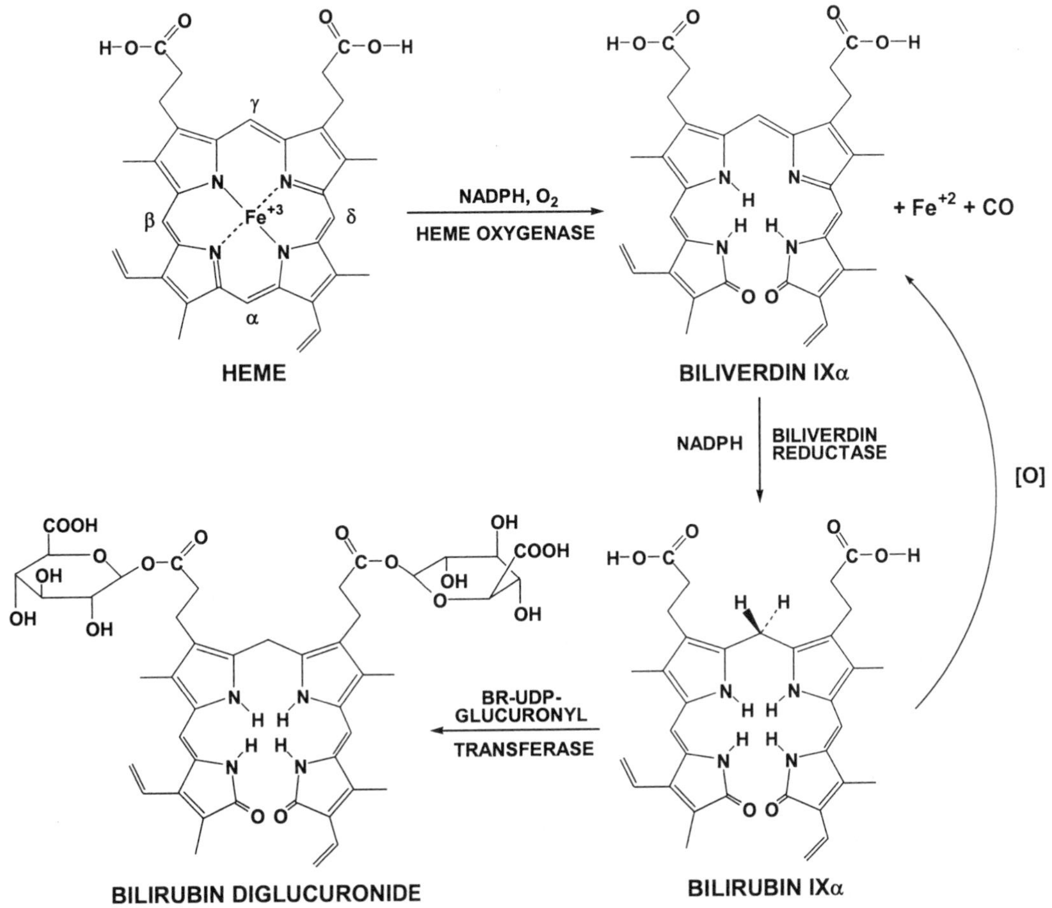

Figure 22-1. Production of bilirubin (BR). The degradation of Fe^{+3}-heme by molecular oxygen and NADPH, catalyzed by microsomal heme oxygenase, produces biliverdin, CO, and Fe^{+2}. Subsequent reduction of biliverdin by NADPH, catalyzed by biliverdin reductase, produces bilirubin. Bilirubin that is produced in phagocytes from degradation of senescent erythrocytes is transported to liver for conjugation with glucuronic acid, catalyzed by bilirubin-UDP-glucuronyltransferase. In some cells, the bilirubin is used as an antioxidant, where it recycles through the biliverdin reductase reaction.

induction of HO-1 and production of CO as part of the cellular response to stress and as a major detoxification/elimination pathway to rid the body of excess bilirubin.

Biliverdin Reductase

The linear tetrapyrrole biliverdin IXα that is a product of the heme oxygenase reaction is the substrate for biliverdin reductase, which catalyzes the NADPH-dependent reduction of biliverdin IXα at the γ–methene bridge to form bilirubin IXα (Fig. 22-1). Many of the pathological problems associated with excess production or diminished elimination of bilirubin are

the result of the low solubility of bilirubin IXα. Other isomers of bilirubin are more soluble than the IXα isomer; however, the IXα isomer is the main product of heme degradation in humans. Bilirubin IXα is much less soluble than biliverdin IXα. This difference in solubility between bilirubin IXα and biliverdin IXα is not obvious from a comparison of their structures (Fig. 22-1). However, bilirubin IXα exists in solution as an intramolecularly H-bonded molecule, as shown in Figure 22-2. This intramolecular H-bonding markedly diminishes the solubility of this bilirubin isomer. Thus, much of the subsequent metabolism of bilirubin involving transport to the liver, conjugation with glucuronic

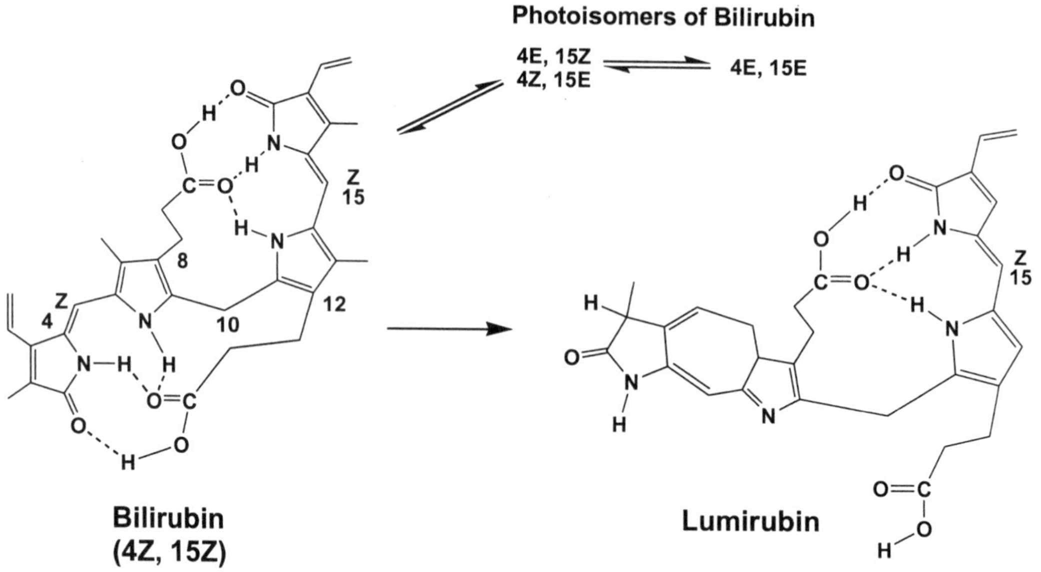

Photoisomers of Bilirubin

Bilirubin
(4Z, 15Z)

Lumirubin

Figure 22-2. Photobilirubins. Light-induced isomerization of bilirubin at the 4- and 15-double bonds produces photoisomers that are water soluble. In addition, bilirubin can be photochemically cyclized to water-soluble lumirubin.

acid, and elimination through the biliary system and intestine is designed to deal with the low solubility of bilirubin and the problems that can arise if bilirubin is not eliminated from the body.

The widespread expression of biliverdin reductase, which parallels the widespread expression of heme oxygenase, suggests that bilirubin may play a special role in particular tissues. Studies suggested that bilirubin is an excellent lipid-soluble antioxidant. Bilirubin reacts with reactive oxygen species (ROS) that oxidize bilirubin back to biliverdin. The biliverdin then is reduced again to bilirubin. This repeated cycling results in the net use of NADPH to protect cells from ROS (Fig. 22-1). This system may be especially important in neurons.

Bilirubin Transport

The bilirubin that is produced in phagocytic cells from degradation of hemoglobin represents the majority of the bilirubin that is produced and must be eliminated. This initially requires transport of bilirubin from the phagocytic cells to the liver. Normally, bilirubin is secreted from phagocytic cells and complexed with albumin for transport to the liver. It is essential that bilirubin is transported through the circulation bound to albumin. The toxicity of

unbound bilirubin, especially that associated with neonatal hyperbilirubinemia, occurs when the binding capacity of serum albumin is exceeded. Unbound bilirubin is readily deposited in skin and other tissue due to its affinity for membrane phospholipids. Unbound bilirubin readily enters the brain, where it can produce bilirubin encephalopathy (kernicterus). Albumin has a high-affinity binding site for bilirubin. A serum albumin concentration of 3 g/dL is sufficient to complex approximately 25 mg/dL bilirubin. The movement of serum through the liver sinusoids allows bilirubin to be transferred from albumin into liver hepatocytes for further metabolism (Fig. 22-3). This is a carrier-mediated process.

Hepatic Metabolism of Bilirubin

Within hepatocytes, bilirubin forms a complex with an abundant cytosolic family of enzymes, the glutathione S-transferases, that have bilirubin-binding sites and function to transport bilirubin to the surface of the endoplasmic reticulum, where one or two glucuronic acid moieties are added to the propionic acid side chains of bilirubin (Fig. 22-1). This reaction, catalyzed by bilirubin-UDP-glucuronyltransferase, involves transfer of glucuronic acid from UDP-glucuronide to bilirubin. The effect of attachment of one or

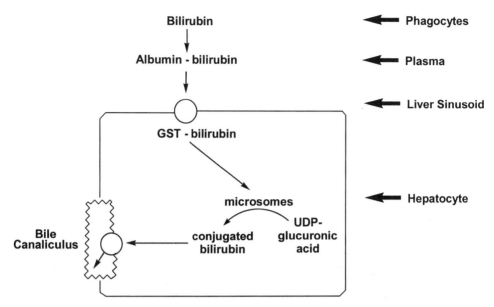

Figure 22-3. Transport and hepatic metabolism of bilirubin. Bilirubin that is produced in phagocytes is transported to liver as an albumin-bilirubin complex. Uptake into the hepatocytes takes place in liver sinusoids. Within the hepatocyte, bilirubin is transported to the endoplasmic reticulum (microsomes) bound to glutathione *S*-transferase (GST). Bilirubin is made water soluble by addition of one or two glucuronic acid moieties obtained from UPD-glucuronic acid, catalyzed by bilirubin-UDP-glucuronyltransferase. The product, conjugated bilirubin, is transported across the bile canalicular membrane for secretion into the biliary system, with subsequent movement into the intestines.

two glucuronic acids to bilirubin is to increase its water solubility and to prepare bilirubin for transfer across the bile cannaliculus (Fig. 22-3).

Bilirubin that contains one or two glucuronic acids is referred to as conjugated bilirubin. Clinically, conjugated bilirubin is called direct-acting bilirubin, and unconjugated bilirubin is called indirect-acting bilirubin. This is related to a colorimetric reaction called the van den Bergh reaction that is sometimes used to quantify the two forms of bilirubin, which is important in differential diagnosis of the causes of hyperbilirubinemia. In the van den Bergh reaction, conjugated bilirubin reacts directly in an azo-dye-coupling reaction. On the other hand, unconjugated bilirubin must first be treated with alcohol to alter some intramolecular H-bonds that prevent the dye-coupling reaction. It is therefore referred to as indirect bilirubin.

Bilirubin-UDP-glucuronyltransferase is one member of a family of glucuronyl transferases that participate in the metabolism of xenobiotics (foreign compounds) by increasing their water solubilities. These enzymes are located on the ER. It is important developmentally that the gene for bilirubin-UDP-glucuronyltransferase not be activated early in fetal development, when it would be undesirable to produce conjugated bilirubin and secrete it into the biliary system. Throughout most of fetal development, bilirubin produced by the fetus is transferred to the maternal circulation. The activity of bilirubin-UDP-glucuronyltransferase increases just before birth and continues to increase after birth, giving the newborn the ability to conjugate and excrete the bilirubin it produces. In premature infants, the activity of bilirubin-UDP-glucuronyltransferase is often low, leading to impaired conjugation and secretion of bilirubin. Therefore, the hyperbilirubinemia associated with premature births is mainly unconjugated bilirubin.

The transfer of conjugated bilirubin in the hepatocyte across the bile canaliculus deposits the conjugated bilirubin along with other hepatic secretions into the biliary system for transport to the small intestine. This transport process is catalyzed by one or more members of the ATP-requiring transporters that belong to the ABC family (ATP binding cassette) of transporters.

Metabolism of Bilirubin in the Intestine

Conjugated bilirubin that is released into the biliary system is concentrated, along with other hepatic and biliary secretions such as bile salts, lecithin and bicarbonate, in the gallbladder and is delivered to the small intestine with the other contents of the gallbladder when the gallbladder contracts. Conjugated bilirubin is absorbed poorly in the intestine. In the lower intestine and colon, bacterial β-glucuronidases remove glucuronic acid to form unconjugated bilirubin. Further metabolism of bilirubin, by bacteria, reduces bilirubin to two colorless compounds, urobilinogen and stercobilinogen. A small amount of urobilinogen is absorbed and enters into the enterohepatic circulation. A minor fraction of the absorbed urobilinogen remains in the circulation, where it is ultimately excreted by the kidney, partly as the oxidized, colored compound urobilin, which imparts the characteristic yellow color of urine. The stercobilinogen is excreted in stool mainly as the oxidized form, stercobilin, which imparts the characteristic color of stool.

Genetic Diseases of Bilirubin Metabolism

A number of genetic diseases are associated with defects in one or more of the enzymes involved in the metabolism of bilirubin. Three of these diseases result in elevated levels of unconjugated bilirubin, and two of these result in elevated levels of conjugated bilirubin. All three of the diseases that produce elevated levels of unconjugated bilirubin are related to defects in the level of expression or in the inherent activity of bilirubin-UDP-glucuronyltransferase (also called UGT1A1). The mildest and most common of these disease is Gilbert syndrome, which is present in about 10% of the Caucasian population.

Gilbert syndrome is the result of the presence of an additional TA in the TATAA box in the proximal promoter of the UGT1A1 gene; this insertion reduces transcription, resulting in bilirubin-UDP-glucuronyltransferase activity that is about 20% of normal in homozygous individuals. This condition is generally benign, with

affected individuals exhibiting mild elevations in unconjugated bilirubin. However, in some individuals with other underlying genetic conditions, such as glucose 6-phosphate dehydrogenase deficiency, there may be much higher levels of unconjugated bilirubin. In addition, some patients with Gilbert syndrome have a problem with hepatic uptake of bilirubin.

The other two diseases related to UGT1A1 are Crigler-Najjar (CN) syndrome types I and II. Many different mutations in UGT1A1 have been identified. CN type I patients express a mutated protein that is essentially devoid of activity. These patients therefore are unable to conjugate bilirubin. Until recently, this condition was lethal in childhood; however, now these patients can be treated with phototherapy (discussed in the next section on Photobilirubin) and liver transplantation. Patients with CN type II express a mutated protein that retains some activity. These patients generally respond to phenobarbital, which increases the transcription of UGT1A1. Both CN types I and II are recessive disorders and rare.

The two genetic diseases associated with elevated levels of conjugated bilirubin are rare and benign diseases that involve altered expression or activity of the ATP-dependent pump that transports conjugated bilirubin across the bile canaliculus. Dubin-Johnson syndrome results in a chronic elevation of conjugated bilirubin and is also characterized by liver histology that shows lysosomal accumulation of a black pigment. Rotor's syndrome is similar in many respects to Dubin-Johnson syndrome except that liver histology is normal. The exact differences that distinguish these diseases are not yet known.

Photobilirubin

For many years, phototherapy has been the standard treatment of neonatal hyperbilirubinemia. The effectiveness of this form of therapy is based on the ability of photons of the appropriate wavelength to convert the intramolecularly H-bonded bilirubin IXα with its low solubility into photoisomers of bilirubin in which the normal Z,Z stereochemistry at the 4- and 15-positions is changed, resulting in photoisomers that are more water soluble. In addition, bilirubin can be converted into the cyclic lumirubin, which is soluble and can be excreted in the urine (Fig. 22-2). Photoproducts can also be excreted through the liver pathway without

Table 22-2. Risk Factors for Neonatal Jaundice

Jaundice in the first 24 hours

Blood group incompatibility

Gestational age less than 38 weeks

Sibling received phototherapy

Cephalohematoma or significant bruising

Exclusive breast-feeding, especially if not going well

Infant of a diabetic mother

Maternal age greater than 25

Male gender

East Asian race

Table 22-3. Stages of Acute Bilirubin Encephalopathy

Early	Middle	Late (Irreversible)
Lethargy	Moderate stupor	Retrocollis-opisthotonos
Hypotonia	Irritability	Shrill cry
Poor suckling	Hypertonia	Refusal to feed
		Apnea
		Fever
		Deep stupor to coma
		Seizures
		Possible death

requiring conjugation. Thus, phototherapy uses photochemical energy to drive the excretion of bilirubin by way of its photoproducts. Blue light (approximately 450 nm), longer wavelength green light, or more commonly, fluorescent white light have been used for phototherapy.

TREATMENT

Treatment begins with prevention and an awareness of risk factors, summarized in Table 22-2. Breast-feeding is now the preferred method of nourishment for infants, and usually frequent nursing is enough to overcome the hydration problems associated with hyperbilirubinemia. However, the combination of low breast milk volume during the first 3 days of life and resultant dehydration affect the level of bilirubin. Interestingly, the addition of water to the feeding of the infant does little to reduce the bilirubin concentration, but the addition of formula is helpful. Knowing the blood type and Rh status of the mother is important and is essential for good prenatal care. In the absence of prenatal care, assessment of these values at the time of birth becomes critical. The use of RhoGAM in Rh-negative mothers is another preventive measure that has improved the outcome of at-risk infants.

Prevention alone is often not enough. Children still become jaundiced even after careful assessment. When this occurs, it is important to assess the risk of developing significant hyperbilirubinemia. The main concern is that the child will develop acute bilirubin encephalopathy, which is caused by the toxicity of bilirubin on the basal ganglia and other brain stem nuclei. There are early, middle, and late stages of acute bilirubin encephalopathy (Table 22-3). The term *kernicterus* is applied to chronic

bilirubin encephalopathy (Table 22-4). Kernicterus occurs most often in infants who have developed the late form of acute bilirubin encephalopathy. However, since it can occur in children with few if any of the signs of acute bilirubin encephalopathy, early diagnosis and treatment are imperative.

Unfortunately, visual assessment has not been correlated with actual bilirubin levels. Therefore, laboratory measurement of the actual total serum bilirubin levels is mandatory. The timing of these measurements becomes important because of the bilirubin load and level of maturation of bilirubin-UDP-glucuronyltransferase.

Acceptable serum bilirubin levels for age have been known for many years, and a nomogram for age versus bilirubin level is available to help the clinician determine severity and define the level of intervention. Most children require careful monitoring only during their hospital stay. However, outpatient monitoring may be needed depending on where they fall on the nomogram. By knowing the age and the bilirubin level, the clinician can predict the rise in bilirubin that will occur for that child. Furthermore, these data also predict which children will require phototherapy or possibly exchange transfusion.

The criteria for use of phototherapy are based on risk factors and a rising bilirubin level that exceeds the rate predicted by the nomogram or levels between 15 and 20 mg/dL The child is at

Table 22-4. Description of Chronic Bilirubin Encephalopathy (Kernicterus)

Severe athetoid cerebral palsy

Auditory dysfunction

Dental-enamel dysplasia

Paralysis of upward gaze

Intellectual handicaps

very high risk if bilirubin levels are greater than 20 mg/dL for a sustained period of time or if the child is not responding to phototherapy, in which case exchange transfusion may be considered. Exchange transfusion replaces the infant's blood volume with blood of the same or compatible type that has a lower bilirubin level. This allows for the equilibration of tissue bilirubin and the removal of antibodies that may lead to hemolysis. The exchange transfusion is done in combination with phototherapy.

Using this approach, the incidence of acute bilirubin toxicity has markedly decreased, and the occurrence of kernicterus is now extremely rare.

BIBLIOGRAPHY

American Academy of Pediatrics Clinical Practice Guideline: Management of hyperbilirubinemia in the newborn infant 35 or more weeks of gestation. *Pediatrics* **114:**297-316, 2004.

Bhutani VK, Johnson L, Sevieri EM: Predictive ability of a predischarge hour-specific serum bilirubin for subsequent significant hyperbilirubinemia in healthy term and near-term newborns. *Pediatrics* **103:**6-14, 1999.

Bosma PJ: Inherited disorders of bilirubin metabolism. *J Hepatol* **38:**107-117, 2003.

Dennery PA, Seidman DS, Stevenson DK: Neonatal hyperbilirubinemia. *N Engl J Med* **344:**581-590, 2001.

Freda VJ, Gorman JG, Pollack W, et al.: Prevention of Rh hemolytic disease—ten-years' clinical experience with Rh immune globulin. *N Engl J Med* **292:**1014-1016, 1975.

Ip S, Chung M, Kulig J, et al.: An evidence-based review of important issues concerning neonatal hyperbilirubinemia. *Pediatrics* **114:**130-153, 2004.

Kaplan M, Hammerman C, Maisels MJ: Bilirubin genetics for the nongeneticist: hereditary defects of neonatal bilirubin conjugation. *Pediatrics* **111:**886-893, 2003.

McDonagh AF: Turning green to gold. *Nature Struct Biol* **8:**198-200, 2001.

Ryter SW, Otterbein LE: Carbon monoxide in biology and medicine. *BioEssays* **26:**270-280, 2004.

Shapiro SM: Bilirubin toxicity in the developing nervous system. *Ped Neurol* **29:**410-421, 2003.

Part IV

Digestion, Absorption, and Nutritional Biochemistry

23

Obesity: A Growing Problem

MIRIAM D. ROSENTHAL and LAWRENCE M. PASQUINELLI

CASE REPORT

T.F. is a 14-year-old girl who came into the office for a well-care examination accompanied by her mother. She had a history of asthma and used albuterol (a bronchodilator) as needed. She was concerned that her weight was too high, and that she was often teased at school by other children. Both T.F. and her mother have been reading about weight loss and exercise; they were ready to make a change to decrease T.F.'s weight.

The patient lived with her mother and her sister. Her father died in a car accident 2 years prior to the visit. Her grandmother had type 2 diabetes and high cholesterol. T.F. ate fast food more than three times a week, drank three 8-ounce cans of nondiet soda each day, and watched about 4 h of television per day. She rarely exercised to break a sweat and did not participate in any sports activities. T.F. was 170 cm tall (90%), weighed 91 kg (>90%), and had a blood pressure of 110/70 mm Hg (normal for her age and height is <125/80 mm Hg).

Her body mass index (BMI) was 31.5 kg/m^2, which is more than 97% of that for her age. Her thyroid was not enlarged, the cardiac examination was normal, and the lung examination was normal without any wheezing (a high-pitched, flutelike noise with expiration often seen with asthma). She had a dark, thick skin rash in the folds on her neck called acanthosis nigricans.

Laboratory studies indicated that her fasting serum glucose level was 85 mg/dL (normal is less than 100). Her serum lipid profile was within the normal range: total cholesterol 168 mg/dL; HDL cholesterol 43 mg/dL; LDL

cholesterol 105 mg/dL; VLDL cholesterol 20 mg/dL; triglycerides 101 mg/dL. She also had normal serum levels of the enzymes AST (aspartate transaminase), ALT (alanine transaminase), and GGT (γ-glutamyl transpeptidase), which are serum markers of liver function.

DIAGNOSIS

Obesity is a common medical condition seen daily by most physicians. BMI is a useful clinical tool to evaluate a patient's size compared with others of the same age. This measure takes into account the patient's height as well as weight. BMI is calculated with either of the following two formulas depending on which measurement system is used:

$$BMI = \frac{\text{Weight (kilograms)}}{\text{Height (meters)} \times \text{Height (meters)}}$$

$$BMI = \frac{\text{Weight (pounds)}}{\text{Height (inches)} \times \text{Height (inches)}} \times 703$$

T.F.'s BMI can be calculated as 31.5 (91 ÷ 1.7 ÷ 1.7); a BMI calculator is provided by the NIH at http://nhlbisupport.com/bmi/bmicalc.htm.

Adults having a BMI between 25.0 and 29.9 kg/m^2 are considered to be overweight; individuals with a BMI greater than or equal to 30 kg/m^2 are classified as obese (Obesity Education Initiative, 1998).

The BMI value can be plotted on a reference BMI curve to determine a child's or adolescent's

CDC Growth Charts: United States

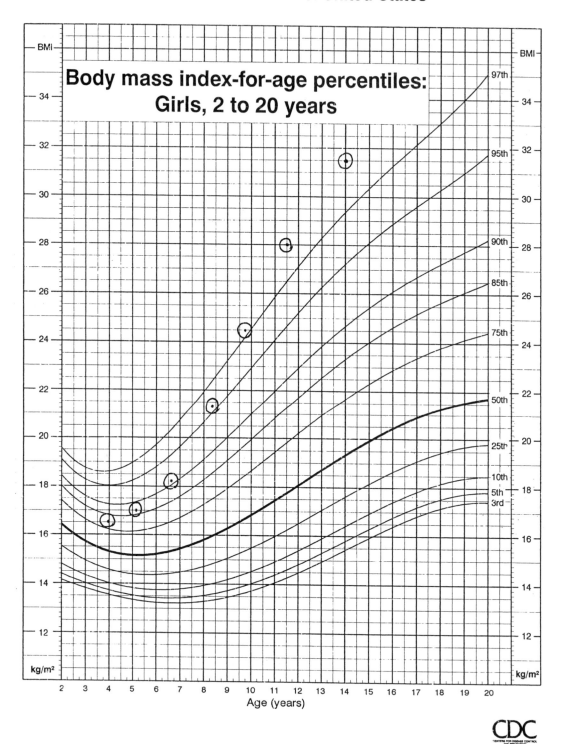

Body mass index-for-age percentiles: Girls, 2 to 20 years

Figure 23-1. T.F.'s body mass index growth curve over time. Plotted on the reference chart of the National Center for Health Statistics, Centers for Disease Control; available at http://www.cdc.gov/nchs/howto/howto.htm.

BMI percentile as a function of age (Fig. 23-1). Children and adolescents with a body mass index percentile of 85% or greater and less than 95% are considered "at risk of overweight"; those with a BMI of 95% or more are considered "overweight." Plotting BMI at the time of medical examinations can be helpful in monitoring growth trends over time. Indeed, plotting BMI for T.F. clearly indicates the progressive development of first overweight and then obesity over a period of many years.

Several methods are available to evaluate a patient's actual body composition rather than total body mass. Skin-fold measurement may be of value in evaluating subcutaneous adiposity (adipose tissue accumulation); proper technique is required for reliable results. Other anthropomorphic measurements such as bioelectrical impedance, dual-energy x-ray absorptiometry, and total body water immersion are also available. These last techniques are often of value in research studies, but it is clinically impractical to use them routinely (Elberg et al., 2004).

For adults, measurement of waist circumference is an easy and accurate indicator of upper body or abdominal adiposity. A waist circumference greater than 102 cm (40 inches) for men and greater than 88 cm (35 inches) for women is indicative of increased risk of cardiovascular disease. Comparable standards are not available for children and teens.

Typically, overweight children are tall for their age when compared with their peers of the same sex and age. If a child is short and overweight, then further studies should be done to exclude a genetically determined problem such as Prader-Willi or Bardet-Biedl syndrome.

Obesity or excess adiposity was relatively rare in earlier centuries. Indeed, an ample belly was often seen as a sign of affluence and prosperity. In the last two decades, however, adult obesity has reached epidemic proportions in the United States and other developed countries. This is strikingly evident from data compiled by the Centers for Disease Control and Prevention (CDC), which estimates obesity rates by state. Data from 1990 indicate that all states had obesity rates (BMI > 30 kg/m^2 or ~ 30 lb overweight) of less than 15%. By contrast, in 2002, every state had an obesity prevalence rate of at least 15%–19%; 29 states had rates of 20%–24%; and the rates in three states were over 25%. Graphic representation of these data, updated annually, is available at http://www.cdc.gov/nccdphp/dnpa/obesity/trend/maps/index.htm.

There has also been a marked increase in childhood obesity in recent years. The above-referenced CDC Web site also includes data on cross-sectional studies on the weight of children. Data from 1963 to 1970 showed that 4% of 6- to 11-year-olds and 5% of 12- to 19-year-olds were overweight. Data from 1999 to 2000 have shown an increased incidence in this number: 15% for 6- to 11-year-olds and 15% for 12- to 19-year-olds.

The chance that an obese child will become an obese adult is estimated to increase from approximately 20% if overweight at age 4 years to approximately 80% if overweight during adolescence (Guo and Chumlea, 1999). Patients who are overweight are at a higher risk for type 2 diabetes, hypertension, and dyslipidemia.

Blood pressure should be measured on overweight patients as part of each physical examination. Based on her height and age, T.F.'s blood pressure should be less than 120/80 mg Hg; her blood pressure (100/70 mm Hg) was acceptable. Blood pressure curves are available that list acceptable blood pressure for patients based on their age and height percentile (http://www.nhlbi.nih.gov/health/prof/heart/hbp/hbp_ped.htm).

Because her BMI is greater than 95%, it puts her at a higher risk for the development of both type 2 diabetes and hypercholesterolemia, fasting plasma glucose and lipid levels were obtained as part of T.F.'s physical examination. In her case, all of the serum levels were within normal limits. If her fasting glucose had been higher than 100 mg/dL, then consideration would have been made for doing a glucose tolerance test to determine how her body manages sugar. A fasting blood glucose level greater than 126 mg/dL is diagnostic for type 2 diabetes and requires treatment. Similarly, if T.F.'s fasting cholesterol had exceeded 170 mg/dL or her triglycerides were greater than 200 mg/dL, then further dietary investigation, testing, nutritional counseling, and possible pharmacological intervention would need to be considered.

T.F. had acanthosis nigricans, a velvety skin rash that mimics the appearance of poorly washed skin and is commonly seen in the neck folds, axilla, or under the breasts. Although this condition may be associated with type 2 diabetes, BMI is a better predicator of risk for the development of type 2 diabetes than the finding of acanthosis nigricans.

Nonalcoholic steatohepatitis (accumulation of triacylglycerol in the liver) or NASH is beginning to be identified more often in overweight individuals. This condition may progress to cirrhosis (fibrosis and loss of normal lobular structure) of the liver. In the case of T.F., measurement of serum levels of AST, ALT. and GGT were used to rule out abnormal liver function.

Patients who are overweight often suffer from depression and poor self-image. Evaluation and screening for these conditions are an essential aspect of caring for patients who are overweight or obese. In addition, although many people are concerned that their increased weight is related to the function of their thyroid gland, it is the cause of obesity in fewer than 1% of patients.

BIOCHEMICAL PERSPECTIVES

Individuals who are overweight or obese primarily have excess adiposity or excess storage of triacylglycerols. The most common cause for patients being overweight is that the individual consumes more calories than are consumed for basic metabolic needs and energy expenditure. For each additional 3500 kcal consumed that are not utilized as fuel, 1 pound of fat is accumulated in the body.

The human organism is well adapted to intermittent availability of food. When we eat, excess energy is stored for future use during intervals of scarcity. Indeed, this fed-fasted cycle is a daily phenomenon, with mobilization of stored fuel used to sustain the individual and maintain critical concentrations of blood sugar during the night.

Most of the body's energy reserves are in the form of fat or triacylglycerol. Estimates are that the reference 70 kg (154 lb) adult male has 15 kg of stored fat compared to a mere 0.2 kg of stored carbohydrate, primarily glycogen. If that same individual were to gain 70 kg in weight and become quite obese, then 65 kg of the increased weight would be triacylglycerol, with the rest comprised of increased fluid and a modest increase in total body protein.

The human diet provides energy primarily from a mixture of carbohydrates and fats, with protein accounting for perhaps 12%–30% of total energy intake. As noted above, the potential for storing carbohydrates is limited. Furthermore, there are no protein stores in the body

per se, although some muscle proteins are readily mobilized during fasting to provide amino acid precursors for gluconeogenesis. Instead, the dietary carbohydrates and protein-derived amino acids not required for the immediate metabolic and biosynthetic needs of the body are converted to triacylglycerol for storage (Fig. 23-2). Similarly, excess dietary fatty acids are esterified into triacylglycerols and stored in adipose tissue.

In the postprandial or fasted state, the body relies on stored triacylglycerols to provide most of its energy needs. As seen in Figure 23-3, the adipocyte triacylglycerols are hydrolyzed by hormone-sensitive lipase, and the released free fatty acids are made available to muscle, liver, heart, and other organs. Some organs, notably brain and red blood cells, cannot utilize free fatty acids as an energy source and are therefore dependent on a continued supply of glucose. The pancreatic hormone glucagon stimulates the release of a modest amount of glucose (up to 70 g) from liver glycogen. Muscle glycogen is unavailable for this purpose. (Muscle cells lack glucose 6-phosphatase, and any glucose-phosphate obtained from glycogenolysis is retained for utilization within the muscle rather than released into the blood.) The liver glycogen stores are, however, insufficient to meet glucose requirements during an overnight fast. Fortunately, when glucagon stimulates glycogen mobilization, it also stimulates gluconeogenesis and thus the synthesis of glucose from glycerol and amino acid precursors (Fig 23-3).

Food energy is usually measured in calories or kilocalories, with 1 kcal representing the amount of heat that is required to raise the temperature of 1 kg of water 1°C. The caloric yield of different energy sources is shown in Table 23-1. The physiological energy yield of protein (4 kcal/g) is less than the 5.7 kcal/g that is observed in a bomb calorimeter; the difference represents the energy required for the synthesis of urea. Note that fats provide more calories per gram than either protein or carbohydrate. Consumption of alcoholic beverages can also provide significant energy, even if they contain relatively few carbohydrates. Dietary ethanol is oxidized to acetyl-CoA, which, depending on the availability of other energy sources, is either further oxidized or utilized for synthesis of fatty acids.

There are two main components of daily energy expenditure: basal or resting energy expenditure and energy expended in exercise.

DIET METABOLISM STORES

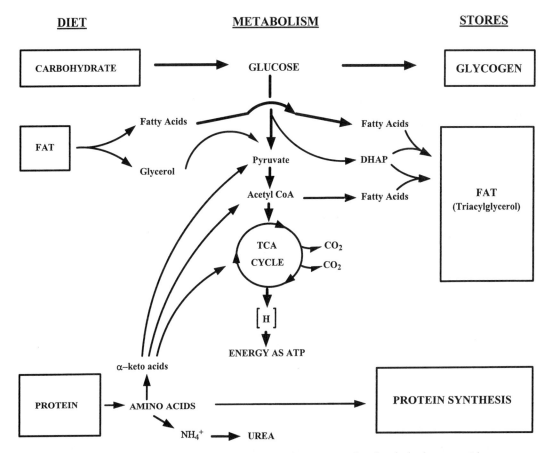

Figure 23-2. Metabolism in the fed state. An adequate supply of carbohydrate provides glucose to replenish glycogen stores. Dietary protein provides amino acids for protein synthesis. Dietary carbohydrates, fats, and proteins can all be metabolized to generate ATP. (For clarity, ATP generation during β-oxidation of fatty acids and substrate-level phosphorylation during glycolysis is not depicted.) Excess dietary carbohydrates and amino acids are converted to fatty acids and, along with excess dietary fatty acids, stored as triacylglycerols. DHAP, dihydroxyacetone phosphate.

For adults, the resting energy expenditure is estimated at about 1800 kcal/day for males and about 1400 kcal/day for females (Recommended Dietary Allowances, 1989). At all ages, resting energy expenditure is closely correlated with lean body mass (amount of actual metabolic tissue); individuals who increase their muscle mass through physical activity actually have a higher energy expenditure at rest.

The other major component of daily energy expenditure is due to physical activity. For most individuals in the United States, physical activity accounts for 15%–30% of the total daily energy. Most people can sustain metabolic rates 8-10 times their resting value (8-10 METS or multiples of the resting metabolic rate) with reasonably strenuous activi-

ties such as running, biking, or fast walking. When estimating energy expenditure due to physical activity, one must consider both the increased metabolic rate per minute and the length of the activity. Thus, individuals who run for 30 minutes per day before going to work at a desk job are still primarily sedentary. Unfortunately, more and more children also lead essentially sedentary lifestyles. Muscle work, independent of sustained physical exercise, can also be a source of significant energy expenditure. When 24-h energy expenditure was studied in a respiratory chamber, much of the differences between individuals were the result of variability in the degree of spontaneous physical activity (i.e., "fidgeting") (Ravussin et al., 1986).

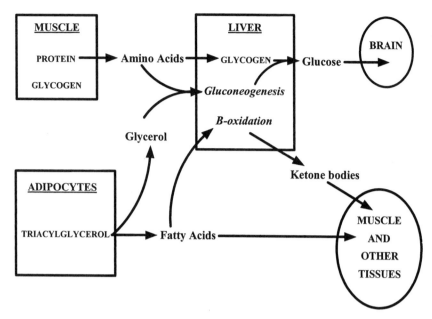

Figure 23-3. Mobilization of fuels during an overnight fast. Adipocyte triacylglycerols are mobilized to provide the major fuel for the body. The released free fatty acids are utilized by muscle and most other tissues. Blood sugar supplies to the brain are maintained by the liver, which releases glucose synthesized by gluconeogenesis as well as from its glycogen stores. Amino acids from catabolism of muscle proteins and glycerol from adipocyte triacylglycerol provide the substrates for gluconeogenesis. Under these conditions, liver utilizes β-oxidation of free fatty acids as a means of generating ATP. The resultant two-carbon moieties from acetyl-CoA are exported as ketone bodies (acetoacetate and β-hydroxybutyrate) and provide an additional fuel supply for muscle. During prolonged fasting, the ketone bodies also become a significant fuel source for the brain, thus sparing glucose.

The accumulation of excess adipose tissue triacylglycerol, which results in development of an overweight status and subsequent obesity, is a gradual process resulting from a long-term, often small imbalance in energy intake and energy expenditure. A modest energy excess intake of 50 kcal/day will add up to 18,250 kcal per year, or approximately 5 lb of additional stored fat (3500 kcal/lb). Similarly, substantial weight loss requires negative energy balance over a prolonged time period. Based on the 3500 kcal/lb of fat, one can reasonably expect that a deficit of 500 kcal/day will result in a weight loss of about 1 lb/week. Consulting the RDA tables (Recommended Dietary Allowances, 1989), one finds the average energy a teenager such as T.F. expends per day is 2200 kcal. If she were to fast completely (which is not medically recommended), then she would not deplete more than about 4 pounds of fat per week. Indeed, much of the initial rapid weight loss on popularized "diets" often reflects depletion of muscle protein for gluconeogenesis or loss of fluids.

The goal of a healthy weight reduction program is the gradual depletion of excess triacylglycerol reserves. This occurs when, over time, the replenishment of triacylglycerol stores after meals is less than the utilization of those stores between meals. Exercise helps this program in several ways. First, exercise increases fuel utilization, with skeletal muscle utilizing a mixture of muscle glycogen, plasma glucose, and plasma free fatty acids. The ratio of glucose to fatty acids oxidized depends on the intensity and duration of the exercise. Since the subsequent meal is then utilized to replenish the glycogen stores as well for triacylglycerol synthesis, the important consideration is the total amount of energy expended rather than the specific fuel mixture. Second, as noted, regular exercise increases the lean muscle mass

Table 23-1. Approximate Energy Values of Metabolic Fuels

Carbohydrate	4 kcal/g
Protein	4 kcal/g*
Fat	9 kcal/g
Ethanol	7 kcal/g

*Net energy yield in human metabolism.

and thus the resting energy expenditure as well.

The medical problems of obesity are severe and multiple. In addition to the obvious increased physical burden to organs such as the heart and joints, obesity is associated with significant metabolic changes. Studies have demonstrated that adipose tissue is not a passive reservoir for energy storage as triacylglycerol but is instead an active endocrine organ (Kershaw and Flier, 2004). Adipocytes produce a variety of bioactive peptides called adipocytokines, which affect metabolism on both the local and systemic level. For example, increased circulating levels of one such adipocytokine, interleukin 6, are associated with impaired glucose tolerance and development of cardiovascular disease. By contrast, adiponectin, a second adipocyte-derived hormone, appears to have an inverse relationship with development of insulin resistance and inflammatory states.

Excess adiposity, particularly the abdominal obesity associated with increased waist circumference, is associated with insulin resistance, hypertension, and proinflammatory states. The prevalence of this complex of comorbidities associated with obesity, now referred to as the metabolic syndrome, is reaching epidemic proportions in the United States (Grundy et al., 2004; Roth et al., 2002). Indeed, increased abdominal adiposity is one of a cluster of factors that are used in the diagnosis of metabolic syndrome. Abdominal tissue in the trunk occurs in several compartments, including subcutaneous and intraperitoneal or visceral fat. Visceral fat in particular appears to contribute to perturbed fuel metabolism by at least two mechanisms. First, hormones and free fatty acids released from visceral fat are released into the portal circulation and impact directly on metabolism of the liver. Second, the visceral adipose depot produces a different spectrum of adipocytokines than that produced by subcutaneous fat (Kershaw and Flier, 2004).

Adipocytes are also a significant source of steroid hormones, including cortisol, andro-gens, and estrogens. Visceral adipocytes appear to be more active than subcutaneous adipocytes in production of glucocorticoids. Excess production of sex steroids by adipocytes has also been linked to problems of polycystic ovary disease, infertility, and dysfunctional uterine bleeding.

Modification of the quantity of energy intake is clearly a primary focus for any approach to prevention or treatment of excess adiposity (Obesity Education Initiative, 1998). Although excess caloric intake, whether carbohydrate, fat, protein, or even ethanol, is readily converted to triacylglycerol for storage, earlier therapies often focused on decreasing total fat in the diet. This was in part because of the high caloric density of fat and the increased caloric content of fried foods and in part because of the established linkage between high saturated fat and cholesterol intake and hypercholesterolemia. With the awareness of the prevalence of hypercholesterolemia and dyslipidemia in overweight individuals, many medical experts use the American Heart Association's guidelines for a prudent diet (limit saturated fat to less than 10% of the patient's total calories, limit total calories from fat to no more than 30%, and limit cholesterol intake to less than 300 mg/day) for their overweight patients (Willett, 2002).

It has become increasingly clear, however, that low fat does not necessarily mean low calorie. Indeed, the increased caloric intake of the American public in the last decade has come primarily from carbohydrates. T.F.'s intake of sugared soda beverages is typical of this situation. Furthermore, epidemiological data have strengthened the link between obesity and type 2 diabetes, including the increased prevalence of this "adult-onset" disease at younger and younger ages. This has led to concern about overall carbohydrate intake, particularly simple sugars and refined carbohydrate foods such as white flour, which have a high glycemic index (or impact on postprandial blood glucose) and thus provoke a high insulin response. While both extreme low-fat and low-carbohydrate advocates have received a lot of popular press, current studies support a more nuanced approach that distinguishes between vegetable oils and saturated animal fats and between whole grain carbohydrate sources and processed sugars (Willett and Stampfer, 2003).

Metabolic research on obesity has also sought to elucidate hormonal and neuroendocrine mechanisms of appetite control. Leptin, a circulating protein produced by adipocytes, contributes to regulation of energy homeostasis through effects on both the hypothalamus and on peripheral tissues. Studies have indicated, however, that leptin's primary role is to serve as a metabolic signal of energy sufficiency rather than excess (Kershaw and Flier, 2004). Indeed, common forms of obesity are neither leptin deficient nor responsive to exogenous leptin. Another molecule that has attracted much research interest is ghrelin, a recently discovered orexigenic (appetite-stimulating) gastric hormone; its production is induced by lack of food in the stomach. There is, however, no compelling evidence that mutations in ghrelin contribute to human obesity (Cowley and Grove, 2004). Furthermore, studies with mice deficient in either ghrelin or its receptor suggest that ghrelin is not essential for normal growth or appetite (Lang, 2004). Further studies on leptin, ghrelin, and other proteins that contribute to metabolic signaling may, however, lead to pharmacological products useful in the treatment of wasting syndromes or morbid obesity.

THERAPY

For most overweight and obese individuals, the primary therapeutic approach involves changing the balance between energy intake and utilization. Efforts need to be made to encourage patients both to decrease the amount of calories consumed and to increase energy expenditure. Programs that incorporate exercise with dietary choice intervention have been more successful in helping patients to lose weight and then to maintain their weight loss (Epstein et al., 1985). Furthermore, identification of the patient's and family's motivation for change is an important step in treatment. Obesity is a family-centered problem, and all members of the family need to be willing to work to help the affected family members. Without this support, long-term success is difficult.

T.F. and her mother were motivated to make behavioral changes to help T.F. lose weight. Setting goals for behavioral change at each visit is important. The goals should be decided by the patient with the family and should be goals that are realistic and achievable. Once the old goals have been met, new goals should be developed. Each visit is an opportunity to meet and to review progress; frequent follow-up in an individual or group setting greatly enhances successful weight loss.

At the visit, T.F. agreed to limit her television watching to less than 2 h a day. For children, limiting the amount of television watching to less than 2 h a day has been associated with weight loss (Robinson, 2001). She also agreed to begin walking in her neighborhood three times a week for 30 min. She would drink only diet soda and try to drink more water. Rather than limiting her eating out at restaurants, she would seek to become aware of portion sizes and try to avoid high-fat, high-sugar meals. She might consider packing lunch for school if the available choices are unsuitable. She and her mother agreed to come back for a follow-up visit in 2 weeks. Her mother agreed to make an effort to increase the availability of foods and snacks with lower caloric density (particularly vegetables and fruits) available at home but to leave actual food choices to T.F.

A realistic weight loss goal should be approximately 0.5 to 1 pound per week, which means that it will require time to reach the patient's personal goal. Weight loss, though important, should not be the sole measure of success. Improvements in how clothing fits or how the patient feels about herself should also be recognized and praised. For younger pediatric patients who are still growing, maintaining the child at a constant weight may allow the child to "grow into" a weight that is appropriate for the child's height.

Effective behavior modification programs also require a long-term approach. It takes time for individuals to acquire appropriate nutritional information and to develop sustainable programs for physical activity. For this reason, T.F. and her mother were referred to a weight management program provided by the local children's hospital. The 7-week program was designed to provide additional education, skills, and tools to assist families as they help their children adopt a healthier lifestyle. The weekly 2-h group sessions, separate for individuals of 8–11 and 12–18 years of age, incorporate physical activity as well as education and peer support. Each patient is also evaluated by a nutritionist, licensed clinical social worker, and a physical therapist.

Unlike T.F., some obese patients have severe medical complications related to their obesity, such as uncontrolled diabetes, severe depression, or sleep apnea. Under these circumstances, more aggressive measures may be necessary. One such measure is a medically supervised very low calorie, ketogenic diet (high protein, very low carbohydrate) for rapid weight loss. Use of a ketogenic diet in children requires intensive family dedication and may require inpatient hospitalization to meet the necessary dietary goals.

A pharmacological approach can also be considered (Therle and Aronne, 2003). Currently, there are few medications available or approved by the Food and Drug Administration for weight loss in children and adolescents. Orlistat, which inhibits pancreatic lipase to decrease fat absorption, and sibutramine, a norepinephrine-, serotonin-, and dopamine-reuptake inhibitor, have been used with some overweight pediatric patients. Current opinion recommends that such medications be used as part of a multicenter research protocol under the supervision of a physician qualified to monitor patients on these medications properly. When patients have life-threatening complications resulting from their obesity or when all other therapies have been exhausted, there may be a role for bariatric surgery, which prevents the patient from eating large quantities of food at a single meal. The surgical procedures are not without risk or potential for complications, including death. Surgical intervention should therefore be the option of last resort, especially in adolescent patients.

QUESTIONS

1. Trying to stay awake to study, a second-year medical student added three 12-oz cans of caffeinated soda a day (~40 g sugar/can) to her diet. She did not otherwise change her diet or physical activity. How much weight would she be expected to gain during the next 6 months?
2. After 6 months, the student described in question 1 now wants to lose the weight she has gained. She decides to switch to diet sodas and starts to walk 3 miles five times per week. She looks up exercise physiology studies and determines that she will burn about 75 kcal/mile walked. How long will it take to lose the added weight?
3. What are the advantages and disadvantages (if any) to utilizing fat rather than carbohydrate as one's primary dietary fuel?
4. What carbohydrate-containing foods would be an important part of a balanced diet for a teenager such as T.F.?
5. What suggestions could you make to a teenager to decrease the caloric density of her diet?
6. What social and economic obstacles might an individual such as T.F. face in trying to control her body weight?

BIBLIOGRAPHY

Cowley MA, Grove KL: Ghrelin—satisfying a hunger for the mechanism. *Endocrinology* **145:** 2604-2606, 2004.

Elberg J, McDuffie JR, Sebring NG, et al.: Comparison of methods to assess change in children's body composition. *Am J Clin Nutr* **80:**64-69, 2004.

Epstein LH, Wing RR, Penner BC, Kress MJ: Effect of diet and controlled exercise on weight loss in obese children. *J Pediatr* **107:**358-361, 1985.

Grundy SM, Brewer HB Jr, Cleeman JI, et al.: Definition of metabolic syndrome: report of the National Heart, Lung, and Blood Institute/American Heart Association conference on scientific issues related to definition. *Circulation* **109:**433-430, 2004.

Guo SS, Chumlea WC: Tracking of body mass index in children in relation to overweight in adulthood. *Am J Clin Nutr* **70**(suppl):145S-148S, 1999.

Kershaw EE, Flier JS: Adipose tissue as an endocrine organ. *J Clin Endocrinol Metab* **89:** 2548-2556, 2004.

Lang L: Studies question role of ghrelin in appetite regulation. *Gastroenterology* **127:**374-375, 2004.

Obesity Education Initiative: *Clinical Guidelines on the Identification, Evaluation, and Treatment of Overweight and Obesity in Adults: The Evidence Report.* 1998. NIH Publication 98-4083. Available at: www.ncbi.nlm.nih.gov/books.

Ravussin E, Lillioja S, Anderson TE, et al.: Determinants of 24-h energy expenditure in man. Methods and results using a respiratory chamber. *J Clin Invest* **76:**1568-1578, 1986.

National Research Council: *Recommended Dietary Allowances.* 10th ed. National Research Council, National Academy Press, Washington, D.C., 1989.

Robinson TN: Television viewing and childhood obesity. *Pediatr Clin North Am* **48:**1017-1025, 2001.

Roth JL, Mobathan S, Clohisy M: The metabolic syndrome: where are we and where do we go? *Nutr Rev* **60:**335-341, 2002.

Thearle M, Aronne LJ: Obesity and pharmacologic therapy. *Endocrinol Metab Clin North Am* **32:**1005-1024, 2003.

Willett WC: Balancing life-style and genomics research for disease prevention. *Science* **296:**695-698, 2002.

Willett WC, Stampfer MJ: Rebuilding the food pyramid. *Sci Am* **288:**64-71, 2003.

24

Protein-Energy Malnutrition

VIJAYAPRASAD GOPICHANDRAN, LIEN B. LAI, and VENKAT GOPALAN

CASE REPORTS

Case 1: Kwashiorkor

A 22-month-old male child was seen in a pediatric clinic in the United States (Carvalho et al., 2001). He had been suffering from intermittent skin eczema since 2 weeks of age. After weaning at 13 months of age, he was given cow's milk, and several episodes of vomiting were observed soon after. Since his parents suspected milk intolerance and were apprehensive about the cow's milk causing a possible worsening of the eczema, he was immediately switched to a lactose-free diet that was primarily a rice milk beverage. This rice drink was extremely low in protein but (somewhat) adequate in caloric content. Although well educated, the parents mistakenly assumed that the beverage, because of its fortified contents and high cost, was a superior food product for their child even though the container stated that the rice milk beverage was not meant for use as an infant formula. Despite normal growth during infancy, poor weight gain was obvious during the second year, when the child was on a daily intake of 1.5 L of the rice drink, which is equivalent to 3 g protein and 790 calories/day (norm for ages 1–3, 16 g protein and 1300 calories/day). In the weeks before admission, he was irritable, was less active, and displayed an increase in skin lesions.

At the time of admission, the child weighed 10.8 kg (10th percentile), and height was 81 cm (5th percentile). His physical examination revealed generalized edema; alternating hyper- and hypopigmented patches in the skin; thin, sparse scalp hair; abdominal distension; and irritability. Laboratory tests of the child's serum revealed 1.0 g/dL albumin (normal is 3.5–5.5 g/dL), less than 0.5 mg/dL urea nitrogen (normal is 2–20 mg/dL), and 2.2 mg/dL phosphorus (optimal is 4.5 mg/dL). Hematological analysis showed normocytic anemia with marked anisocytosis (variation in cell size). The white blood cell (WBC) count of 11,500 cells/mm^3 was normal.

A diagnosis of kwashiorkor was made after a detailed workup to rule out other causes of hypoproteinemia such as proteinuria (loss of proteins in urine) and protein-losing enteropathy (loss of serum proteins through the gut). As there was severe anorexia, gradual refeeding was started using a nasogastric tube. A soy-based, protein-rich formula was initiated at the rate of 80 mL/kg/day and gradually increased to 120 mL/kg/day. Potassium, phosphorus, zinc, folate, and other vitamins were supplemented. The child also received a 10-day course of oral cotrimoxazole (a broad-spectrum antibiotic) for his otitis media (acute inflammation of the middle ear) with effusion. He was subsequently switched to a milk-based nutritional supplement since soybeans are relatively deficient in methionine, an essential dietary amino acid. Within 3 weeks of treatment, rising serum albumin levels and resolution of the edema were observed. After 2 months, his body weight of 11.5 kg placed him in the 20th percentile. The 1-year follow-up revealed normal development after having been maintained on a milk-based pediatric nutritional supplement containing micronutrients.

Case 2: Marasmus

A 10-month-old male child was examined during a health-screening camp for women and children in a developing country. The mother complained that her child was always hungry and crying for food and was having loose stools for the past 1 month. The striking feature about this irritable and constantly crying child was the emaciated appearance, with gross wasting of all muscle groups. The skin was hanging in loose folds and lacked the normal shine and texture.

The child's height was 70 cm, and weight was 5 kg, which were in the 10th and below the 5th percentile, respectively, of normal height and weight for his age. There was no edema. The midarm circumference (MAC) was 10 cm, and the triceps skinfold thickness (TSF) was 5 mm. The midarm muscle circumference (MAMC), defined as (MAC, cm) − [π (TSF, mm)/10], was calculated be to 8.5. All these anthropometric values, when compared to standard tables for age group and sex, were below the 5th percentile and indicated wasting, low fat, and low protein reserve.

On further evaluation in a referral center, the child's laboratory test results were as follows: 60 mg/dL fasting blood glucose (normal is 70-100 mg/dL); 174 mg/dL 2-h postprandial blood glucose (normal is 120 mg/dL); 1.8 g/dL serum albumin (normal is 3.5-5.5 g/dL); 8 mg/dL serum prealbumin or transthyretin (normal is 16-40 mg/dL); 0.6 mmol/day urine creatinine (normal is 1-1.3 mmol/day). The urinary creatinine-to-height index (CHI) was 46% as calculated by the formula CHI (%) = [(Actual 24-hr creatinine excretion)/(Expected 24–hr creatinine excretion for height)] × 100. The WBC count of 3,500 cells/mm^3 was low (normal is 4,500-10,000 cells/mm^3). The T-cell count at 300 cells/mm^3 was significantly below the expected value (i.e., 8%-22% of the normal WBC count). A routine stool examination revealed plenty of fat globules, pus cells, and red blood cells (10-12/hpf (high-power field)).

The child was diagnosed as suffering from malnutrition of the marasmus type. Cotrimoxazole was given twice daily to treat the intestinal infection. Nutritional refeeding was initiated with a liquid gruel containing 1 g egg protein/kg ideal body weight, wheat flour equivalent to 1000 calories/day, and plenty of vegetables and fruits to replace the vitamins and minerals. Vitamins A and D were given as oral supplements. A follow-up analysis 6 months later revealed a nearly complete recovery as reflected in the anthropometric measurements and biochemical tests.

DIAGNOSIS

Signs and Symptoms

The signs and symptoms of protein-energy malnutrition (PEM) depend on various factors, including the duration of the nutritional inadequacy, age at onset, and frequency/types of concomitant infections. Figure 24-1 shows children diagnosed with kwashiorkor and marasmus and outlines some of the diagnostic features discussed in this section (Scrimshaw and Behar, 1961).

A hallmark of kwashiorkor (absent in marasmus) is the rotund appearance caused by generalized edema in the hands, feet, and abdomen (Fig. 24-1; Hendrickse, 1991). While low body weight for height is always found in children with marasmus, fluid retention and edema frequently lead to increased weight in kwashiorkor and tend to mask growth failure. Children with kwashiorkor usually have lower serum albumin values than those diagnosed with marasmus. "Flaky paint" dermatitis, discolored and brittle hair devoid of natural sheen and curl, enlarged fatty liver, growth retardation, and apathy are features associated with kwashiorkor. The easy peeling of the epidermis results in infections of the underlying tissues. Periodic variations between poor and acceptable nutritional status lead to the multicolored hair that looks like a "striped flag" with alternating depigmented and pigmented portions. According to Hendrickse (1991), the mental state and behavior of those with kwashiorkor are distinguished by extreme irritability and the absence of a smile.

Children with marasmus are likely to have been weaned early and look extremely thin due to loss of muscle mass and body fat. The disease of hunger is portrayed most poignantly in the skeletal spectre of marasmic children. The head appears disproportionately large, with bones and joints jutting out prominently. The facial fat (i.e., the buccal pad) is usually retained even when subcutaneous fat elsewhere is being consumed rapidly. These facial features lend the children an elderly appearance. Muscle wasting, weight loss, modest irritability,

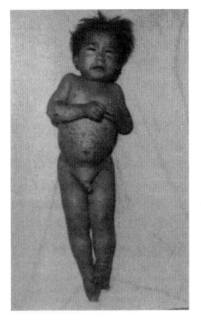 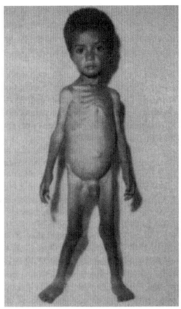

Features	Kwashiorkor	Marasmus
Edema	Present	Absent
Weight	60-80% of expected body weight	<60% expected body weight
Skin	Hyperpigmented patches "Flaky paint" dermatitis	Loose and inelastic Dry and lusterless
Hair	Thin, brittle, pluckable A "striped-flag" appearance due to alternating pigmentation	None noticeable
Psychomotor Behavior	Apathetic	Hungry and eager

Figure 24-1. Typical features found in children with kwashiorkor and marasmus. Photographs reprinted with permission from Scrimshaw and Behar (1961). © 1961, AAAS.

frequent infections, an absence of edema, and a grossly shrunken appearance typify marasmus.

Since children suffering from PEM exhibit growth retardation, lower scores on developmental measures, and weak cognitive performance, it is imperative for the diagnosis to be made as early as possible to remedy nutritional inadequacies and ensure appropriate developmental progress. In addition, even though PEM is usually associated with developing countries or those who are at war or facing famine, it has been found elsewhere. In many instances, food fads and fallacies in developed countries lead to PEM, and many of these cases may remain either undetected or unreported as there is little clinical suspicion of PEM.

General Nutritional Assessment

The tools for nutritional assessment include medical history and screening aides, physical examination and anthropometric measurements, biochemical assessment, and tests of immune function. A general health assessment and medical history are required to rule out causes of secondary malnutrition such as poor oral health, chronic illness, disease, and medication. Malnutrition is influenced by lifestyle, which includes alcohol usage in adults, food preference, eating habits, social interactions, and economic status. Various screening tools, such as the DETERMINE checklist (White et al., 1991), are available to assess the risk of malnutrition.

The physical examination in children concentrates on anthropometric measurements such as height, weight, and calculation of the percentile of the height and weight for age (Gurney and Jelliffe, 1973). Signs of associated vitamin and mineral deficiencies may also be detected. The TSF and MAMC values indicate the body fat and protein reserve, respectively. In adults and the elderly, anthropometrics include weight, height, and body mass index, which is calculated as (Weight in kg)/(Height in m)^2. Taken together, these patient data, when compared to the average normal values, can help draw inferences of stunting, wasting, or both.

PEM is frequently associated with changes in serum markers such as protein, lipid, and nitrogen (Hendrickse, 1991). Decreased serum albumin levels have been used as a standard PEM indicator. Since albumin has a long half-life of 18 days in the plasma and a large pool size that decreases in various illnesses (such as hepatic insufficiency and nephrosis), it is not a specific marker for recent nutritional inadequacies. Prealbumin (or transthyretin), by virtue of its higher catabolic rate (half-life = 1.9 days) and small pool size, is a very sensitive and fairly specific indicator of acute malnutrition and short-term responses to nutritional replacements in patients of all ages (Bernstein and Ingenbleek, 2002).

While low serum cholesterol levels have been observed in malnourished patients, largely as a result of decreased synthesis of lipoproteins in the liver, hypocholesterolemia occurs later in the course of malnutrition and is therefore not useful as a screening test. PEM usually results in low serum urea nitrogen (BUN), urinary urea, and total nitrogen. Estimation of 24-h urine creatinine excretion is also a valuable biochemical index of muscle mass (when there is no impairment in renal function). The urinary CHI is correlated to lean body mass and anthropometric measurements. In edematous patients, for whom the extracellular fluids contribute to body weight and spuriously high body mass index values, the decreased CHI values are especially useful in diagnosing malnutrition.

Yet another indication of PEM is usually obtained from an analysis of the immunodeficiency of the patient. An atrophied thymus in malnourished patients results in a lower T-cell count. In addition, macrophages from PEM individuals have decreased interleukin 1 activity, for which a sensitive (albeit expensive) assay is available.

BIOCHEMICAL PERSPECTIVES

The word "marasmus" is derived from the Greek word *marasmos*, which means to waste away. Marasmus represents the severe arrest in growth that accompanies the sustained deprivation of nutrients and is the most common form of malnutrition. Pursuant to Cicely Williams' documentation of kwashiorkor (which means "sickness of weaning concomitant with birth of the next child" in the Ga language) in Ghana in the 1930s, marasmus and kwashiorkor were considered distinct for several years until the realization that both are associated with malnutrition. Since protein supplementation alone did not significantly reduce the unfortunately high occurrence of malnutrition-associated deaths in different parts of the world, the term protein-energy or -calorie malnutrition (PEM or PCM) was coined to emphasize factors other than protein in the diet (Golden, 2002). PEM now encompasses three clinical phenotypes: marasmus, marasmic-kwashiorkor, and kwashiorkor.

The finding of kwashiorkor in parts of the world where starchy, watery gruels derived from cassava, maize, plantain, and yam are used as infant foods (immediately after weaning) led to the view that kwashiorkor results from high-carbohydrate diets, rich in calories but poor in protein. It is becoming increasingly evident that factors other than nutritional deficiency might dictate the onset and progression of kwashiorkor (Golden, 2002; see Etiology section). In contrast, marasmus is clearly associated with a diet deficient in calories but balanced in nutrient composition.

Metabolic Alterations and Causative Hormonal Changes in Protein-Energy Malnutrition

When food intake decreases, the utilization of fat and protein reserves in the body enables various essential metabolic processes to continue during the nutritional inadequacy. In the early stage of fasting or starvation, glucose requirements of the brain and nervous system are fulfilled by mobilization of glycogen in the liver. This short-term adaptation lasts only a day until glycogen stores are exhausted. Gluconeogenesis is then initiated in the liver, using as precursors carbon backbones obtained from deamination of amino acids, which in turn were obtained from the breakdown of muscle proteins.

Adaptation to decreased food intake also activates a hormone-sensitive lipase, which hydrolyzes triglyceride reserves in fat cells to generate fatty acids and glycerol. The fatty acids provide substrate for the citric acid cycle and furnish the carbon backbone for the synthesis of ketone bodies in liver. Once their levels stabilize, ketone bodies can serve, in part, as an alternative fuel in place of glucose for the brain, and muscle protein is no longer degraded as extensively to furnish precursors for gluconeogenesis. Since unremitting muscle protein loss (particularly in respiratory tissue) will be fatal, the utilization of ketone bodies by the brain helps to spare lean body mass until the subcutaneous fat tissue in the body is depleted. Decreased resting energy expenditure also serves to minimize protein turnover in PEM (Jackson, 2003).

Although the proportionate shortage of all macronutrients in marasmus ensures homeostasis to a large extent, there is a severe metabolic derangement in kwashiorkor. Since the diet in kwashiorkor is deficient in protein, it is not surprising that decreased *de novo* protein synthesis grossly affects the functioning of various organs. In the liver, the failure to synthesize transport proteins results in the deprivation of lipids, vitamins, and other micronutrients to peripheral tissues. Deficiency in key metabolic enzymes also impairs several hepatic processes, including fatty acid oxidation, bile salt formation, and detoxification of xenobiotics. Moreover, the absence of pancreatic digestive enzymes leads to poor digestion, and malabsorption of fat and fat-soluble vitamins manifests as loose stools (steatorrhea). These drastic changes do not occur in marasmus (except after prolonged starvation) since the amino acid pool derived in part from muscle catabolism and in part from the modest dietary intake provides precursors for synthesis of key hepatic proteins such as albumin and lipoproteins.

The hormonal fluxes that orchestrate metabolism among various organs and tissues also vary between these two forms of PEM and contribute to their respective clinical phenotypes (Torun and Chew, 1999). In the case of marasmus, the overall decreased food intake (i.e., reduced concentration of blood glucose and free amino acids) causes a decline in insulin levels with a concomitant increase in catabolic hormones such as glucagon, epinephrine, and cortisol. Glucagon activates glycogenolysis and helps increase blood glucose concentration. Epinephrine activates lipolysis in adipocytes to supply fatty acids for oxidation in other tissues and glycerol for gluconeogenesis. In the liver, fatty acid oxidation provides acetyl-CoA as a substrate for the synthesis of ketone bodies. Cortisol triggers proteolysis, specifically of muscle protein, to generate amino acids for use by the liver as precursors for gluconeogenesis and for *de novo* synthesis of serum proteins. High cortisol levels also cause diminished sensitivity of the tissues to insulin as well as a decrease in glucose utilization by directly inhibiting glucose transport.

The carbohydrate-rich, protein-deficient diet of kwashiorkor causes, at least initially, an increase in the anabolic hormone insulin, an undesirable situation in a malnourished state. Despite an energy shortage, insulin inhibits lipolysis and promotes lipogenesis (fatty acid synthesis) using the excess carbohydrate in the diet as precursors. The increase in insulin is accompanied by dampening of the adrenergic response that prevents fat and protein breakdown and by a decreased mobilization of much needed precursors for *de novo* serum protein synthesis. Although initially stimulated, insulin secretion decreases after prolonged protein deficiency in kwashiorkor due to exhaustion and atrophy of the pancreatic beta cells. Glucose intolerance is therefore observed in kwashiorkor but not in marasmus. The decreased insulin results in palliative endocrine changes (such as increased glucocorticoid levels) that stimulate increased lipolysis and muscle protein catabolism. However, muscle wasting with little or no dietary intake of essential amino acids cannot entirely ameliorate decreased hepatic protein synthesis in kwashiorkor.

Both forms of PEM are associated with hypercortisolemia. The level of cortisol in kwashiorkor is lower, however, than in marasmus, likely due to decreased adrenocortical function caused by low protein intake (and not adrenal failure). If a sufficiently high level of cortisol is not maintained, then adequate muscle protein is not mobilized to sustain hepatic protein synthesis. Indeed, hypoproteinemia, evident by the decreased serum albumin and transferrin levels, is more acute in kwashiorkor than marasmus.

The reduced levels of serum lipoproteins needed for lipid transport also contribute to the "fatty liver" usually observed in kwashiorkor.

Pathophysiology

In conserving energy, cellular processes are compromised, aggravating the effects of malnutrition. Decreased rate of cellular replication causes atrophy of the intestinal mucosal cells and leads to both bacterial colonization of the gut and poor bioavailability of nutrients. When ATP-requiring reactions are downregulated, processes such as the transport of nutrients across the intestinal lumen or pumping of ions across the cell membrane are perturbed significantly. In the absence of an active Na^+/K^+ ATPase pump, the concentration gradient favors potassium efflux and sodium influx as borne out by the increased intracellular sodium and decreased potassium that are observed in PEM. Membrane leakiness due to alteration of lipid composition may also underlie this change. In fact, recently designed rehydration regimens for PEM patients provide less sodium and more potassium on account of this imbalance (see Therapy section). Economizing energy also invokes oxidative stress. Due to reduced synthesis of new red blood cells (RBC) and ferritin during PEM, the iron released from degraded RBC is not sequestered. The resulting free iron promotes the dangerous generation of free radicals.

During the last four decades, the interdependence between malnutrition, decreased immunity, and infection has become increasingly clear (Jolly and Fernandes, 2000). Since PEM was initially attributed entirely to dietary insufficiencies, it was thought that enrichment of the diet was the key. It soon became clear, however, that food consideration alone could not adequately explain all facets of malnutrition. In 1959, Scrimshaw and coworkers proposed that malnutrition makes a person susceptible to infections, which in turn perpetuates the malnutrition state. In fact, the high mortality observed in PEM has been attributed to the increased susceptibility to infections arising from immunodeficiency. These observations have led to a two-prong therapeutic modality for children with malnutrition: stem the infection while enhancing the nutritional status. Advances in immunology have now facilitated a comprehensive understanding of the defense mechanisms of the body and placed decreased immunity in the vicious triangle concomitant with malnutrition.

Malnutrition causes a breakdown in the seemingly invincible array of defense mechanisms and renders the host highly susceptible to frequent infections and even malignancies. There is a dramatic atrophy of the thymus and a decrease in the number of functionally mature and differentiated T cells (Jolly and Fernandes, 2000). Moreover, lower cytokine activity results in reduced proliferation of T cells. Although circulating B-lymphocyte levels are usually normal, response to vaccine antigens is low in PEM, as might be expected from the reduced antigen presentation by T cells. The breakdown in mucosal immunity, as reflected in the decreased secretory immunoglobulin A levels, might account for the increased risk of respiratory and gastrointestinal tract infections usually observed in PEM. There is also a reduction in the components of the complement system in PEM and as a consequence the ability of macrophages to phagocytose various pathogens is impaired.

How does infection exacerbate malnutrition? Infection is a catabolic state accompanied by various metabolic alterations. Calorigenesis (increased caloric usage), required for producing fever, utilizes the already limiting stores of glucose, fats, and amino acids. Infection leads to increased inflammation and repair, which demand further use of reserves and causes nutrient losses. The liver uses valuable amino acids from muscle breakdown to synthesize acute-phase reactants, such as the tumor necrosis factor, instead of serum proteins. The acute-phase reactants also lead to cachexia (general wasting and decrease in body mass). Albeit counterintuitive, malnourished individuals also lose appetite for food, allowing the cycle of infection and malnutrition to be self-perpetuating. Halting cytokine-induced cachexia merits consideration as a future pharmacological approach to circumvent this problem.

The synergy between illness and malnutrition is clear. Malnutrition does not merely arrest development but is life threatening for children in many developing countries. In fact, recent studies examining the risks of dying from underweight and malnutrition concluded that a large number of deaths from pneumonia, diarrhea, malaria, and measles could be prevented by eradication of undernutrition among children.

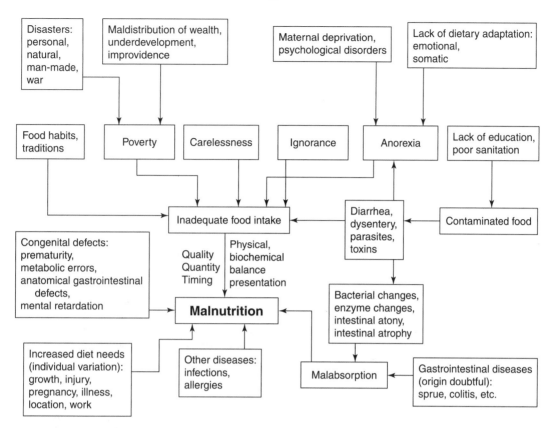

Figure 24-2. Multiple etiologies of protein-energy malnutrition. Reprinted from Williams (1986) with permission from Elsevier.

Etiology

PEM arises due to a negative energy balance, that is, a combined intake of proteins and calories less than that required for body expenditure. Inadequate food intake in PEM may have multiple causes, ranging from secondary malnutrition to sociopolitical problems (Fig. 24-2).

There has been considerable debate over the pathogenesis of kwashiorkor and marasmus (Golden, 2002). The edema unique to kwashiorkor was initially attributed to the low plasma protein content and the resulting decrease in plasma oncotic pressure. Results from various studies in the last few decades challenged this notion and suggested consideration of a multifactorial basis for the etiology of kwashiorkor (reviewed by Golden, 2002). Yet, the concept of an acute protein deficiency with normal caloric intake as the underlying basis survived due to the absence of a substitute paradigm.

In 1968, Gopalan (who does not share antecedents with an author of this chapter) pro-

posed a new theory of "dysadaptation" and was prescient in drawing early attention to the possible role of nondietary factors in the etiology of kwashiorkor. Finding no significant difference in the dietary patterns between kwashiorkor and marasmic children in India, he concluded that only children with kwashiorkor suffer from a form of dysadaptation to the unfavorable environment, and that amino acids were being shunted from synthesis of visceral proteins to synthesis of acute-phase reactants. The resulting decrease then causes reduced plasma oncotic pressure and edema. Other challenging findings include observations such as the inability to induce kwashiorkor in animals fed low-protein diets, the cure of children with kwashiorkor by a low-protein diet and with complete resolution of edema in the absence of an increase in serum albumin levels, and breast-fed infants suffering from kwashiorkor despite healthy mothers.

The observation that glutathione, a free-radical scavenger, was reduced in the erythrocytes of children with kwashiorkor but not marasmus led Golden and Ramdath (1987) to propose a new pathogenesis model in which oxidative stress was ascribed a central role. They postulated an overproduction of reactive oxygen species and inadequate scavenging of these free radicals in kwashiorkor. The sophisticated antioxidant system designed to counter the adverse effects of free radicals was hypothesized to fail in its objective largely due to the unavailability of protein, micronutrients, and vitamins. In light of this model, it is of interest to examine the oxidative stress in the two forms of PEM.

Although glutathione is specifically decreased in kwashiorkor, blood levels of selenium-dependent glutathione peroxidase (a scavenger of peroxides) and vitamins A, C, and E (all members of the antioxidant machinery) are lower in both kwashiorkor and marasmus (Ashour et al., 1999). Why then are marasmic children, also deficient in some antioxidants, spared the oxidative stress? Does a weakened antioxidant defense manifest as a serious threat only in the presence of pro-oxidant activities of the type encountered in kwashiorkor? What is a possible trigger for the increase in free radicals, and how might this account for some of the phenotypic alterations in kwashiorkor?

Unlike marasmic or well-nourished children, those with kwashiorkor have low transferrin levels and detectable free iron in the plasma (Sive et al., 1996). Uncomplexed iron is extremely toxic due to its ability to generate free radicals by the Haber-Weiss and Fenton reactions. The onslaught of opportunistic infections in the malnourished also elicits production of free radicals and accentuates the oxidative stress.

Free radicals through lipid peroxidation can cause membrane damage, induce electrolyte imbalance and edema. Indeed, children with kwashiorkor display low levels of polyunsaturated fatty acids (e.g., linoleic acid) in the erythrocyte membrane compared to the marasmic children, presumably due to increased lipid peroxidation (Leichsenring et al., 1995). Interestingly, cysteinyl leukotrienes, which can cause edema by altering capillary permeability, are also enhanced in those with kwashiorkor but not marasmic children (Mayatepek et al., 1993).

Studies indicated that cysteine supplementation is beneficial in restoring glutathione levels in children with severe edematous malnutrition (Badaloo et al., 2002). If the reduced rate of glutathione synthesis in kwashiorkor is convincingly attributed to a shortage of protein in the diet, then the new findings on oxidative stress could indeed be gratifyingly integrated with the long-held belief that kwashiorkor is at least attributable in part to a protein deficit.

Despite the advances enumerated in this section, the conundrum posed by Gopalan (1968) regarding whether the same diet could lead to both kwashiorkor and marasmus remains. Profitable future investigations might entail an examination of the genetic contributions to oxidative stress and the consequent phenotypic sequelae while on an inadequate diet.

THERAPY

The high mortality rate observed with severe malnutrition has been attributed to errors of management precipitated by the lack of an integrated treatment for the various problems. A primary and unfortunately frequent mistake has been the injudicious approach of correcting weight loss without managing illness and repairing the highly damaged cellular machinery. The advances in our understanding of PEM together with the documented failures from prior approaches have led the World Health Organization (WHO) to issue a manual for managing severe malnutrition. The principles of clinical management elaborated by WHO consist of 10 steps that encompass an initial treatment phase aimed to resolve life-threatening situations and a subsequent rehabilitation phase that focuses on reestablishing good nutritional status and catching up lost growth (Table 24-1).

Resolving Life-Threatening Situations: The Initial Treatment Phase

PEM is often associated with two specific sets of physiological problems: (1) infections, hypothermia, and hypoglycemia; and (2) fluid and electrolyte derangements (Jackson, 2003). Treatment of infection plays an important role in PEM management. Broad-spectrum antibiotics like cotrimoxazole should be used for addressing gut, respiratory, or urinary infections. In addition to immunization for measles, antihelminthic tablets (e.g., mebendazole) for deworming the gut and antimalarial tablets (e.g., chloroquine) for combating malarial parasites are prescribed in the tropical countries. Loss of body mass contributes to reduced thermal insulation. The malnourished patient presenting with a body

Table 24-1. Time Frame for Management of a Child with Severe Malnutrition

Activity	Initial Treatment		Rehabilitation	Follow-up
	Days 1-2	*Days 3-7*	*Weeks 2-6*	*Weeks 7-26*
Treat or prevent:				
Hypoglycemia	$\longrightarrow$			
Hypothermia	$\longrightarrow$			
Dehydration	$\longrightarrow$			
Correct electrolyte imbalance		$\longrightarrow$		
Treat infection		$\longrightarrow$		
Correct micronutrient deficiencies	$\longleftarrow$ Without iron $\longrightarrow$		$\longleftarrow$ With iron $\longrightarrow$	
Begin feeding		$\longrightarrow$		
Increase feeding to recover lost weight ("catch-up growth")				$\longrightarrow$
Stimulate emotional and sensorial development		$\longrightarrow$		
Prepare for discharge			$\longrightarrow$	

Reproduced with permission from World Health Organization (1999).

temperature less than 35.5°C is in imminent danger and needs to be immediately warmed. The depletion of glucose that results either from combating infections or increasing body temperature causes hypoglycemia and reduces the supply of glucose to the brain. A multiprong approach of combating infections, reducing the heat loss and supplying glucose by intravenous/oral means is absolutely essential to rescue the patient from the medical emergency caused by severe malnutrition.

The signs of malnutrition can occasionally mask the clinical signs of hypovolemia (decreased volume of circulating blood). For example, the laxity of skin, which is a good marker of hypovolemia, cannot be relied on in the case of the marasmic child, who has an inelastic skin. Valuable indicators of hypovolemia include exaggerated thirst, dry mouth, decreased urinary output, tachycardia (abnormally rapid heartbeat) with a thready pulse, hypotension with orthostasis (dizziness caused only on standing), and declining levels of consciousness. Rehydration should be initiated with a modified version of the original WHO-recommended oral rehydration salt (ORS) solution that has an osmolarity of 300 mOsm/L and contains 125 mM glucose, 45 mM sodium, 40 mM potassium, 70 mM chloride, 7 mM citrate, 3 mM magnesium, 0.3 mM zinc, and 0.045 mM copper. For infants, breast-feeding should be continued during rehydration. The fluid replacement should continue at the rate of 70–100 mL ORS/kg body weight until a urinary output of 200 mL/day in

children (and 500 mL/day in adults) is reached. If the patient has incessant vomiting and is unable to tolerate ORS, then nasogastric fluid replacement should be considered.

Reestablishing Nutritional Status: The Rehabilitation Phase

The atrophied gut mucosa and the pancreatic insufficiency will contribute to an intolerance of rapid and vigorous refeeding regiments. In fact, it is well documented that malabsorption caused the high mortality among prisoners of war who were starved for long durations and subjected to rapid refeeding on release. Nutritional replacement is best done orally and in two stages: the therapy stage, which starts with low doses of foods to restore vital cellular functions, and the rehabilitation stage, which aims at catching up and regaining nutritional adequacy.

Formula diets F-75 and F-100 are comprised of defined amounts of dried skimmed milk, sugar, cereal flour, oil, minerals, and vitamins designed both for the initial (F-75, 75 kcal/ 100 mL) and the rehabilitation (F-100, 100 kcal/ 100 mL) stages. While the initial stage should entail caloric intake of 80–100 kcal/kg body weight/day, the rehabilitation stage should begin with about 130 kcal and gradually increase to 150–200 kcal/kg body weight/day. The return of a normal appetite signals the clearance of infections and the end of the initial stage and permits the switch to rehabilitation. Judicious and careful refeeding is essential for ensuring a speedy and complete recovery. Food should be given in small amounts and frequently; the recommended intakes can be found in the WHO manual.

If formula diets are not used, then the type of protein used is important due to considerations of biological value and digestibility. Milk, animal proteins, egg, certain legumes, and soy products are appropriate, rich sources. If lactose intolerance is encountered, then milk should be replaced with soy-based feeds or an alternative. Fish and vegetable oils are good sources of fats as they provide generous amounts of essential fatty acids and long-chain unsaturated fatty acids.

In addition to proteins and calories, the patients with PEM must be replenished with respect to vitamins and micronutrients especially to enhance antioxidant status. Due to heavy vitamin A losses that occur during infections and PEM, vitamin A supplements are necessary to prevent blindness. Selenium, zinc, manganese, and cobalt are important micronutrients deficient in patients with PEM and therefore need to be replaced. These micronutrients play a vital role in the function of several enzymes (e.g., selenium in glutathione peroxidase). Iron must be excluded from the diet in the initial stage since early administration increases the risk of free-radical production and infection.

Psychosocial Support

Children with PEM frequently do not realize their full mental and developmental potential and display mental apathy, lethargy, and psychomotor retardation. Developmental and psychosocial rehabilitation are needed together with restoration of nutritional status. Modest physical activity that helps in rebuilding lean mass and stimulatory activities that facilitate recovery of brain function should be pursued after the patient has been rescued from the initial emergency phase. A caring and supportive environment is absolutely necessary for ensuring the emotional well-being and expediting recovery to normalcy.

QUESTIONS

1. Is it necessary to identify and differentiate between the two types of PEM while formulating a plan of treatment? Explain your reasoning.

2. Draw a comparison between energy metabolism in a child with PEM and another fed with excess carbohydrates and proteins.

3. For the adverse factors complicating malnutrition such as oxidative stress discussed in the chapter, explain what genetic factors would further exacerbate the problem.

4. Postulate biochemical mechanisms for the deterioration of health that occurs after rapid refeeding of a child with PEM.

5. If a child is fed a diet that is poor in proteins but rich in carbohydrate and antioxidants, would the edema associated with kwashiorkor be prevented?

6. Do you expect hibernating animals to show signs of PEM under any circumstances?

BIBLIOGRAPHY

Ashour MN, Salem SI, El-Gadban HM, et al.: Antioxidant status in children with protein-energy malnutrition living in Cairo, Egypt. *Eur J Clin Nutr* **53:**669-673, 1999.

Badaloo A, Reid M, Forrester T, et al.: Cysteine supplementation improves the erythrocyte glutathione synthesis rate in children with severe edematous malnutrition. *Am J Clin Nutr* **76:** 646-652, 2002.

Bernstein LH, Ingenbleek Y: Transthyretin: its response to malnutrition and stress injury. Clinical usefulness and economic implications. *Clin Chem Lab Med* **40:**1344-1348, 2002.

Carvalho NF, Kenney RD, Carrington PH, et al.: Severe nutritional deficiencies in toddlers resulting from health food milk alternatives. *Pediatrics* **107:**E46, 2001.

Golden MHN: The development of concepts of nutrition. *J Nutr* **132:**2117S-2122S, 2002.

Golden MHN, Ramdath D: Free radicals in the pathogenesis of Kwashiorkor. *Proc Nutr Soc* **46:**53-68, 1987.

Gopalan C: Kwashiorkor and marasmus: evolution and distinguishing features, *in* McCance RA, Widdowson EM (eds): *Calorie Deficiencies and Protein Deficiencies.* Little, Brown and Company, Boston, 1968, pp. 49-58.

Gurney JM, Jelliffe DB: Arm anthropometry in nutritional assessment: normograms for rapid calculation of muscle circumference and cross sectional muscle and fat mass. *Am J Clin Nutr* **26:**912-915, 1973.

Hendrickse RG: Protein-energy malnutrition, *in* Hendrickse RG, Barr DGD, Matthews, TS (eds): *Paediatrics in the Tropics.* Blackwell Scientific, Oxford, UK, 1991, pp. 119-131.

Jackson AA: Severe malnutrition, *in* Warrell DA, Cox TM, Firth JD, et al. (eds): *Oxford Textbook of Medicine.* 4th edition Oxford University Press, Oxford, UK, pp. 1054-1061, 2003.

Jolly CA, Fernandes G: Protein-energy malnutrition and infectious disease, *in* Gershwin ME, German JB, Keen CL (eds): *Nutrition and Immunology: Principles and Practice.* Humana Press, Totowa, NJ, 2000, pp. 195-202.

Leichsenring M, Sutterlin N, Less S, et al.: Polyunsaturated fatty acids in erythrocyte and plasma lipids of children with severe protein-energy malnutrition. *Acta Paediatr* **84:**516-520, 1995.

Mayatepek E, Becker K, Gana L, et al.: Leukotrienes in the pathophysiology of kwashiorkor. *Lancet* **342:**958-960, 1993.

Scrimshaw NS, Behar M: Protein malnutrition in young children. *Science* **133:**2039-2047, 1961.

Scrimshaw NS, Taylor CE, Gordon JE: Interactions of nutrition and infection. *Am J Med Sci* **237:** 367-372, 1959.

Sive AA, Dempster WS, Malan H, et al.: Plasma free iron: a possible cause of oedema in kwashiorkor. *Arch Dis Child* **76:**54-56, 1996.

Torun B, Chew F: Protein-energy malnutrition, *in* Shils ME (ed): *Modern Nutrition in Health and Disease.* 9th ed. Lippincott, Williams and Wilkins, Baltimore, MD, 1999, pp. 963-988.

White JV, Ham RJ, Lipschitz DA, et al.: Consensus of the Nutrition Screening Initiative: Risk factors and indicators of poor nutritional status in older Americans. *Journal of the American Diabetic Association* **91**:783-787, 1991.

Williams SR: Nutritional deficiency diseases, *in* Williams SR (ed): *Nutrition and Diet Therapy.* 5th ed. Elsevier, Philadelphia, 1985, pp. 327-350.

World Health Organization: *Management of Severe Malnutrition: A Manual for Physicians and Senior Health Workers.* WHO, Geneva, Switzerland, 1999.

25

Lactose Intolerance

MARCY P. OSGOOD and ABIODUN O. JOHNSON

CASE REPORT

A 6-year-old African American boy presented with a 6-month history of nausea, abdominal discomfort, and diarrhea with three to four watery stools a day associated with passage of much gas. These complaints began soon after he started first grade when he was required to drink 2 cups of milk with his school lunch. The symptoms occurred after lunch, and he felt much better after having a bowel movement. No blood was noted in the stool. He was mostly symptom free on weekends, when he rarely drinks milk. There has been no fever or no weight loss, and his appetite has remained good.

In general, the boy has been healthy since birth at full term. He was breast-fed for 6 months, at which time he was weaned to regular infant formula, and started taking solids in the form of rice cereal. He began eating table food at 1 year of age. Neither parent drinks much milk. He is the only child of both parents, and there are no other family health concerns.

The patient was brought to the clinic for evaluation directly from school and soon after lunch. Physical examination revealed a pleasant and healthy looking young boy. His growth and development were appropriate, with both his height and weight in the 50th percentile on the growth chart. He had a normal temperature, pulse and respiratory rates, and blood pressure. The only positive findings on systematic examination were in the abdomen, which was mildly distended with increased bowel sounds and tympanicity on percussion (the abdomen is resonant when tapped with fingers or an instrument because of distension of the abdomen with air or gas). There was no tenderness. Neither the liver nor the spleen was palpable, and no other mass was palpated. There was mild perianal excoriation (destruction and loss of the surface of the skin around the anus), and rectal examination revealed loose stool in the rectum. The stool was negative on testing for occult blood (blood present in such small quantities that it can only be detected by chemical testing). Further examination of a stool specimen in the laboratory showed no red or white blood cells, Rotazyme stool testing for rotavirus was negative, and no bacterial pathogen was identified on stool culture. The stool pH was 5.5, and Clinitest (for detecting reducing sugar in stool) was positive. Blood cell count and serum electrolytes were normal.

As this patient's history indicated that his problems began soon after he started taking 2 cups of milk with lunch at school and his physical examination and stool examination findings suggested he had carbohydrate malabsorption, a diagnosis of lactose intolerance was made. It was recommended that his milk intake at lunch be decreased to half a cup (about 4 oz). His symptoms improved considerably and almost immediately. His milk intake was then gradually increased such that he was ultimately able to take up to 8 oz of milk without much complaint, especially when the milk was taken with other foods.

DIAGNOSIS

It is necessary to confirm the clinical impression of lactose intolerance by specific tests based on measurement of products of lactose digestion or fermentation. Such tests demonstrate lactose maldigestion and malabsorption and may be direct or indirect. In the direct test, lactase activity in a small intestinal mucosal specimen is determined by enzymatic assay. The small intestinal specimen is obtained by biopsy. However, because this test is invasive, it has no place in routine clinical management; it is used now essentially in research situations. The indirect tests include testing for stool acidity and presence of lactose, a reducing sugar; measurement of blood glucose levels in the lactose tolerance test; and the determination of breath hydrogen levels.

In the lactose tolerance test, an oral dose of 2 g lactose per kilogram body weight (maximum dose of 50 g in adults) is administered to the patient after an overnight fast and after drawing venous blood for fasting blood sugar baseline. Serial venous blood samples are then taken every half hour for 2 h for measurement of blood glucose levels. The test is positive if the blood glucose level increases less than 20 mg/dL above the fasting level, indicating the lack of hydrolysis of lactose to glucose and galactose and therefore little or no transport of glucose into the bloodstream from the small intestine. Also, symptoms of lactose intolerance may occur during the test, but this is not necessary to make the diagnosis.

False-positive and false-negative results occur in up to 20% of subjects due to variable gastric emptying times and individual differences in glucose metabolism. It is sometimes necessary to demonstrate that the lactose tolerance test is truly positive because of failure to hydrolyze lactose and not due to a mucosal absorptive disorder. This is done by repeating the test after the patient drinks an aqueous solution containing half of the carbohydrate dose as glucose and the other half as galactose. The blood sugar level should now rise at least 20 mg per dL above the fasting level.

The hydrogen (H_2) breath test is generally considered the diagnostic method of choice because it is sensitive, noninvasive, and relatively inexpensive. Normally, humans exhale very little H_2 gas as H_2 is not a product of human metabolism. However, H_2 and other gases are produced when undigested lactose in the colon is fermented by bacteria. The H_2 is absorbed and carried through the bloodstream to the lungs, where it is exhaled and can be detected. Raised H_2 levels in exhaled air indicate insuffi-

cient digestion of lactose in the small intestine or the presence of unusually large numbers of H_2-producing bacteria in the colon. After an overnight fast, a baseline sample of exhaled breath is collected in a balloonlike collection bag. The patient then drinks an aqueous solution of lactose at a dose of 2 g/kg body weight (maximum dose 50 g). Serial 15-min breath samples are then collected, and the H_2 level in each collection bag is determined by gas chromatography. A rise in breath H_2 concentration greater than 20 ppm over the baseline level suggests hypolactasia. The hydrogen breath test is positive in about 90% of patients with lactose malabsorption. Gastrointestinal symptoms and a positive H_2 breath test have been shown to be strongly correlated (Hermans et al., 1997).

A false-negative test can occur in the absence of colonic bacteria (often due to recent use of antibiotics or a high colonic enema), absence of any H_2-producing colonic bacteria, or overabundance of methane-producing bacteria in the gut. Sleep deprivation, exercise, use of aspirin, gum, or mouthwash, or smoking may increase breath H_2 secretion independent of lactose load or hypolactasia. Again, a stool pH equal to or less than 5.6 and the presence of reducing sugar in the stool by Clinitest are important ancillary diagnostic findings needed for diagnosis.

Our patient manifested most of the above clinical and laboratory findings, which improved when the amount of milk (and lactose) he ingested was reduced. He had tolerated both breast milk and cow milk-based formula in infancy and developed symptoms only when he was induced to drink relatively large amounts of regular milk at one sitting. Thus, he had the very common primary, hereditary, late-onset type of lactose intolerance. This type is even more pronounced in adults, resulting in the common nomenclature, "adult-type" lactose intolerance, which is really a misnomer since this condition can start anytime after the weaning period. Our patient was gradually able to tolerate about 1 cup of milk a day with his meal.

Because the symptoms of lactose intolerance are nonspecific, lactose intolerance needs to be differentiated from other common disorders causing diarrhea and abdominal pain or discomfort. These differential diagnoses include milk protein allergy, gastroenteritis, colitis, and irritable bowel syndrome. Allergy or sensitivity to one or more of cow's milk proteins characteristically occurs in formula-fed infants, and although no age is exempt, it is rare in the older child and in adults. Gastroenteritis is commonly caused by toxins or by infections by viruses or bacteria. In infectious gastroenteritis, the stool contains white blood cells and may contain gross or occult blood, especially if it is caused by an invasive bacterial pathogen such as *Shigella, Salmonella,* or enteroinvasive *Escherichia coli.* These pathogens can be cultured from the stool. In colitis, the stools are loose, mucousy, and bloody, and the characteristic intermittent crampy lower abdominal pain is often relieved by defecation. Irritable bowel syndrome is characterized by the alternation of diarrhea and constipation.

The diagnosis of lactose intolerance should be strongly suspected ahead of any of these other differential diagnoses when a patient presents with the characteristic symptoms enunciated above following ingestion of lactose-containing drinks or foods such as milk, particularly if the patient belongs to an at-risk population.

BIOCHEMICAL PERSPECTIVES

General Biochemistry of Lactose as a Dietary Sugar

Carbohydrates in various forms make up a significant portion of the human diet in most parts of the world. Dietary carbohydrates range from the simple polyhydroxy aldehydes and ketones such as glucose, galactose, and fructose, to the large polysaccharides of glucose, starch, and glycogen. Also important are the dietary disaccharides, which include lactose (β-D-galactopyranosyl-(1→4)- α-D-glucopyranose), the main carbohydrate in mammalian milk (Fig. 25-1); sucrose (α-D-glucopyranosyl-(1→2)-β-D-fructofuranoside) from sugar beet and sugar cane; maltose (α-D-glucopyranosyl-(1→4)- α-glucopyranose) from corn syrup and naturally occurring in several fruits; and, less commonly, trehalose (α-D-glucopyranosyl-(1→1)-α-D-glucopyranoside) from mushrooms, insects, and some seaweeds.

Sugars capable of reducing ferric or cupric ion are called reducing sugars; lactose, which has a free anomeric carbon (not involved in a glycosidic bond), is a reducing sugar, as is maltose. Sucrose and trehalose, both of which have no free anomeric carbon, are nonreducing sugars. Reduced digestion, transport, or absorption of any of the dietary carbohydrates can cause

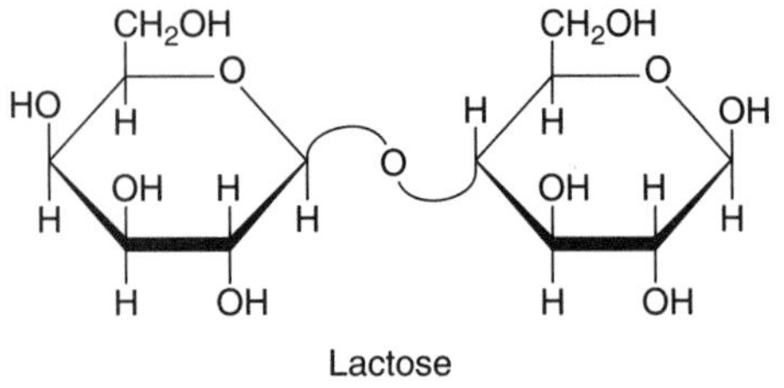

Figure 25-1. Lactose.

mild-to-severe symptoms of carbohydrate malabsorption.

Lactose is only found in high quantities in mammalian milk, which is an essential food for suckling mammals. Lactose milk concentration varies from almost undetectable in the milks of some marine mammals to as much as 7 g/100 mL in mature human milk. Once ingested, lactose is digested to its component monosaccharides by the enzyme lactase, which is located in the brush border (microvilli) of the small intestine mucosal cell (enterocyte). Transport of the released glucose and galactose occurs through sugar transporters on the small intestine brush border (Fig. 25-2).

Forms of Lactose Intolerance

Lactase deficiency leading to lactose intolerance may be congenital, primary (hereditary, delayed onset, adult), or acquired. Congenital lactase deficiency is a very rare condition in newborn babies, and it is inherited by an autosomal recessive mechanism. It is characterized by total absence of intestinal lactase activity (alactasia). Diarrhea and gaseous abdominal distension occur soon after the newborn is fed breast milk or milk-based infant formula. Because lactase activity is vital in all baby mammals in order to digest the lactose in milk, an infant's inability to utilize its primary food (milk) and the dehydration and discomfort caused by the lactose malabsorption can lead to a severe illness that can be fatal if not diagnosed promptly and if lactose is not excluded from further feedings. Cases of congenital alactasia have been reported mostly in Finland, and it is one of the "Finnish recessive disorders" (Jarvela et al., 1998).

Primary, hereditary delayed-onset, or adult lactose intolerance (also referred to as lactase nonpersistence) is the most familiar form of this condition. Lactase nonpersistence is actually much more common worldwide than adult

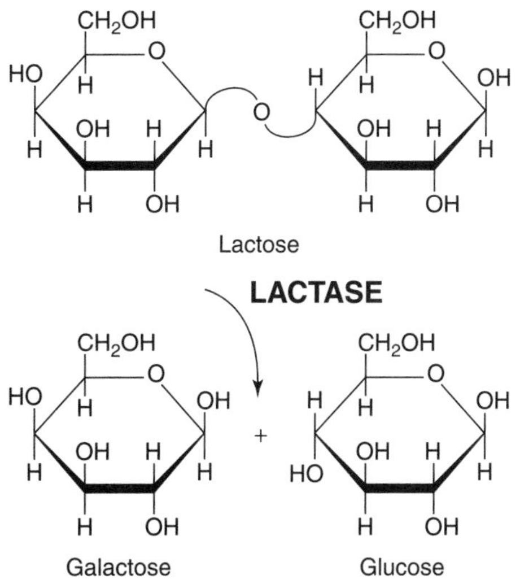

Figure 25-2. Hydrolysis of lactose to component monosaccharides by the enzyme lactase.

lactase persistence. Developmental expression of lactase is tightly controlled. Intestinal lactase activity rises relatively late in the fetus, reaching optimal levels at term; thus, the preterm newborn has reduced lactase levels, and the more premature the baby is, the greater the risk of reduction in lactase level. Intestinal lactase activity remains at peak levels from birth in the full-term baby through infancy and early childhood, when the diet is mostly milk and lactose-containing milk products. Lactase activity falls gradually with reduction in milk intake and the introduction of non-lactose-containing weaning foods. Intestinal lactase levels become quite low after the child is well established on cereals and by the time weaning is complete. The ability to digest lactose becomes compromised thereafter, and this type of lactose intolerance is well established by 3–7 years of age depending on the weaning practices of the particular population (Scrimshaw and Murray, 1988). As lactase is not an inducible enzyme (Gilat et al., 1972), the fall in lactase activity with weaning in most of the world's population is ultimately genetic. Thus, this state of lactase insufficiency (hypolactasia) is normal in all suckling mammals, including humans. However, populations of northern European descent and some nomadic tribes in Africa and Asia have retained the ability to digest lactose past the weaning period (Saavedra and Perman, 1989; Scrimshaw and Murray, 1988; Thomas et al., 1990).

Finally, lactose intolerance may be secondary to disorders that damage the normal formation and functioning of the small intestinal mucosa. These may be due to acute diarrheal diseases (e.g., enteritis), parasitic infestations (e.g., giardiasis), enteropathies (e.g., celiac disease), chronic inflammatory bowel disease (e.g., Crohn's disease), ionizing radiation, antimetabolite medications, and intestinal surgery or resection.

Physiological Effects of Lactase Insufficiency

Carbohydrates that reach the large intestine provide a metabolic resource to other nonmammalian organisms, specifically certain types of colonic bacteria; to these, lactose is a fermentable substrate. Microbial fermentation occurs when appropriate substrates are available and oxygen is excluded from the environment (i.e., under anaerobic conditions). Metabolic end products of fermentation vary according to the specific organisms present but can include short-chain acids and alcohols and various gases. The presence of fermentation products in the colon does not necessarily lead to discomfort. However, in the absence of sufficient, or sufficiently active, lactase in the small intestine, significant amounts of unhydrolyzed lactose enter the large intestine. The disaccharide osmotically draws fluid into the bowel lumen, increasing the volume and fluidity of the gastrointestinal contents. The accumulation of water in the lumen produces watery stools, resulting in fluid and electrolyte loss from the gastrointestinal tract and hemoconcentration of the blood. In addition, bacterial hydrolysis of the lactose in the large intestine splits the disaccharide into its component monosaccharides, which cannot be absorbed by the colonic mucosa, thereby further increasing the osmotic load. Bacterial fermentation of the glucose and galactose leads to the evolution of carbon dioxide, hydrogen, and methane gases. The osmotic imbalance and increase in concentration of fermentation end products results in the gastrointestinal symptoms of lactose intolerance: excessive gas, bloating, increased bowel sounds (borborygmi), abdominal pain, and acidic diarrheal stools containing reducing sugar. However, not all individuals with lactase insufficiency (lactose maldigesters) have symptoms of lactose intolerance; and not all lactose-intolerant people are lactose maldigesters (Carrocio et al., 1998; Johnson et al., 1993a) (Figure 25-3).

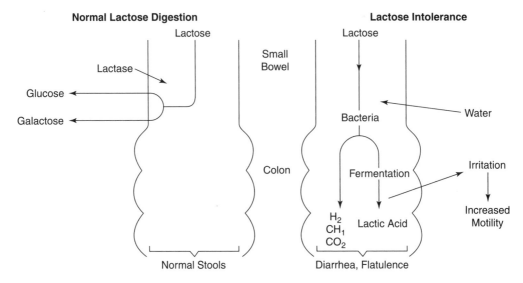

Figure 25-3. Genesis of symptoms in lactose malabsorption.

Lactase

Lactase (lactase phlorizin hydrolase [3.2.1.23]) has two activities: β-galactosidase activity, which catalyzes the hydrolysis of lactose, and a β-glucosidase activity, which is responsible for hydrolyzing phlorizin, a disaccharide found in some seaweeds and in the roots and bark of plants of the family Rosaceae.

In the small intestine mucosal cells (enterocytes), lactase is synthesized as a propolypeptide that is proteolytically cleaved inside the cell. The mature enzyme has an apparent molecular weight of approximately 160,000. Lactase has a carboxy-terminal, membrane-spanning domain that acts to anchor the enzyme, but the bulk of the enzyme projects into the lumen of the intestine. The protein dimerizes on the brush border membrane of the small intestine to form the active enzyme. Like all brush border hydrolases and transporters, lactase is glycosylated. There is evidence of both N- and O-glycosylation, and there are person-to-person differences in these terminal glycosylations related to the ABH blood group antigens (Grand et al., 2003; OMIM; Swallow et al., 2001) (Fig. 25-4).

Primary Hypolactasia

Primary hypolactasia results in up to 75% of dietary lactose passing unhydrolyzed through the small intestine into the colon, where it is rapidly metabolized by colonic bacteria. The gas-

trointestinal symptoms that result vary from patient to patient and are related to the quantity of lactose ingested, the relative hypolactasia, and the patient's pain or discomfort tolerance level. They occur between half an hour and 2 h after ingestion of lactose, depending in part on whether lactose is taken by itself (e.g., in an aqueous solution) or as part of a meal with other nutrients (such as fat) ingested at the same time. The amount of lactose required to produce symptoms also varies, ranging from 4.5 to 18 g (3–12 oz milk). Severity of symptoms can be directly related to the osmotic pressure caused by the presence of unhydrolyzed lactose in the colon.

Ingestion of larger amounts of the disaccharide, faster gastric emptying time, and faster intestinal transit time all contribute to more severe symptoms. In general, since an increase in the fat content of food slows the rate of gastric emptying, lactose intolerance symptoms would be expected to decrease with ingestion of higher-fat milk. However, symptoms reported by lactose maldigesters were not different after ingestion of fat-free compared to full-fat milk (Vesa et al., 1997).

A common misconception is that lactose malabsorption and lactose intolerance symptoms are caused by an allergy to milk or other dairy products. Milk allergy is an immunologically mediated reaction to milk proteins that may involve single systems (e.g., the gastrointestinal tract, skin, respiratory tract) or multiple

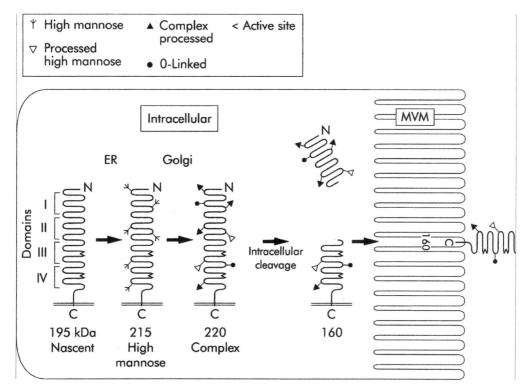

Figure 25-4. Model of the molecular forms of lactase during synthesis and processing in the human villus enterocyte. MVM, microvillus membrane.

systems (systemic anaphylaxis). Also, milk protein allergy may be an immediate or delayed type hypersensitivity reaction. A recent study showed that children who are hypersensitive to cow's milk (that is, are allergic to milk proteins) are tolerant of lactose even from bovine sources, clearly delineating the two conditions (Fiocchi et al., 2003).

Bacterial Fermentation of Lactose in the Colon

The catabolism of any organic energy source (carbohydrates, lipids, amino acids) involves its oxidation: the transfer of electrons from the energy source to an electron acceptor. The electrons released during fuel oxidation are transferred to NAD^+ (or other electron carriers) to form the reduced NADH. But, NADH must be reoxidized to NAD^+ for the catabolic pathway to continue operating, either through the process of cellular respiration, using oxygen (or nitrate or sulfate in some bacteria) as a terminal electron acceptor or through the process of fermentation.

In anaerobic environments like the colon,

where oxygen is not available as a final electron acceptor, fermentative bacteria transfer electrons from NADH to some organic compound as the mechanism to regenerate NAD^+. The redox reactions occur in the cytosol of the microorganism, and ATP is produced through substrate-level phosphorylation. There are a number of variations of microbial fermentation, but all need to have an acceptor for the electrons produced during the oxidations. So, fermentations are characterized by excretion of relatively large quantities of reduced organic compounds, including alcohols (such as ethanol) and organic acids (such as lactic, acetic, propionic, and butyric acids).

For example, lactic acid bacteria are a large and heterogeneous group of gram-positive bacteria whose sole or major fermentation product from carbohydrates is lactate. Lactobacilli and bifidobacteria are two groups of lactic acid bacteria normally found in the human colon. In homofermentative lactate fermentation, glucose is oxidized to pyruvate via the 10 steps of glycolysis. The NADH produced in the oxidation step of glyceraldehyde 3-phosphate to 1,3-bisphosphoglycerate is used to reduce pyruvate to lactate; NAD^+ is regenerated concurrently. Those lactic acid bacteria that utilize what is known as heterofermentative lactate fermentation generate lactate using the decarboxylation and transferase reactions of the pentose phosphate pathway. Lactate is ultimately created from the reduction of pyruvate to regenerate NAD^+, and ethanol is also produced in other NADH-using, NAD^+-regenerating reactions.

Frequently, hydrogen gas is also a fermentation end product; in some bacterial species, protons can be used as electron acceptors by enzymes known as hydrogenases, which catalyze reactions that essentially reduce protons to hydrogen gas: $NADH + H^+ \rightarrow H_2 + NAD^+$. Hydrogen gas is therefore a product only of particular bacterial fermentative processes and not of human metabolism.

The excreted end-products of fermentations, including hydrogen gas, can be used by other anaerobic bacteria, and what is known as an anaerobic food chain develops. At the "bottom" of the food chain are the archaeal methanogens, different species of which convert hydrogen gas, carbon dioxide, or acetate to CH_4. The process of methanogenesis from H_2 and CO_2 occurs as follows:

$$4H_2 + HCO_3^- + H^+ \rightarrow CH_4 + 3\ H_2O$$

Methanogenesis from acetate occurs as follows:

$$CH_3COO^- + H_2O \rightarrow CH_4 + HCO_3^-$$

Therefore, the colonic hydrolysis of lactose to glucose and galactose, the fermentation of these monosaccharides to various organic acids and alcohols and H_2, and the further conversion of these end products to CO_2, and CH_4 require the combined action of several types of bacteria.

Because of this sequential catabolism, the presence or absence of certain types of microorganisms in the mixed populations of the colon can have a significant effect on the symptoms experienced by lactase-nonpersistent patients and even on the accuracy of measurement of symptoms. Billions of microorganisms are present in each gram of feces, and these include organisms from many different bacterial families. The exact balance of individual species of bacteria within the total flora can change rapidly according to diet, colonic conditions such as pH, and interactions between the various guilds that range from syntrophic to competitive.

Three examples illustrate how the microbial ecology of the small and large intestine can influence the symptoms of lactose intolerance. First, the absence of H_2-producing bacterial guilds, which would result in less H_2 gas produced, or the presence of large numbers of methanogens, which would result in more H_2 gas consumed, can alter the net amount of gas in the colon, with or without the presence of lactose as a fermentable substrate. Methane production consumes 4 mol of H_2 to reduce 1 mol of CO_2 to CH_4 (Pelletier et al., 2001; Vernia et al., 2003). A second example of how the microbial ecology of the gut can influence the symptoms of lactose intolerance has to do with the presence of lactic acid bacteria. Lactic acid bacteria that are ingested with food (e.g., *Lactobacillus bulgaricus* and *Streptococcus thermophilus* in yogurt) may contribute their own lactase and thereby increase lactose hydrolysis and improve lactose absorption in the small intestine. Ingestion of yogurt by lactase-nonpersistent patients has in fact been shown to reduce H_2 production beyond that expected simply because of the reduced lactose content of yogurt (25%–50% less than in the same amount of milk) due to its fermented state. Such a beneficial effect of a bacterial food supplement is called a *probiotic effect* (Hove et al., 1999; Pelletier et al., 2001). Finally, exposing the colon to increasing amounts of lactose over time can change the numbers and types of bacteria present, so that the colonic flora becomes better suited to processing undigested lactose entering from the small intestine (Hertzler and Savaiano, 1996; Johnson et al., 1993b; Pribila et al., 2000).

Prevalence

As mentioned earlier, primary late-onset hereditary (adult) hypolactasia is developmentally the "normal" state. The level of expression of lactase is controlled by a genetically determined regulatory polymorphism that shows large differences in allele frequencies in human populations and results in the widely varying prevalence of hypolactasia among ethnic backgrounds. Estimates range from 2%–5% hypolactasia in persons of northern European descent to nearly 100% hypolactasia in adult Asians and Native Americans of North America. African Americans and Ashkenazi Jews have hypolactasia prevalences of 60%–80% and Latinos 50%–80%. In North America alone, it is estimated that about 50 million people are lactose intolerant.

While lactase nonpersistence is the more common phenotype worldwide, lactase persistence tends to be the most frequent in populations where fresh milk historically has been a significant part of the adult diet, specifically in northern Europeans and in some pastoral nomadic tribes of Africa and Asia. The very high frequency of the lactase persistence allele in these populations has resulted from positive selection over time for a mutation that provided a selective advantage by opening up the enzymatic opportunity to benefit from the high nutritional content of milk. Human cultural evolution influenced this molecular evolution. About 40,000 years ago, humans domesticated milk-producing animals, and about 9,000–10,000 years ago the pastoralist age began. The pastoralists were nomads who traveled with their herds from one pasture to another. They continued to hunt and gather other foods but complemented their diet with the milk of their animals, often in the form of cheese and fermented milks. The presence of lactose in the diet after weaning was a nutritional windfall, and those with lactase persistence who could take advantage of it benefited and passed on the opportunity to their descendents. Recent population genetics evidence suggests that the persistence of lactase activity in certain populations represents one of the strongest signals of recent positive selection so far documented in the human genome (Bersaglieri et al., 2004).

It appears that the allele for lactase persistence has coevolved with certain cattle milk protein genes. Distribution of the allele for human lactase persistence is most frequent in north central Europe, and this closely matches the area of high allelic richness and genetic distinctiveness of cattle milk proteins. It is speculated that the advantages conferred by milk consumption led to the keeping of larger herds of cattle and artificial selection within those herds for increased yields and altered milk protein composition. Geographic co-presence of certain cattle milk protein genes with the human lactase persistence allele represents a rare example of cultural-genetic coevolution between humans and another species. Previously, instances of coevolution were documented for human genes and genes of parasites (e.g., *Plasmodium*); this was the first non-disease-related example, emphasizing the importance of animal domestication in shaping human genomes as well as societies (Beja-Pereira et al., 2003).

Molecular Basis of Lactase Persistence/Nonpersistence Polymorphism

Lactase is coded for by the gene designated LCT on chromosome 2q21. It is made up of 17 exons, about 49-kb long, and the mRNA transcribed from it is a little more than 6 kb after processing. For many years, a sort of molecular mystery surrounded the lactase persisstence/nonpersistence phenomenon; although it has been assumed that regulation of gene transcription was the mechanism of control, the gene that encodes lactase did not appear to be different in people with these differing conditions. But, studies done in 2002 on nine extended Finnish families found variations in the DNA located outside the lactase gene itself that were correlated to the differences in ability to digest lactose (Ennatah et al., 2002).

This and subsequent work (Kuokkanen et al., 2003; Troelsen et al., 2003) showed that the phenotypic polymorphism of lactase persistence or nonpersistence into adult life is associated with two single nucleotide polymorphisms (SNPs) that occur upstream of the LCT gene. One of these SNPs, a T/C polymorphism at position −13910, is perfectly associated with lactase persistence/nonpersistence. All individuals in the group studied who had low lactase levels (nonpersistent) were homozygous for C at this site; those who were lactase persistent had C/T or T/T genotypes. The other SNP in the upstream region is at position −22018; this is a G/A polymorphism. Its association with the condition is not perfect but very high (97%). G/G was the genotype in those patients with lactase nonpersistence and G/A or A/A in those with the persistent phenotypes. The genotypes correlated with the level of the disaccharidase activities in intestinal biopsies.

The −13910 T/C SNP is located in a strong enhancer region. Functional studies using luciferase reporter constructs showed that these regions of DNA in both lactase-persistent and -nonpersistent people have enhancer activity, but the −13910 (T) variant enhances the lactase gene promoter approximately four times more than the −13910 (C) variant. Control over the LCT gene promoter regulates the transcription of the lactase gene and thus the level of lactase produced. Functional evidence for the nonpersistent −13910 (C) and persistent −13910 (T) allele was also obtained by relative quantitation of the expressed lactase alleles; several times higher expression of the lactase mRNA in the intestinal mucosa is found in individuals with the T allele compared to that found in individuals with the C allele, confirming regulation of the lactase gene at the transcriptional level.

The SNPs identified and a role for differential activity of an enhancer in lactase persistence/nonpersistence do not, however, explain how those individuals with the genotype leading to adult lactase nonpersistence were able to produce sufficient lactase in infancy. There are developmental questions that remain to be answered. Congenital lactase deficiency has been localized to a separate region, also on chromosome 2q21 but not within the LCT gene (Jarvela et al., 1998).

Interestingly, the lactase-persistent phenotype found in some pastoral groups in sub-Saharan Africa is not correlated with the −13910 (T) genotype as it is in northern European populations. This implies that the −13910 SNP is not a causative mutation or not the only causative mutation influencing lactase persistence. There is speculation that other variants may be involved in this region of the DNA and are yet to be identified (Bersaglieri et al., 2004; Mulcare et al., 2004; OMIM).

Health Consequences of Lactose Intolerance

The gastrointestinal manifestations of primary hereditary delayed-onset hypolactasia, while uncomfortable, are not life threatening and can be completely eliminated by dietary manipulation. Is lactose intolerance a serious health issue or just a nuisance? In certain circumstances, specifically at the extremes of life (infancy and old age) lactose maldigestion may have grave health consequences.

When substantial carbohydrate maldigestion occurs in infants, it can lead to diarrhea. This is most often seen when the infant has experienced some other insult that has damaged the small intestine enterocytes, producing a secondary hypolactasia. This is more so when the infant has a rotavirus infection, and rotavirus is the most important cause of gastroenteritis in infancy. Rotavirus infects only mature enterocytes,

in which it induces apoptosis with consequent loss of lactase, as well as resulting in defective mucosal absorption (Boshuizen et al., 2003). The small size, relatively large body surface area, and small circulating blood volume of infants place them at greater risk of significant dehydration, hypotension, and metabolic acidosis from severe diarrhea. Although these can be life-threatening complications, they are quite uncommon complications of isolated lactose intolerance.

Old age represents the other extreme of life during which lactose intolerance can present dangerous consequences. A severe bout of lactose-induced osmotic diarrhea in a frail elderly person may interfere with already precarious glucose regulation. Lactose maldigestion and malabsorption result in reduced energy (glucose) intake, which can lead to hypoglycemia. This in turn may produce dizziness, a potential cause of a fall. Because the frail elderly person often has brittle bones and fragile vascular walls, a fall can result in bone fractures or head injuries with intracranial bleeding. The elderly also commonly have hemodynamic instability. Significant diarrhea from lactose maldigestion in this population may therefore also result in hypovolemia and circulatory collapse or reduced arterial perfusion and ischemia (Solomons, 2002).

Connection Between Lactose Intolerance and Other Diseases

Studies from Sardinia and Finland have raised the possibility of an association between lactase persistence genotypes, lactase activity, and diabetic mellitus. Even though the findings of these studies are presently inconclusive, these studies are important because Sardinia and Finland represent areas with populations with the highest incidence of type I diabetes in the world, and Finland has the highest annual consumption of milk products, with an average of 220 kg milk products/capita (Enattah et al., 2004; Meloni et al., 2001). Also, the genetic predisposition for adult lactose intolerance significantly affects calcium intake, bone density, and likelihood of fractures in postmenopausal women. Whether lactose intolerance in young adults prevents the achievement of adequate peak bone mass and predisposes to severe osteoporosis remains controversial (Di Stephano et al., 2002; Kudlacek et al., 2002; Obermayer-Pietsch et al., 2004; Prentice, 2004).

Public Health and Cultural Concerns

The public health and political/cultural aspects of lactose intolerance may be more complicated than the simple biochemistry of the condition. For example, the U.S.-based consumer advocate group Physicians Committee for Responsible Medicine has challenged the U.S. Department of Agriculture in a legal action over the issue of the Food Pyramid and its recommendation for a range of daily servings of dairy foods and for their inclusion of these foods in government-sponsored feeding programs such as school lunches. They argue that the African American population (and other minorities) tend to have genetic lactase nonpersistence and that milk-based beverages can produce intolerance symptoms (Solomons, 2002). Since lactase nonpersistence is known to be the biological norm, why do most nutrition programs in the United States still treat it as a disease? Many schools require a physician's note before they will provide an alternate beverage. The national School Lunch Program reimburses for cow's milk in a lunch but not for soy or rice milk (Barnard, 2003).

On the other hand, some diseases for which African Americans are at greater risk, such as hypertension and stroke, may be made worse by a low intake of calcium. Average intake of calcium in African American, Hispanic, and Asian populations are at the threshold (600–700 mg/day) below which bone loss and hypertension can result. Though many members of these groups are lactase nonpersistent, intolerance symptoms can be reduced to acceptable levels with commonsense dietary practices that still allow sufficient intake of dairy products for health. Partial reduction of national health disparities between ethnic groups may be possible by overcoming the "barrier of lactose intolerance" (Jarvis and Miller, 2002).

THERAPY

Lactose intolerance can be readily managed by ensuring that the amount of lactose ingested is restricted to the amount the individual can tolerate, which is related to the individual's level of residual intestinal lactase activity. Lactose maldigesters can determine their individual threshold for the occurrence of lactose intoler-ance symptoms and adjust their lactose intake accordingly (Johnson et al., 1993b). Indeed, most adult lactose maldigesters know from experience how much milk (and lactose) they can handle, and consuming smaller servings of milk at a time improves tolerance. Total elimination of milk and dairy products from the diet is unnecessary and is nutritionally unwise because such a management excludes intake of important and essential nutrients, including high-quality protein, calcium, vitamins A and D, and riboflavin.

Tolerance to lactose can be improved by slowly increasing intake of lactose-containing dairy products. As lactase is not an inducible enzyme, this adaptation is likely to be due to qualitative or quantitative changes in colonic bacterial flora (Johnson et al., 1993b). Also, consuming lactose-containing foods as part of a meal improves tolerance to lactose. In addition to the amount of lactose, the type of dairy food consumed influences symptoms of lactose intolerance in lactose maldigesters (Scrimshaw and Murray, 1988). Also, chocolate milk appears to be better tolerated than unflavored milk by lactose maldigesters (Lee and Hardy, 1989). Yogurt and buttermilk are fermented milk products that may be better tolerated than milk in individuals with lactose intolerance. The enhanced efficiency of lactose digestion from yogurt is attributed to the activity of a β-lactosidase (lactase) enzyme contained in bacteria (*S. thermophilus, L. bulgaricus*) present in yogurt. The bacterial lactase survives passage through the stomach and is released in the small intestine, where it aids the digestion of the yogurt's lactose (Martini et al., 1991). Kefir is a fermented milk beverage that contains different cultures than yogurt; ingestion of this beverage was shown to lower levels of breath hydrogen and the perceived severity of flatulence (Hertzler and Clancy, 2003).

If specific treatment is considered necessary, supplemental lactase can be provided as replacement therapy. This is derived from specific species of yeast or fungus and is available as caplets, tablets, and drops. Whole milk pretreated with lactase is marketed in some states as Lactaid and can be used by lactose maldigesters. The availability of the replacement enzyme has made unnecessary the use of the lactose-free diet, which can be nutritionally unsound, as discussed. Also, since lactose is common in many foods and drinks and is used in compounding some drugs, compliance with a lactose-free diet is likely to be difficult even if advisable.

QUESTIONS

1. Explain the pathophysiological basis of the common manifestations (symptoms) of lactose intolerance.
2. All patients with lactase insufficiency have symptoms of lactose intolerance. Discuss why this statement is false.
3. Describe the biochemistry behind the following diagnostic tests: stool pH of 5.5; positive stool test for presence of reducing sugar (what other sugars besides lactose would give a positive test?).
4. How are H_2, CO_2, and methane produced in the human gut? Why is expired CO_2 *not* used as a measure of bacterial fermentation?
5. Why is an overnight fast required before the lactose tolerance test or the breath hydrogen test is administered?
6. What is the point (to the fermenting bacteria) of producing alcohols, acids, and H_2 gas?
7. From your general understanding of how biomolecules interact with each other, how could change of a single nucleotide alter transcriptional activity? Describe possible bonds/interactions that could be altered by C→T or G→A changes in a DNA sequence.
8. Many lactose-intolerant patients can, over time, increase the amount of lactose ingested without an increase of symptoms. What is the mechanism of this "tolerance"? Is there a limit to its extent?
9. Discuss the clinical consequences of lactose intolerance.

BIBLIOGRAPHY

Barnard ND: The milk debate goes on and on and on! *Pediatrics* **112:**448, 2003.

Beja-Pereira A, Luikart G, England PR, et al.: Gene-culture coevolution between cattle milk protein genes and human lactase genes. *Nat Genet* **35:**311–313, 2003.

Bersaglieri T, Sabeti PC, Patterson N, et al.: Genetic signatures of strong recent positive selection of the lactase gene. *Am J Hum Genet* **74:**1111–1120, 2004.

Boshuizen JA, Reimerink JH, Korteland-van Make AM, et al.: Changes in small intestinal homeostasis, morphology, and gene expression during rotavirus infection of infant mice. *J Virol* **77:** 13005–13016, 2003.

Carrocio A, Montalto G, Cavera G, et al.: Lactose intolerance and self-reported milk intolerance: relationship with lactose maldigestion and nutrient intake. *J Am Coll Nutr* **17:**631–636, 1998.

Di Stephano M, Veneto G, Malservisi S, et al.: Lactose malabsorption and intolerance and peak bone mass. *Gastroenterology* **122:**1793–1799, 2002.

Enattah NS, Forsblom C, Rasinpera H, et al., The FinnDiane Study Group: The genetic variant of lactase persistence C (−13910) T as a risk factor for type I and II diabetes in the Finnish population. *Eur J Clin Nutr* 1–4, 2004.

Enattah NS, Sahi T, Savilahti E, et al.: Identification of a variant associated with adult-type hypolactasia. *Nat Genet* **30:**233–237, 2002.

Fiocchi A, Restani P, Gualtiero L, et al.: Clinical tolerance to lactose in children with cow's milk allergy. *Pediatrics* **112:**359–362, 2003.

Gilat T, Russo S, Gelman-Malachi E, et al.: Lactase in man: a nonadaptable enzyme. *Gastroenterology* **62:**1125–1127, 1972.

Grand RJ, Montgomery RK, Chitkara DK, et al.: Changing genes; losing lactase. *Gut* **52:**617–619, 2003.

Hermans MM, Brummer RJ, Ruijgers AM, et al.: The relationship between lactose tolerance test results and symptoms of lactose intolerance. *Am J Gastroenterol* **92:**98–104, 1997.

Hertzler SR, Clancy SM: Kefir improves lactose digestion and tolerance in adults with lactose maldigestion. *J Am Diet Assoc* **103:**582–587, 2003.

Hertzler SR, Savaiano DA: Colonic adaptation to daily lactose feeding in lactose maldigesters reduces lactose intolerance. *Am J Clin Nutr* **64:**232–236, 1996.

Hove H, Norgaard H, Mortensen PB: Lactic acid bacteria and the human gastrointestinal tract. *Eur J Clin Nutr* **53:**339–350, 1999.

Jarvela I, Enattah NS, Kokkonen J, et al.: Assignment of the locus for congenital lactase deficiency to 2q21, in the vicinity but separate from the lactase-phlorizin hydrolase gene. *Am J Hum Genet* **63:**1078–1085, 1998.

Jarvis JK, Miller GD: Overcoming the barrier of lactose intolerance to reduce health disparities. *J Natl Med Assoc* **94:**55–66, 2002.

Johnson AO, Semenya JG, Buchowski MS, et al.: Correlation of lactose maldigestion, lactose intolerance, and milk intolerance. *Am J Clin Nutr* **57:**399–401, 1993a.

Johnson AO, Semenya JG, Buchowski MS, et al.: Adaptation of lactose maldigesters to continued milk intakes. *Am J Clin Nutr* **58**:879–881, 1993b.

Kudlacek S, Freudenthaler O, Weissboeck H, et al.: Lactose intolerance: a risk factor for reduced bone mineral density and vertebral fractures? *J Gastroenterol* **37**:1014–1019, 2002.

Kuokkanen M, Enattah NS, Oksanen A, et al.: Transcriptional regulation of the lactase-phlorizin hydrolase gene by polymorphisms associated with adult-type hypolactasia. *Gut* **52**:647–652, 2003.

Lee CM, Hardy CM: Cocoa feeding and human lactose intolerance. *Am J Clin Nutr* **49**:840–844, 1989.

Martini MC, Kukielka D, Savaiano DA: Lactose digestion from yogurt: influence of a meal and additional lactose. *Am J Clin Nutr* **53**:1253–1258, 1991.

Meloni GF, Colombo C, La Vecchia C, et al.: High prevalence of lactose absorbers in Northern Sardinian patients with type 1 and type 2 diabetes mellitus. *Am J Clin Nutr.* **73**:582–585, 2001.

Mulcare CA, Weale ME, Jones AL, et al.: The T allele of a single-nucleotide polymorphism 13.9 kb upstream of the lactase gene (LCT)(C-13.9kbT) does not predict or cause the lactase-persistence phenotype in Africans. *Am J Hum Genet* **74**:1102–1110, 2004.

Obermayer-Pietsch BM, Bonelli CM, Walter DE, et al.: Genetic predisposition for adult lactose intolerance and relation to diet, bone density and bone fractures. *J Bone Miner Res* **19**:42–47, 2004.

OMIM Online Mendelian Inheritance in Man. www.ncbi.nlm.nih.gov/entrez.

Pelletier X, Laure-Boussuge S, Donazzolo Y: Hydrogen excretion upon ingestion of dairy products in lactose-intolerant male subjects: importance of the live flora. *Eur J Clin Nutr* **55**:509–512, 2001.

Prentice A: Diet, nutrition and the prevention of osteoporosis. *Public Health Nutr* **7**:227–243, 2004.

Pribila BA, Hertler SR, Martin BR et al.: Improved lactose digestion and intolerance among African-American adolescent girls fed a dairy-rich diet. *J Am Diet Assoc.* **100**:524–528, 2000.

Saavedra JM, Perman JA: Current concepts in lactose malabsorption and intolerance. *Annu Rev Nutr* **9**:475–502, 1989.

Scrimshaw NS, Murray EB: The acceptability of milk and milk products in populations with a high prevalence of lactose intolerance. *Am J Clin Nutr* **48**:1083–1159, 1988.

Solomons NW: Fermentation, fermented foods, and lactose intolerance. *Eur J Clin Nutr* **56**:S50–55, 2002.

Swagerty DL, Walling AD, Klein RM: Lactose intolerance. *Am Family Phys* **65**:1845–1850, 2002.

Swallow DM, Poulter M, Hollox EJ: Intolerance to lactose and other dietary sugars. *Drug Metab Dispos* **29**:513–516, 2001.

Thomas S, Walker-Smith JA, Senewiratne B, et al.: Age dependency of the lactase persistence and lactase restriction phenotypes among children in Sri Lanka and Britain. *J Trop Pediatr.* **36**:80–85, 1990.

Troelsen JT, Olsen J, Moller J, et al.: An upstream polymorphism associated with lactase persistence has increased enhancer activity. *Gastroenterology* **125**:1686–1694, 2003.

Vernia P, Di Camillo M, Marinaro V, et al.: Effect of predominant methanogenic flora on the outcome of lactose breath test in irritable bowel syndrome patients. *Eur J Clin Nutr* **57**:1116–1119, 2003.

Vesa TH, Lember M, Korpela R: Milk fat does not affect the symptoms of lactose intolerance. *Eur J Clin Nutr* **51**:633–636, 1997.

Vesa TH, Marteau P. Korpela R: Lactose intolerance. *J Am Coll Nutr* **19**:165S–175S, 2000.

White D: *The Physiology and Biochemistry of Prokaryotes.* Oxford University Press, New York, 1995.

26

Pancreatic Insufficiency Secondary to Chronic Pancreatitis

PETER LAYER and JUTTA KELLER

CASE REPORT

A 45-year-old male patient presented with diarrhea and weight loss (12 kg during the past year; his current body weight was 63 kg, height was 181 cm, and Body Mass Index (BMI) was 19.2 kg/m² [normal is 19.2-24.9]). He reported that his stools were bulky, loose, and odorous, particularly following large meals rich in fat. During the last 15 years, the patient had suffered from recurrent attacks of abdominal pain. Most episodes were self-limited and subsided after 1-3 days. In time, the patient found that avoiding food intake during acute attacks was helpful. In association with one attack, a peptic ulcer was suspected, and the patient was treated unsuccessfully with an acid-suppressing drug (possibly a proton pump inhibitor), the name of which he did not remember; upper gastrointestinal endoscopy and ultrasound were not performed.

The patient had observed a gradual decrease over time of both frequency and intensity of acute attacks and therefore did not pursue a systematic diagnostic workup. On further inquiry, the patient admitted to substantial, continuous alcohol consumption over the last 20 years of about 2-3 L of beer per day (on weekends and "special occasions" even more) as well as hard liquor. He did, however, abstain from alcohol during acute attacks. Thus, his mean daily consumption can be estimated as about 120 g pure alcohol. Moreover, the patient was a heavy smoker, smoking 20-30 cigarettes per day for nearly 30 years.

Physical examination indicated poor nutri- tional status (BMI 19.2 kg/m²) and reduced general condition but otherwise normal results. Routine laboratory examinations showed macrocytosis (mean corpuscular volume of erythrocytes increased to 105 fL; normal is 82-101 fL) and elevated γ-glutamyltransferase (152 U/L; normal is 5-39 U/L) compatible with ongoing alcohol abuse and liver damage. Fasting blood glucose concentrations and serum concentrations of amylase and lipase were normal. Abdominal ultrasound showed a fatty liver, nonhomogeneous pancreatic tissue with evidence of calcifications, and a widened and irregular pancreatic duct (Fig. 26-1). A plain abdominal radiogram confirmed pancreatic calcifications. Endoscopic ultrasound revealed no evidence of a pancreatic tumor but confirmed structural changes as observed on abdominal ultrasound.

Quantitative fecal fat excretion was markedly increased (28 g/day; normal is <7 g/day), and fecal elastase 1 concentration was reduced to 24 µg/g (lower level of normal is 200 µg/g). The patient was diagnosed with severe pancreatic exocrine (but not endocrine) insufficiency due to alcoholic chronic calcifying pancreatitis and advised to stop alcohol and cigarette consumption.

The patient also was advised to change his dietary habits by avoiding large meals and eating several smaller or medium meals. He was treated with pancreatin, a medication containing a mixture of porcine pancreatic enzymes, including lipase, amylase, and proteases, with the dosage determined by units of lipase activity (Layer and

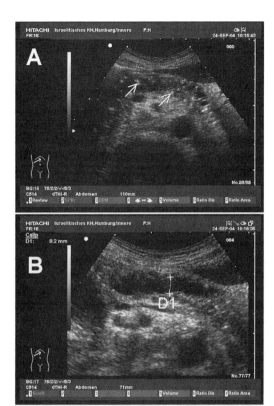

Figure 26-1. Abdominal ultrasound showing pathological alterations typical of chronic pancreatitis, i.e. a nonhomogenous pancreatic tissue with calcifications (*A*; several calcifications are marked with an arrow) and a widened and irregular pancreatic duct (*B*; diameter of pancreatic duct D1 is 8.2 mm, upper limit of normal is 3 mm). Courtesy C. Pachmann, MD.

Keller, 2003). The initial dosage (25,000 U lipase with each small meal or snack and 50,000 units with a medium meal) resulted in partial improvement. Symptoms virtually disappeared with subsequent doubling of enzyme dosage. In particular, stools became normal, and the patient gained 4 kg of weight within 3 months.

DIAGNOSIS

Pancreatic exocrine insufficiency with nutrient maldigestion as described in the case report is both a classical complication and a defining leading symptom of chronic pancreatitis. Therefore, taking a careful history provides the key for the diagnosis.

In the majority of patients, pancreatic exocrine insufficiency develops as a late complication, mostly in the second decade following first onset of symptoms. Its typical manifestation is insidious, with gradual progression. Thus, it is necessary to consider this diagnosis in patients in whom weight loss, usually associated with steatorrhea (fat in the stool, perceived by the patient as bulky, loose, odorous stools) develops following a long-standing history of abdominal pain and/or known chronic pancreatitis. As a further clue, pancreatic exocrine insufficiency may be associated with diabetes mellitus, in which there is destruction of endocrine as well as exocrine pancreatic parenchyma. Diabetes mellitus is a late consequence in more than 60% of patients with pancreatic exocrine insufficiency.

It is important to keep in mind, however, that not all patients with chronic pancreatitis develop clinical pancreatic exocrine insufficiency; approximately 25% of patients still have sufficient exocrine function after 25 years of disease. On the other hand, it is also important to note that 10%–15% of patients with chronic pancreatitis have primary painless disease; in these patients, pancreatic exocrine insufficiency may be the first (and possibly only) clinical manifestation. Thus, the absence of pain or a history of pancreatitis does not exclude the diagnosis (DiMagno et al., 1993).

Irreversible destructive morphological changes (such as ductal alterations, calcifications, scarring, pseudocysts, etc.) are essential features of chronic pancreatitis and are therefore usually, albeit not invariably, detectable in pancreatic exocrine insufficiency by imaging methods, that is, morphological investigations. These include plain abdominal x-ray, sonography, computed tomography (CT), endosonography, endoscopic retrograde cholangiopancreatography (ERCP), and magnetic resonance imaging (MRI)/magnetic resonance cholangiopancreatography (MRCP). (ERCP involves endoscopic injection of a radioopaque solution and radiological imaging of the pancreatic duct system. Magnetic resonance cholangiopancreatography uses specific resonance properties of compartmentalized fluid within the pancreatic duct system for visualization.) It has to be kept in mind, however, that imaging findings may provide evidence for chronic pancreatitis but do not prove pancreatic exocrine insufficiency (with the possible future exception of functional MRI techniques). Hence, in order to diagnose pancreatic exocrine insufficiency, secretory function needs to be assessed.

Pancreatic function tests are therefore indicated if and when one or more of the following aspects need be clarified: Is a symptom or sign caused by pancreatic exocrine insufficiency? Has pancreatic exocrine insufficiency developed in the course of chronic pancreatitis? Does a patient require enzyme supplementation treatment?

To be of value in routine clinical practice, any pancreatic function test is required to be not only precise and reliable, but also uncomplicated and inexpensive. However, due to the peculiarities of pancreatic anatomy and physiology, no currently available test meets all these criteria. Indeed, despite astounding developments in virtually every other diagnostic field (including pancreatic imaging), pancreatic exocrine function is estimated today by using very much the same principles and even methods as three decades ago.

In principle, pancreatic function can be tested by quantifying exocrine secretory output directly by duodenal intubation, juice aspiration, and measurement of enzymes under defined stimulatory conditions, usually by intravenous application of cholecystokinin and/or secretin. ERCP-guided direct cannulation and collection of pure pancreatic juice is, however, not a routine procedure due to its substantial inherent risk of iatrogenic pancreatitis. Pancreatic enzymes can also be quantified indirectly by measuring a representative enzyme in a stool sample.

The other approach is indirect, namely, to measure not enzymes as such, but their physiological biochemical efficacy. This can be achieved by oral administration of a composite test substance, which is hydrolyzed ("digested") into its components exclusively by a specific pancreatic enzyme and subsequently absorbed and eliminated by the renal or the respiratory system. Ideally, the urinary excretion/respiratory exhalation of a metabolite of the test substance is proportional to its hydrolysis in the small intestine, which in turn is directly dependent on the quantity of pancreatic enzymes present.

BIOCHEMICAL PERSPECTIVES

Physiology of Human Pancreatic Enzyme Secretion

Depending on nutrient intake, the human pancreas secretes about 3 L of alkaline juice per day. Pancreatic juice contains hydrolytic enzymes (or their precursors, see below) for digestion of complex carbohydrates, proteins, and lipids, with the most important ones α-amylase, trypsin, chymotrypsin, lipase, and colipase. In addition, elastases, carboxypeptidases, phospholipase A_2, carboxylester lipase, and ribo- and deoxyribonucleases are also secreted. Some of the enzymes are present in more than one form (e.g., cationic and anionic trypsinogen). The principal inorganic components of pancreatic juice are water, potassium, chloride, and bicarbonate. The high bicarbonate content of pancreatic juice is responsible for its alkaline pH. This serves to protect enzymes from acidic denaturation and increases enzymatic activity within the intestinal lumen (pH optima within the alkaline range). α-Amylase and lipase are secreted in active form, whereas proteases enter the duodenum as inactive zymogens (Rinderknecht, 1993). Within the duodenum, trypsinogen is partly converted to trypsin by the duodenal enzyme enterokinase. Subsequently, trypsin has an autocatalytic effect and also activates the other proteases (Fig. 26-2).

Under physiological circumstances, two distinctive secretory patterns are observed: During the fasting state, the healthy human pancreas secretes low amounts of pancreatic juice; pancreatic secretion is cyclical and integrated with upper gastrointestinal motility, gastric acid secretion, and entry of bile into the duodenum (Keller and Layer, 2002). One cycle takes 90–120 min and consists of a period of secretory and motor quiescence (phase I) followed by irregular secretion and motility (phase II, about 80% of time). Maximal interdigestive secretion rates (about 50% of maximum) occur at the end of phase II and just before onset of phase III (motility), in which the motility in the duodenum is characterized by regular and aborally propagated contractions at maximum frequency. This motor pattern has a strong propulsive effect and is thought to clean the small intestine of residual nutrients and endogenous substances. The clearing effect is enhanced by the high volumes of pancreatic juice and bile secreted just prior to it. Pancreatic secretion declines during duodenal phase III. A short phase of irregular motor activity (phase IV) may follow phase III before onset of the next phase I (DiMagno and Layer, 1993).

The digestive pattern is initiated by stimulation of pancreatic exocrine secretion due to imagination, sight, smell, and taste of food (i.e., the so-called cephalic phase of pancreatic

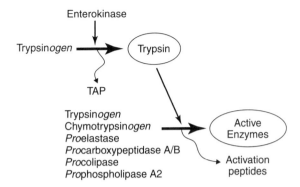

Figure 26-2. The pancreatic enzyme cascade. Pancreatic proteases enter the intestinal lumen as inactive zymogens. Within the duodenum, a specific enzyme of the duodenal mucosa, enterokinase, activates trypsinogen by releasing the trypsinogen activation peptide (TAP). Subsequently, active trypsin activates the other zymogens and acts autocatalytically.

exocrine secretion). Distention of the stomach (gastric phase) may also increase pancreatic secretion via vagal reflexes. However, the most important stimulatory mechanism of prandial pancreatic exocrine secretion is nutrient exposure of the duodenal mucosa. There is experimental evidence that digestive products of enzymatic hydrolysis (such as free fatty acids) rather than intact macromolecules (such as triglycerides) evoke neurohormonal stimulation of the physiological enzyme response to a meal. The most important stimulatory hormones are cholecystokinin and secretin. Both are peptide hormones produced and released by the enterochromaffin cells of the proximal small intestinal mucosa. Cholecystokinin is the strongest physiological stimulator of enzyme secretion. By contrast, secretion of bicarbonate is stimulated by secretin, which is released mainly in response to duodenal acid exposure (Owyang and Logsdon, 2004). Following a regular meal, the digestive pattern will prevail for about 4–7 h. Thus, with three or more meals per day, the interdigestive pattern will usually only occur during nighttime (DiMagno and Layer, 1993).

Sufficient absorption of macronutrients to maintain energy supply requires prior hydrolysis by pancreatic enzymes. Thus, complete absence of pancreatic enzymes (e.g., due to pancreatectomy) is, if untreated, incompatible with life. Normally, however, in healthy individuals the cumulative postprandial pancreatic enzyme response exceeds by far (10- to 15-fold) the quantity required to prevent overt maldigestion. In particular, lipid digestion is fast and

highly efficient under physiological circumstances. Hydrolysis of dietary triacylglycerols depends on an intricate interplay among pancreatic lipase, colipase, and bile salts. Pancreatic lipase binds to the oil-water interface of oil droplets and hydrolyzes triacylglycerol to two fatty acid molecules and a monoacylglycerol, with the fatty acid esterified at position 2; both bile salts and colipase are important to achieve its full lipolytic activity: Bile salts enhance the emulsification of triacylglycerols and form micelles, which remove fatty acids and monoacylglycerol from the oil-water interface. In the presence of bile salts, colipase forms a complex with lipase that acts to anchor the lipase and allows its action in a more hydrophilic environment. After incorporation into micelles, the fatty acids, and monoacylglycerol are absorbed, incorporated into chylomicrons, and transported to the liver.

In healthy humans, up to 80% of lipids may be absorbed during duodenal transit (i.e., before reaching the ligament of Treitz (Holtmann et al., 1997)). In exocrine pancreatic insufficiency, on the other hand, 7%–10% of normal prandial secretory rates may be enough to prevent elevated fecal fat excretion. Still, even in healthy human subjects, digestion and absorption of nutrients after a regular meal is incomplete, and substantial nutrient quantities regularly escape intestinal absorption and pass the ileocecal junction. Nutrient exposure of these intestinal sites inhibits upper gastrointestinal secretory and motor functions (Layer et al., 1990; Read et al., 1984). This mechanism is called *ileal brake*. In addition, malabsorbed

Table 26-1. Clinically Important Differential Diagnoses of Steatorrhea

Pathophysiology	Disease
Pancreatic exocrine insufficiency	
Decreased intraluminal fat digestion	Chronic pancreatitis
	Cystic fibrosis
Disturbed secretion of bile acids	
Impaired fat solubilization, decreased	Primary biliary cirrhosis
formation of micelles	Primary sclerosing cholangitis
Malabsorption	
Reduced absorptive capacity of intestinal	Celiac disease
mucosa due to inflammation	Morbus Whipple
	Crohn's disease
	Parasitosis
Nutrient unavailability	
Abdominal surgery, radiation therapy	
Loss of absorptive surface	Short-bowel syndrome
Bypass	Enteroenteric fistual
Nutrient unavailability, deconjugation	Bacterial overgrowth
of bile acids	
Disturbed solubilization of lipids,	Loss of bile acids
decreased formation of micelles	

nutrients serve as exogenous energy supply of the colonic microflora.

After having been secreted intraluminally, enzymatic activity decreases during small intestinal transit. The rate of inactivation differs between enzymes because they have different stability against degradation (Layer et al., 1986). For example, about 60% of duodenal protease activities reach the jejunum and between 20% and 30% reach the ileum. It should be noted that trypsin's hydrolytic activity survives better than its immunoreactivity, which suggests that complete structural integrity may not be required for its enzymatic action. Pancreatic amylase is rather stable because it is not easily proteolyzed and consequently has been found to have a high duodeno-ileal survival rate. By contrast, lipase is inactivated very rapidly, particularly in the absence of triglycerides, and only a small proportion may reach the distal small bowel. Chymotrypsin appears to be of particular importance for destroying lipase activity.

Pancreatic Exocrine Insufficiency in Chronic Pancreatitis

Nutrient maldigestion due to pancreatic exocrine insufficiency is a classical complication of chronic pancreatitis. In most cases, it occurs late in life because of the enormous functional reserve of the gland described above. In alcoholic pancreatitis, its manifestation usually develops within the second decade of clinical disease, but it may also appear more rapidly.

Steatorrhea, the clinical result of insufficient intraluminal lipid hydrolysis, is the most important digestive malfunction in pancreatic exocrine insufficiency. As a rule, concomitant malabsorption of the lipid-soluble vitamins A, D, E, and K must be suspected in these patients. Naturally, potential differential diagnoses have to be considered in patients who present with steatorrhea (Table 26-1). The pivotal role of fat malabsorption in chronic pancreatitis is due to several interacting mechanisms:

1. In progressive chronic pancreatitis, acinar synthesis and release of lipase decrease earlier and more markedly compared with proteases.
2. Pancreatic bicarbonate secretion is also diminished in exocrine pancreatic insufficiency. There may thus be insufficient intraduodenal buffer protection for enzymes against denaturation by gastric acid emptied with postprandial chyme. Indeed, intraluminal pH may decrease below 4.0, which results in irreversible destruction of lipase.

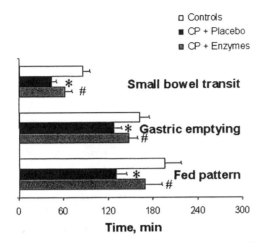

Figure 26-3. Patients with severe pancreatic exocrine insufficiency (n = 14, mean ± SE) show marked alterations of gastrointestinal functions with shortened small bowel transit time, 90% gastric emptying time, and duration of the fed pattern. These alterations are corrected by enzyme replacement therapy (*$P < .05$ vs. controls, # $P < .05$ vs. placebo) (Layer et al., 1997).

3. During small intestinal transit, lipase is proteolyzed more rapidly than other enzymes.
4. Extrapancreatic lipolytic mechanisms (such as gastric lipase) play only a minor role and cannot compensate for the loss of pancreatic lipase.

Protein and starch digestion, on the other hand, have potent nonpancreatic compensatory mechanisms. Due to the compensatory action of salivary amylase and brush border oligosaccharidases, a substantial proportion of starch digestion can be achieved without pancreatic amylase. Similarly, protein denaturation and hydrolysis is initiated by gastric proteolytic activity (acid and pepsin) and continued by intestinal brush border peptidases, and is thus partly maintained even in the absence of pancreatic proteolytic activity.

The coefficient of fat absorption is defined as the amount of fat absorbed as a percentage of the ingested amount. This coefficient normally exceeds 93% and is used (rather than crude fecal fat excretion) to indicate efficacy of luminal fat digestion following different dietary lipid intakes. By contrast, fecal carbohydrate measurements do not fully reflect the extent of starch malabsorption because carbohydrates are metabolized by the intracolonic microbial flora. Since intracolonic metabolism of carbohydrates

produces H_2, starch malabsorption can be measured by determining hydrogen breath concentrations.

In addition to steatorrhea and nutritional deficiencies, patients with pancreatic exocrine insufficiency also develop symptoms such as postprandial pain, cramps, bloating, and distention. These are caused by profound alterations of upper gastrointestinal secretory and motor functions in response to increased nutrient delivery to the distal small intestine, particularly the ileum. In the first 5–10 years of chronic pancreatitis, overt malabsorption is usually neither detected nor a major clinical problem, although enzyme output may decrease by 60%–90%. Still, there is evidence that, even in the early stages of chronic pancreatitis, the site of maximal nutrient digestion and absorption is shifted from the duodenum to the more distal small intestine.

Moreover, recent studies suggest that gastric emptying and small intestinal transit are markedly accelerated in patients with untreated pancreatic insufficiency (Fig. 26-3) (Layer et al., 1997). The available time for digestion and absorption is therefore markedly decreased in these patients, which may contribute further to malabsorption. Disturbance of both digestion and gastrointestinal transit are corrected by enzyme replacement, suggesting that malabsorption is not only a consequence but also a cause of abnormal motor function. In turn, this pathophysiological mechanism explains the alleviating effects on pain and dyspepsia of pancreatic enzyme supplementation in a subset of patients.

Direct Pancreatic Function Tests

The gold standard for measuring pancreatic exocrine function is direct measurement of pancreatic enzyme and bicarbonate output in response to a specific and defined hormonal stimulus such as cholecystokinin (or an analogue such as cerulein) alone or in combination with secretin (secretin-cerulein [SC] test). Because sensitivity and specificity of this test both exceed 90%, it is the only method apt to diagnose mild-to-moderate pancreatic insufficiency reliably. Unfortunately, the test is invasive, demanding, costly, and not standardized across expert centers. It requires placement of a double-lumen nasoduodenal tube for continuous elimination of gastric juice and complete collection of duodenal juice in ice at 10- to 15-min intervals during intravenous infusion of secretin and cerulein. Analyses of the samples include measurements of volume, bicarbonate, trypsin, chymotrypsin, lipase, and amylase outputs.

The Lundh test also includes intestinal intubation and direct measurement of enzyme output in duodenal juice but uses a standardized test meal as a pancreatic stimulus. Because this test requires release of physiological regulatory mediators from the duodenal mucosa, it is less specific than the SC test and may render false-positive results in intestinal diseases such as celiac sprue.

Although all pancreatic enzymes are inactivated during intestinal transit, fecal outputs of several enzymes correlate with pancreatic enzyme secretion. Fecal chymotrypsin activity, which is comparatively stable in the lumen as well as in extracorporal fecal samples, can be measured by a commercially available photometric test kit. When performed on three consecutive days, this test detects severe pancreatic exocrine insufficiency, but sensitivity and specificity are low in mild-to-moderate cases. In addition, the test does not differentiate between porcine and human chymotrypsin, so that pancreatin supplements need to be discontinued 5 days prior to the test. For this reason, however, the test is able to monitor a patient's compliance in severe pancreatic insufficiency apparently refractory to enzyme treatment. Patients

who still suffer from steatorrhea although they take the pancreatin as prescribed will have high fecal chymotrypsin activities, whereas those who fail to ingest their medication will have low chymotrypsin activities.

Fecal elastase 1 concentration can be measured by an ELISA test kit using an antibody specific for the human enzyme; pancreatin supplements do not interfere with this pancreatic function test and need not be discontinued. Although measurement of fecal elastase 1 excretion appears to be somewhat more sensitive than fecal chymotrypsin, its specificity and positive predictive value are similarly low, and false-positive results can be expected in patients with intestinal diseases. Conversely, mild-to-moderate stages of pancreatic exocrine insufficiency cannot be diagnosed reliably.

Small quantities of pancreatic enzymes are released from the pancreas into the bloodstream even physiologically and are detectable as low serum activities and/or concentrations of lipase, amylase, trypsinogen, and chymotrypsinogen, respectively. Since progressive destruction of the organ occurs in chronic pancreatitis, this should theoretically be reflected by decreased serum enzymes, but so far these tests are not clinically useful because of their low accuracy.

Indirect Pancreatic Function Tests

Measurement of stool weight and quantitative fecal fat excretion on three consecutive days during a balanced diet are common screening tests for both pancreatic insufficiency and other pathologies that result in malabsorption. However, these tests are insensitive and nonspecific for pancreatic malfunction: Steatorrhea occurs only after loss of more than 90% of exocrine parenchyma, and other causes of malabsorption (e.g., celiac sprue or Crohn's disease) may also induce abnormal fecal fat excretion of more than 7 g/day or more than 5 g/100 g.

Orally administered fluorescein is readily absorbed in the small intestine. By contrast fluorescein coupled to dilaurate cannot be absorbed unless the composite molecule is cleaved intraduodenally by the pancreatic cholesterol esterase to form lauric acid and (absorbable) fluorescein. After its absorption, fluorescein is partly glucuronidated in the liver and then excreted in urine, predominantly as fluorescein diglucuronide. Thus, in pancreatic-insufficient

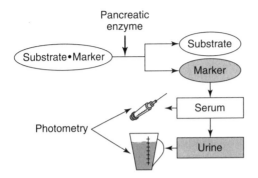

Figure 26-4. Principle of the Pancreolauryl® and the NBT-PABA (*N*-benzoyl-L-tyrosyl-*P*-aminobenzoic acid, bentiromide) test. The composite molecule consisting of a substrate and a marker molecule cannot be absorbed but can be cleaved intraduodenally by pancreatic enzymes (cholesterol esterase and chymotrypsin, respectively), leading to release of an absorbable marker substance. Following absorption and hepatic conjugation, the marker is excreted in urine. In pancreatic-insufficient patients, decreased secretion of pancreatic enzymes results in incomplete cleavage of the composite molecule. This results in decreased absorption and subsequent excretion of the marker, which can be measured photometrically.

patients, decreased secretion of cholesterol esterase results in incomplete cleavage and decreased generation and absorption of free fluorescein (Fig. 26-4). The Pancreolauryl® test involves ingestion of a standard breakfast together with 0.5 mmol of fluorescein dilaurate. Urine is collected for 10 h postprandially for determination of fluorescein excretion. After a washout period of at least 24 h, the protocol is repeated with free fluorescein instead of fluorescein dilaurate; this procedure serves to control for individual differences in postdigestive processing of free fluorescein. Results are expressed as the ratio of fluorescein excreted on the test and the control days in percentage (normal is > 30%, abnormal is < 20%, equivocal is 20%–30%).

The test is valid for diagnosing severe pancreatic exocrine insufficiency but has the sensitivity limitations described above with respect to detecting mild impairment of pancreatic function. Conversely, despite the inclusion of the control test, false-positive results may occur in patients with intestinal and biliary diseases, as well as following gastric resection or Y-en-Roux procedures. In the latter patients, intraluminal lack of pancreatic enzymes (despite normal secretory

capacity of the pancreas) is caused predominantly by postprandial asynchrony of pancreatic secretory output and chyme delivery and subsequent impaired mixing of enzymes and nutrient macromolecule substrates, as well as reduced release of stimulatory mediators. However, the test may be useful in such patients because it reflects the efficacy of postprandial intraluminal nutrient digestion as well as the effects of enzyme therapy.

The test principle of the NBT-PABA (*N*-benzoyl-L-tyrosyl-*P*-aminobenzoic acid, bentiromide) test very much resembles the Pancreolauryl® test (Fig. 26-4). Again, the unsplit molecule NBT-PABA cannot be absorbed, and absorption of its metabolite PABA depends on prior hydrolysis by chymotrypsin within the intestinal lumen. Subsequently, PABA undergoes conjugation in the liver and is excreted in the urine. In healthy subjects, at least 50% of the administered dose is excreted in the urine during 6 h postprandially.

A noninvasive and simple H_2 breath test has been suggested for measurement of pancreatic function based on the principle that undigested starch will pass into the colon, be metabolized by the colonic flora, and thus lead to an increase in breath H_2 exhalation. However, numerous mechanisms for false-positive (e.g., bacterial overgrowth) and -negative (e.g., insufficient H_2 production by colonic bacteria) limit its validity.

Several breath tests using ^{13}C-labeled lipids have been developed for measurement of pancreatic exocrine function. They are based on the common principle that intestinal triglyceride absorption requires prior hydrolysis by pancreatic lipase to produce free fatty acids and monoacylglycerol. These metabolites are incorporated into micelles, absorbed, and transported to the liver. Further degradation by hepatic enzymes and β-oxidation results in formation of $^{13}CO_2$, which is absorbed into the bloodstream, transported to the lungs, and exhaled (Fig. 26-5). Thus, an increase in $^{13}CO_2$ concentration in breath correlates with intestinal lipid digestion as a marker of pancreatic exocrine function. Measurements are performed by mass spectrometry or isotope-selective infrared spectrometry. Varying test modifications have been developed using ^{13}C-tripalmitin, ^{13}C-triolein, ^{13}C-Hiolein® (a mixture of physiological long-chain triglycerides), ^{13}C-trioctanoin, or so-called ^{13}C-mixed triglycerides [1,3-distearyl, 2(carboxyl-^{13}C)octanoyl glycerol] as substrates.

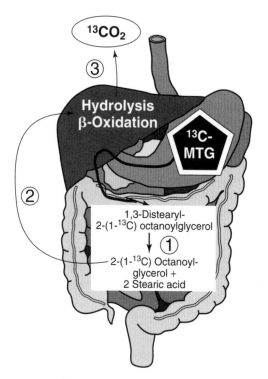

Figure 26-5. Principle of the ^{13}C-mixed triglyceride breath test. Absorption of ^{13}C-mixed triglycerides requires prior hydrolysis by pancreatic lipase (1), which leads to production of free fatty acids (stearic acid) and monoacylglycerol [2-(1-^{13}C)octanoylglycerol]. These metabolites are incorporated into micelles, absorbed, and transported to the liver (2). Further degradation by hepatic enzymes and β-oxidation results in formation of ^{13}CO$_2$, which is absorbed into the bloodstream, transported to the lung, and exhaled (3). Thus, exhalation of ^{13}CO$_2$ reflects intestinal lipolysis and is a marker of pancreatic exocrine function.

The breath test using ^{13}C-mixed triglycerides is best established because it offers several advantages over other substrates. Octanoic acid as a medium-chain fatty acid is metabolized faster and therefore allows a shorter test duration than substrates with long-chain fatty acids. Since a normal diet contains only low amounts of octanoic acid, the marker is not diluted by unmarked substrate. Furthermore, maximal and cumulative ^{13}C-exhalation are higher with ^{13}C-mixed triglycerides than with long-chain triglycerides because incorporation of carbon atoms from octanoate into the fatty tissue is lower (Vantrappen et al., 1989). Most current protocols report sensitivities of about 90% for

severe but less than 60% for mild pancreatic exocrine insufficiency, which is similar to other indirect pancreatic function tests.

Differential Use of Pancreatic Function Tests

Direct tests of secretory function such as fecal chymotrypsin and elastase 1 are the tests of first choice if the main diagnostic goal consists of noninvasive confirmation of chronic pancreatitis. Indirect tests may be preferred, however, if the main goal is to verify maldigestion (which needs not be due to loss of pancreatic secretory capacity) or to optimize enzyme treatment. For patients for whom noninvasive direct or indirect tests are negative or equivocal and diagnosis or exclusion of pancreatic exocrine insufficiency appears relevant, the invasive secretin-cerulein (SC) test should be considered.

THERAPY

Basis of Enzyme Treatment

To restore nutrient digestion in exocrine pancreatic insufficiency, sufficient enzymatic activity must be administered into the duodenal lumen simultaneously with meal substrates. Intraluminal lipid digestion in postprandial chyme requires lipase activity of at least 40–60 IU/mL throughout the digestive period, which translates into 25,000 to 40,000 IU intraduodenal lipase for digestion of a regular meal. Because plain enzyme preparations undergo rapid lipase inactivation due to acid and proteolytic destruction, it is necessary to administer up to 10-fold more lipase orally to achieve these quantities within the duodenum.

Pharmaceutical inhibition of gastric acid output (proton pump inhibitor, H$_2$ receptor blocker) may have beneficial effects when combined with an unprotected pancreatin preparation, not only by protection of enzymes during their gastric passage, but also by increasing duodenal pH and thereby improving enzymatic action. (Note that, in chronic pancreatitis, duodenal pH is lower due to impairment of pancreatic bicarbonate secretion, see above).

Coating of pancreatin preparations with polymers that resist acidic pH but allow disintegration and release of enzymes at pH 5.5 to 6.0 can be used to protect exogenous enzymes from premature acidic denaturation. However,

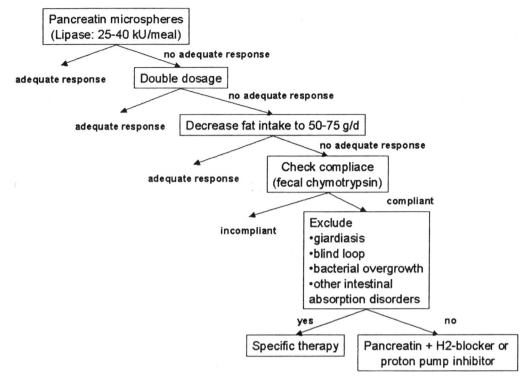

Figure 26-6. Therapeutic algorithm in pancreatic exocrine insufficiency.

solid particles that cannot be reduced to pieces less than 2 mm by gastric contractions are not emptied prandially. Instead, they are retained in the stomach until the return of the interdigestive motor pattern. Consequently, acid-resistant coating of a capsule containing pancreatin protects enzymes from acidic denaturation but leads to dissociation between duodenal delivery of enzymes and nutrients (Keller and Layer, 2003). Thus, modern pancreatin preparations consist of acid-resistant coated pancreatin microspheres with diameters not exceeding 2 mm. These mix intragastrically with the meal and are emptied intact into the duodenum simultaneously with the meal. In the duodenum, increasing pH causes release and hydrolytic action of enzymes.

Although the small, coated pancreatin preparations have been shown to be superior compared with unprotected pancreatin extracts, it should be noted that enzyme release requires several minutes after exposure to the intestinal milieu. This may further delay digestive action and shift the site of maximal absorption more distally; this pathophysiological mechanism is exacerbated by accelerated gastrointestinal transit characteristic for pancreatic exocrine insufficiency. For this reason, the physicochemical properties of the microsphere coating are crucial for the efficacy of enzyme therapy.

Practical Enzyme Supplementation

Enzymes for Steatorrhea

At present, the majority of patients with exocrine pancreatic insufficiency are treated with pH-sensitive pancreatin microspheres taken with each meal. To reduce steatorrhea to less than 15 g of fat per day, a minimal dose of 25,000–40,000 IU of lipase per meal are required (Fig. 26-6) (Keller and Layer, 2003). It is recommended that, for small meals or snacks, 1 tablet/capsule (containing 10,000–25,000 IU of lipase) should be swallowed with the start of the meal, and that for larger meals, a second dose should be taken during the meal. In many cases, these doses must be doubled (case report).

Efficacy of treatment is checked by clinical criteria, mainly by monitoring body weight and consistency of feces. In treatment-refractory cases, enzyme dosage should be further increased, and the patient should be advised to distribute nutrient intake over five or six smaller meals. If the steatorrhea still does not respond, then the compliance of the patient should be checked by fecal chymotrypsin measurement; low activities suggest an insufficient intake of enzymes.

A dose-dependent risk of developing stenotic fibrosing colonopathy (colonic strictures and marked submucosal fibrosis) has been observed in patients with cystic fibrosis taking ultrahigh doses of pancreatin. Although the mechanism remains controversial and may be specific for cystic fibrosis, and there is no evidence that patients with chronic pancreatitis also have an increased risk, we therefore do not generally recommend dosages of more than 75,000–100,000 IU of lipase per meal. In refractory cases, pathophysiological and therapeutic alternatives should be considered.

Following gastric or intestinal resections, bacterial overgrowth or mucosal infections such as *Giardia lamblia* as well as other intestinal absorption disorders may further compromise absorption. Patients with accelerated gastric emptying due to gastric resections or gastroenterostomies should be supplemented with pancreatin granule or powder preparations. Similarly, patients lacking gastric acid secretion, including those continuously receiving acid blockers, can be treated successfully with conventional unprotected pancreatin preparations. If patients are treated with enzyme supplementation, then use of medium-chain triglycerides as a dietary adjunct does not further enhance lipid absorption.

Enzymes for Pain Treatment

There is evidence that, in humans, a luminal, protease-mediated, negative feedback system may be operative under certain circumstances (Slaff et al., 1984), but it is controversial whether (and rather unlikely that) this mechanism contributes to the pathogenesis of pain in patients with chronic pancreatitis. Several controlled therapeutic trials in patients with chronic pancreatitis have yielded conflicting results. Moreover, experimental data suggest that hormonally-induced inhibition of pancreatic secretion alone is ineffective in painful pancreatitis. It is more likely that amelioration of pain following enzyme administration originates from correction of disturbed motor function, such as ileal brake mechanisms (inhibition of upper gastrointestinal functions by ileal nutrient exposure), induced by maldigested nutrients.

QUESTIONS

1. How is digestive pancreatic exocrine secretion induced?
2. Why is steatorrhea the most important digestive malfunction in pancreatic exocrine insufficiency in chronic pancreatitis?
3. What proportion of normal pancreatic exocrine secretion is needed to prevent steatorrhea?
4. Which pancreatic function tests are indirect tests?
5. Which hormonal mediators stimulate pancreatic exocrine secretion and are used for direct pancreatic function testing?
6. Why are pancreatin microspheres with acid-resistant coating usually more effective in reducing steatorrhea than identical lipase doses provided as either plain pancreatin powder or monolithic capsules or tablets with acid-resistant coating?

Acknowledgmens: Our studies cited in this article were supported by the German Research Foundation (DFG, grants La 483/5) and the Anna-Lorz-Foundation.

BIBLIOGRAPHY

Chowdhury RS, Forsmark CE: Review article: pancreatic function testing. *Aliment Pharmacol Ther* **17:**733–750, 2003.

DiMagno EP, Clain CE, Layer P: Chronic pancreatitis, *in* Go VL (ed): *The Pancreas: Biology, Pathobiology and Disease.* Raven Press, New York, 1993, pp. 665–706.

DiMagno EP, Layer P: Human exocrine pancreatic enzyme secretion, *in* Go VL (ed): *The Pancreas: Biology, Pathobiology and Diseases.* Raven Press, New York, 1993, pp. 275–300.

Holtmann G, Kelly DG, et al.: Survival of human pancreatic enzymes during small bowel transit: effect of nutrients, bile acids, and enzymes. *Am J Physiol* **273:**G553–G558, 1997.

Keller J, Layer P: Circadian pancreatic enzyme pattern and relationship between secretory and motor activity in fasting humans. *J Appl Physiol* **93:**592–600, 2002.

Keller J, Layer P: Pancreatic enzyme supplementation therapy. *Curr Treat Options Gastroenterol* **6:**369–374, 2003.

Layer P, Go VL, DiMagno EP: Fate of pancreatic enzymes during small intestinal aboral transit in humans. *Am J Physiol* **251**:G475–G480, 1986.

Layer P, Keller J: How to make use of pancreatic function tests, *in* Buechler M (ed): *Chronic Pancreatitis: Novel Concepts in Biology and Therapy.* Blackwell Science, Oxford, UK, 2002, pp. 233–242.

Layer P, Keller J: Lipase supplementation therapy: standards, alternatives, and perspectives. *Pancreas* **26**:1–7, 2003.

Layer P, Peschel S, et al.: Human pancreatic secretion and intestinal motility: effects of ileal nutrient perfusion. *Am J Physiol* **258**:G196–G201, 1990.

Layer P, von der Ohe MR, Holst JJ, et al.: Altered postprandial motility in chronic pancreatitis: role of malabsorption. *Gastroenterology* **112:** 1624–1634, 1997.

Owyang C, Logsdon CD: New insights into neurohormonal regulation of pancreatic secretion. *Gastroenterology* **127:**957–969, 2004.

Read NW, McFarlane A, Kinsman RI, et al.: Effect of infusion of nutrient solutions into the ileum on gastrointestinal transit and plasma levels of neurotensin and enteroglucagon. *Gastroenterology* **86:**274–280, 1984.

Rinderknecht H: Pancreatic secretory enzymes, *in* Go VL (ed): *The Pancreas: Biology, Pathobiology and Disease.* Raven Press, New York, 1993, pp. 219–251.

Slaff J, Jacobson D, Tillman CR, et al.: Protease-specific suppression of pancreatic exocrine secretion. *Gastroenterology* **87:**44–52, 1984.

Vantrappen GR, Rutgeerts PJ, et al.: Mixed triglyceride breath test: a noninvasive test of pancreatic lipase activity in the duodenum. *Gastroenterology* **96:**1126–1134, 1989.

27

Abetalipoproteinemia

PAUL RAVA and M. MAHMOOD HUSSAIN

CASE REPORT

A 28-year-old man who immigrated to the United States a few years ago saw his primary care physician for mild recurrent abdominal discomfort and diarrhea. Past medical history was benign except for what the patient referred to as "occasional abdominal distress." Further discussion revealed this to include diarrhea, flatus, and abdominal pains. He described the stool during these episodes to be greasy, pale, and foul smelling. Family history was unremarkable. Both of his parents, as well as three siblings, had no history of abdominal symptoms. The patient had been diagnosed with celiac disease and treated with a gluten-free diet at a previous visit. Even though he was compliant with dietary instructions, symptoms continued for the next year. The patient noted that he had experienced these symptoms periodically throughout his life, but that they had worsened since his arrival in the United States. He had not traveled since his immigration and had no pets or recent animal exposures, and there was no association between his abdominal discomfort and specific foods. He denied past or present use of drugs or alcohol and took no medications. Concerned that celiac disease may have been a misdiagnosis, a physical examination, blood tests, and a diagnostic procedure were performed.

Physical inspection revealed a healthy adult male, 1.8 m in height and weighing 76.5 kg. He was hemodynamically stable. Noticeable bruises were observed on his thighs. The patient attributed them to bumping into furniture, "not an uncommon event," as he sometimes left the lights off on entering the house to avoid disturbing his wife. Further examination revealed a mild peripheral neuropathy with numbness, decreased proprioception, and dulled response to painful as well as vibratory stimuli in the extremities. Deep tendon reflexes were also reduced. Muscle strength was preserved bilaterally. He had a positive Romberg sign (loss of balance while standing eyes closed) and slight ataxic gait. Fundoscopic examination revealed pigmented retinopathy.

Blood tests were performed and had the following results: hematocrit 33% (normal is 38%–45%); reticulocyte count 2.0% (normal is 0.5%–1.5%); mean corpuscular volume 90 (normal). A decreased erythrocyte sedimentation rate and a prothombrin time (PT) of 15 s (normal 11–13 s) were noted. A complete blood cell count; values for total protein and albumin, ALT, and AST, fasting glucose, Hb-A1c, as well as amylase and lipase were within normal range. Plasma levels of vitamins A and K were below normal, and there was near absence of vitamin E. Dysmorphic red blood cells (RBC) with multiple thorny projections (acanthocytes) were present on a blood smear. All other laboratory tests and findings were within normal limits.

Lipid analysis revealed low plasma cholesterol. A fasting lipid profile showed total cholesterol was 1 mmol/L (normal is 3.5–5.0 mmol/L). On fractionation, HDL was found to be normal while LDL was undetectable. Postprandial electrophoresis of plasma lipoproteins demonstrated the presence of HDL, but absence of chylomicrons, VLDL, and LDL. Plasma levels of apolipoprotein B (apoB) were well below the sensitivity of the test used for their measurement and determined to be absent, while those of apoA1 were only moderately reduced.

Examination of a stool sample revealed steatorrhea (foul-smelling stool with high fat content). Stool was negative for fecal occult blood, leukocytes, ova, parasites, and cultures. An endoscopic procedure was performed. Macroscopically, the small intestine was atypically white/yellow in appearance. Microscopy of a biopsy specimen taken from the jejunum showed normal villous architecture, high fat content in epithelial cells visible on staining with Oil-Red O, and no evidence of inflammation, ulceration, or parasites. On reviewing the findings, a diagnosis of abetalipoproteinemia (ABL) was made, and the patient was treated accordingly.

DIAGNOSIS

Abetalipoproteinemia (ABL) is a rare, autosomal recessive disease first described by Bassen and Kornsweig in 1950. It is characterized by the absence of plasma apoB lipoproteins, fat-soluble vitamin deficiencies (A, E, and K), and the presence of acanthocytosis (Table 27-1). Other signs include fat malabsorption presenting as steatorrhea, flatus, abdominal discomfort, and progressive ataxic neuropathy. The key diagnostic feature is an extremely low plasma total cholesterol and absence of all apoB lipoproteins (chylomicrons, VLDL, and LDL).

Three disorders of lipoprotein metabolism share these characteristics: familial hypobetalipoproteinemia, chylomicron retention disease, and ABL (Table 27-2). The presence or absence of specific plasma apoB lipoproteins, as well as their mode of inheritance, can be useful when attempting to differentiate between these disorders. Symptoms associated with familial hypobetalipoproteinemia are usually milder than for the other two and are inherited as dominant traits, that is, symptoms are observed in at least one parent of an affected offspring. Chylomicron retention disease is an autosomal recessive disorder with a severe phenotype commonly presenting soon after birth. Plasma lipoprotein analysis from affected individuals shows a specific absence of chylomicrons (apoB48) but normal amounts of VLDL and LDL (apoB100). In our patient, evidence of recessive inheritance and absence of all apoB-containing lipoproteins implicates ABL as the most likely diagnosis.

Malabsorption, an early nonspecific clinical sign of ABL, is commonly encountered in many

Table 27-1. Abetalipoproteinemia

Signs and symptoms associated with
 abetalipoproteinemia
    Malabsorption syndrome (steatorrhea, diarrhea,
     flatus, failure to thrive)
    Spinocerebellar disease
     Ataxia, positive Romberg sign
     Decreased proprioception and vibratory senses
     Loss of deep tendon reflexes
    Night blindness

Laboratory and other diagnostic findings
    Low plasma cholesterol levels
    Absence of plasma apoB lipoproteins (chylomicrons,
     VLDL, and LDL)
    Fat-soluble vitamin (A, E, and K) deficiencies
    Pigmented retinopathy
    Acanthocytosis
    Normocytic anemia with compensatory
     reticulocytosis
    Decreased erythrocyte sedimentation rate
    Hepatic steatosis
    Gelee blanche intestine by endoscopic evaluation
    Histological presentations: normal villi, absence of
     inflammation, accumulation of neutral lipids

diseases of the gastrointestinal tract. It can be loosely defined as the intestine's inability to absorb lumenal contents (i.e., sugars, nutrients, fat, water, and/or carbohydrates). Presenting symptoms of malabsorption are abdominal discomfort and diarrhea. Some major causes of acute and chronic malabsorption are listed in Table 27-3.

In ABL, fat malabsorption is responsible for the diarrhea and flatus. Symptoms are prominent in affected newborns with the severity coupled to their lipid-rich diets. Chronic diarrhea results in nutrient wasting and, in some cases, failure to thrive. Since fat malabsorption is responsible for the initial gastrointestinal symptoms, it is not uncommon for affected individuals to restrict dietary fat independent of medical advice, alleviating the frequency of diarrhea and flatus. Occasional exacerbations still occur, but not serious enough to provoke a clinical visit. As a result, affected individuals often develop normally, unaware of their disease, until a gross secondary neuropathy becomes symptomatic toward the third decade of life or even earlier.

The patient described in the case report is a textbook example of this. His history suggests the presence of chronic malabsorption since birth and a self-discipline resulting in alleviation of gastrointestinal symptoms before his move

Table 27-2. Prominent Genetic Disorders with Decreased or Absent Plasma apoB Lipoproteins

Disease	Gene/Mode of Inheritance	Defective Assembly Step	Symptoms/ Diagnostic Features	Plasma Lipoproteins
Abetalipoproteinemia (ABL)	*mttp/* recessive	Biosynthesis of apoB lipoproteins particle	Fat malabsorption, fat-soluble vitamin deficiencies, spinocerebellar disease, retinitis pigmentosa, acanthocytosis, galee blanche intestine, fatty liver	Absence of all apoB lipoproteins (chylomicrons, VLDL, and LDL)
CMRD/Anderson disease	*sar1b/* recessive	Budding of vesicles containing nascent lipoproteins from ER of intestinal cells	Similar to ABL, absence of fatty liver, failure to thrive in infancy, no acanthocytosis	Absence of chylomicrons; VLDL and LDL present
CMRD-MSS	*sar1b/* recessive	Same as CMRD	Same as CMRD; also congenital cataracts, mental deficiency, and cerebellar atrophy	Similar to CMRD
Hypobetalipo-proteinemia	*apob/* dominant	Synthesis of apoB peptide	Presents only in a homozygous or complex heterozygous state with symptoms similar to ABL	Low to absent apoB lipoproteins

CMRD, chylomicron retention disease; CMRD-MSS, CMRD with Marinesco Sjogren syndrome.

to the United States. The likely reason for the reappearance in severity of diarrhea and overall discomfort was the introduction to a high-fat Western diet. This clearly demonstrates the importance of fat restriction in the treatment of ABL symptoms.

ABL is frequently misdiagnosed due to a multitude of nonspecific and unrelated symptoms, as well as rarity of the disease. An initial diagnosis of celiac disease, a more common malabsorptive disorder, is therefore frequently made. Celiac disease also presents as abdominal discomfort and diarrhea with frequent remissions and exacerbations. Its etiology is unknown, but there is a clear association with gliadin, a constituent of most grains, as well as an undefined immunological component. Symptoms of celiac disease often abate when the individual is placed on a gluten-free diet, whereas those associated with ABL do not, as this patient clearly demonstrated.

Endoscopic analysis and intestinal biopsies are useful to rule out other diseases of the intestine and to confirm ABL. In ABL, the intestinal lumen has a "gelee blanche" or white frothy appearance from massive accumulation of lipids within the mucosa, which persists even in the setting of a low-fat diet. On microscopic evaluation of a biopsy sample taken from this region, inflammation commonly observed in other malabsorption syndromes is usually ab-

sent, and villi have normal appearance. Inspection of individual cells shows distension with cytoplasmic lipid droplets that stain positive for neutral lipids (triglycerides and cholesterol esters). Variable-size droplets, which may or may not be surrounded by membranes, have been noted by electron microscopy (Berriot-Varoqueaux et al., 2000).

Neurological problems are also diagnostic features of ABL and are consequences of prolonged

Table 27-3. Causes of Diarrhea

Acute
  Bacterial, parasitic, and viral infections
  Food poisoning
  Medications (antibiotics, chemotherapy, laxatives, nonsteroidal anti-inflammatory drugs etc.)
  Ingestion of large amount of nonabsorbable sugar
  Intestinal ischemia

Chronic
  Irritable bowel syndrome
  Inflammatory bowel disease (i.e., Crohn's disease)
  Chronic infection
  Radiation enteritis
  Medications
  Local cancer/lymphoma
  Previous surgery (i.e., gastrectomy)
  Endocrine causes (diabetes, hypo- and hyperthyroidism, etc.)
  Malabsorption syndromes (i.e., celiac disease, abetalipoproteinemia, etc.)

vitamin E deficiency. The function of vitamin E in nervous tissue is largely undefined, but general consensus is that it plays an important antioxidant role preventing membrane lipid oxidation, especially of myelin. One of the first symptoms to present is the loss of deep tendon reflexes. Proprioception, vibratory senses, and development of an ataxic gait soon follow. A Romberg sign is usually present in older individuals as long-term untreated disease severely affects the dorsal columns. Paraethesias, in a stocking-and-glove distribution, may also be observed. Autopsy results from patients with ABL have revealed demyelination within the central and peripheral nervous systems with loss of large myelinated fibers (Sorbrevilla and Goodman, 1964). Electromyography reveals a slow conduction velocity in patients, again suggesting demyelination in ABL.

The spinocerebellar degenerative symptoms observed in ABL are often confused with Friedreich ataxia. Friedreich ataxia is also an autosomal recessive disease, but involves expansion of trinucleotide (GAA) repeats within the frataxin gene. Like ABL, presenting symptoms include progressive ataxia and loss of vibratory senses beginning around the second decade of life owing to ordered regression of large myelinated axons in the peripheral as well as central nervous systems. Friedreich ataxia, however, does not show malabsorption symptoms.

Plasma levels of vitamin A, and to a lesser extent vitamin K, are also below normal in ABL. Vitamin A deficiency presents as progressive night blindness. This could explain the bruises on the patient's thighs resulting from decreased visual acuity in the dark, and thus leading to excessive bumping into furniture. Individuals with chronic low levels may also complain of difficulty in driving at night. Pigmented retinopathy is also associated with vitamin A deficiency but is not specific to ABL.

Low levels of vitamin K cause hemostatic abnormalities and hemorrhage. A prolonged prothrombin time (PT) is a measurable evidence of this. PT is commonly elevated in liver diseases, anticoagulant therapies, inborn or acquired deficiencies in the clotting pathways, and severe vitamin K deficiency. In ABL, vitamin K deficiency symptoms are either generally mild or absent. Nonetheless, spontaneous gastrointestinal bleeding can occur in some individuals.

Other nonspecific findings in ABL include acanthocytosis and associated abnormalities resulting from it. Acanthocytosis is the appearance of dysmorphic, "starry-shaped" RBC on a smear. These peculiar looking cells are believed to result from decreased cholesterol content and abnormal cholesterol:phospholipid ratio in cell membranes. Acanthocytes are fragile and prone to increased destruction. A mild normocytic anemia (hematocrit < 38% and a normal mean corpuscular volume) with compensated reticulocytosis is indicative of this destruction. Acanthocytes also contribute to the decreased erythrocyte sedimentation rates observed in ABL. Normal RBC tend to aggregate under *in vitro* conditions, forming clusters referred to as rouleaux and sediment more quickly. Acanthocytes decrease the structured formation of rouleaux, in effect slowing the rate of erythrocyte sedimentation.

BIOCHEMICAL PERSPECTIVES

Lipoprotein Assembly and Microsomal Triglyceride Transfer Protein

Apolipoprotein B (apoB) is an essential structural component of triglyceride-rich lipoproteins. These apoB lipoproteins are responsible for plasma transport of lipids and fat-soluble vitamins, including triglycerides, phospholipids, and cholesterol esters, as well as vitamins A, E, and K (Hussain et al., 1996; Kane et al., 1995). A single *apob* gene is inherited from both parents; however, two tissue-specific, liver (apoB100) and intestine (apoB48), forms of the protein exist (Fig. 27-1). ApoB100 (100%, full-length single polypeptide of 4536 amino acids), expressed mainly in hepatocytes, is the essential structural component of VLDL, IDL, and LDL. In contrast, differentiated intestinal cells produce apoB48, a vital element of chylomicrons. Production of apoB48 is accomplished through the activity of an intestinal cell-specific nuclear cytosine deaminase, apobec-1. Apobec-1 deaminates deoxycytosine to deoxyuracil at position 6666 of the apoB mRNA, resulting in the generation of a stop codon (UAA) in place of the glutamine codon (CAA) present in apoB100 mRNA. The stop codon terminates apoB mRNA translation in the intestine, producing a stable and functional single polypeptide of 2152 amino acids, apoB48.

Translation of apoB mRNA initiates on free ribosomes in the cytoplasm. On production of an

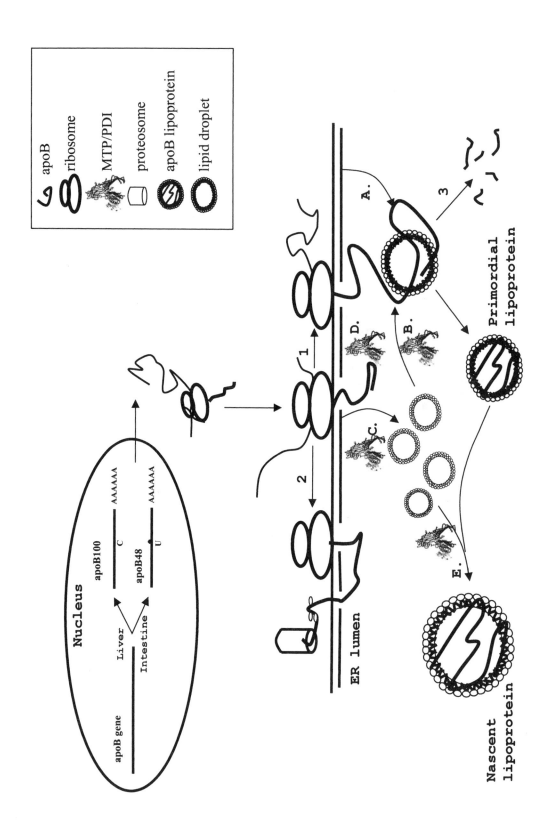

Nucleus

apoB gene

Liver → apoB100 — C — AAAAAA

Intestine → apoB48 — U — AAAAAA

apoB
ribosome
MTP/PDI
proteosome
apoB lipoprotein
lipid droplet

ER lumen

A.
B.
C.
D.
E.

Primordial lipoprotein

Nascent lipoprotein

1
2
3

Figure 27-1. Schematic diagram of apoB lipoprotein assembly. In the nucleus, the apoB gene is transcribed into a 15-kb mRNA. In the intestine, this mRNA undergoes posttranscriptional editing, resulting in deamination of cytosine$_{6666}$ to uracil, converting a glutamine codon into a stop codon. In the liver, no such editing occurs. The apoB mRNA is transported from the nucleus to cytosol, where its N-terminal signal sequence is translated. On the binding of the signal sequence to the signal recognition particle, the translation of the mRNA is stalled, and the complex is translocated to the ER. After binding to the ER membrane, translation of the apoB mRNA resumes. Complete translation of apoB mRNA results in the synthesis of apoB48 and apoB100 in intestine and liver, respectively. The newly translated apoB can either be used for lipoprotein assembly (1) or be degraded (2) by endoplasmic reticulum-associated degradation (ERAD) involving proteosomes. Microsomal triglyceride transfer protein (MTP) plays a critical role in the lipoprotein assembly (1) by different mechanisms: (A) MTP can transfer lipids either from membrane to the nascent apoB, forming a primordial lipoprotein. (B) MTP can transfer lipids from lipid droplets to nascent apoB. (C) MTP can import triglycerides into the ER lumen that can be used for lipoprotein assembly or lipid droplet formation. (D) MTP can interact with the nascent apoB and help in early folding and lipidation of the molecule leading to the synthesis of a primordial lipoprotein particle. (E) MTP may facilitate the fusion of lipid droplets and the primordial lipoprotein resulting in the synthesis of a nascent lipoprotein. Incompletely assembled apoB lipoproteins are degraded in the ER (3) by mechanisms other than ERAD. PDI, protein disulfide isomerase.

N-terminal ER signal sequence, the complex is escorted to the rough ER by cytoplasmic chaperones, where protein synthesis continues. Proper folding, disulfide bond formation, and acquisition of lipids (phospholipids, triglycerides, and cholesterol) accompany cotranslational translocation of the growing peptide into the lumen. Defects in any of these events lead to degradation of the nascent apoB polypeptide. Since apoB mRNA is constitutively produced, degradation of the nascent peptide significantly influences lipoprotein assembly and secretion. ApoB lipoprotein assembly begins with an initial highly dense "primordial lipoprotein" and culminates with a larger "nascent lipoprotein" particle (Hussain et al., 2003). Quality control processes monitoring apoB lipoprotein assembly are extremely efficient. Secretion is only allowed to occur upon apoB obtaining an appropriately folded structure and sufficient lipid content.

In ABL, an early step in apoB lipoprotein assembly shared by intestinal and liver cells is defective. The net result is near absence of all plasma apoB lipoproteins. ApoB synthesis from a mRNA transcript occurs, but its successful assembly into the mature lipoprotein particle does not. The inability to assemble apoB into lipoproteins was shown to be due to a defect in the *mttp* gene in affected individuals (Wetterau et al., 1992). Its translational product is an 894-amino acid, 97-kd, polypeptide that exists in the ER complexed with a 55-kd protein disulfide isomerase which is believed to maintain solubility, physiologic activity, and ER retention of the 97-kd peptide. The heterodimeric complex of the 97-kd and 55-kd subunits is referred to as microsomal triglyceride transfer protein (MTP) (Wetterau et al., 1992).

Several functions of MTP have been identified; all have been implicated in coordinating successful lipoprotein assembly (Fig. 27-1). MTP transfers lipids between vesicles *in vitro*, and this activity is likely to be its major function. MTP can pick up lipids from membrane (step A) or vesicles and droplets (step B) and transfer them to the nascent apoB. In addition, the lipid transfer activity of MTP has been implicated in the accretion of neutral lipids from the cytosol into the ER lumen (step C). Compounds that inhibit *in vitro* transfer activity of MTP decrease apoB secretion by cells, indicating that this activity is essential for apoB lipoprotein secretion. Apart from transferring lipids, MTP has been shown to interact physically with apoB (step D). This activity

also appears important since inhibition of MTP-apoB binding results in decreased apoB secretion. Last, MTP can also associate with lipid droplets in the ER and may stabilize these particles. It may also help in the fusion (step E) of lipid droplets and primordial lipoproteins, resulting in the formation of nascent, triglyceride-rich lipoproteins (Hussain et al., 2003).

Biochemical Explanation for Symptoms

Chronic malabsorption does not fully explain the different extents of fat-soluble vitamin deficiencies associated with ABL. More specifically, why are plasma vitamin E levels more severely affected than those of vitamins A or K? The answer for this can be traced to apoB lipoprotein biosynthesis and catabolism (Fig. 27-2). Just as observed for lipids, hydrophobic, fat-soluble vitamins require apoB lipoproteins as vehicles for plasma transport. The reliance of each fat-soluble vitamin on apoB lipoproteins varies, and this variable dependency is directly related to the severity of symptoms observed in ABL.

Vitamin E, like neutral lipids, requires apoB lipoproteins at every stage of its transport (Fig. 27-2). Dietary vitamin E becomes emulsified in micelles produced during the digestive phase of lipid absorption and permeates the intestinal epithelium, similar to fatty acids and cholesterol. Uptake of vitamin E by enterocytes appears to be concentration dependent. Within intestinal cells, vitamin E is packaged into chylomicrons and secreted into lymph. During blood circulation of chylomicrons, some vitamin E may be released to the tissues as a consequence of partial lipolysis of these particles by endothelial cell-anchored lipoprotein lipase. The rest remains associated with chylomicron remnants. Remnant particles are mainly endocytosed by the liver and degraded, resulting in the release of fat-soluble vitamins.

In hepatocytes, vitamin E can take two routes. A fraction of it is packaged as VLDL and reenters the circulation, while excess is excreted in the bile. Plasma lipolysis of the VLDL particle again results in release not only of lipids, but also of vitamin E, with the remainder left with the LDL particles. This fraction can be further distributed to tissues via LDL receptor-mediated endocytosis or transferred between lipoproteins, mainly to HDL, by plasma lipid transfer proteins. Thus, mobilization of vitamin E from intestinal and liver

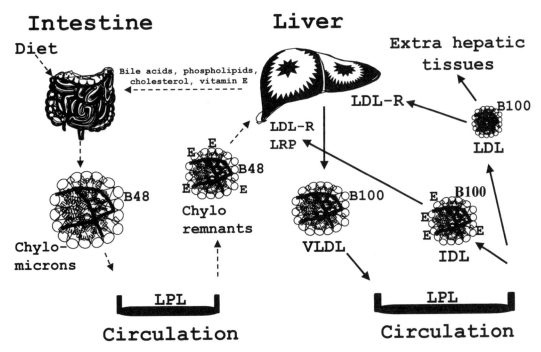

Figure 27-2. An overview of lipoprotein metabolism. Intestine and liver are two major organs that play crucial roles in transporting dietary and endogenous lipids. *Intestine* (dashed lines): Dietary triglycerides, phospholipids, and cholesterol esters are hydrolyzed in the lumen of the intestine and are absorbed by enterocytes. In the intestinal cells, fat is resynthesized and assembled into particles referred to as chylomicrons. During lipoprotein assembly, fat-soluble vitamins are also incorporated into these particles. Assembly of these particles requires apoB48 and microsomal triglyceride transfer protein (MTP). In the circulation, chylomicorns are hydrolyzed by endothelial cell-bound lipoprotein lipase (LPL), and adjacent cells take up the released free fatty acids. The lipoproteins left after hydrolysis, called chylomicron (chylo) remnants, contain significant amounts of dietary lipids and fat-soluble vitamins. These particles acquire apoE (E) from plasma, which is a high affinity ligand for LDL receptors (LDL-R) and LDL receptor-related protein (LRP). Recognition of apoE by these receptors results in the internalization and degradation of lipoprotein particles. *Liver* (solid lines): In hepatocytes, lipids are resynthesized and packaged into lipoproteins called very low density lipoproteins (VLDL). The VLDL contain apoB100, lipids, and vitamin E. In the circulation, these particles are also hydrolyzed by the endothelial cell-bound lipoprotein lipase-generating intermediate-density lipoproteins (IDL) and low-density lipoproteins (LDL). IDL acquire apoE, similar to chylomicron remnants, and are cleared rapidly from plasma by receptor-mediated endocytosis. LDL do not acquire apoE; however, apoB100 present in these particles is recognized by LDL receptors expressed in liver and other peripheral tissues. Since apoB100 has a lower affinity for the receptor than does apoE, LDL are removed slowly with a plasma half-life of about 24 h.

cells is critically dependent on apoB lipoprotein assembly and secretion.

Uptake of vitamin A by intestinal cells is carrier mediated at low concentrations. If higher amounts are present, then it enters intestinal cells via diffusion. Like vitamin E, it also exploits chylomicrons as a vehicle to exit the enterocytes and reaches the liver as a component of the remnant particles. In the liver, the metabolisms of vitamin A and vitamin E diverge. Here, unlike vitamin E and triglycerides, vitamin A is either stored in Ito cells or secreted bound to retinol-binding protein for plasma transport and further tissue distribution.

The ultimate dependence of vitamin E for transport by liver and intestinal cells via apoB lipoproteins may explain the severe vitamin E deficiency observed in ABL. In contrast, apoB lipoprotein assembly is required only for the mobilization of dietary vitamin A by the intestinal cells; liver distributes the endogenous vitamin A to other tissues by retinol-binding protein. Unlike vitamins E and A, dietary vitamin K may only partially depend on apoB lipoproteins for its transport across the intestinal epithelial cells and tissue targeting and may explain why bleeding diathesis is rarely observed in ABL.

THERAPY

Presently, ABL is not a curable disease, but the associated morbidity and premature death are preventable. Thus, early diagnosis and treatment are essential to avoid secondary neurological and ophthalmic pathologies and to provide an opportunity of a normal life for affected individuals. Initiation of treatment, after delayed diagnosis and symptomatic development, can prevent further progression of symptoms.

To treat the malabsorption and subsequent diarrhea, lipid-poor diets (<5 g/day) should be implemented with a restriction of triglycerides containing long-chain fatty acids. Medium-chain fatty acids rely on other protein carriers besides apoB (i.e., albumin) for plasma transport, making them an ideal lipid substitute. However, long-term supplementation should be cautioned as associated hepatic fibrosis could occur. Diets should also contain increased protein and carbohydrate content to compensate for caloric loss from fat restriction.

Most of the neurological pathologies are preventable even in the setting of chronic malabsorption associated with ABL. Lifelong supplementation is required to treat vitamin deficiencies, especially that of vitamin E. Oral routes are effective. However, large doses are required to overcome the inefficiency of alternate transport pathways (e.g., albumin and HDL). Prescription of large doses of vitamin E (100–300 mg/kg/day) results in only a moderate increase in plasma levels (<50% of the normal range), yet this appears sufficient to prevent development and progression of the associated symptoms.

Vitamin A should be supplemented at 5000 IU/day by the oral route with routine blood work to monitor plasma levels. Toxicity due to excess vitamin A is not common but is potentially fatal. Acute toxicity presents as vertigo, diplopia, seizures, and exfoliative dermatitis. Chronic toxicity manifests very differently (i.e., dry skin, alopecia, amenorrhea, symptoms of liver fibrosis, etc.). It is imperative to monitor plasma vitamin A levels regularly, especially in the setting of the large doses required to treat ABL.

Since vitamin K deficiency varies among patients, not all will require supplementation. When it is needed, the recommended oral dose is 1–2 mg/day. Toxicity from dietary vitamin K has not been described in adults, but a parenteral dose may cause hemolytic anemia in infants; therefore, caution should be taken when administered to such patients.

In summary, ABL is a rare, often-misdiagnosed disease, presenting initially as severe fat malabsorption and later with predominantly neurological sequelae. The symptoms and findings are nonspecific except for the complete absence of plasma apoB lipoproteins and below normal plasma total cholesterol. Before widespread use of cholesterol screening, this treatable disease was easily overlooked or misdiagnosed. Treatment includes dietary restriction of long-chain fatty acids as well as lifelong supplementation of vitamins A, E, and K.

QUESTIONS

1. Why do abetalipoproteinemia (ABL), chylomicron retention disease, and homozygous hypobetalipoproteinemia present so similarly? How would one differentiate between them?
2. Acanthocytosis is associated with ABL, but not with chylomicron retention disease. Explain.
3. Hypobetalipoproteinemia presents clinically only in the homozygous state. Why does it sometimes present similar to ABL with absent plasma apoB lipoproteins and at other times as a much milder phenotype?
4. Of the fat-soluble vitamins (A, D, E, and K), only vitamin D deficiency is not associated with ABL and is not a required supplement. Why?
5. Why has the use of MTP lipid transfer activity inhibitors been unsuccessful as

a treatment for hypercholesterolemia? (Hint: think of possible adverse affects *in vivo*.)

6. A nonfunctional MTP gene/protein causes ABL. What are the possible affects on lipid levels and cardiovascular pathology if this protein is overexpressed?

Acknowledgment: National Institutes of Health grants DK46900 and HL64272 partially supported this work.

BIBLIOGRAPHY

Bassen FA, Kornzweig AL: Malformation of the erythrocytes in a case of atypical retinitis pigmentosa. *Blood* **5:**381–387, 1950.

Berriot-Varoqueaux N, Aggerbeck LP, et al.: The role of the microsomal triglyceride transfer protein in abetalipoproteinemia. *Annu Rev Nut.* **20:**663–697, 2000.

Chan L, Chang HJ, Nakamuta M, et al.: Apobec-1 and apolipoprotein B mRNA editing. *Biochim Biophys Acta* **1345:**11–26, 1997.

Hussain MM, Kancha RK, Zhou Z, et al.: Chylomicron assembly and catabolism: role of apolipoproteins and receptors. *Biochim Biophys Acta* **1300:**151–170, 1996.

Hussain MM, Shi J, Dreizen P: Microsomal triglyceride transfer protein and its role in apoB-lipoprotein assembly. *J Lipid Res* **44:**22–32, 2003.

Kane JP, Havel RJ: Disorders of the biogenesis and secretion of lipoproteins containing the B apolipoproteins, *in* Scriver CR, Beaudet AL, Sly WS, Valle D (eds): *The Metabolic and Molecular Basis of Inherited Diseases.* McGraw-Hill, New York, 1995, pp. 1853–1886.

Sorbrevilla LA, Goodman ML: Demyelinating CNS disease, macular atrophy and acanthocytosis (Bassen-Kornzweig syndrome). *Am J Med* **37:** 821–832, 1964.

Wetterau JR, Aggerbeck LP, Bouma M, et al.: Absence of microsomal triglyceride transfer protein in individuals with abetalipoproteinemia. *Science* **258:**999–1001, 1992.

28

Vitamin B₁₂ Deficiency

DOROTHY J. VANDERJAGT and DENIS M. McCARTHY

CASE REPORT

The patient, an 84-year-old male resident of a veteran's home, was admitted to the hospital following a fall in which he had sustained a fracture of his left radius and several lacerations. Physical examination on admission revealed a well-nourished elderly male in no great distress (body mass index (BMI), 22.5 kg/m²). He was moderately confused but with prompting was oriented to time, place, and person. There was no obvious pallor, cyanosis, or jaundice, and his skin and mucous membranes were unremarkable apart from the injuries he sustained in the fall. His right lower extremity was swollen and tender, and he walked cautiously and with a pronounced limp.

His blood pressure was 145/85 mm Hg (normal is 120/80 mm Hg). His pulse rate was 80 beats per minute (normal is 75 beats per minute), and his respiratory rate was 16 per minute (normal is 12-14 per minute). His temperature was 98.2°F (normal is 98.4°F). Except for a soft systolic ejection murmur in the neck and in the left parasternal area, his cardiovascular, respiratory, abdominal, and genitourinary systems were all normal. The neurological examination was normal except for impaired cognitive function, a positive Romberg sign, and equivocal plantar responses. (A patient is considered to have a positive Romberg sign when, in a standing position, the patient is more unsteady with eyes closed than with eyes open. This indicates a loss of proprioceptive control.) There were no signs of head injury.

The director of the veteran's home stated that the patient's memory had been gradually failing over the past 2 years. His balance had also become mildly impaired, which resulted in the fall and associated injuries. His medical history revealed that the patient had been a heavy smoker, but he stopped smoking 20 years ago. It also revealed that he had suffered from numerous recurrences of a duodenal ulcer that was managed with diet, antacids, and H₂ receptor antagonist drugs. However, he has had no recurrences of ulcer symptoms since age 70 years.

Laboratory investigations yielded the following results: hemoglobin 148 g/L (normal is 140-180 g/L); hematocrit 45% (normal 42% is 52%); mean corpuscular volume 98 fL (normal is 80-100 fL); red cell distribution width 14% (normal is 11%-13 %); reticulocytes 1% (normal is 0.5%-1.5%); white blood cell count 7.8 × 10³/mm³ (normal is 4-8 × 10³/mm³) with a normal differential count; platelets 230 × 10³/mm³ (normal is 140-460 × 10³/mm³); prothrombin time 12 s (normal or control is 11.9-14.8 s). The following analytes were all within the normal range: blood urea nitrogen (BUN), creatinine, electrolytes, calcium, phosphorus, magnesium, glucose, TSH, total protein, albumin, lactate dehydrogenase (LDH), and liver function markers, including alkaline phosphatase. Serum iron and folate concentrations were also within the normal range; serum cobalamin (vitamin B₁₂) was 230 pg/mL, at the lower end of the normal range (normal is 200-850 pg/mL). Holotranscobalamin II (holo-TCII) was undetectable. The low normal serum vitamin B₁₂ and undetectable holo-TCII indicated deficient intake of vitamin B₁₂. However, serum 25-hydroxyvitamin D, vitamin C, carotene, and trace minerals were all within normal limits.

Chest x-ray showed mild unfolding of the aortic arch and scattered calcifications in the area of the aortic valve. There was no change in cardiac size. To exclude the presence of subdural hematoma, a CT of the head was obtained but showed no focal abnormalities. However, there was mild diffuse bilateral cortical atrophy, especially in the frontal areas.

On the day of admission, the patient had developed a deep venous thrombosis in his right calf, a site not involved in the injury. In investigating the underlying cause of the deep venous thrombosis, serum homocysteine was measured and found to be 17.4 μmol/L (normal is < 14 μmol/L). To distinguish between folic acid and vitamin B_{12} deficiencies, a serum methylmalonic acid (MMA) assay was performed; it yielded a result of 0.59 μmol/L MMA (normal is < 0.30 μmol/L). This confirmed the presence of vitamin B_{12} deficiency, despite a serum B_{12} concentration that was within the normal range.

DIAGNOSIS

Most often, the classical vitamin B_{12}-deficient patient is an elderly subject who presents with insidious onset of nonspecific symptoms of anemia (e.g., lack of energy, easy fatigability, deterioration in work ability). If the anemia is severe, then cardiovascular symptoms such as dyspnea on exertion may also be evident. Depending on the etiology of the condition, other signs of malnutrition or some other underlying disease (e.g., Crohn's disease) may also be present. At this late stage of the disease (now rarely seen), neurological symptoms predominate, notably paresthesias such as "tingling," "pins and needles," "numbness," and other sensory loss manifesting as a "glove-and-stocking" distribution involving fingers and toes. These symptoms usually start in the lower limbs. Physical examination reveals marked pallor, with a pale lemon yellowish tint to the skin, conjunctivae, and mucous membranes. The tongue is painful, atrophic, and pale, but only rarely ulcerated. Neurologically, there may be loss of vibration sense, diminished reflexes (especially in the ankles), and a positive Romberg sign or other evidence of involvement of the posterior or lateral columns of the spinal cord.

In pernicious anemia (PA), the urine contains excess urobilinogen, and gastric analysis reveals histamine-fast achlorhydria. Laboratory examination reveals a low serum B_{12} (usually under 200 μg/mL) and the presence of a severe macrocytic anemia in the peripheral blood, with a high mean corpuscular volume (MCV, usually 110–125 fL) and a blood smear showing anisocytosis, poikilocytosis, a few nucleated red cells, normoblasts, rarely even megaloblasts, and few or no reticulocytes. There is also leukopenia involving granulocytes, and the polymorphs present are mature and hypersegmented and show 3–7 nuclei per cell; platelets are moderately reduced (Fig. 28-1). When the cause of the vitamin B_{12} deficiency is classical PA, the patient's serum may also contain antibodies directed against parietal cells or intrinsic factor (IF). Such patients may also show serological or clinical features of a variety of other autoimmune diseases such as type 1 diabetes, hypothyroidism, primary biliary cirrhosis, hypoadrenalism, or myasthenia gravis.

Over the past 50 years, the presentation of vitamin B_{12} deficiency has changed considerably, at least in developed countries, where megaloblastic anemia has become less common and is usually detected and treated before these relatively late hematological and neurological features develop. It is widely accepted that neurological and psychiatric features can develop in the absence of anemia (Lindenbaum et al., 1988), especially in patients receiving folate supplements, and can be accompanied by serum vitamin B_{12} concentrations within normal limits, albeit at the low end of the normal range. At the other end of the socioeconomic scale, in areas where malnutrition is widespread, there is mounting concern about the need for vitamin B_{12} supplements, at least in vulnerable groups (e.g., young pregnant women, infants, and the elderly). As recently as 1992, an outbreak of myeloneuropathy in Cuba due to dietary vitamin B_{12} deficiency involved more than 50,000 patients (Roman, 1994).

In North America and the United Kingdom, there is growing concern that many elderly subjects with mild or no anemia and normal serum B_{12} concentrations are suffering from preventable and correctable vitamin B_{12} deficiency disease. Today, in economically advanced countries, as many as 75% of vitamin B_{12}-deficient patients present with various neurological symptoms, including somatic and autonomic neuropathies, myelopathies, cortical atrophy, and dementia (Carranza, 2002). In addition, vitamin B_{12}-depleted subjects may develop postoperative myeloneuropathy when exposed to anesthesia

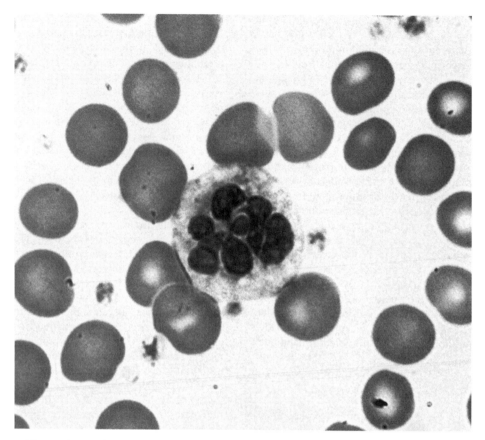

Figure 28-1. Characteristic features of vitamin B_{12} or folate deficiency in the peripheral blood include larger-than-normal mature red blood cells (oval macrocytes with an elevated mean corpuscular volume) and large hypersegmented neutrophils (1 neutrophil with six nuclear lobes or more than 5% neutrophils with five nuclear lobes). These characteristics are associated with megaloblastic changes in the bone marrow and are the result of fewer cell divisions due to impaired DNA synthesis.

with nitrous oxide (Metz, 1992). In the absence of screening tests, many individuals institutionalized for senile dementia or Alzheimer disease may actually have treatable vitamin B_{12} deficiency (Carranza, 2002). The reversibility of such neuropsychiatric illnesses following vitamin B_{12} therapy is still under debate; it is clear that reversibility deteriorates with delay in instituting therapy. Because screening is not readily available and testing is expensive, most geriatricians in the United States today simply prescribe monthly or 3-monthly injections or oral dietary supplements of vitamin B_{12} for all patients over age 65 years.

Vitamin B_{12} status is usually determined by measuring vitamin B_{12} concentrations in serum by competitive protein-binding radioimmunoassay. In such an assay, the vitamin B_{12} in the patient's serum and the unlabeled B_{12} in the standard compete with the radioactive tracer (^{57}Co) for binding sites on purified intrinsic factor (binding protein). Because of the relationship between folate and vitamin B_{12} metabolism, folate and vitamin B_{12} should both be assayed simultaneously in the patient's serum using radioactive tracers and binding proteins specific for each vitamin. Normal values for serum vitamin B_{12} are 200–835 pg/mL (148–616 pmol/L). However, low or normal serum vitamin B_{12} concentrations may be present in clinically apparent vitamin B_{12} deficiency.

Direct assays for vitamin B_{12}, such as the competitive protein-binding immunoassays, detect all forms of vitamin B_{12} in the serum, including physiologically inactive analogues. The vitamin B_{12} bound to transcobalamin II (TCII) has been shown to be the physiologically relevant pool of vitamin B$_{12}$, and a decrease in holo-TCII concentrations is one of the early signs of deficient intake of vitamin B$_{12}$ (Herzlich and Herbert, 1988). Methods have been developed to measure holotranscobalamin (Nexo et al., 2002). (Holotranscobalamin refers to transcobalamin that has B$_{12}$ bound to it.) The expected concentration range of holo-TCII in healthy adults is between 40 and 150 pmol/L.

Indirect indicators of vitamin B$_{12}$ deficiency include measurements of the metabolites homocysteine and methylmalonic acid (MMA) in serum and MMA in urine (see the Biochemical Perspectives section). Whereas the serum homocysteine concentration increases during folate or vitamin B$_{12}$ deficiencies, the serum and urine MMA concentrations increase only in vitamin B$_{12}$ deficiency. Therefore, MMA determinations can be used to differentiate vitamin B$_{12}$ deficiency from folate deficiency. The normal concentration of MMA in serum ranges from 0.08 to 0.28 µmol/L. MMA is quantified using gas-liquid chromatography and mass spectrometry. Elevated concentrations of MMA and homocysteine in serum may precede the development of hematological abnormalities and reductions in serum vitamin B$_{12}$ concentrations. One should be aware that other conditions, including renal in sufficiency and inborn errors of metabolism, can also result in elevated serum levels of MMA.

BIOCHEMICAL PERSPECTIVES

A severe anemia now known to be due to vitamin B$_{12}$ deficiency was first described in 1855 by the English physician Thomas Addison. Shortly thereafter, it was discovered that this anemia was linked to severe macroscopic and microscopic atrophy of the gastric mucosa. Because of its usually fatal outcome, the condition was named *pernicious anemia* (PA) in 1872 by the German physician Anton Biermer. Addisonian pernicious anemia was the subject of the first definitive description of the disease by Gardner and Osler in 1877, who pioneered the use of microscopy to describe the unique appearance of strange, large, nucleated red blood cells (*macro-ovalocytes*) in the peripheral blood. These patients had mild jaundice (a lemon-yellow color to their skin), severe peripheral neuropathy, and progression to death within 1 year from the time of onset of neurol-

gical complications and anemia. In 1880, Ehrlich coined the descriptor *megaloblastic* for the appearance of the circulating blood cells; however, another half century passed before it was discovered that feeding patients large amounts of animal liver was curative.

This observation led to the discovery that a dietary compound (extrinsic factor) was absorbed only after combination with a protein secreted by the normal stomach (intrinsic factor [IF]), and that the IF was missing from the secretions of the atrophic stomach found in patients with PA. The extrinsic factor, later named vitamin B$_{12}$, was obtained in crystalline form in 1948, and its structure was defined by x-ray crystallography by Dorothy Hodgkins, an accomplishment for which she received the Nobel Prize for Chemistry in 1964.

Over the next 20 years, it was learned that the gastric mucosal and glandular atrophy were principally due to an autoimmune gastritis accompanied by circulating antibodies directed against parietal cells, IF, and other antigens. These antibodies damaged the patient's mucosa and abolished the secretion of hydrochloric acid and IF, both of which were believed to originate from parietal cells in humans. Thus, in some definitions, the use of the term *pernicious anemia* is restricted to those cases of vitamin B$_{12}$ deficiency anemia caused by absent secretion of IF as a result of autoimmune gastropathy.

Other causes of gastric atrophy, such as those due to *Helicobacter pylori*, AIDS, or radiation injury, can lead to a similar outcome but from different pathogenic mechanisms. Therefore, vitamin B$_{12}$ deficiency, resulting in neurological, psychiatric, metabolic, and hematological disorders, can arise from any one of the many causes listed in Table 28-1. For this reason, the term pernicious anemia (PA) is used here to describe only the classical disease that is associated with IF deficiency due to autoimmune gastritis.

Some authors use the term *adult onset pernicious anemia* to distinguish this condition from rare disorder subdivisions of "pernicious anemia" due to congenital defects in IF secretion or structure or to various types of enterocyte cobalamin malabsorption. In all other situations, the term vitamin B$_{12}$ deficiency is used, and an associated anemia, if consequent on it, is called megaloblastic anemia, bearing in mind that identical appearances of the peripheral blood and the bone marrow may be

Table 28-1. Differential Diagnosis of the Causes of Vitamin B_{12} Deficiency

1. Dietary deficiency of vitamin B_{12}
   Vegetarian diets, especially in vegans
   Prolonged severe malnutrition

2. Gastric disorders involving intrinsic factor
   Autoimmune Addisonian pernicious anemia (major)
   Severe gastric atrophy due to *Helicobacter pylori* infection
   Congenital abnormalities of intrinsic factor
   Total gastrectomy

3. Inadequate gastric release of food-bound vitamin B_{12}
   Atrophic gastritis with achlorhydria/deficient proteases (*H. pylori* [major], AIDS and other causes)
   Partial gastrectomy, gastroenterostomy
   Sustained hypochlorhydria due to drugs (proton pump inhibitors, high dose H_2-receptor antagonists)*

4. Impaired degradation of R-proteins in intestine
   Pancreatic enzyme deficiency*
   Zollinger-Ellison syndrome*

5. Competition for vitamin B_{12} with host
   Bacterial overgrowth syndromes in various diseases (diabetes,* scleroderma, jejunal diverticulosis, blind loops)
   Tape worms (*Diphyllobothrium latum*)

6. Absent or diseased ileal mucosa
   Resection of at least 3 feet of terminal ileum for any reason
   ileal bypass operations, ileal loop bladders
   Diseases of ileal mucosa (Crohn's or Bechet's disease, TB, actinomycosis, lymphoma, ulcerative ileo-jejunitis [due to
      sprue], radiation enteritis, HIV enteropathy, *Yersinia* enteritis)

7. Impaired translocation of vitamin B_{12} or vitamin B_{12}–F complex
   Absent ileal IF receptor
   Transcobalamin II deficiency
   Imerslund-Grasbeck syndrome
   Metformin therapy,* possibly colchicine*

*Although these have been linked to malabsorption of B_{12} (e.g., cause abnormal Schilling tests), they have not been associated with megaloblastic anemia or neuropsychiatric diseases. Intrinsic factor is normally secreted in amounts greatly in excess of normal requirements, so that so that a 90% reduction in intrinsic factor secretion may be of little or no consequence.
IF, intrinsic factor.

observed in patients deficient in folic acid, as described below.

The prevalence and impact of vitamin B_{12} deficiency vary in different groups, races, and geographic areas (Stabler and Allen, 2004). In North America, true autoimmune PA is uncommon, far less common than vitamin B_{12} deficiency as a whole, especially in the elderly population. Older studies, mainly from Scandinavia, indicated a prevalence of PA in the population of 0.1%–0.2%, but a study of people over 60 years of age in Los Angeles found 2.3% of subjects affected, of whom most (1.9%) were undiagnosed (Carmel, 1996). The prevalence of undiagnosed PA was 2.7% in women and 1.4% in men; the rates were 4.3% in black women, 4.0% in white women, but lower in women of other races. These figures refer to patients who had characteristic antibody profiles and whose disorder corrected with administration of IF. Vitamin B_{12} deficiency *per se* was not assessed (Carmel, 1996). Other studies in subjects over

60 years of age also suggest a prevalence of PA of 1%–3% (Stopeck, 2000).

However, there has been a growing awareness that gastric atrophy from *H. pylori* infection, particularly when there is long-term use of proton pump inhibitors (PPIs) in infected patients and the organism has not been eliminated, are causing much of the problem. Reports suggested that about 15% of over 40 million elderly people living in the United States have metabolic or clinical evidence of vitamin B_{12} deficiency, and the number of elderly at risk is projected to grow to 65 million by the year 2050 (Dharmarajan and Norkus, 2005), a number much higher than the currently estimated 800,000 cases of PA in the United States (Carmel, 1996).

Among the remaining cases of B_{12} deficiency, food-cobalamin malabsorption due to achlorhydria or hypochlorhydria caused by *H. pylori* gastritis, even in the absence of atrophy or the widespread use of proton pump inhibitors or

H$_2$ receptor antagonists for various acid peptic disorders, accounts for much of the clinical and subclinical deficiency. Such individuals usually have sufficient IF to absorb low doses of aqueous vitamin B$_{12}$. Malabsorption of vitamin B$_{12}$ in subjects with *H. pylori* gastritis reverses with eradication of the infection without therapeutic administration of B$_{12}$ (Avcu et al., 2001; Kaptan et al., 2000), as does the malabsorption associated with abnormal bacterial colonization of the stomach or small intestine. Nevertheless, there are numerous current investigations examining whether *H. pylori*, through mechanisms of molecular mimicry or through the perpetuation of autoimmune gastritis, may also play some part in the genesis of classical PA.

Lacking large, prospective national studies that screen for inadequate vitamin B$_{12}$ intake with serum holo-TCII assays and for subclinical or clinical disease using either urinary or serum assays of MMA, the true magnitude of vitamin B$_{12}$ deficiency remains unknown. It is clear that screening based on serum vitamin B$_{12}$ measurement is inadequate to the task of detecting neurological and psychiatric disease, and unknown numbers of cases with reversible neuropathy, cognitive impairment, and dementia are being left untreated or undetected until it is too late for successful therapy. Screening defined populations for vasculotoxic and neurotoxic concentrations of homocysteine in serum raises a number of additional issues, some of which also involve deficiencies of folic acid. Vitamin B$_{12}$ deficiency in the U.S. population is further complicated by U.S. Food and Drug Administration regulations that mandate folate fortification of the diet and, by preventing megaloblastic anemia, mask or exacerbate B$_{12}$ deficiency states other than anemia. Similar issues arise in other countries where malnutrition is common, affecting particularly pregnant women and children; where meat is scarce; and where there are large populations of vegetarians or subjects consuming parasite-infested fish.

The term *vitamin B$_{12}$ (cobalamin)* is used to describe a family of compounds that contain a planar corrin ring with a single cobalt atom at the center. The structure of vitamin B$_{12}$ is shown in Figure 28-2. The corrin ring system, which resembles the porphyrin rings of heme, is composed of four reduced pyrrole rings linked by three methylene bridges and a single saturated bond between rings 3 and 4. The cobalt atom is coordinated to each of the nitrogen atoms of the four pyrrole rings, a dimethyl-

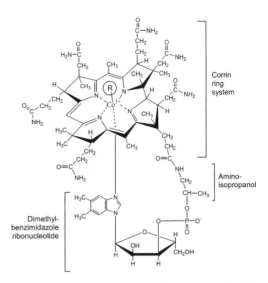

Figure 28-2. The structure of vitamin B$_{12}$ (cobalamin). Vitamin B$_{12}$ is composed of a planar corrin ring containing a cobalt atom at the center. The corrin ring system is composed of four pyrrole rings and is similar to porphyrin in heme. The cobalt atom is coordinated to the nitrogens of each pyrrole ring and to a dimethylbenzimidazole group. The R group attached to the sixth coordination site of the cobalt atom in vitamin B$_{12}$ can be a –CN, –OH, –CH$_3$, or adenosyl group.

benzimidazole group, and a sixth ligand, which may be a cyanide, hydroxyl, methyl, or adenosyl moiety.

The vitamin B$_{12}$ that occurs in nature is produced almost entirely by bacterial synthesis in animals but not in humans (Battersby, 1994). The richest dietary sources of vitamin B$_{12}$ are organ meats, such as liver and kidney. Lesser amounts are present in shellfish, chicken, fish, muscle meats, and dairy products (the principal source in lacto-vegetarians). Plants contain no vitamin B$_{12}$ unless they are contaminated by bacteria, and foods that contain microorganisms often provide the only source of vitamin B$_{12}$ for strict vegetarians, such as the vegans of southern India.

The ligand attached to the cobalt atom determines the activity of vitamin B$_{12}$ in human enzymatic reactions. The two active coenzyme forms are methyl-cobalamin and 5'-adenosylcobalamin, the primary form of vitamin B$_{12}$ in tissues. Cyanocobalamin, the therapeutic form of vitamin B$_{12}$ contained in vitamin supplements, is produced by the cleavage of the unstable link between the 5'-deoxyadenosyl group and the cobalt ion in adenosylcobalamin that occurs during its isolation from liver. The adenosyl group is replaced by a molecule of cyanide that is leached from the charcoal columns used in the purification procedure. Cyanocobalamin, which is not physiologically active, is readily hydrolyzed in tissues to hydroxycobalamin. Hydroxycobalamin is converted in the body to adenosylcobalamin by successive reactions involving two flavoprotein-dependent reductases, which reduce Co^{3+} sequentially to Co^{1+}. Co^{1+}, a powerful nucleophile, then attacks the 5'-carbon of ATP, expelling a triphosphate anion and resulting in the synthesis of 5'-adenosylcobalamin.

In the diet, vitamin B_{12} is bound to proteins. Although some release of protein-bound vitamin B_{12} begins in the mouth, most of the release occurs in the stomach on exposure of food to gastric acid (HCl) and the proteolytic enzyme pepsin. For this reason, either hypochlorhydria (abnormally low concentration of HCl in gastric fluid) or achlorhydria (the absence of HCl in gastric fluid) may decrease the availability of dietary vitamin B_{12} for absorption by preventing the activation of pepsinogen to pepsin, the principal enzyme responsible for proteolysis in the stomach. Achlorhydric patients with adequate production of IF may have low normal or subnormal serum B_{12} concentrations because of failure to liberate B_{12} bound to food.

Vitamin B_{12} is absorbed primarily by an active transport process in the ileum and by simple diffusion at high doses, although with lower efficiency. The receptor-mediated intestinal absorption of vitamin B_{12} and delivery of the vitamin to tissues requires a series of vitamin B_{12} carrier proteins (Fig. 28-3). These include R proteins (also referred to as haptocorrins), IF, and the transcobalamins (TCI, II, III). The two vitamin B_{12}-binding proteins present in the stomach are IF and R proteins (Neale, 1990). The R proteins consist of a family of glycoproteins that can be fractionated on the basis of their sialic acid content (sialic acid is a nine-carbon acidic sugar). They were designated R proteins on the basis of their more rapid migration relative to IF during electrophoresis.

R proteins are synthesized primarily in granulocytes but are also present in saliva, plasma, bile, tears, and milk. The affinity of R proteins for vitamin B_{12} at pH 2.0 is about 50 times greater than that of IF. At low pH, the R protein-B_{12} complex is resistant to proteolytic

degradation by pepsin. Thus, most vitamin B_{12} is bound to R proteins during transit through the stomach.

Intrinsic factor (IF) is a 60,000-d glycoprotein that is synthesized and secreted by gastric parietal cells in humans. It is highly specific for vitamin B_{12} and does not bind other nonfunctional cobalamin analogues ingested in food or excreted in the bile. IF secretion is stimulated by several endogenous agents, including insulin, gastrin, histamine, and acetylcholine. The average concentration of IF in gastric fluid is 1 µg/mL, an amount approximately 50 times in excess of that estimated to be needed for physiological purposes.

When the gastric contents reach the duodenum and the pH of the chyme is raised to neutrality, the haptocorrins (R proteins) become susceptible to degradation by pancreatic proteolytic enzymes (e.g., trypsin), causing vitamin B_{12} to be released (Fig. 28-3). The free vitamin B_{12} is then immediately bound to IF. In the presence of pancreatic disease, the lack of proteolytic enzymes to degrade the B_{12}-R protein complex can result in malabsorption of vitamin B_{12}. In the duodenum, gastric contents are mixed with bile, which contains approximately 0.5 nmol/L cobalamins secreted by the liver. Intrinsic factor is thus available in duodenal contents to bind not only recently ingested vitamin B_{12} but also any physiologically active cobalamin excreted in bile. In this way, about 90% of the physiologically active, nontoxic metabolites of vitamin B_{12} in bile are reabsorbed. Thus, the enterohepatic recirculation provides for efficient conservation of vitamin B_{12} and, together with the fact that large amounts are stored in the liver, accounts for the fact that vitamin B_{12} deficiency does not occur rapidly even in the prolonged absence of vitamin B_{12} intake. Anemia in most cases takes 5 to 7 years to develop after the onset of reduced vitamin B_{12} intake or absorption. An exception to this generalization occurs with individuals who are infested with the fish tapeworm *Diphyllobothrium latum*, which absorbs and uses large amounts of vitamin B_{12}. In tapeworm infestation, anemia can develop in less than 3 years.

IF has two binding sites, one for vitamin B_{12} and one for the ileal receptor cubulin, which recognizes the IF-vitamin B_{12} complex. Cubulin is synthesized by epithelial cells lining the terminal ileum and other absorptive tissues. It is coexpressed with megalin, a multiligand transmembrane endocytic receptor. The vitamin B_{12}-IF

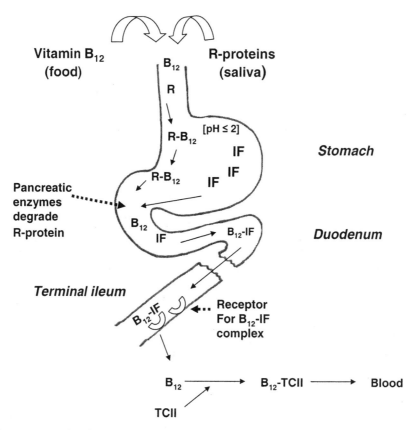

Figure 28-3. The absorption of vitamin B$_{12}$ in humans. The sequence of transitions between protein-bound dietary vitamin B$_{12}$ and circulating B$_{12}$ bound to TCII. R, R proteins, haptocorrins; IF, intrinsic factor; TCII, transcobalamin II.

complex (ligand) binds to cubulin (receptor), and the ligand-receptor complex is internalized via clathrin-coated pits and coated vesicles. The vitamin B$_{12}$-IF ligand is dissociated in the acidic vesicles, and cubulin and megalin return to the membrane for reuse. After dissociation from the cubulin-megalin complex, the vitamin B$_{12}$-IF complex is transferred to lysosomes, where IF is degraded and vitamin B$_{12}$ is released. After it is dissociated from the IF, vitamin B$_{12}$ is transferred to TCII for transport to tissues.

TCII is a 50,000-d β-globulin synthesized in the ileum and the liver. It is the transport protein for recently absorbed vitamin B$_{12}$. About 20% of the plasma vitamin B$_{12}$ is bound to TCII; the remainder of the vitamin B$_{12}$ in plasma is transported by TCI and TCIII, primarily in the form of 5-methylcobalamin. Normal serum contains 0.7–1.5 nmol/L of TCII, which is capable of binding 600–1300 ng of vitamin B$_{12}$; however, only about 15% of its binding capacity is used at any one time. Unlike TCI and TCIII, the

other serum proteins that transport vitamin B$_{12}$, TCII is not a glycoprotein. The specific functions of TCI and TCIII have not been determined; however, they are believed to transport potentially toxic vitamin B$_{12}$ analogues to the liver for excretion in the bile (Fig. 28-4).

The absence of TCI and TCIII is clinically benign; however, the prolonged absence of TCII results in the typical hematological, neurological, and metabolic symptoms that characterize vitamin B$_{12}$ deficiency. Infants who have a genetic defect resulting in a nonfunctional form of TCII show evidence of vitamin B$_{12}$ deficiency within a few months following birth.

The TCII-vitamin B$_{12}$ complex is recognized by specific high-affinity plasma membrane receptors present on the cells that utilize vitamin B$_{12}$. After internalization, the complex is transferred to lysosomes, where TCII is rapidly degraded, and the hydroxycobalamin is released into the cytosol and methylated. The hydroxycobalamin that enters the mitochondria

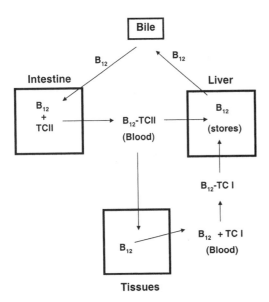

Figure 28-4. The enterohepatic circulation of vitamin B_{12}. TCII (transcobalamin II) is the transport protein that carries newly absorbed dietary vitamin B_{12} from the intestine to tissues. Approximately 20% of circulating vitamin B_{12} is transported by TCII; the remainder of vitamin B_{12} is bound to TCI. THF, tetrahydrofolate.

is converted to the adenosyl form by the enzyme adenosyl transferase. Vitamin B_{12} present in plasma in excess of the binding capacity of the transport proteins is excreted in the urine. Exogenous radiolabeled vitamin B_{12} can be used to determine glomerular filtration rate in humans.

In the early stages of reduced vitamin B_{12} absorption, the amount of vitamin B_{12} bound to TCII decreases rapidly (10–21 days) without any decrease in the total serum B_{12} level. The total vitamin B_{12} concentration begins to decline only when the saturation of TCII falls below 5%. Reduced saturation of TCII is thus one of the earliest indicators of reduced intake of vitamin B_{12} and is detectable in advance of clinical disease. This makes holo-TCII particularly valuable for use as a screening test in susceptible populations. Elevated serum and urine concentrations of homocysteine and MMA occur somewhat later and represent early evidence of cellular dysfunction that occurs when body (liver) stores have been greatly depleted.

The total body pool of vitamin B_{12} in humans ranges from 2 to 5 mg, most of which is stored in the liver. Daily losses of vitamin B_{12} are usually 1–3 μg or approximately 0.1% of total body stores. These losses occur primarily through excretion of vitamin B_{12} in bile and through sloughing of gastrointestinal epithelial cells. Although a dietary intake of 1 μg/day is probably sufficient to meet the needs of most adults, the recommended dietary allowance is 2 μg/day to allow for individual variability and to ensure maintenance of body stores (Herbert, 1987). The average American diet contains 5–30 μg/day of vitamin B_{12}. Regularly scheduled vitamin B_{12} injections are generally preferred by clinicians since measurement of IF and TCII are expensive and are not readily available.

The total serum B_{12} concentration reflects body stores of B_{12} only when liver concentrations fall below 0.6 μg/g, wet weight (normal is 0.6–1.5 μg/g, wet weight). Moderately low serum vitamin B_{12} concentration (110–148 pmol/L) may not be specific for vitamin B_{12} deficiency; however, serum vitamin B_{12} concentrations below 74 pmol/L are almost always associated with clinical manifestations of B_{12} deficiency, except in vegans or strict vegetarians.

Vitamin B_{12} is required by only two enzymes in human metabolism: methionine synthetase and L-methylmalonyl-CoA mutase. Methionine synthetase has an absolute requirement for methylcobalamin and catalyzes the conversion of homocysteine to methionine (Fig. 28-5). 5-Methyltetrahydrofolate is converted to tetrahydrofolate (THF) in this reaction. This vitamin B_{12}-catalyzed reaction is the only means by which THF can be regenerated from 5-methyltetrahydrofolate in humans. Therefore, in vitamin B_{12} deficiency, folic acid can become "trapped" in the 5-methyltetrahydrofolate form, and THF is then unavailable for conversion to other coenzyme forms required for purine, pyrimidine, and amino acid synthesis (Fig. 28-6). All folate-dependent reactions are impaired in vitamin B_{12} deficiency, resulting in indistinguishable hematological abnormalities in both folate and vitamin B_{12} deficiencies.

The catabolism of certain amino acids (e.g., valine, isoleucine, methionine) and odd-chain fatty acids (17:0) produces propionyl-CoA. Propionyl-CoA enters the TCA (citric acid) cycle following conversion to succinyl-CoA, as shown in Fig. 28-7. Propionyl-CoA is first carboxylated to produce D-methylmalonyl-CoA, which in turn is then racemized to L-methylmalonyl-CoA. In an intramolecular rearrangement reaction catalyzed by L-methylmalonyl-CoA mutase, a vitamin B_{12}-

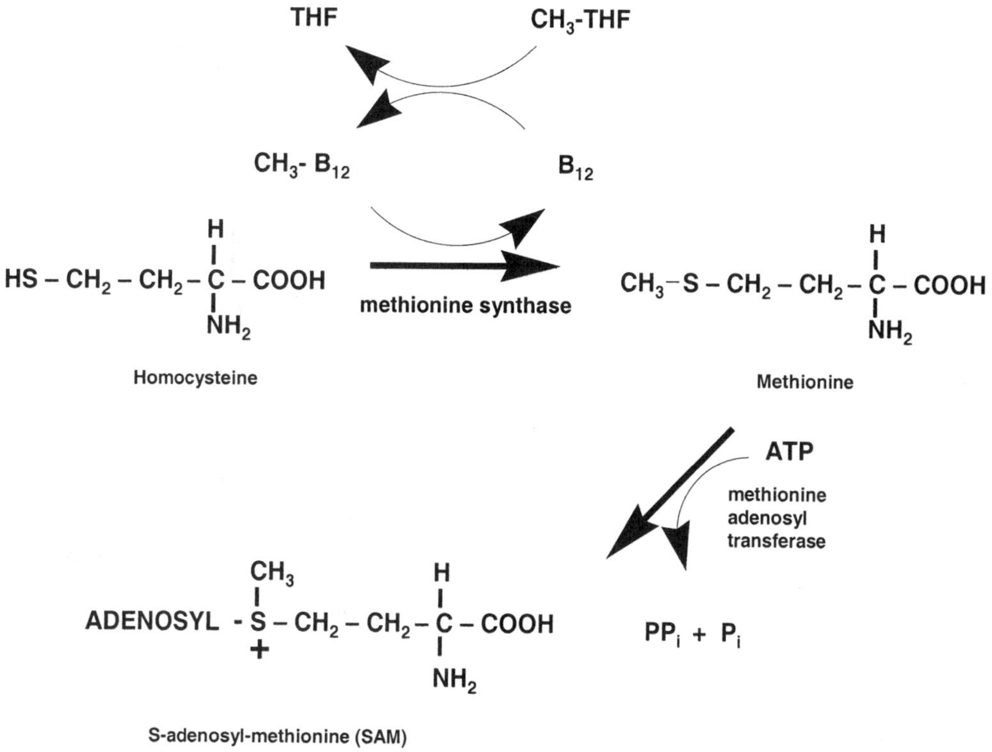

Figure 28-5. The reaction catalyzed by methionine synthase, a vitamin B₁₂-requiring enzyme. In this reaction, homocystine is converted to methionine, with the simultaneous production of tetrahydrofolate (THF) from 5-methyltetrahydrofolate. Methionine can then be converted to *S*-adenosylmethionine (SAM), the universal methyl-group donor.

requiring enzyme, methylmalonyl-CoA, is converted to succinyl-CoA. In vitamin B₁₂ deficiency, cellular levels of both propionyl-CoA and methylmalonyl-CoA increase. Propionyl-CoA can then substitute for acetyl-CoA in fatty acid synthesis, leading to the production of fatty acids comprised of odd numbers of carbon atoms. Similarly, methylmalonyl-CoA can substitute for malonyl-CoA in fatty acid synthesis, resulting in the synthesis of branched-chain fatty acids.

Myelination is essential to the normal function of sensory neurons. Because the synthesis of normal myelin is dependent on the availability of specific fatty acids, the inclusion of abnormal fatty acids (e.g., odd-chain, branched-chain fatty acids) in myelin may alter neural function or cause premature demyelination. This hypothesis has been put forth to explain the neurological impairment observed in vitamin B₁₂ deficiency (Shevell and Rosenblatt, 1992).

Methionine, through subsequent conversion to *S*-adenosylmethionine (see Fig. 28-4), is also required for the synthesis of choline and

choline-containing phospholipids and for the methylation of myelin basic protein, a major protein component of myelin. Although the mechanisms responsible for the development of neurological impairment resulting from vitamin B₁₂ deficiency have not been precisely defined, defective methionine metabolism may also contribute to neurological complications in vitamin B₁₂-deficient patients.

THERAPY

In the setting of established B₁₂ deficiency, treatment is usually by parenteral injection, with 1000 µg given daily for the first 5 days. Thereafter, cyanocobalamin (1000 µg) is given monthly by intramuscular or deep subcutaneous injection. While orally administered drug is not recommended in most patients who have a B₁₂ deficiency due to malnutrition or achlorhydria (failure to release food-bound B₁₂), 1000 µg oral vitamin B₁₂ can be administered daily. A

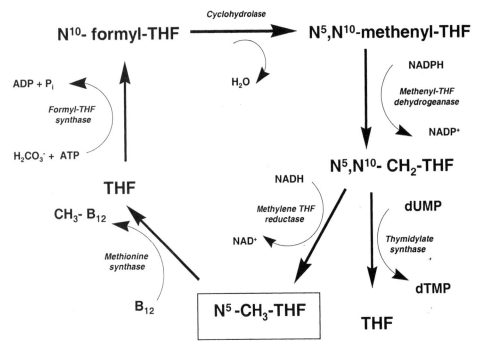

Figure 28-6. The "folate trap."

transnasal vitamin B_{12} preparation is available (Nascobal) that can be used by the patient in a dose of 500 μg/week, thereby obviating the need for injection. The transnasal drug is more expensive but avoids indirect costs such as needles, syringes, patient and nursing time, travel, and office expenses that are part of injection therapy and greatly dwarf the cost of the injected drug. Although most patients could be taught self-injection, this form of therapy remains little used.

For prevention of disease in the elderly, the pregnant, or other susceptible groups, national fortification of food with vitamin B_{12} appears sensible and inexpensive but at present is not used and, in the absence of population screening, is unlikely to be mandated by governmental edict. In general terms, the hematological manifestations of vitamin B_{12} deficiency are rapidly and fully correctable, although deficiencies of other micronutrients such as iron, folic acid, pyridoxine, copper, or vitamin C may be unmasked in the process and may limit the bone marrow's response until they are also corrected.

Therapy of patients with megaloblastic anemia should always start with vitamin B_{12} replacement and never with folic acid; giving

folate before adequate vitamin B_{12} replacement has occurred is dangerous, not only because it may mask vitamin B_{12} deficiency, but also, more importantly, because it may promote utilization of vitamin B_{12} by bone marrow, leading to critical deterioration of vital neurological functions. The likelihood that the neurological functions will recover, even slowly, depends on the duration of the vitamin B_{12} deficiency before therapy: If less than 1 year, the prognosis is good; if over 2 years, it is poor; and if only 1–2 years, it may be partial or incomplete. While the treatment may appear simple, for many reasons compliance is often poor, needed therapy is discontinued, and the patient ends up with inadequate vitamin B_{12} replacement and deteriorating disease, an unfortunate outcome.

QUESTIONS

1. What metabolites in serum and urine can be used to differentiate between a folate deficiency and a vitamin B_{12} deficiency?
2. How does a vitamin B_{12} deficiency cause a decrease in the hematocrit and hemoglobin concentration?

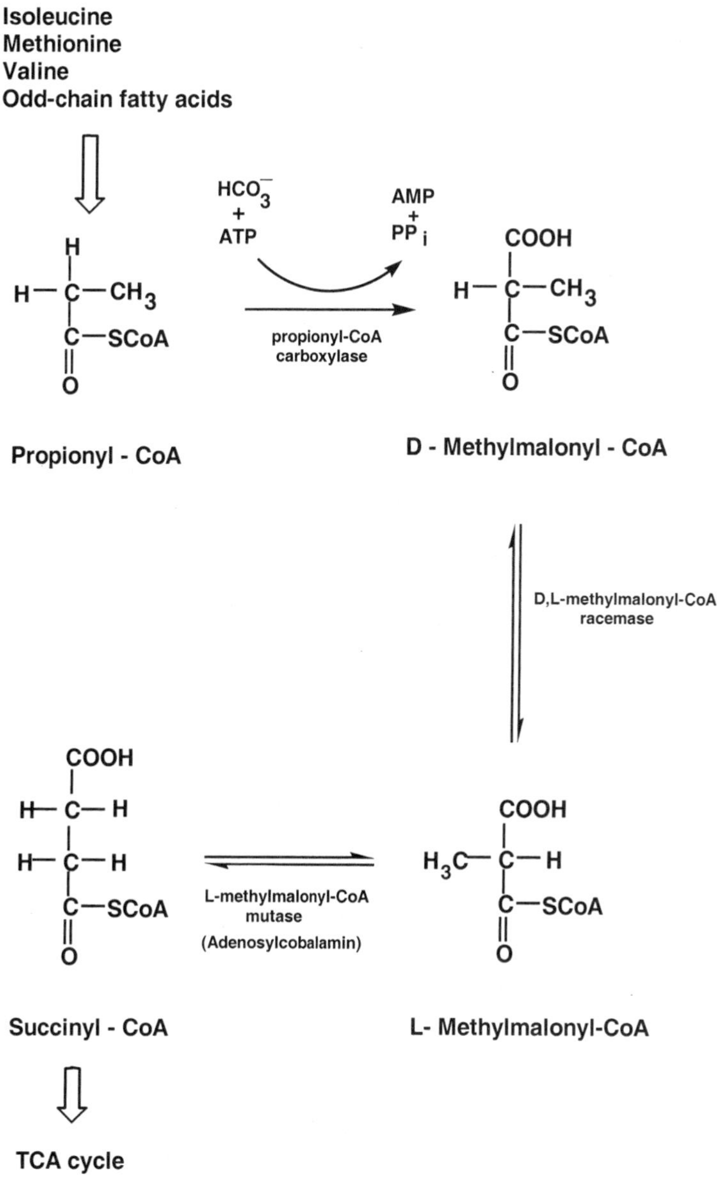

Isoleucine
Methionine
Valine
Odd-chain fatty acids

Figure 28-7. The metabolism of branched-chain amino acids and odd-chain fatty acids via propionyl-CoA. Propionyl-CoA is converted to D-methylmalonyl-CoA by propionyl-CoA carboxylase. D,L-Methylmalonyl-CoA racemase catalyzes the conversion of D-methylmalonyl-CoA to L-methylmalonyl-CoA. L-methyl malonyl-CoA mutase, an adenosylcobalamin-requiring enzyme, converts L-methylmalonyl-CoA to succinyl-CoA. TCA cycle is citric acid cycle or Kreb's cycle.

3. How can pancreatic insufficiency contribute to the development of vitamin B$_{12}$ deficiency despite the presence of adequate intake of vitamin B$_{12}$ and normal secretion of intrinsic factor?

4. How can a deficiency of intrinsic factor develop?

5. What are the metabolic and clinical consequences of using folic acid to treat macrocytic anemia caused by a vitamin B$_{12}$ deficiency?

6. What are the most common causes of vitamin B$_{12}$ deficiency in elderly nursing home residents?

BIBLIOGRAPHY

Avcu N, Avcu F, Beyan C, et al.: The relationship between gastric-oral *Helocobacter pylori* and oral hygeine in patients with vitamin B_{12}-defciency anemia. *Oral Surg Oral Med Oral Pathol Oral Radiol Endod* **92:**166-169, 2001.

Battersby AR: How nature builds the pigments of life: the conquest of vitamin B_{12}. *Science* **264:** 1551-1557, 1994.

Carmel R: Prevalence of undiagnosed pernicious anemia in the elderly. *Arch Int Med* **156:** 1097-1100, 1996.

Carranza E: The neurological manifestations of vitamin B_{12} deficiency, *in* Herbert V (ed): *Vitamin B12 Deficiency.* Royal Society of Medicine, Round Table Series 66, RSM Press, London, pp. 21-26, 2002.

Dharmarajan TS, Pais W, Norkus EP: Does anemia matter? Anemia, morbidity, and mortality in older adults: Need for greater recognition. *Geriatrics* **60:**22-27, 2005.

Dharmarajan TS, Ugalino JT, Kanagala M, et al.: Vitamin B_{12} status in hospitalized elderly from nursing homes and the community. *J Am Med Dir Assoc* **1:**21-24, 2000.

Herbert V: Recommended dietary intake (RDI) of vitamin B_{12} in humans. *Am J Clin Nutr* **45:** 671-678, 1987.

Herzlich B, Herbert V: Depletion of serum holo-transcobalamin II. An early sign of negative vitamin B_{12} balance. *Lab Invest* **58:**332-337, 1988.

Kaptan K, Beyan C, Ural AU, et al: *Helicobacter pylori*—is it a novel causative agent in vitamin B^{12} deficiency? *Arch Int Med* **160:**1349-1353, 2000.

Lindenbaum J, Healton EB, Savage DG, et al.: Neuropsychiatric disorder caused by cobalamin deficiency in the absence of anemia or macrocytosis. *N Engl J Med* **318:**1720-1728, 1988.

Metz J: Cobalamin deficiency and the pathogenesis of nervous system disease. *Annu Rev Nutr* **12:**59-79, 1992.

Neale G: B_{12} binding proteins. *Gut* **31:**59-63, 1990.

Nexo E, Christensen A-L, Hvas A-M, et al.: Quantification of holo-transcobalamin, a marker of vitamin B_{12} deficiency. *Clin Chem* **48:**561-562, 2002.

Roman GC: An epidemic in Cuba of optic neuropathy, sensorineural deafness, peripheral sensory neuropathy and dorsolateral myeloneuropathy. *J Neurol Sci* **127:**11-28, 1994.

Shevell MI, Rosenblatt DS: The neurology of cobalamin. *Can J Neurol Sci* **19:**472-486, 1992.

Stabler SP, Allen RH: Vitamin B_{12} deficiency as a worldwide problem. *Annu Rev Nutr* **24:**299-326, 2004.

Stopeck A: Links between *Helicobacter pylori* infection, cobalamin deficiency, and pernicious anemia. *Arch Int Med* **160:**1229-1230, 2000.

29

Vitamin A Deficiency in Children

NUTTAPORN WONGSIRIROJ, EMORN WASANTWISUT,
and WILLIAM S. BLANER

CASE REPORTS

Case 1

A boy aged 3 years and 8 months was admitted to a local hospital in Thailand with the following symptoms: high fever, difficulty breathing, and diarrhea with approximately 10 episodes per day lasting 1 week. The child showed eye symptoms (see Fig. 29-1), including Bitot's spot and corneal xerosis, that were consistent with the early stages of xerophthalmia, the clinical syndrome associated with vitamin A deficiency. (The clinically defined stages of xerophthalmia are provided in Table 29-1.) Night blindness was also identified through interview of the parents using the local term for night blindness. (For cultures in which vitamin A deficiency has been common, there is often a specific term in the local language for night blindness.) Concomitant with vitamin A deficiency, the child was diagnosed as experiencing protein-energy malnutrition type 2 (moderate), pneumonia, and chronic diarrhea. The boy spent 14 days in the hospital and was treated with vitamin A capsules (200,000 IU/day) on days 1, 2, 3, and 14 as well as with standard antibiotics for the infections. Following treatment with vitamin A, the child's eye symptoms disappeared, and his vision returned to normal. He continued to receive vitamin A capsules providing 200,000 IU every 3–6 months throughout his childhood.

Case 2

A 3-year-old boy was admitted to a hospital with a high temperature, vomiting, and diarrhea that had persisted for over 2 weeks. On examination of his eyes, he showed keratomalacia (see Table 29-1) in both eyes. In addition, he refused to eat and to drink milk. One week before coming to the hospital, the boy had red eyes and eye pain and cried frequently. His parents indicated that, at the onset of symptoms, the boy had experienced night blindness and had become inactive. He subsequently developed a high fever and refused his normal food and milk. On evaluation, the child was diagnosed as experiencing protein-energy malnutrition type 3 (severe), keratomalacia, diarrhea, and sepsis. The boy was treated with an intramuscular injection of water-miscible vitamin A (200,000 IU) and standard antibiotics. He continued to receive vitamin A capsules (200,000 IU) every 3–6 months throughout his childhood. Owing to this bout with vitamin A deficiency, the boy developed a corneal scar in both eyes (see Fig. 29-2) that will remain throughout his life.

DIAGNOSIS

Vitamin A deficiency remains a major public health problem in the developing world. Data compiled in 2002 by the World Health Organization (WHO) suggest that worldwide as many as 21% of children in the age range 0.5 to 5 years suffer from vitamin A deficiency. Extrapolations from these data indicate that as many as 140 million children under the age of 5 years and more than 7 million pregnant women experience vitamin A deficiency every year (West, 2002).

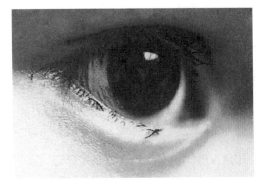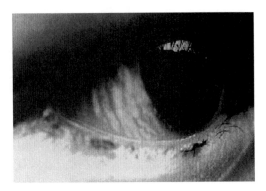

Figure 29-1. Two views of eye symptoms for a boy aged 3 years and 8 months with vitamin A deficiency (case study 1). Bitot's spot and corneal xerosis are present in these views. Following treatment with vitamin A for 14 days, the eye symptoms returned to normal.

Vitamin A deficiency in preschool children is now rare in Thailand due to public health programs that have been implemented since the early 1970s. In rare instances, it still can be found in remote areas of northern Thailand (Wasantwisut, 2002). From 1995 to 1999, there were 39 cases of malnutrition with vitamin A deficiency reported. (It should be noted that vitamin A deficiency is usually associated with other nutritional deficiencies, especially protein-energy malnutrition.) Two of these cases are presented in this chapter.

The eradication of vitamin A deficiency in Thailand did not arise from a government program focused specifically on vitamin A deficiency but rather from a comprehensive national program to promote primary health care in local communities. Vitamin A supplements were administered only to children who showed eye symptoms but not to all children deemed to be at risk of vitamin A deficiency. The program was aimed at improving the quality of health care available in communities, food availability and quality, and community awareness of the symptoms of malnutrition and associated illness. Educational programs were put into place to train and motivate community members to identify children experiencing malnutrition (especially protein-energy malnutrition and micronutrient deficiencies) and/or infection. In addition to a marked reduction in the observed rates of vitamin A deficiency in children, the program was also successful in bringing about the virtual elimination of protein-energy malnutrition and broke the downwardly reciprocating relationship between malnutrition and infection. Hence, the success of the program in Thailand is credited primarily to improved public health measures, including educational programs and empowerment of local communities to recognize and act effectively to prevent and treat malnutrition and its associated infections in children

Table 29-1. Clinical Classification of Xerophthalmia

Xerophthalmia Classification		*Symptom*
XN	Night blindness	Cannot see properly in dim light
X1A	Conjunctival xerosis	Dryish, sandylike change in the conjunctiva
X1B	Bitot's spot	Foamy and cheeselike patches on the whites of the eyes
X2	Corneal xerosis	Drying of the cornea, scaly appearance
X3A	Corneal ulceration/keratomalacia	Formation of holes on the cornea (involving less than a third of corneal surface)
X3B	Corneal ulceration keratomalacia	Cornea becomes cloudy and soft (involving a third or more of the corneal area)
XS	Corneal scar	Scar on the cornea
XF	Xerophthalmia fundus	Structural damage to the rods in retina, followed by degeneration of the both rods and cones

From Sommer and West (1996).

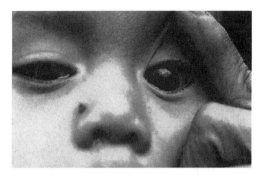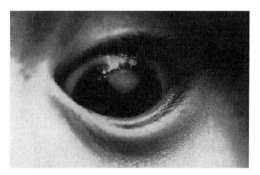

Figure 29-2. Residual corneal scarring following administration of vitamin A therapy to a 3-year-old who had experienced vitamin A deficiency (case study 2).

Serum retinol concentrations are used as a measured index for assessing vitamin A status. Routinely, serum retinol levels in the range of 0.35–0.69 μM (10–20 μg/dL) define moderate vitamin A deficiency, whereas levels below 0.35 μM (<10 μg/dL) indicate severe vitamin A deficiency (see Table 29-2). The clinical symptoms of xerophthalmia, the name of the syndrome associated with vitamin A deficiency, are most evident in the eye and progress initially from night blindness (stage XN) to the development of Bitot's spot (stage X1B), corneal ulceration and keratomalacia (stage X3), and formation of a corneal scar (stage XS) and ultimately result in xerophthalmia fundus (stage XF). The full clinical classifications of the stages of xerophthalmia are listed in Table 29-1. The early stages of xerophthalmia are readily reversible on administration of vitamin A to the patient; however, the later stages commencing with the formation of a corneal scar are irreversible.

Subclinical vitamin A deficiency results in an increased risk of morbidity and mortality arising primarily from impaired immunity (Sommer and West, 1996). Serum levels of retinol in the range of 0.70–1.05 μM (20–30 μg retinol/dL serum) should be taken to indicate an at-risk population for subclinical vitamin A deficiency.

BIOCHEMICAL PERSPECTIVES

Vitamin A is an essential fat-soluble compound acquired from the diet. The parent form of vitamin A is all-*trans*-retinol. Vitamin A is needed to maintain normal vision, normal reproduction (including spermatogenesis, conception, and placenta formation), and normal cell differentiation (including bone remodeling, maintenance of differentiated epithelial linings and skin, em-

bryogenesis, and immune system function) (Gudas et al., 1994). Because vitamin A is important to so many essential processes in the body, vitamin A deficiency results in severe consequences for the health of human beings. The body is able to store substantial quantities of vitamin A, primarily in liver, and this stored vitamin A is used to maintain (defend) blood vitamin A levels. Adults normally acquire enough vitamin A over their lifetime to have stores that provide protection from developing vitamin A deficiency in times of dietary insufficiency. Since tissue vitamin A stores are relatively low at birth, young children, especially those born to mothers with poor vitamin A reserves, are vulnerable to developing vitamin A deficiency.

When vitamin A stores are adequate, the liver secretes retinol bound to retinol-binding protein (RBP) into the circulation to provide tissues with a constant supply of vitamin A. In the circulation, the retinol-RBP complex is found bound to another circulating protein of hepatic origin, transthyretin (TTR). TTR also binds thyroid hormone and consequently plays a role in the transport of both vitamin A and thyroid hormone. The molecular size of the retinol-RBP complex is quite small, and the formation of the

Table 29-2. Classification of Vitamin A Status by Serum Retinol Levels

Serum Retinol Level		
μg/dL	μM (μmole/L)*	*Vitamin A Status*
≥30	≥1.05	Normal
20–30	0.7–1.05	At risk
10–20	0.35–0.69	Moderate
<10	<0.35	Severe

From sommer and West (1966).

*1 μM equals 28.6 μg/dL.

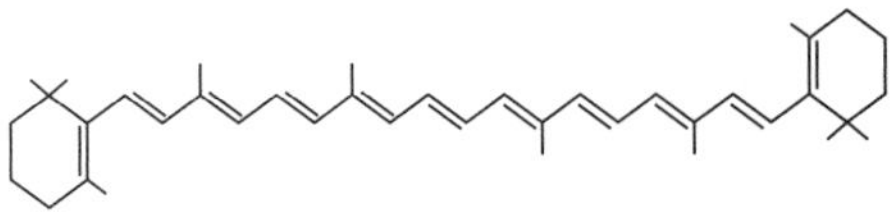

(I) all-trans β-Carotene

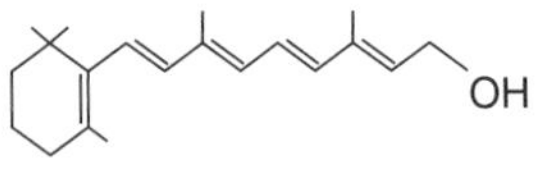

(II) all-*trans* Retinol

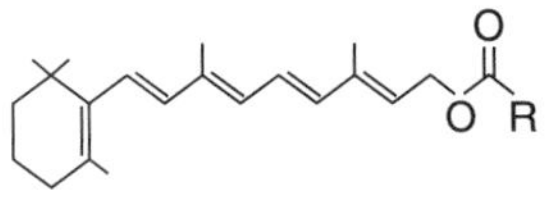

(III) Retinyl Ester (R = Acyl Chain)

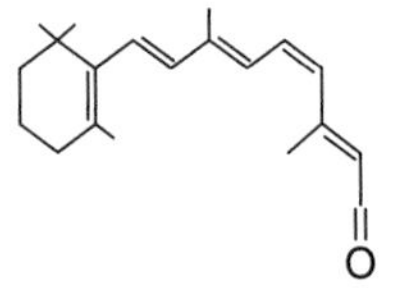

(IV) 11-*cis* Retinal

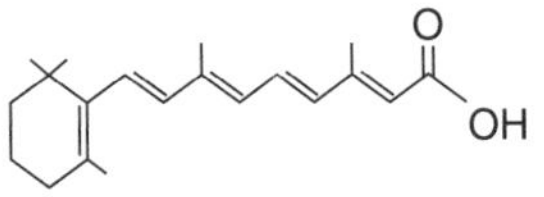

(V) all-*trans* Retinoic Acid

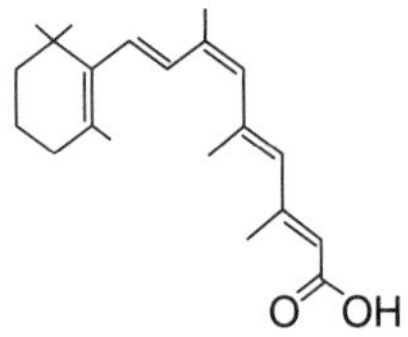

(VI) 9-*cis* Retinoic Acid

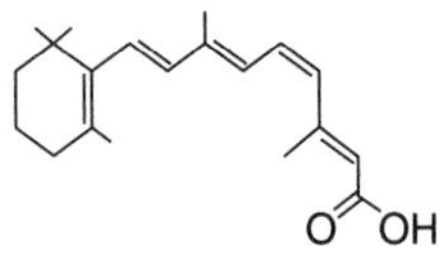

(VII) 13-*cis* Retinoic Acid

Figure 29-3. Chemical structures of important vitamin A species and the provitamin A carotenoid β-carotene. All-*trans*-β-carotene (I) is the most important provitamin A carotenoid, which can be converted to all-*trans*-retinal and then all-*trans*-retinol (II), which by definition is vitamin A. All-*trans*-retinol can be esterified with long-chain fatty acids to form retinyl ester (III), the storage form of vitamin A in the body. The active form of vitamin A in vision is 11-*cis*-retinal (IV). The transcriptionally active forms of vitamin A are all-*trans*-retinoic acid (V) and 9-*cis*-retinoic acid (VI). 13-*cis*-Retinoic acid (VII) has poor transcriptional regulatory activity but is used clinically as isotretinoin to treat skin diseases.

retinol-RBP-TTR complex serves to prevent renal filtration of retinol-RBP. When hepatic stores of vitamin A become depleted, retinol-RBP is no longer secreted from the liver, and consequently blood levels of retinol decline. The retinol bound to RBP is measured diagnostically (see Diagnosis section) to assess the vitamin A status of a patient. Low blood retinol levels indicate insufficient vitamin A stores. However, normal blood retinol levels are not a good indicator for assessing liver stores since the liver secretes retinol-RBP until the stores are completely exhausted.

Chemistry, Biochemistry and Nutrition of Vitamin A

The term *retinoid* refers to any naturally occurring or synthetic compound bearing a struc-

tural resemblance to all-*trans*-retinol with or without the biological activity of vitamin A (O'Byrne and Blaner, 2004). The structures of some important vitamin A species as well as the most active provitamin A carotenoid, all-*trans*-β-carotene, are shown in Figure 29-3.

Structurally, vitamin A and many synthetic retinoids consist of a β-ionone ring, a polyunsaturated polyene chain, and a polar end group. The polar end group can exist in several oxidation states, as retinol, retinal, or retinoic acid. Retinol and retinyl esters are the most abundant vitamin A forms found in the body (Blaner and Olson, 1994). Retinol can be esterified with long-chain fatty acids (mainly palmitate, oleate, and stearate) to form retinyl esters, which are the body's storage form of vitamin A. Retinol also can undergo oxidation to retinal, which can be oxidized further to retinoic acid. The active form of vitamin A in vision is 11-*cis*-retinal (see more details in the Vision section) (Wald, 1968). Outside of vision, vitamin A acts by regulating gene transcription (Chambon, 1994; Mangelsdorf et al., 1994). The preponderance of the biological activity of vitamin A arises from effects on gene expression. The transcriptional regulatory actions of vitamin A are mediated by all-*trans*-retinoic acid and 9-*cis*-retinoic acid (see section on Transcriptional Regulation). A large number of synthetic retinoids have been generated and used in clinical trials as potential treatments for many different diseases, especially cancers and skin diseases.

All vitamin A present in the body must be acquired from the diet (O'Byrne and Blaner, 2004; Vogel et al., 1999). Two forms of vitamin A are available in the diet, preformed vitamin A and provitamin A carotenoids. The preformed vitamin A consists primarily of retinol and retinyl ester that have been consumed in animal food products. Provitamin A carotenoids like β-carotene are consumed in dark green and yellow fruits and vegetables (mangoes, papaya, carrots, dark green leafy vegetables, and red palm oil are some rich dietary sources of provitamin A carotenoids). Dietary provitamin A carotenoids are converted in the intestine and other tissues to vitamin A by the actions of the enzyme β-carotene-15,15'-monooxygenase (also called carotene cleavage enzyme). Once dietary provitamin A carotenoid has been converted in the body to vitamin A, it is metabolically and functionally indistinguishable from vitamin A originating in the diet as preformed vitamin A.

The vitamin A content of foods is often given in terms of the international unit (IU). One IU of vitamin A is defined as 0.3 µg of all-*trans*-retinol. The term *retinol equivalent* (RE) is used to convert all sources of vitamin A and carotenoids in the diet to a single unit. One RE is by definition 1 µg of all-*trans* retinol, 12 µg of β-carotene, or 24 µg of other (mixed) provitamin A carotenoids. The recommended dietary allowance for vitamin A ranges from 375 µg RE/day for infants to 1,000 RE/day for adults.

Excessive intake of vitamin A (hypervitaminosis A), like too little intake, can result in adverse health consequences. Approximately 60%–80% of vitamin A is stored in the liver in hepatic stellate cells (also called Ito cells and fat-storing cells). Retinyl esters are the main storage form of vitamin A in the liver and are found in lipid droplets present in the hepatic stellate cells (Fig 29-4). Both the size and number of these lipid droplets increase in response to vitamin A intake. Initially, hypervitaminosis A promotes cheilitis (dryness and cracking of the lips) as well as dryness of nasal mucosa, eyes, and skin; hair loss; and nail fragility. Later clinical indicators of vitamin A toxicity include bone pain, nausea, vomiting, and hepatomegaly. Some cases of excessive vitamin A intake have resulted in irreversible liver damage.

Biochemical Actions of Vitamin A

Vision

The form of vitamin A required in vision is 11-*cis*-retinal. In the retina, the initiating event of vision occurs when a photon of light excites a molecule of 11-*cis*-retinal that is covalently bound to the protein opsin (11-*cis*-retinal bound to opsin is known as rhodopsin or the visual pigment) (Saari, 1999). As shown in Figure 29-5, when rhodopsin is struck by a photon of light, the 11-*cis*-retinal undergoes photoisomerization to all-*trans*-retinal, thus initiating a signal transduction cascade that results in transmission of the visual impulse to the brain. This action of vitamin A involves a large number of very well characterized enzymatic and nonenzymatic processes that arise ultimately as the result of the photoisomerization of 11-*cis*-retinal to all-*trans*-retinal. These vitamin A-dependent processes are known as the visual cycle of vitamin A and are unique to the eye and vision (Saari, 1999).

Transcriptional Regulation

Outside of vision, the physiological actions of vitamin A arise through the regulation of vitamin A-dependent gene expression (Chambon, 1994; Mangelsdorf et al., 1994). More than 500 different genes may be responsive to vitamin A (Balmer and Blomhoff, 2002). The genes reported to be responsive to vitamin A are quite diverse and include ones encoding transcription factors, peptide hormones, growth factors, growth factor receptors, protein kinases and phosphatases, and enzymes involved in intermediary metabolism and the regulation of this metabolism.

Vitamin A acts to regulate gene expression through interactions with its specific ligand-dependent transcription factors, which are sometimes referred to as nuclear receptors (Chambon, 1994; Chawla et al., 2001; Mangels-

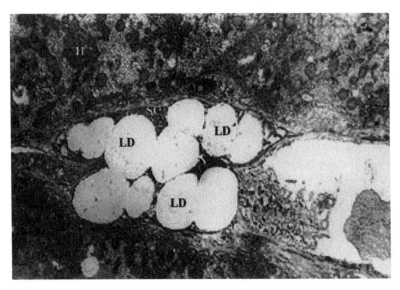

Figure 29-4. Stellate cell lipid droplets present in a biopsy obtained from the liver of a patient experiencing vitamin A toxicity. Image obtained from electron microscopy of a biopsied human liver showing the characteristic lipid droplets (LD) found in hepatic stellate cells (SC). These lipid droplets are highly enriched in vitamin A, and the size and number of lipid droplets is influenced by dietary vitamin A intake and nutritional status. In this image of a human stellate cell, the nucleus (N) is compressed by the surrounding lipid droplets, and very little cell cytoplasm within the stellate cell can be seen in this view. Adjoining the stellate cell are two hepatocytes (H).

dorf et al., 1994). The vitamin A-dependent transcription factors consist of three retinoic acid receptors (RARs) and three retinoid X receptors (RXRs). The RARs and RXRs are members of the large steroid/thyroid/retinoid superfamily of ligand-dependent transcription factors that regulate hormone- and nutrient-dependent gene expression. Thus, vitamin A functions biochemically within the body in a manner that is very similar to steroid hormones and thyroid hormone.

The form of vitamin A that is needed for regulating vitamin A-dependent gene expression is retinoic acid. All-*trans*-retinoic acid can interact with each of the three RARs (RARα, RARβ, and RARγ) and each of the three RXRs (RXRα, RXRβ, and RXRγ). 9-*cis*-Retinoic acid binds and effectively transactivates only the RXRs. The RARs and the RXRs recognize well-defined *cis*-acting response elements, termed retinoic acid response elements (RAREs) and retinoid X response elements (RXREs) that are present in the promoter regions of responsive genes. The RARs and RXRs bind to RAREs and/or RXREs as dimers, either homodimers or heterodimers.

When bound to a response element, the vitamin A-dependent nuclear receptors are able to interact with coactivators and corepressors present in the nucleus either to stimulate or to repress transcriptional activity. Interactions with coactivators or corepressors will result respectively in transcriptional activation or repression. Thus, retinoic acid availability as a ligand for binding to RARs and/or RXRs and the ability of these receptors to bind alternatively to either coactivators or corepressors provides a mechanism through which genes can be either activated or repressed by retinoic acid. It is this gene regulatory mechanism that accounts for the great majority of vitamin A action in the body.

Vitamin A has a very important role in regulating the actions of other hormone- and nutrient-dependent genes because the RXRs can interact with other nuclear receptors to form heterodimers that are able to bind and regulate hormone and nutrient responsiveness. The RXRs are able to heterodimerize with the vitamin D receptor, the thyroid hormone receptors, the peroxisome proliferator activated

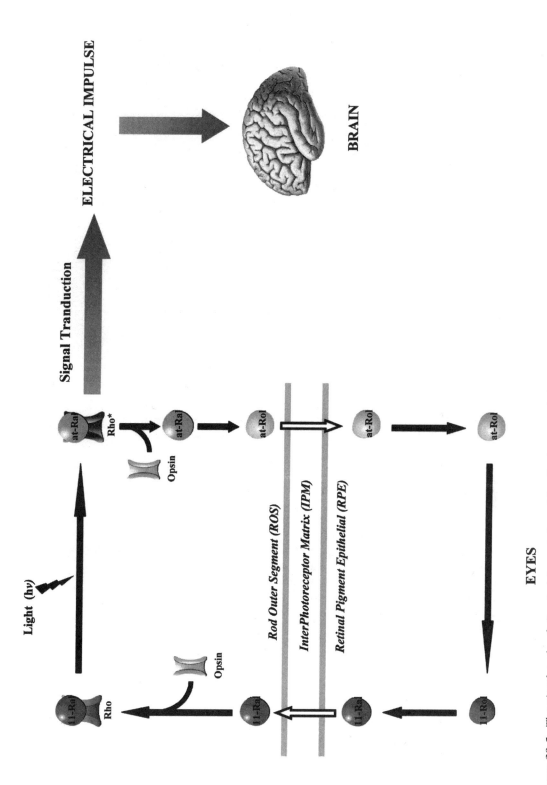

Figure 29-5. The visual cycle of vitamin A is central to vision. In the retina, light stimulates the conversion of 11-*cis*-retinal, part of rhodopsin (Rho), to all-*trans*-retinal and activates rhodopsin (Rho*).This initiates the first step of the signal transduction cascade that results in the transmission of the visual signal to the brain. The visual cycle involves biochemical and metabolic events in both the photoreceptors (rods) and the retinal pigment epithelium.

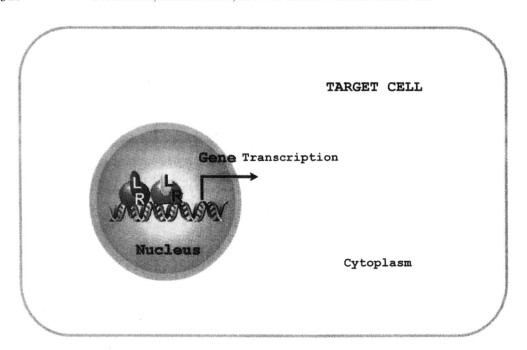

Receptor (R)	Ligand (L)
Retinoid X Receptor (RXR)	9–cis–retinoic acid
Retinoic Acid Receptor (RAR)	all–*trans*–retinoic acid
Thyroid Hormone Receptor (TR)	Triiodothyronine (T_3)
Vitamin D Receptor (VDR)	1,25–$(OH)_2$–Vitamin D
Peroxisome Proliferator Activated Receptor (PPAR)	Fatty Acid Metabolite

Figure 29-6. Gene transcription is regulated by retinoic acid. All-*trans*-retinoic acid and 9-*cis*-retinoic acid are ligands for retinoic acid receptors (RARs) and retinoid X receptors (RXRs), respectively. The RXRs can form heterodimers with RARs and with the thyroid hormone receptors (TRs), the vitamin D receptor (VDR), and the peroxisome proliferator-activated receptors (PPARs) and a number of other hormone- and nutrient-responsive transcription factors to moderate gene transcription. Because of the ability of RXR to form heterodimers with other nuclear receptors, vitamin A has abroad effect on many hormonally and nutrient-responsive genes.

receptors, as well as a number of other hormone-/nutrient-dependent transcription factors (Chawla et al., 2001). Through this interaction, vitamin A and the RXRs can regulate a broad spectrum of hormonally or nutrient-responsive genes. These receptors and their ligands are illustrated in Figure 29-6.

The Biochemical Basis for the Clinical Manifestations of Vitamin A Deficiency

The initial effects of vitamin A deficiency on child health are subclinical and manifested as an increased risk of morbidity and mortality

Table 29-3. Vitamin A Supplement According to WHO Guidelines

Age	Treatment Dose (IU)
<6 months of age	50,000
6–12 months of age	100,000
>12 months of age	200,000

From WHO/UNICEF/IVAGG (1997).

arising primarily from gastrointestinal and respiratory infections. This results from a diminished immune response and disruption of the intestinal barrier. Vitamin A is needed to ensure normal cell proliferation and differentiation of both white blood cells and the intestinal epithelium. Thus, retinoic acid and the transcriptional regulatory actions of the RARs and RXRs are needed to ensure optimal immune cell action and maintenance of an intact intestinal barrier.

The first clinical sign of vitamin A deficiency is night blindness. This arises because too little 11-*cis*-retinal is produced in the retina to support normal night vision and the visual cycle. As the effects of xerophthalmia progress from night blindness through Bitot's spot and corneal xerosis to keratomalacia, the clinical effects of vitamin A deficiency result from impairments of vitamin A-dependent gene expression. Corneal xerosis is thought to arise from inappropriate expression of collagenase genes that are normally repressed by retinoic acid. In the absence of retinoic acid, these genes become activated and collagenases are produced. This leads to digestion of connective tissue needed to maintain the structural integrity of the eye. Ultimately, if vitamin A deficiency is not recognized and treated it will result in death owing to impaired immunity and infection.

THERAPY

Patients presenting with any stage of xerophthalmia should immediately be given high-dose vitamin A supplements according to WHO treatment dosing guidelines (Table 29-3). This dose should be repeated the next day and 1–4 weeks later (WHO/UNICEF/IVACG, 1997).

Because of the potential teratogenic effects of high-dose vitamin A, caution must be taken in the treatment of severe vitamin A deficiency among pregnant women as well as women of reproductive age. Women of reproductive age should be treated with 200,000 IU only when they display active corneal xerophthalmia. For milder eye signs (night blindness or Bitot's spot), women should be given 5,000–10,000 IU per day but less than 25,000 IU per week for 4 weeks or longer.

The preferred form and route of administration is retinyl palmitate in oil given orally. The full dosing schedule should be given for all stages of xerophthalmia, aside for pregnant women and women of reproductive age. In cases of severe diarrhea or vomiting, which may prevent ingestion and absorption, an intramuscular injection of water-miscible vitamin A (at the same doses) may be administered. A recent field trial in Ethiopia (Biesalski et al., 1999) indicated that an aerosol of retinyl palmitate for inhalation resulted in well-absorbed vitamin A through the respiratory tract and may in the future become the preferred treatment option for patients with severe diarrhea or vomiting.

QUESTIONS

1. A measure of an individual child's serum retinol level may not be a good indicator of the vitamin A status of the child. Why is this?
2. What protocols should be followed in providing vitamin A to a child who is suspected of being either subclinically or clinically vitamin A deficient?
3. Although vitamin A must be acquired from the diet, why might it be thought of as being hormonelike?
4. Clinical signs of vitamin A deficiency (xerophthalmia) are often diagnosed together with infections such as pneumonia and diarrhea. Why?
5. What would be the recommended treatment for pregnant women with night blindness? Explain the basis for such a recommendation.
6. For a preventive measure, high-dose vitamin A is administered every 4–6 months. What is the biochemical basis behind this periodic regime?

BIBLIOGRAPHY

Balmer JE, Blomhoff R.: Gene expression regulation by retinoic acid. *J Lipid Res* **43**:1773–1808, 2002.

Biesalski H, Reifen R, Furst P, et al.: Retinyl palmitate supplementation by inhalation of an aerosol improves vitamin A status of preschool children in Gondar (Ethiopia). *Br J Nutr* **82:** 179-182, 1999.

Blaner WS, Olson JA: Retinol and retinoic acid metabolism, *in* Sporn MB, Roberts AB, Goodman DS (eds): *The Retinoids: Biology, Chemistry, and Medicine*. 2nd ed. Raven Press, New York, 1994, pp. 229-256.

Chambon P: The retinoid signaling pathway: molecular and genetic analysis. *Cell Biol.* **5:**115-125, 1994.

Chawla A, Repa JM, Evans RM, et al.: Nuclear receptors and lipid physiology: opening the X-files. *Science* **294:**1866-1870, 2001.

Gudas LJ, Sporn MB, Roberts AB: Cellular biology and biochemistry of the retinoids, *in* Sporn MB, Roberts AB, Goodman DS (eds): *The Retinoids, Biology, Chemistry and Medicine*. 2nd ed. Raven Press, New York, 1994, pp. 443-520.

Mangelsdorf DJ, Umesono K, Evans RM: The retinoid receptors, *in* Sporn MB, Roberts AB, Goodman DS (eds): *The Retinoids, Biology, Chemistry and Medicine*. 2nd ed. Raven Press, New York, 1994, pp. 319-350.

O'Byrne SM, Blaner WS: Introduction to retinoids, *in* Packer L, Kraemer K, Obermueller U, Sies H (eds): *Carotenoids and Retinoids*. AOCS Press, Champaign, IL, 2005, pp. 1-22.

Saari JC: Retinoids in mammalian vision, *in* Nau H, Blaner WS (eds): *The Handbook of Experimental Pharmacology, Retinoids: The Biochemical and Molecular Basis of Vitamin A and Retinoid Action*. Vol. 139. Springer-Verlag, Heidelberg, 1999, pp. 563-588.

Sommer A, West K: *Vitamin A Deficiency: Health Survival and Vision*. Oxford University Press, New York, 1996.

Vogel S, Gamble MV, Blaner WS: Retinoid uptake, metabolism and transport, *in* Nau H, Blaner WS (eds): *The Handbook of Experimental Pharmacology, Retinoids: The Biochemical and Molecular Basis of Vitamin A and Retinoid Action*. Springer-Verlag, Heidelberg, 1999, pp. 31-96.

Wald G: Molecular basis of visual excitation. *Nature* **219:**800-807, 1968.

Wasantwisut E: A combined approach to vitamin A deficiency in Thailand. *Sight Life Newsl* **3:**63-67, 2002.

West KP Jr: Extent of vitamin A deficiency among preschool children and women of reproductive age. *J Nutr* **132:**2857S-2866S, 2002.

WHO: *The World Health Report 2002: Reducing Risks, Promoting Healthy Life*. World Health Organization, Geneva, 2002.

WHO, UNICEF, IVACG Task Force: *Vitamin A Supplements. A Guide to Their Use in the Treatment and Prevention of Vitamin A Deficiency and Xerophthalmia*. 2nd ed. World Health Organization, Geneva, 1997.

30

Calcium-Deficiency Rickets

DOROTHY J. VANDERJAGT and ROBERT H. GLEW

CASE REPORT

The patient was a 3-year-old female who lived with her family in a rural village in northern Nigeria that was situated 40 miles distant from the nearest urban center. She was the fifth of eight children. Her parents were subsistence farmers who grew millet and maize that, together with a small vegetable garden, provided most of the family's diet. Because of their high cost, dairy products were rarely consumed by the parents or children.

The patient was brought by her mother to the local community health clinic because the child had a bacterial infection on her knee. The infection was successfully treated with a 10-day course of antibiotics. During that clinic visit, the physician noted that the patient's legs were severely bowed (genu varum) (Fig. 30-1) and advised the mother that it would be beneficial for the child to receive a more thorough examination at the teaching hospital in the nearby city. She also noticed that the patient's 6-year-old brother had a pronounced "K-leg" (rotation of knees toward one another, genu valgum). However, the youngest of the eight children, a 1.5-year-old girl who accompanied the mother and who was still being breast-fed, exhibited no evidence of outstanding skeletal problems.

The physician at the rural clinic made arrangements to transport the child and her mother to the teaching hospital in the nearby city. At the hospital, she was given a complete examination by a physician in the Department of Family Medicine, and blood and urine samples were obtained. The weight of the patient (14.8 kg) was above the 50th percentile for fe-

males in her age range according to World Health Organization (WHO) standards (z score = +0.66) (WHO, 1983). A z score is a method used to compare an individual's own data to a reference population. The z score is calculated as the difference between the individual's value and the corresponding mean of the reference population at the same age and gender divided by the standard deviation for the corresponding reference population. The patient's standing height was 80 cm, which corresponds to a z score of −2.1. The patient was otherwise in good health. The mother reported that the child cried when she was required to walk for even a short distance, and that she carried her daughter a good part of the time.

Stereotypical signs of rickets were evident in the patient, including bowed legs and the presence of a "rachitic rosary" (palpable beadlike enlargement of the costochondral junctions or ribs). X-rays of the long bones of the patient revealed widening of the growth plates and metaphyseal cupping and fraying. The metaphysis is a growth area of bone located between the diaphysis (the shaft of long bone) and the epiphysis, which is the section of bone beyond the growth plate. During growth, endochondral ossification, the process by which cartilage is transformed into bone, occurs at the growth plate of the long bones. This results in lengthening of bone. There was severe osteomalacia, as evidenced by increases in the volume, surface area, and thickness of the osteoid, and a reduced calcification front.

The results of the laboratory analyses are summarized in Table 30-1. The serum total calcium concentration was low (7.9 mg/dL; normal

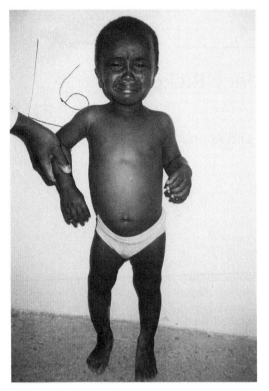

Figure 30-1. A 3-year-old child in Nigeria with evidence of rickets, specifically genu varum.

is 8.8–10.8 mg/dL), as was the phosphorus concentration (4.4 g/dL; normal is 4.5–5.5 g/dL). Serum albumin was 41 g/L (normal is 38–54 g/L). The intact parathyroid hormone (PTH) concentration (283 pmol/L; normal is 1.05–6.84 pmol/L)

and serum alkaline phosphatase activity (1500 U/L; normal is 160–320 U/L) were both elevated. Urinary calcium excretion was below the normal range (normal is 50–100 mg/24 h), but urinary phosphate excretion was increased (1.9 g/24 h; normal is 0.4–1.3 g/24 h). Analysis of a serum sample that had been sent to a laboratory in the United States revealed that the child's serum 25-hydroxyvitamin D level was normal but at the lower end of the reference range (46 nmol/L; normal is 35–150 nmol/L); however, her serum 1,25-dihydroxyvitamin D level was above the upper limit of the reference range for children (250 pmol/L; normal is 42–169 pmol/L).

The laboratory also measured biochemical markers of bone metabolism. The urinary excretion of deoxypyrolidone, a marker of bone resorption, was elevated (128 nmol/mmol creatinine; normal is 31–110 nmol/mmol creatinine). Bone-specific alkaline phosphatase, a marker of bone synthesis, was also elevated at 400 U/L (normal is 70–139 U/L for girls between 3 and 8 years of age) (Tsai et al., 1999). The concentration of another marker of bone resorption, NTx (N-teleopeptide), in the patient's serum was elevated (110 nmol BCE/L; normal is 20–68 nmol BCE/L [bone collagen equivalents]).

DIAGNOSIS

The clinical presentation and laboratory data for this patient are consistent with the bone

Table 30-1. Summary of the Laboratory Analyses for the Patient

Parameter	Patient Before Therapy	After Therapy (3 months)	Normal Range
Total calcium (mg/dL)	7.9	9.2	8.8–10.8
Phosphorus (mg/dL)	4.4	5.0	4.5–5.5
Albumin (g/L)	41	43	38–54
iPTH (pmol/L)	283	8	1.05–6.84
Alkaline phosphatase activity (U/L)	1500	300	160–320
Urinary calcium (mg/24 h)	n.d.	45	50–100
Urinary phosphorus (mg/24 h)	2.0	0.8	0.4–1.3
25-Hydroxyvitamin D (nmol/L)	46	52	35–150
1.25-Dihydroxyvitamin D (pmol/L)	250	165	42–169
Urinary deoxypyrolidone (nmol/mmol creatinine)	128	60	31–110
Bone-specific alkaline phosphatase (U/L)	400	145	70–139
Serum NTx (BCE/L)	110	67	20–68

n.d., not detectable; PTH, intact parathyroid hormone; BCE, bone collagen equivalents; NTx, N-teleopeptide.

disorder known as rickets (Wharton and Bishop, 2003). Nutritional rickets can be caused by a deficiency of calcium (calcipenic rickets) or phosphate (phosphopenic rickets). Calcium-deficiency results from an inadequate calcium intake or a deficiency of vitamin D, the main regulator of calcium homeostasis. Vitamin D occurs as vitamin D_3 (cholecalciferol), which is produced endogenously in the skin, or as vitamin D_2 (ergocalciferol), which is synthesized by the irradiation of ergosterol from yeast and plants (Holick, 2004). When vitamin D is expressed without a subscript, it is referring to a combination of the two forms. Other nonnutritional causes of rickets in children are related to genetic defects in the kidney enzyme 1α-hydroxylase, which converts 25-hydroxyvitamin D to 1,25-dihydroxyvitamin D (type 1 vitamin D-deficient rickets) or a mutation in the vitamin D receptor (type 2 vitamin D-resistant rickets).

The principal method of diagnosis of rickets is radiographic (Jergas and Genant, 2002). Cupping and fraying of the metaphysis and longitudinal widening of the growth plates are hallmarks of rickets and are common to vitamin D-deficiency and calcium-deficiency rickets. Bone consists of two phases: an osteoid protein phase composed primarily of collagen produced by osteoblasts on which the mineral phase (calcium and phosphorus) is deposited as a crystal (hydroxyapatite). Rickets is characterized by an increase in demineralized osteoid. In adults, in whom the growth plate has closed, decreased mineralization of the osteoid is referred to as osteomalacia. Proper mineralization of the osteoid matrix in the growth plate requires adequate calcium and phosphate to allow crystal formation. If inadequate calcium is provided in the diet of a growing child, then the osteoid will not be sufficiently mineralized, resulting in soft bones that can bend due to the weight of the child. This is the basis of the bow-leg or knock-knee seen in rickets.

The site and type of bone deformity seen in rickets depend on the age of the child. In a small infant, deformities of the forearms and anterior bowing of the distal tibias are more common. Clinical features such as craniotabes (areas of thinning and softening in the bones of the skull), hypotonia, and tetany are common in vitamin D-deficiency rickets, which occurs more frequently in infants 1 year old or younger. These features may be absent in calcium-deficiency rickets, which usually presents after the age of 1 year or after the child has been weaned from the breast and begins consuming food that is low in calcium (Thacher, 2003). An exaggeration of the normal bowing of the legs (genu varum) may be more common in a toddler, whereas an older child may present with K-leg (genu valgum) or windswept deformity (valgus deformity of one leg and a varus deformity of the other).

In rickets and adult osteomalacia, the ratio of unmineralized to mineralized bone is increased. This is in contrast to osteoporosis, where the ratio of unmineralized to mineralized bone is normal. Osteoporosis is characterized by a decrease in bone mass caused by an imbalance in bone formation relative to reabsorption but is not associated with changes in the histological appearance of bone.

The biochemical features of calcium-deficiency and vitamin D deficiency are very similar. Both disorders result in a low-to-normal serum calcium concentration, an elevated PTH level, a decreased or normal phosphorus concentration, and increased alkaline phosphatase activity. The serum concentration of 25-hydroxyvitamin D is normal or slightly decreased in calcium-deficiency rickets but is markedly decreased in vitamin D deficiency. On the other hand, the serum concentration of 1,25-dihydroxyvitamin D is greatly elevated in calcium-deficiency rickets but is normal or even slightly decreased in vitamin D-deficiency rickets.

The dietary history and laboratory findings for this patient pointed to calcium-deficiency as the cause of her rickets: a low serum calcium within the normal range; secondary hyperparathyroidism with an elevated serum concentration of PTH; and a normal serum concentration of 25-hydroxyvitamin with an elevated serum concentration of 1,25-dihydroxyvitamin D, the active hormone form of vitamin D. The patient's calcium-deficiency was due to the fact that she did not have access to milk because of the expense and the lack of adequate storage facilities for fresh dairy products in the home.

Therapy for this patient consisted of a daily supplement of elemental calcium (1000 mg) in the form of calcium carbonate. Because of the elevated concentration of 1,25-dihydroxyvitamin D and the normal concentration of 25-hydroxyvitamin D, vitamin D supplements were not prescribed for this child. The subject of this case report responded well to calcium supplementation. After 3 months of supplementation, there was radiographic evidence of healing, and the serum calcium concentration rose to within normal limits. She no longer had evidence of pain when walking. The mother was advised to continue giving the child calcium supplements for another 3 months and then bring the child back to the hospital 6 months later for an examination. After 6 months of calcium therapy, the patient's serum 1,25-dihydroxyvitamin D decreased to 165 pmol/L, which is in the normal range (Table 30-1). The concentrations of the two markers of bone turnover were also measured and found to be within normal limits: The serum bone-specific alkaline phosphatase was 145 U/L, and the serum NTx was 67 BCE/L. The older brother was also diagnosed with calcium-deficiency rickets, and he also received calcium supplements.

Because the younger child was ready to be weaned from the breast, the mother was given nutritional counseling by a dietitian in the Dietetics Department of the teaching hospital to prevent the younger child from also developing calcium-deficiency rickets. The mother was also provided information regarding how to increase calcium in the diet of the entire family using locally available foods such as dried fish and baobab leaf, which contain high amounts of calcium.

BIOCHEMICAL PERSPECTIVES

Calcium accounts for 2%–4% of the gross body weight in humans. Approximately 99% of the total body calcium is in bones and teeth. Calcium, in the form of hydroxyapatite $[Ca_{10}(PO_4)_6(OH)_2]$, accounts for approximately 40% of the bone mass and, in combination with the protein components of bone, contributes to bone strength. Type 1 collagen is the most abundant extracellular protein present in bone. In addition to its role as a structural component in bone, calcium serves as an intracellular signaling molecule and is required for the normal neural excitation and relaxation of muscles. Insufficient ionized calcium in the extracellular fluid (ECF) results in tetany (continuous excitation of muscle due to hypocalcemia). Approximately 1 g of calcium is contained in the plasma and ECF bathing the cells, and about 6–8 g are found in the tissues, primarily in storage vesicles (e.g., sarcoplasmic reticulum). Serum calcium is maintained within a narrow concentration range (8.8–10.8 mg/dL) and is in

Table 30-2. Adequate Intakes* of Calcium and Vitamin D at Different Ages

Age	Calcium (mg/day)	Vitamin D[†] (µg/day)
0–6 month	210	5
7–12 month	270	5
1–3 year	500	5
4–8 year	800	5
9–18 year	1300	5
19–50 year	1000	5
51–70 year	1200	10
>70 year	1200	15
Pregnancy		
≤ 18 year	1300	5
19–50 year	1000	5
Lactation		
≤ 18 year	1300	5
19–50 year	1000	5

From Food and Nutrition Board (2000).

*Adequate intake is believed to cover the needs of all individuals in the group; lack of data prevent the ability to specify with confidence the percentage of individuals covered by this intake.

[†]In the absence of adequate exposure to sunlight; 1 µg vitamin D = 40 IU vitamin D.

equilibrium with the ECF calcium, which is on the order of 5 mg/dL. The calcium concentration of the ECF is less than that of plasma due to the lower concentration of proteins in the ECF. It is the calcium concentration in the ECF that is regulated by the vitamin D/parathyroid endocrine system.

The main sources of dietary calcium are milk and dairy products. In the United States, it is estimated that 73% of calcium is obtained from milk products, 9% from fruit and vegetables, 5% from grains, and about 12% from all other sources combined. The optimal intake of dietary calcium depends on age, gender, and physiological status and is summarized in Table 30-2.

Calcium is absorbed in the intestine by two distinct mechanisms, an active process that is vitamin D dependent and another that is vitamin D independent. When the dietary intake of calcium is low, the intestinal uptake of calcium occurs by an active transport process that is vitamin D dependent. Active transport is most efficient in the duodenum and proximal jejunum, areas of the intestine that have a pH close to 6.0 and where calbindin, a calcium transport protein, is present. However, the amount of calcium absorbed in the ileum may be greater than that absorbed in the duodenum and jejunum

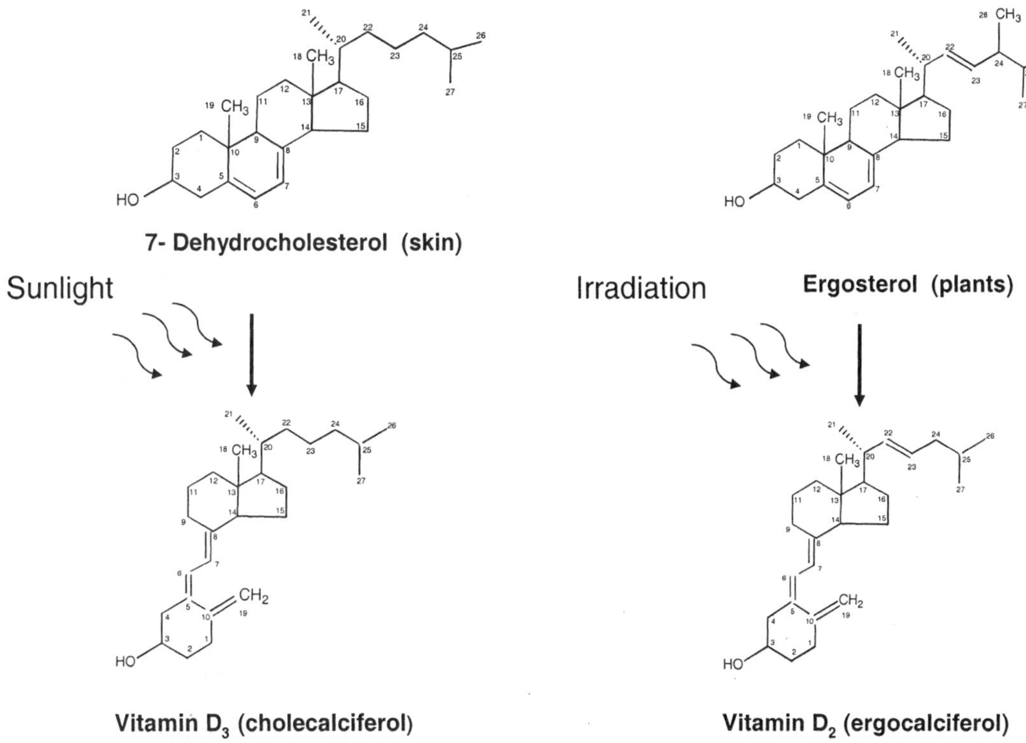

Figure 30-2. Structures of vitamin D_2 and vitamin D_3 and their precursors.

due to the longer transit time of food in this portion of the intestine. Calbindin, which is regulated by 1,25-dihydroxyvitamin D, binds two molecules of calcium on the surface of the intestinal cell. The calbindin-calcium complex is internalized via endocytosis into a lysosome, after which calcium is released in the acidic environment of the lysosome and calbindin is recycled to the cell surface. Calcium then leaves the cell via the basolateral membrane of the enterocyte and enters the blood.

When the luminal content is high, such as when a calcium supplement or food high in calcium is ingested, calcium is absorbed mainly by a nonsaturable paracellular process that is vitamin D independent. Although theoretically paracellular transport is bidirectional, the predominant direction of calcium flux is from the intestinal lumen to the blood. The rate of transport depends on the calcium load and the tightness of the intracellular junctions in the enterocyte. Water may carry calcium through the intracellular junctions by solvent drag. Citrate, when present in the intestinal lumen simultaneously with calcium, is thought to enhance the passive transport of calcium.

Both the active and passive modes of calcium transport are increased during pregnancy and lactation. This is probably due to the increase in calbindin and serum PTH and 1,25-dihydroxyvitamin D concentrations that occur during normal pregnancy. Intestinal calcium absorption is also dependent on age, with a 0.2% per year decline in absorption efficiency starting in midlife. The fractional absorption of calcium depends on the form and dietary source. Absorption rates are 29% for the calcium in cow's milk, 35% for calcium citrate, 27% for calcium carbonate, and 25% for tricalcium phosphate. Other factors that limit the bioavailability of calcium in the intestine are oxalates and phytates, which are found in high quantities in vegetarian diets and which chelate calcium.

Vitamin D is a fat-soluble vitamin; its main function is the maintenance of normal plasma levels of calcium and phosphorus (Zittermann, 2003). Vitamin D_3 is synthesized in the skin from 7-dehydrocholesterol on exposure to sunlight (290–315 nm) (Fig. 30-2). The UV light causes a rearrangement of the 5,7 diene bonds in the B ring of 7-dehydrocholesterol, resulting in a break in the B ring to form previtamin D_3.

Previtamin D_3 is thermodynamically unstable and rearranges its double bonds to form the more thermodynamically stable vitamin D_3. After synthesis, vitamin D_3 is transported to the liver by a vitamin D-binding protein, which is an α-globulin.

The efficiency of vitamin D_3 synthesis depends on the melanin content of skin and age. Melanin, a skin pigment, reduces the efficiency of vitamin D_3 synthesis in the skin because it absorbs UV light in the same region as 7-dehydrocholesterol. Although increased skin pigmentation can decrease the amount of vitamin D_3 synthesized, melanin may also protect the vitamin D which is synthesized from being destroyed as a result of sunlight exposure. Because vitamin D_3 is also converted to inactive products such as lumisterol, tachysterol, and other sterols when exposed to UV light, vitamin D_3 production in the skin plateaus after 30 min of sunlight exposure (Hollick, 1994). Therefore, extended sunlight exposure does not result in the production of toxic amounts of vitamin D_3. Approximately 80% of the required vitamin D_3 can be provided by endogenous synthesis; however, vitamin D_3 synthesis in the skin may be reduced by as much as 75% by the age of 70 years (Holick et al., 1989).

In the absence of inadequate endogenous synthesis, vitamin D must be obtained from dietary sources or from supplements. Few foods contain vitamin D except for the flesh of fatty fish (salmon, mackerel, sardines), fish liver oils, and eggs from hens fed feed enriched with vitamin D. In the United States, all commercially produced milk is fortified with vitamin D_2 at a level of 400 IU/L (1 IU = 0.025 μg of vitamin D_3). Therefore, in the United States (and other economically advanced countries) most dietary vitamin D is obtained from milk and other vitamin D_2-fortified foods. Both vitamin D_2 and vitamin D_3 are converted at the same rate to 25-hydroxyvitamin D by a hydroxylase in the liver and are equally active as a prohormone. Because dietary uptake of vitamin D is dependent on normal fat absorption, conditions in which fat malabsorption is present can result in vitamin D deficiency. Because breast milk contains little vitamin D, vitamin D deficiency can occur in infants who are solely breastfed, are not exposed to adequate sunlight, and are not receiving vitamin D supplements. The adequate intake of vitamin D for children is 5 μg/day (200 IU/day) (Table 30-2).

Although vitamin D_3 toxicity cannot be

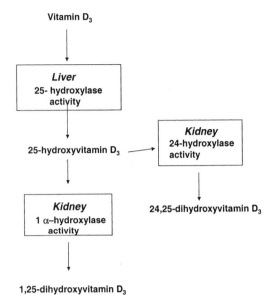

Figure 30-3. Metabolism of vitamin D.

caused by extensive exposure to sunlight, excessive dietary intake of vitamin D can result in deleterious concentrations of vitamin D. Vitamin D toxicity is characterized by hypercalcemia (elevated serum calcium concentration) and hyperphosphatemia (elevated serum phosphate concentration). The end result of hypervitaminosis D is calcinosis (calcification of soft tissues) of the kidney, heart, and lungs. Calcification of the tympanic membrane of the ear can result in deafness. The tolerable upper limit of vitamin D intake is 1000 IU/day for infants and 2000 IU/day for children and adults.

Vitamin D that is taken up by the liver is converted to 25-hydroxyvitamin D by a microsomal hydroxylase (Fig. 30-3). 25-Hydroxyvitamin D is the main circulating form of vitamin D in the serum and the best indicator of vitamin D status. Normal serum levels are 14–60 ng/mL (35–150 nmol/L). When serum calcium concentrations decline, 25-hydroxyvitamin D is converted to 1,25-dihydroxyvitmin D by 1α-hydroxylase, a mixed-function oxidase that is located in the inner mitochondrial membrane in kidney tissue and whose expression is regulated by parathyroid hormone (PTH). The main function of 1,25-dihydroxyvitamin D is to increase the intestinal absorption of dietary calcium and phosphorus. When serum concentrations of calcium and phosphorus are normal or when large doses of vitamin D are administered, 25-hydroxyvitamin D is metabolized to 24,25-dihydroxyvitamin D in the renal

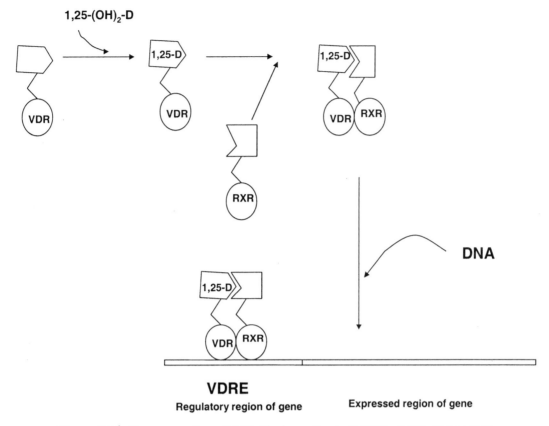

Figure 30-4. Hormone action of 1,25-dihydroxyvitamin D. VDR, vitamin D receptor; RXR, retinoic acid receptor; VDRE, vitamin D response element.

cortex. Normal levels of 24,25-dihydroxyvitamin D in the circulation are between 1 and 4 ng/mL but are not detectable in patients with vitamin D deficiency.

Tissues contain two types of receptors for 1,25-dihydroxyvitamin D: a classic steroid hormone nuclear receptor and a putative membrane receptor. 1,25-Dihydroxyvitamin D interacts with the nuclear receptor to form a receptor-ligand complex (Fig. 30-4). This complex then interacts with other nuclear proteins, such as the retinoic acid receptor (RXR) to form a functional transcription complex. The main effect of this transcription complex is to alter the amount of mRNAs coding for selected proteins such as calbindin, the calcium transport protein in the intestine, and the vitamin D receptor. In concert with PTH, 1,25-dihydroxyvitamin D acts to mobilize calcium from bone. As a consequence, serum calcium and phosphate homeostasis is maintained by a combination of 1,25-dihydroxyvitamin D stimulation of intestinal absorption and bone turnover.

Calcium homeostasis is maintained by a regulatory system comprised of vitamin D, PTH, and various feedback mechanisms (Fig. 30-5). The concentration of calcium in the ECF is monitored by a calcium receptor (CaR) present in the parathyroid gland and renal tubular cells. The CaR is a 120-kd G-protein-coupled receptor that is responsive to the concentration of extracellular calcium. At normal or elevated serum calcium concentrations, the receptor is inactive, and PTH release from the parathyroid gland is inhibited. Conversely, reducing the ECF ionized calcium concentration below the set point for CaR activation removes this inhibition and triggers PTH release. If the serum calcium concentration falls below the set point for the receptor, CaR undergoes a conformational change that removes the inhibitory pathway that triggers PTH release.

Chief cells in the parathyroid gland synthesize, store, and secrete PTH. PTH is synthesized as a pre-pro PTH precursor. The pre- and pro- segments are cleaved enzymatically during

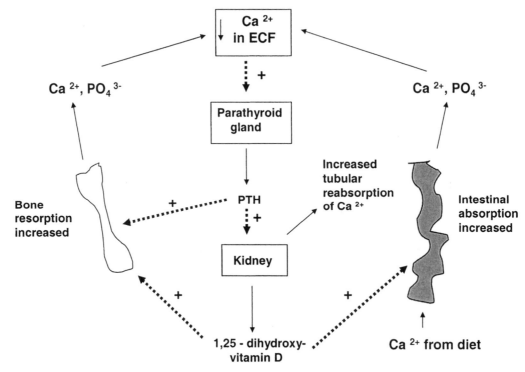

Figure 30-5. Regulation of calcium homeostasis by the combined action of 1,25-dihydroxyvitamin D and parathyroid hormone (PTH). ECF, extracellular fluid.

intracellular synthesis and processing in the Golgi apparatus. PTH is then secreted, stored, or degraded. The mature intact PTH molecule that is secreted is a 9.5-kd, 84-amino acid peptide with a half-life of less than 5 min. Intact PTH is metabolized by the liver and kidneys to generate the metabolically active 2.5-kd fragment that contains the amino terminal portion of the intact peptide, and the inactive carboxy terminal fragment, which is excreted in urine. Intact PTH accounts for only 5%–25% of the total circulating PTH.

PTH interacts with receptors located on the plasma membrane of target cells such as bone and kidney, where it increases the cAMP concentration, resulting in an increase in intracellular calcium. This increase in intracellular calcium initiates a cascade of intracellular events mediated by phospholipase C acting on phosphatidylinositol bisphosphate. Phospholipase C catalyzes the hydrolysis of phosphatidylinositol bisphosphate to diacylglycerol and inositoltrisphosphate. The primary role of PTH is to increase bone turnover to increase blood calcium. In bone, the osteoblast is the primary target of PTH. PTH regulates gene expression in

the osteoblast, promoting synthesis of matrix proteins required for new bone formation and proteins associated with matrix degradation and turnover.

Chronic exposure to PTH increases bone resorption by altering the number and activity of osteoblasts (bone-forming cells) and osteoclasts (bone-resorbing) cells. The effect of PTH on osteoclasts is indirect and is exerted through the release of local mediators produced by the osteoblast or released from the bone matrix. PTH decreases collagen synthesis in osteoblasts and increases osteclastic bone resorption, resulting in a net increase in calcium and phosphate release from bone into the ECF. The serum calcium concentration is restored to normal, but hypophosphatemia persists, and results in impaired minneralization of bone. In the absence of disease, an increase in serum calcium reduces PTH secretion through a negative-feedback loop to maintain homoeostasis.

PTH also activates renal 1α-hydroxylase, increasing the amount of the active form of vitamin D (1,25-dihydroxyvitamin D), which in turn enhances intestinal calcium absorption. In

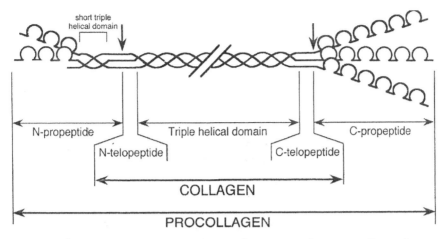

Figure 30-6. Schematic diagram of type 1 collagen. Vertical arrows indicate cleavage sites between the mature collagen molecule, the N-propeptide, and the C-propeptide. Reproduced with permission from Rossert J and de Crombrugghe B (2002).

the kidney, PTH increases calcium reabsorption in the distal tubules and decreases reabsorption of phosphate in the proximal tubule, thereby promoting phosphaturia. Approximately 85% of renal phosphorus reabsorption occurs in the proximal tubule. PTH synthesis and secretion are controlled not only by the extracellular calcium concentration but also by negative feedback inhibition by 1,25 dihydroxy-vitamin D.

Rickets can also be the result of hypophosphatemia. Because a dietary deficiency of phosphorus is very rare, hypophosphatemia is usually the result of excess phosphate excretion in the urine due to one of several rare inherited disorders such as X-linked hypophosphatemic rickets or autosomal dominant hypophosphatemic rickets. These disorders share common features, including renal phosphate wasting, low 1,25-dihydroxyvitamin D concentrations, short stature, bone pain, rickets, and osteomalacia. Mutations in the product of the PHEX gene (phosphate-regulating gene with homologies to endopeptidase on the X chromosome) have been identified as the cause of X-linked hypophosphatemic rickets. These mutations result in an excess of the hormonelike phosphatonin protein, leading to urinary phosphate leakage and ultimately hypophosphatemia (Schiavi and Kumar, 2004).

Bone is a dynamic tissue in which both bone modeling and remodeling occur. Bone modeling occurs during skeletal growth and results in an increase in bone mass. Remodeling occurs after skeletal growth has ceased and is the response to stress on the skeleton and changes in

diet (e.g., low calcium intake). Bone remodeling is also necessary for repair of minor fractures that occur in bones over time. It has been estimated that, at any one time, approximately 4% of bone is undergoing remodeling. Remodeling is initiated by the activation of osteoclasts by various cytokines that are produced by osteoblasts. Prolonged calcium deprivation results in increased recruitment of osteoclasts which catalyze the release of calcium phosphate and peptides from the bone matrix, including collagen-derived hydroxyproline and the pyridinoline collagen cross-links discussed in the next paragraph. Prolonged exposure of osteoblasts to the increased PTH level associated with calcium-deficiency eventually leads to increases in the serum concentrations of biochemical markers of bone synthesis, such as alkaline phosphatase and osteocalcin.

The principal protein in bone is type 1 collagen, a triple helix comprised of two identical α_1-chains and one α_2-chain. Collagen is synthesized as precursor type 1 procollagen, containing both N- and C-terminal extensions (Fig. 30-6). Procollagen undergoes posttranslational processing reactions that include hydroxylation of proline and lysine residues, glycosylation, and formation of interchain disulfide bonds. After it is secreted, procollagen is converted to collagen by extracellular processing involving enzymatic cleavage of the N- and C-propeptides (Fig. 30-7). Three amino acid side chains react to form a trivalent amino acid structure that contains a pyridinium ring. Deoxypyridinoline is formed from two hydroxylysyl residues

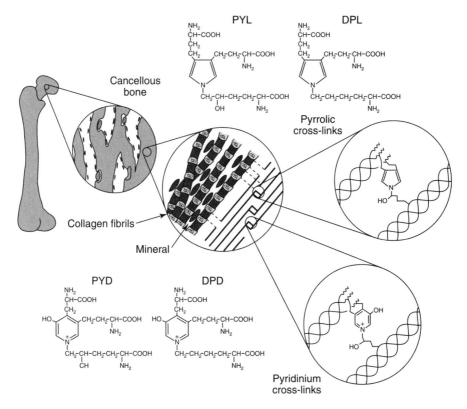

Figure 30-7. Stabilization of bone matrix by pyridinium and pyrroline cross-links. PYD, pyridinoline cross-link; DPD, deoxypyridinoline cross-link. Reproduced with permission from Rossert J and de Crombrugghe B (2002).

and one lysyl residue, whereas pyridinoline is formed when three hydroxylysyl moieties combine to form a cross-link. Deoxypyridinoline occurs in bone, dentine, ligaments, and aorta, whereas pyridinoline is more widespread in hard connective tissues that also contain large amounts of soft cartilage. Since these cross-links are formed in mature collagen and are not further metabolized after bone resorption, they can be used as markers of bone turnover.

Markers of bone resorption can be measured in serum or urine, whereas bone formation markers, such as bone-specific alkaline phosphatase, are usually measured in serum. Measurement of bone markers allows for real-time assessment of bone resorption or formation and can be used to monitor therapy (Ravn et al., 2003). The pyridonolines (deoxypyridinoline and pyridinoline) and the N- and C-teleopeptides are the most frequently measured markers of bone resorption. Pyridinoline and teleopeptides (NTx and CTx) are increased in individuals with metabolic bone diseases associated with increased bone resorption, such as osteomalacia and primary hyperparathyroidism, and they are decreased in individuals with hypoparathyroidism.

Alkaline phosphatases from liver, bone, and kidney are members of an isozyme family. Tissue-specific isoforms are produced by tissue-specific posttranslational processing. Because osteoblasts are the source of bone-specific alkaline phosphatase (BSAP) and serum levels of this isoenzyme reflect osteoblast activity, BSAP can be used as a marker of bone formation. It has a relatively long half-life (1–2 days) and is unaffected by diurnal variation. Reference intervals for adults are 7–30 U/L and are dependent on age and gender. Children have much higher levels of BSAP activity, especially during growth spurts.

THERAPY

The type of therapy for rickets depends on the specific cause of the disease. For patients with pure vitamin D deficiency due to lack of exposure to sunlight or inadequate dietary intake, treatment with oral preparations of vitamin D or natural sources rich in the vitamin, such as fish oil, can be used. Conventional treatment consists of the administration of 2000–5000 IU/day of vitamin D until the serum alkaline phosphatase levels returns to normal or radiology shows signs of bone healing. This usually takes from 2 to 10 weeks. Thereafter, maintenance is achieved with 400 IU/day vitamin D or 800–1200 IU/day if the patient is also taking anticonvulsants. Assuming laboratory facilities are available, one can monitor serum levels of calcium, phosphate, and alkaline phosphatase. Alternatively, but less commonly, the 25-hydroxy form of vitamin D (20–50 μg/day) or 1,25-dihydroxivitamin D (0.5–1 μg/day) can be given. For type 1 vitamin D-deficiency rickets, the treatment consists of 1,25-dihydroxyvitamin D. Patients with type 2 vitamin D-resistant rickets, are treated with large doses of calcium supplements.

In West Africa and many other regions of sub-Saharan Africa where lack of adequate dietary calcium is the main cause of rickets, the goal of immediate therapy is to provide the rachitic child with 1000–1500 mg of calcium per day for 6 months to promote bone healing. This can be accomplished through calcium replacement therapy using daily calcium carbonate supplements or three to four glasses of milk per day, depending on which is more economically feasible. Each 250 mL of milk provides 300 mg calcium. The effectiveness of the calcium therapy should be monitored weekly, as described in the Diagnosis section.

The major emphasis should be the prevention of rickets by providing adequate calcium and vitamin D in the diet, particularly if exposure to sunlight is restricted. One teaspoon (4 mL) of cod-liver oil provides 360 IU of vitamin D. In developing countries where dairy products are prohibitively expensive, local foods such as dried fish containing small soft bones can add to the calcium intake (Larsen et al., 2000).

QUESTIONS

1. Assume that you are a public health official in northern Nigeria. What actions might you take at the population level to reduce the risk and incidence of calcium-deficiency rickets in the region?

2. How would you distinguish if a child's rickets was caused by inadequate dietary calcium versus a deficiency of vitamin D?

3. Assume that a 30-year-old man who had been in good health previously develops an ectopic PTH-producing tumor. What are the biochemical and pathological changes you would expect to find in this patient?

4. What are the consequences of a genetic deficiency of 1α-hydroxylase on the bone status of an individual, and what treatment would be appropriate for a patient with this disorder?

5. How would a mutation that inactivates the parathyroid calcium receptor (CaR) affect calcium homeostasis?

6. How can biochemical markers be used to assess the therapeutic efficacy of drugs to treat osteoporosis?

BIBLIOGRAPHY

Food and Nutrition Board: *Dietary Reference Intakes: Applications in Dietary Assessment*. Institute of Medicine, National Academy Press, Washington, DC, 2000.

Hollick MF: Vitamin D: importance in the prevention of cancers, type 1 diabetes, heart disease, and osteoporosis. *Am J Clin Nutr* 79:362–371, 2004.

Holick MF, Matsuoka LY, Wortman J: Age, vitamin D and solar ultraviolet. *Lancet* 2:1104–1105, 1989.

Holick MF: McCollum Award Lecture, Vitamin D: new horizons for the 21st century. *Am J Cin Nutr* 60:619–630, 1994.

Jergas M, Genant HK: Radiologic imaging of metabolic bone disease, *in* Coe FL, Favus MJ (eds): *Disorders of Bone and Mineral Metabolism*. Lippincott Williams and Williams, Philadelphia, 2002, pp. 428–447.

Larsen T, Thilsted SH, Kongsback K, et al.: Whole small fish as a rich calcium source. *Br J Nutr* 83:191–196, 2000.

Ravn P, Thompson DE, Ross PD, et al.: Biochemical markers for prediction of 4-year response in bone mass during bisphosphonate treatment for prevention of postmenopausal osteoporosis. *Bone* 33:150–158, 2003.

Rossert J, de Crombrugghe B: Type 1 collagen: structure, synthesis, and regulation, *in* Bilezikian JP, Raisz LG, Rodan GA (eds): *Principles of Bone Biology*. Academic Press, San Diego, CA, 2002, pp. 189–210.

Schiavi SC, Kumar R: The phosphatonin pathway: new insights in phosphate homeostasis. *Kidney Int* 65:1–14, 2004.

Thacher T: Calcium-deficiency rickets. *Endocr Dev* 6:105–125, 2003.

Tsai K-S, Jang M-H, Hsu S H-J, et al.: Bone alkaline phosphatase isoenzyme and carboxy-terminal propeptide of type 1 procollagen in healthy Chinese girls and boys. *Clin Chem* **45:**136–138, 1999.

Wharton B, Bishop N: Rickets. *Lancet* **362:**1389–1400, 2003.

World Health Organization: *Measuring Changes in Nutritional Status.* World Health Organization, Geneva, Switzerland, 1983.

Zittermann A: Vitamin D in preventive medicine: are we ignoring the evidence? *Br J Nutr* **89:**552–572, 2003.

31

Hereditary Hemochromatosis

SCOTT A. FINK and RAYMOND T. CHUNG

CASE PRESENTATION

A 46-year-old Caucasian man was referred to the gastroenterology clinic for evaluation of abnormal liver chemistries. The patient had initially presented to his primary care physician 1 month earlier complaining of new-onset fatigue, impotence, and diminished libido. He denied any abdominal pain, confusion, or change in skin color. He did note a recent 10-pound weight loss.

The patient had recently immigrated to the United States from Scotland. He claimed only social use of alcohol and denied any illicit drug use. He worked at a bank and denied exposure to toxic materials.

His primary care physician obtained the following serum tests, which indicated liver damage: alanine aminotransferase 103 U/L (reference 10-55 U/L); aspartate aminotransferase 967 U/L (reference 10-55 U/L); alkaline phosphatase level 125 U/L (reference 45-115 U/L); and total bilirubin 0.8 mg/dL (reference 0-1.0 mg/dL). In addition, the serum glucose level was 711 mg/dL (reference 30-100 mg/dL). Decreased levels of follicle-stimulating and luteinizing hormones were also noted.

On further testing, the patient displayed the biochemical signs of iron overload. He had a serum iron of 197 mg/dL (reference 30-360 µg/dL), a total iron binding capacity of 202 µg/dL (reference 228-428 µg/dL), and a ferritin level of 4890 ng/mL (reference 30-300 ng/mL). His serum transferrin saturation was calculated to be 97.5% (reference 20%-50%).

A liver biopsy was performed and revealed advanced-stage cirrhosis and hemosiderosis with marked iron deposition in hepatocytes, Kupffer cells, and bile ducts. Hepatic iron concentration was determined to be 37,880 µg/g dry weight (reference 200-2400 µg/g dry weight).

A diagnosis of hemochromatosis was established, and the patient was tested for HFE gene mutations. He was homozygous for the C282Y mutation.

The patient was begun on a phlebotomy program, a therapy in which whole blood is taken from the patient intravenously, to remove the excess iron from his blood, eventually leading to iron equilibrium. His libido improved, he has achieved better glycemic control, and he normalized his liver chemistries.

Given the diagnosis of hereditary hemochromatosis (HH), his two siblings were tested for HFE mutations. Both were heterozygous for the C282Y mutation and showed no evidence of iron overload.

DIAGNOSIS

Abnormally high systemic iron levels can lead to cirrhosis of the liver, diabetes mellitus, and heart failure. Although a number of disease processes can lead to iron overload, this chapter focuses on hereditary hemochromatosis, the prototypical disease of iron overload.

The most common Mendelian genetic disorder in Caucasians, HH is estimated to occur with a prevalence of approximately 1 in 200. Among Caucasians, cases are concentrated in those of northern European origin, specifically individuals of Nordic or Celtic ancestry (Tavill, 2001).

Iron stores are maintained in a delicate balance, controlled primarily at the level of absorption. It is hypothesized that an increase in the iron regulatory "set point" promotes excessive dietary iron absorption in individuals with HH despite already elevated iron stores (Parkkila, 2001).

Patients with HH who have developed iron overload can present with fatigue, malaise, abdominal pain, arthralgias, and impotence. However, the majority of patients are asymptomatic at the time that serum indices of iron overload are first seen (Bacon, 2001).

Once iron overload has been present for many years, organ damage occurs. Patients develop arthritis, cirrhosis, congestive heart failure, increased skin pigmentation, cardiac arrhythmias, and diabetes as a result of pancreatic islet cell infiltration. Physical examination of patients with mild iron overload is generally benign. Those with full-blown hemochromatosis often exhibit hepatomegaly; stigmata of chronic liver disease, including characteristic skin lesions; splenomegaly; and in patients with cardiomegaly, findings associated with congestive heart failure. In addition, patients whose endocrine system is affected may have testicular atrophy or signs of hypogonadism and hypothyroidism (Bacon, 2001).

The diagnosis of HH is established based on serum transferrin saturation (TS), defined as serum iron divided by total iron binding capacity (TIBC). Since serum iron and ferritin levels lack specificity for diagnosis when used alone, measurement of fasting TS is currently recommended as a first screen to detect iron overload. TS is the best indirect biochemical marker of iron stores. A fasting TS of greater than 45% will detect over 98% of all cases of phenotypic hemochromatosis (Tavill, 2001).

Once serum TS is determined to be greater than 45% and the serum ferritin elevated, a polymerase chain reaction (PCR) based gene test for HH is recommended. Two genotypic profiles are consistent with the diagnosis of HH: homozygosity for the C282Y mutation or compound heterozygosity with a C282Y/H63D genotype. If homozygosity for the C282Y mutation is detected, then PCR testing should be offered to first-degree relatives of the proband (Tavill, 2001).

If liver disease is suggested either biochemically or clinically, then the liver should be biopsied to establish the presence of advanced fibrosis or cirrhosis, to rule out iron overload in the liver when serum markers of iron overload are equivocal, or to investigate other causes of liver disease (Tavill, 2001).

BIOCHEMICAL PERSPECTIVES

The French pathologist Trousseau first described a patient with hemochromatosis in 1865. Four years later, the German pathologist Von Recklinghausen (1889) coined the phrase hemochromatosis when describing a patient with pigmentation ("chrom") thought to be caused by a factor in the bloodstream ("hemo").

Not until 1996 did Feder and colleagues identify a novel major histocompatibility complex (MHC) class I-like gene in which homozygosity for specific mutations were found in 83% of patients with hemochromatosis.

In 1998, Zhou and colleagues used an HFE knockout mouse model to elegantly bring together the pathophysiological and molecular aspects of the disease. Even when fed a standard diet, the knockout mice showed abnormally high transferrin saturations and excessive iron deposition in the liver and passed these traits on in an autosomally recessive manner.

A perspective on normal iron metabolism is necessary for understanding the biochemistry of HH. The healthy adult body has a total iron content of 3–5 g of iron, two thirds of which is incorporated in erythrocytes and precursors in their lineage (Pietrangelo, 2002). Only 1–2 mg of iron, 10% of the total ingested from the diet, is absorbed daily (Parkkila et al., 2001). Each day, 1–2 mg of iron leaves the body through processes such as menstruation and sloughing of skin (Pietrangelo, 2002).

Approximately 20 mg of iron is required daily for erythropoiesis. The iron requirements are supplied by recycled iron and from residual body iron stores. One major store is in hepatocytes where 0.5–1 g of iron is bound to specialized proteins such as ferritin and hemosiderin. Ferritin is a large, 440-kd cellular storage protein for iron. Measurement of plasma ferritin is seen as a reflection of the cellular ferritin stores, which in turn reflects cellular iron stores. Body stores of iron are maintained by recycling: Senescent erythrocytes are ingested by macrophages, and their iron is taken up by serum transferrin. The iron is delivered to the bone marrow, where it once again will be incorporated into erythrocytes (Pietrangelo, 2002).

Iron levels are tightly regulated through control of dietary absorption of iron. The duodenum and upper jejunum are the only areas of the body where this occurs. Since nonheme iron forms insoluble complexes when ingested, it must first be converted into soluble complexes. This is accomplished on the apical surface of duodenal villus enterocytes by duodenal ferric reductase, which converts insoluble duodenal ferric (Fe^{3+}) iron into soluble and absorbable ferrous (Fe^{2+}) iron. Iron is then transported across the membrane to the cytoplasm through a transporter known as the divalent metal transporter 1 (DMT-1), a proton symporter (Harrison and Bacon, 2003).

Once absorbed, iron becomes part of the cellular iron pool, either stored as ferritin or transported across the basolateral membrane of the enterocyte into the circulation by an iron transporter called ferroportin 1. Hephaestin, a basolateral membrane ferroxidase, oxidizes the ferrous iron back to its ferric form, thus completing the absorption process (Harrison and Bacon, 2003).

In the bloodstream, ferric iron binds tightly to circulating plasma transferrin (TF) to form diferric transferrin (FeTF). Absorption of iron into erythrocytes depends on basolateral membrane receptor-mediated endocytosis of FeTF by transferrin receptor 1 (TfR 1). FeTF binds to TfR 1 on the surface of erythroid precursors. These complexes invaginate in pits on the cell surface to form endosomes. Proton pumps within the endosomes lower pH to promote the release of iron into the cytoplasm from transferrin. Once the cycle is completed, TF and TfR 1 are recycled back to the cell surface. TF and TfR 1 play similar roles in iron absorption at the basolateral membrane of crypt enterocytes (Parkilla et al., 2001; Pietrangelo, 2002).

Iron transport across the intestinal cell occurs at both the apical and basolateral interfaces. Figure 31-1 highlights the importance of this polarity in both iron transport into the cell and the sensing of iron stores in both the villus and crypt enterocytic apical and basolateral interfaces. The apical membrane is specialized to transport heme and ferrous iron into the cell through three major pathways. The first is via DMT-1, which transports ferrous iron and divalent metal ions into the enterocyte. Iron can also be absorbed as the intact heme moiety,

which after easily passing through the brush border of the apical membrane intact, is broken down by heme oxygenase into elemental iron. Finally, intestinal mucins and other proteins such as mobilferrin, integrins, and ferric reductase can transport iron directly across the apical membrane (Parkkila et al., 2001).

The need for iron by erythrocytes dictates the direction of body iron stores and is the body's iron supply priority. Duodenal epithelial cells must be kept programmed to respond to these requirements and to the status of the body's iron deposits (Pietrangelo, 2002). The defect in the molecular iron absorptive machinery in HH is thought to be localized within the interplay between the enterocyte and body iron stores. The "stores regulator" hypothesis describes a pathway that would facilitate a slow accumulation of dietary iron and would prevent iron overload after iron stores are deemed adequate. Potentially involving TF-bound iron, serum ferritin, and serum TF, the stores regulator is thought to be impaired in individuals with HH. It has been shown, for example, that after phlebotomy in patients with HH, there is an increase in intestinal absorption of iron that persists even after adequate iron stores are replenished. This implies that the defect rests not with abnormally functioning absorptive machinery, but with abnormal feedback from the body's stores regulator, which either is unable to recognize the replenishment of adequate iron stores or cannot communicate this information to the small intestine (Parkkila et al., 2001).

The HFE gene, mutations of which are responsible for HH, codes for a novel MHC class I-like protein that requires interaction with β_2-microglobulin for normal presentation to the cell surface (Bacon, 2001). Located on the short arm of chromosome 6, it has been detected by immunohistochemistry in small-intestinal cryptal enterocytes (Parkilla et al., 2001).

The protein encoded by the HFE gene is a 343-amino acid protein consisting of a 22-amino acid signal peptide, a large extracellular domain, a single transmembrane domain, and a short cytoplasmic tail (Fig. 31-2). As Figure 31-2 shows, the extracellular domain includes three loops (α_1, α_2, and α_3) with intramolecular disulfide bonds within the second and third loops, a structure similar to other MHC class I proteins (Feder et al., 1996).

The two most common mutations, C282Y and H63D, are in the extracellular domain. The

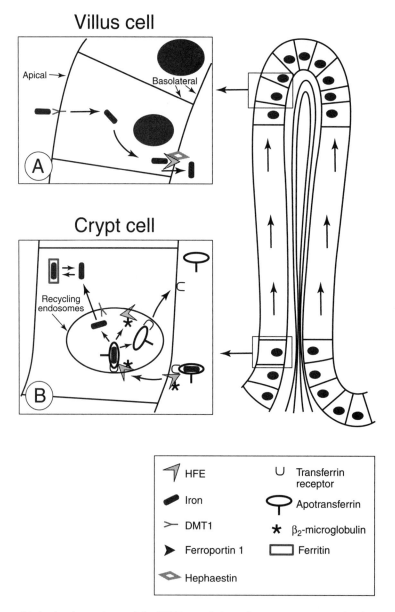

Figure 31-1. A schematic model of HFE regulation of iron transport in duodenal enterocytes. *A* and *B* correspond to villus and cryptal enterocytes, respectively. As noted, HFE lies at the center of regulation of iron absorption through its role in sensing body iron stores in the villus enterocyte. It communicates this information to the crypt enterocyte indirectly through regulation of development of ferroportin and DMT-1. Reprinted with permission from Parkkila et al. (2001). © 2001, American Gastroenterological Association.

C282Y mutation represents a change from cysteine to tyrosine at amino acid 282, while the H63D mutation is a substitution of aspartate for histidine at amino acid 63 (Feder et al., 1996). It has been estimated that 83%–100% of patients with HH are homozygous for C282Y (Bacon and Briton, 2003).

Ten to fifteen percent of Caucasians of European ancestry are heterozygous for the C282Y mutation. It has been suggested that

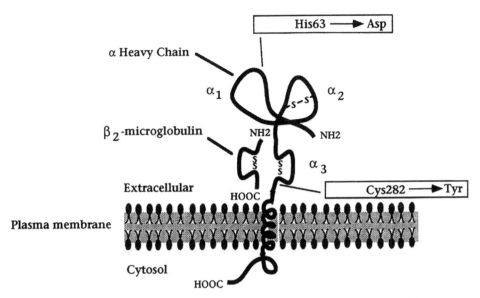

Figure 31-2. Model of HFE protein. The HFE protein shares structural similarities to other MHC class I proteins. The locations of the two most common mutations are noted. Reprinted with permission Feder et al. (1996).

the mutation originated in Celts and spread to northern Europe, perhaps imparting an advantage at a time when dietary iron availability was either poor or impaired by parasitic infection (Bacon and Britton, 2003).

The HFE protein interacts with TfR 1, a protein known to be involved in iron metabolism, at the HFE-β_2 microglobulin complex (Parkilla 2001). By abolishing a disulfide bond in the α_3 loop of HFE's transmembrane domain, the C282Y mutation interferes with this interaction (Feder et al., 1996). HFE binds TfR 1 with an affinity similar to that of transferrin (Pietrangelo, 2002). While binding to TfR 1 is not required for targeting of HFE to the basolateral membrane, it is required for HFE to be transported to transferrin-positive endosomes for regulation of intracellular iron homeostasis (see Fig. 31-1). The biological effect of HFE on TfR may be exerted in the endosomal compartment, where iron is released from the TfR-TF complex (Parkkila et al., 2001).

As the primary site of iron absorption, the duodenum shows a distinctive pattern of HFE expression: HFE is highly expressed in crypt but not villus duodenal cells (Parkilla et al., 2001). As the absorption of ferrous iron from the diet is principally mediated by DMT-1 at the villus tip, a connection between abnormal HFE and overexpression of DMT-1 has been hypothesized. While the DMT-1 protein is expressed

primarily in villus cells, mRNA expression for DMT1 begins in crypt cells. Mutated HFE may lead to decreased uptake of plasma iron by crypt cells, thus diminishing the intracellular iron pool. This might in turn result in increased expression of mRNA for DMT-1 and ferroportin 1 in villus enterocytes that mature from crypt enterocytes. This hypothesis would link dysfunctional HFE in crypt cells to overabsorption of iron in villus cells (Bacon, 2001).

An intriguing question has been what role, if any, the liver plays in sensing and regulating iron absorption. As the liver also expresses the HFE protein and is a major iron-storing organ, a defective signaling mechanism related to abnormal HFE has been postulated as a cause of iron overabsorption. For many years, however, there was little understanding of possible mechanisms for signaling between the liver and the small intestine.

Recent studies have characterized a 25-amino acid, 2- to 3-kd circulating peptide of hepatic origin called hepcidin. Hepcidin is thought to have anti-inflammatory properties perhaps related to its ability to downregulate iron stores. It has been shown that hepatic expression of hepcidin mRNA is significantly lower in patients with hemochromatosis when compared with controls. Hepcidin mRNA expression has also been shown to be decreased in HFE knockout mice. These data suggest that

$$LH + R^{\cdot} \rightarrow L^{\cdot} + RH$$

$$L^{\cdot} + O_2 \rightarrow LOO^{\cdot}$$

$$LOO^{\cdot} + LH \rightarrow LOOH + L^{\cdot}$$

$$LOOH + Fe^{2+}/Fe^{3+} \rightarrow alkanes$$

alkanals

alkenals

4-hydroxyls

Figure 31-3. Free radicals resulting from the reaction of ferric iron with hydrogen peroxide can progress to damage cell membranes through lipid peroxidation (Britton, 1996). LH = polyunsaturated fatty acid; R = free radical; LOO = lipid peroxyl radical; LOOH = lipid peroxide.

circulating hepcidin produced in the liver may play a role in inhibiting iron absorption in the small bowel, and that this effect is suppressed in patients with HFE mutations (Bridle et al., 2003).

Without a mechanism for its excretion, iron accumulates in vital organs (Pietrangelo, 2002). Because the liver binds both circulating nontransferrin and transferrin-bound iron, the liver is at particular risk for iron overload. Excess iron causes damage to hepatocytes primarily through induction of oxidative stress (Parkilla et al., 2001).

During a cell's normal life cycle under aerobic conditions, some of the consumed oxygen is reduced to highly reactive molecules called reactive oxygen species (ROS). Transition metal ions such as iron, with their frequently unpaired electrons, act as excellent catalysts for the creation of ROS. The body's inability to modulate "free iron" availability creates an environment prone to the formation of ROS and free-radical induced cellular damage in the event of iron overload. The "classical" reaction between Fe^{3+} and superoxide ($O_2^{\cdot-}$) is known as the Haber-Weiss reaction:

$$Fe^{3+} + O_2^{\cdot-} \rightarrow Fe^{2+} + O_2$$

$$H_2O_2 + Fe^{2+} \rightarrow OH\bullet + OH^- + Fe^{3+}$$

Figure 31-3 shows the common biochemical reactions responsible for the initiation of free radicals (Pietrangelo, 2002). ROS are highly heterogeneous in terms of half-life and reactivity against cellular targets. Common ROS include H_2O_2, singlet molecular oxygen ($^1O_2$), hydroxyl (OH•), superoxide ($O_2^{\cdot-}$), alkoxyl (RO•), peroxyl (ROO•), and nitric oxide radicals (NO•). ROS play important physiological roles in normal signal transduction pathways, mitochondrial respiration, and transcriptional factor activity (Pietrangelo, 1998).

These free radicals are extremely reactive and capable of attacking cell constituents. Polyunsaturated fatty acids found in membrane phospholipids, proteins, and nucleic acids are all vulnerable targets (Pietrangelo, 1998). Cellular antioxidant defenses exist to breakdown ROS. Owing to these defenses, a severe iron burden is necessary to cause damage (Pietrangelo, 2002).

Fibrosis of the liver is caused by the excessive accumulation of extracellular matrix (ECM) components. These include interstitial collagens, noncollagenous glycoproteins such as fibronectin, laminin, undulin, entactin, vitronectin, and proteoglycans. They normally provide cohesiveness for cells, promote normal tissue architecture, and play roles in normal cell function and differentiation. Chaotic expansion of the ECM leads to pathological disruption of the histological architecture of the liver and replacement of hepatocytes and bile ductules with ECM. Cytokines, growth hormones, and other biological peptides promote expansion of the ECM (Pietrangelo, 1998).

During the fibrogenic process, Kupffer cells and invading monocytes stimulate fibrogenesis through release of soluble factors such as transforming growth factor β (TGF-β), platelet-derived growth factor (PDGF), and chemokines, which activate a subpopulation of cells called hepatic stellate cells as shown in Figure 31-4. Once activated, hepatic stellate cells undergo a myofibroblastlike transformation. Iron can directly promote activation of hepatic stellate cells by accumulating in monocytes and Kupffer cells (Pietrangelo, 1996).

In addition to its effects on the promotion of ROS formation and fibrogenesis, iron is directly toxic to hepatocytes and causes hepatocellular necrosis (sideronecrosis). Iron also acts as a cofactor in the promotion of fibrogenesis by other hepatotoxins such as alcohol and viruses (Pietrangelo, 1998).

Iron damages hepatocellular organelles. Mitochondria exposed to excessive iron show increased fragility, increased volume, increased pH, decreased fluidity, and increased lipid peroxidation (Britton, 1996). Lysosomes exposed to iron overload show increased fragility and

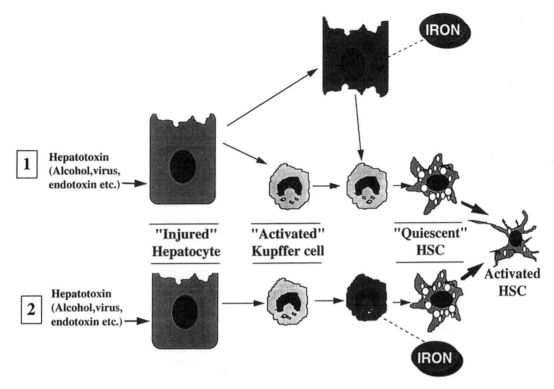

Figure 31-4. Hepatic stellate cell activation. Iron-induced injury to hepatocytes can activate Kupffer cells through the release of soluble growth factors that contribute to scarring of the liver through activation of hepatic stellate cells (HSC). Reprinted with permission from Pietrangelo (1998). © 1998, European Association for the Study of the Liver.

release of hydrolytic enzymes directly into the cytoplasm, further promoting cellular damage.

THERAPY

Hereditary hemochromatosis evolves clinically in a series of stages. In the first stage, from 0 to 20 years of age, there is clinically insignificant iron accumulation of less than 5 g of parenchymal iron. After 20–40 years of life, approximately 10–20 g of iron accumulates, and iron overload is evident in the bloodstream. Disease is still not evident clinically. Finally, after approximately 40 years of iron accumulation, more than 20 g of iron accumulates, and the patient progresses to the stage of iron overload with organ damage. In its final stages, HH can lead to decompensated cirrhosis, hepatocellular carcinoma, diabetes mellitus, and cardiomyopathy (Tavill, 2001).

Once iron overload is established, current recommendations are to proceed with phlebotomy. Ideally, phlebotomy should be initiated before the onset of clinically significant disease. Once symptoms set in, the malaise, fatigue, skin pigmentation, and abdominal pain can be reversed with phlebotomy. However, hemochromatosis-associated arthropathy, hypogonadism, and cirrhosis are less responsive to therapeutic phlebotomy.

As with other end-organ damage, diabetes mellitus can be prevented if phlebotomy is initiated prior to pancreatic damage. It is important to note that, while phlebotomy may reduce insulin requirements, hemochromatosis-associated diabetes with onset prior to initiation of phlebotomy will likely continue (Tavill, 2001). Diabetes mellitus remains a major cause of death in patients with noncirrhotic HH, occurring seven times more frequently in patients with HH when compared with normal controls (Niederau et al., 1985).

Routine therapeutic phlebotomy, with a goal of the removal of 500 mL of whole blood (approximately 200–250 mg of iron) weekly or biweekly, should be continued until iron-limited erythropoiesis develops. This is marked by the failure of hemoglobin and hematocrit to re-cover before the next phlebotomy. Transferrin saturation and ferritin levels are monitored peri-odically to predict the return to normal iron stores (Tavill, 2001).

QUESTIONS

1. What organs are most commonly affected in patients with HH?
2. What are the genetics of hereditary of HH?
3. How does the HFE protein normally con-tribute to maintenance of iron stores at normal levels, and how could mutations affect this?
4. Describe the mechanisms by which iron may by toxic to the liver.
5. What are ROS, and how does iron func-tion as a cofactor in their development?
6. How is HH treated?

BIBLIOGRAPHY

Bacon BR: Hemochromatosis: diagnosis and man-agement. *Gastroenterology* **120**:718–725, 2001.

Bacon BR, Britton RS: Hemochromatosis and other iron storage disorders, *in* Schiff ER, Sorrell MF, Maddrey WC, et al. (eds): *Schiff's Diseases of the Liver*. Philadelphia, Lippincott Williams and Wilkins, 2003, pp. 1187–1205.

Bridle KR, Frazer DM, Wilkins SJ, et al.: Disrupted hepcidin regulation in HFE-associated he-mochromatosis and the liver as a regulator of iron homeostasis. *Lancet* **361**:669–673, 2003.

Britton RS. Metal-induced hepatotoxicity. *Sem Liver Dis* **16**:3–12, 1996.

Feder JN, Gnirke A, Thomas W, et al.: A novel MHC class-1-like gene is mutated in patients with hereditary haemochromatosis. *Nat Genet* **13**:399–408, 1996.

Harrison SA, Bacon BR: Hereditary hemochromato-sis: update for 2003. *J Hepatol* **38**:S14–S23, 2003.

Niederau, Fischer R, Sonnenberg A, et al.: Survival and causes of death in cirrhotic and in noncir-rhotic patients with primary hemochromatosis *N Engl J Med* **313**:1256–1262, 1985.

Parkkila S, Niemela O, Britton RS, et al.: Molecular aspects of iron absorption and HFE expression. *Gastroenterology* **121**:1489–1496, 2001.

Pietrangelo A: Metals, oxidative stress, and hepatic fibrogenesis. *Sem Liver Dis* **16**:13–30, 1996.

Pietrangelo A: Iron, oxidative stress, and liver fibro-genesis. *J Hepatol* **28**:8–13, 1998.

Pietrangelo A: Physiology of iron transport and the hemochromatosis gene. *Am J Physiol Gastroin-test Liver Physiol* **282**:G403–G414, 2002.

Pietrangelo A: Non-HFE hemochromatosis. *Semin Liver Dis* **25**:450–460, 2005.

Tavill AS: Diagnosis and management of hemochro-matosis. *Hepatology* **33**:1321–1328, 2001.

Trousseau A: Glycosurie, diabete sucre, *in Clinique medicale de l'Hotel-Dieu de Paris*. Vol. 2, 2nd ed. Balliere, Paris, 1865, p. 663.

Von Recklinghausen FD: Uber hamochromatose. Tageblatt der Versammlung Deutsch. *Natur-forsch Arzte Heidelberg* 324–325, 1889.

Zhou XY, Tomatsu S, Fleming RE, et al.: HFE gene knockout produces mouse model of hereditary hemochromatosis. *Proc Natl Acad Sci USA* **95**:2492–2497, 1998.

Part V

Endocrinology and Integration of Metabolism

32

Type 1 Diabetes Mellitus

SRINIVAS PANJA, ARUNA CHELLIAH, and MARK R. BURGE

Diabetes mellitus is a group of metabolic diseases characterized by hyperglycemia. This can result from defects in insulin secretion, defects in insulin action, or both. Because glucose is a chemically reactive molecule, the chronic hyperglycemia of diabetes is associated with long-term damage, dysfunction, and, ultimately, failure of various organs. These include the eyes, the kidneys, the nervous system, and the cardiovascular system. Several pathogenic processes are involved in the development of diabetes. These range from autoimmune destruction of the β-cells of the pancreas with consequent insulin deficiency (type 1 diabetes, about 10% of cases) to poorly characterized abnormalities that result in resistance to insulin action combined with inadequate insulin secretion (type 2 diabetes, about 90% of cases). Regardless of mechanism, the ultimate basis of known abnormalities in carbohydrate, fat, and protein metabolism in diabetes is the deficient action of insulin on target tissues.

CASE REPORT

Initial Presentation

A 19-year-old girl was brought to the emergency department by her parents who reported that she had been vomiting and feeling weak for 24 h. The patient complained of feeling lethargic and fatigued for a few weeks. She had lost weight despite having a good appetite. Despite drinking large volumes of water, she continued to feel thirsty all the time. She also complained of an increased frequency of urination during the day and at night. Her parents said that she had been having a mild fever and a sore throat for 2–3 days, and that the day before she had started vomiting and had not been able to get out of bed by herself.

Her past medical history was unremarkable, and she was not currently taking any medications. She had regular menstrual periods and denied smoking, alcohol use, or recreational drug use. The patient's father had type 2 diabetes, and he was concerned that some of her symptoms were similar to what he experienced at the time his diabetes was diagnosed.

Physical Examination

The patient was a young girl lying in bed, breathing rapidly. Her pulse was 108 beats per minute (normal is less than 80), and her blood pressure was 94/56 mm Hg supine and 72/48 mm Hg sitting (normal is less than 140/90 with no decrease on postural adjustment). Her temperature was 97.4°F (normal is 98.6°F), and she was breathing at a rate of 34 breaths per minute (normal is less than 20). Her reported height was 5 ft 6 inches, and she presently weighed 110 pounds, but her usual weight was 125 pounds. She had poor skin turgor and dry mucous membranes. She had a fruity odor on her breath. There was no thyromegaly (enlargement of the thyroid gland), and the cardiopulmonary examination was unremarkable. Her abdomen was diffusely tender, but pelvic examination was normal. She responded to questions appropriately, although she was slow to answer. There were no neurological

Table 32-1. Laboratory and Radiological Evaluation of Case Study*

Capillary blood glucose in the emergency department: "High"

Arterial blood gas:

   pH = 7.15 (7.35–7.45)

   pO_2 = 84 mm Hg (83–108)

   pCO_2 = 24 mm Hg (32–48)

   HCO_{3-} = 14 mmol/L (22–28)

White cell count: 19,500/mm³

Sodium: 128 mmol/L (134–148)

Potassium: 5.0 mmol/L (3.5–5.0)

HCO_{3-}: 15 mmol/L (22–28)

Chloride: 90 mmol/L (96–106)

Plasma glucose: 28.2 mmol/L (3.6–6.1)

BUN: 8.9 mmol/L (2.6–6.43)

Creatinine: 176.8 µmol/L (80–132)

Serum ketones: Strongly positive

HbA_{1C}: 12.6% (4.4%–5.8%)

Urinanalysis: Glucose +5, ketones +3

Chest radiograph: Normal

*Numbers in parentheses indicate the normal range.

deficits. Results of the laboratory evaluation are shown in Table 32-1.

DIAGNOSIS

The patient was suffering from newly diagnosed type 1 diabetes and one of its common metabolic decompensations, diabetic ketoacidosis (DKA).

The diagnosis of type 1 diabetes is made by a combination of typical clinical features and laboratory tests. The American Diabetes Association (ADA) and World Health Organization diagnostic criteria for diabetes mellitus are shown in Table 32-2. The diagnosis of diabetes mellitus can be made on the basis of classic symptoms, including polyuria (frequent urination), polydipsia (frequent water drinking), and weight loss in addition to an unequivocal elevation of fasting or postprandial plasma glucose concentrations. The vast majority of patients with newly presenting type 1 diabetes will meet these criteria (as in our illustrative case). In the absence of these classical findings (i.e., when random plasma glucose values are less than 11.1 mmol/L) or in the absence of classic symptoms, the most useful diagnostic tests are a

Table 32-2. Diagnostic Criteria for Diabetes Mellitus

1. Symptoms of diabetes plus a casual plasma glucose concentration ≥11.1 mmol/L (200 mg/dL). Casual is defined as any time of day without regard to the time since the last meal. The classic symptoms of diabetes include polyuria, polydipsia, and unexplained weight loss. Or

2. Fasting plasma glucose ≥7.0 mmol/L (126 mg/dL). Fasting is defined as no caloric intake for at least 8 h. Or

3. Two-hour postload glucose ≥11.1 mmol/L (200 mg/dL) during a standardized oral glucose tolerance test (OGTT). The test should be performed using a glucose load containing the equivalent of 75 g of anhydrous glucose dissolved in water.

In the absence of unequivocal hyperglycemia, these criteria should be confirmed by repeat testing on a different day. The third measure (OGTT) is not recommended for routine clinical use.

fasting plasma glucose or an oral glucose tolerance test (OGTT) (ADA, 2004a).

Oral Glucose Tolerance Test

For the OGTT, subjects are given a syrupy beverage containing 75 g of glucose after an 8- to 14-h fast. Plasma glucose is sampled prior to the glucose load and again 2 h after the glucose load. Table 32-3 gives the guidelines for interpreting OGTT results.

Glycated Hemoglobin and Hemoglobin A_{1C}

Glycated hemoglobin is formed continuously in erythrocytes as the product of a nonenzymatic reaction between hemoglobin (HgA) and glucose, first forming the labile Schiff base (or pre-HbA_{1C}), then the more stable Amadori product (Fig. 32-1A). HbA_{1C} specifically refers to the Amadori product of the N-terminal valine of each β-chain of HbA with glucose. The basic chemical structure of an advanced glycation end product, as shown in Figure 32-1B, demonstrates how

Table 32-3. Guidelines for Interpreting the 75-g Oral Glucose Tolerance Test (OGTT)

- 2-h postload glucose < 7.8 mmol/L (140 mg/dL) = normal glucose tolerance

- 2-h postload glucose 7.8–11.0 mmol/L (140–199 mg/dL) = impaired glucose tolerance

- 2-h postload glucose ≥11.1 mmol/L (200 mg/dL) = provisional diagnosis of diabetes

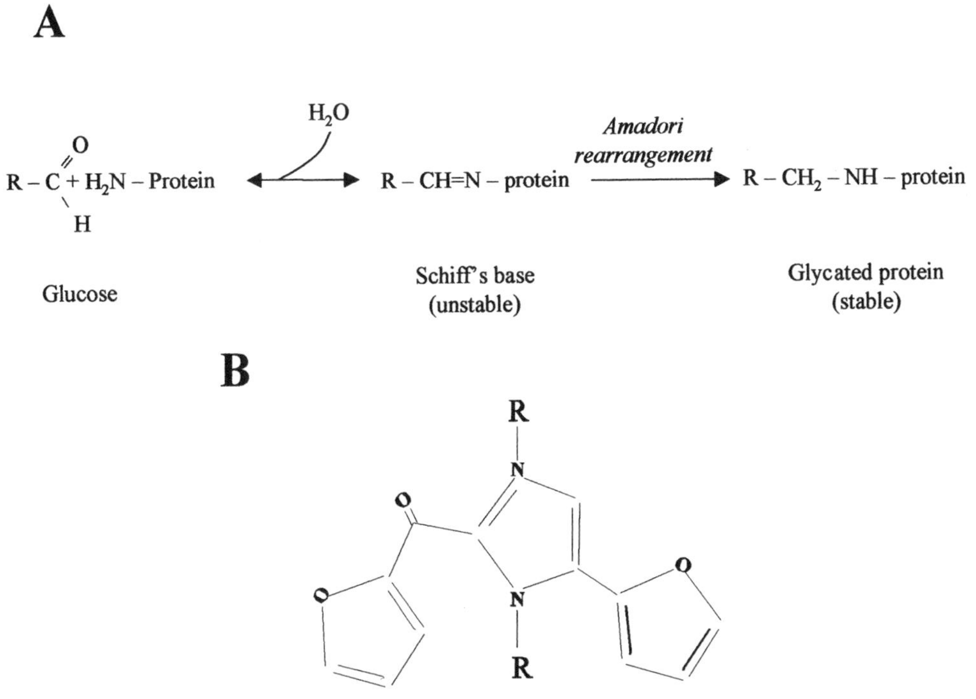

A

$$R - \overset{\overset{\displaystyle O}{\|}}{\underset{\underset{\displaystyle H}{\diagdown}}{C}} + H_2N - \text{Protein} \quad \overset{H_2O}{\longleftrightarrow} \quad R - CH{=}N - \text{protein} \quad \xrightarrow{\substack{\textit{Amadori} \\ \textit{rearrangement}}} \quad R - CH_2 - NH - \text{protein}$$

Glucose   Schiff's base (unstable)   Glycated protein (stable)

B

2-(2-furoyl)-4-(5)-(2-furanyl)-1H-imidazole

Figure 32-1. (*A*) Schematic representation of the nonenzymatic glycation of proteins, including hemoglobin, resulting in glycated HbA$_{1C}$. (*B*) Chemical structure of advanced glycation end products in tissues exposed to chronic hyperglycemia. The R groups designate tissue proteins that have become cross-linked and frequently become dysfunctional as a result of this process. Adapted from Brownlee (1992).

chronic exposure to hyperglycemia can result in permanent chemical modifications to collagen and connective tissue. This process accounts for many of the end-stage complications of diabetes.

HbA$_{1C}$ makes up about 80% of the glycated HbA$_1$. The HbA$_{1C}$ fraction represents hemoglobin molecules that have undergone irreversible glycation. The proportion of hemoglobin molecules that have undergone such a reaction is a direct reflection of the average prevailing blood glucose concentration during the life of the hemoglobin molecule (i.e., about 3 months). Measuring HbA$_{1C}$ proves to be an accurate and reliable method for estimating glycemic control over the preceding 2–3 months. Current guidelines do not allow for HbA$_{1C}$ to be used as a diagnostic test for diabetes, but it is an essential tool for assessing the effectiveness of diabetes treatment. Current treatment guidelines recommend an HbA$_{1C}$ level of 6. 5%–7.0% for patients with well-controlled diabetes (ADA, 2004b).

C-Peptide

The connecting peptide, a 31-amino acid chain between the α- and β-chain of the insulin molecule, is an excellent measure of endogenous insulin secretion in healthy individuals. However, C-peptide concentrations are difficult to interpret in the setting of new diabetes because of considerable overlap between normal individuals and those with type 1 or type 2 diabetes, depending on the duration and degree of metabolic control of the disease. The vast majority of children with type 1 diabetes do not produce any detectable C-peptide 2 years after diagnosis. A diagram showing how C-peptide is derived from proinsulin during the production of insulin is shown in Figure 32-2.

Antibodies

Antibodies to islet cells, insulin, and glutamic acid decarboxylase are present in many patients with newly diagnosed type 1 diabetes. In

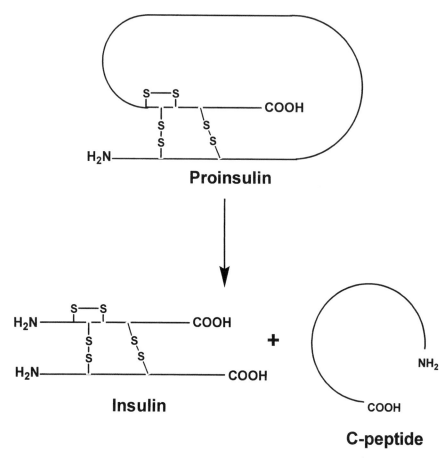

Figure 32-2. A schematic representation of the production of insulin and C-peptide from proinsulin in the pancreatic β-cell. C-peptide acts as an indicator of endogenous insulin secretion, even in people who inject exogenous insulin.

combination, they can be very sensitive and specific in predicting the risk of disease, but they are currently limited only to research applications and are not routinely used in clinical practice.

BIOCHEMICAL PERSPECTIVES

Glucose Homeostasis

An understanding of the symptoms and biochemical results in the illustrative case requires an overview of the homeostatic mechanisms regulating blood glucose concentration. Plasma glucose concentrations are tightly controlled by a balance between the actions of hormones, enzymes, and substrates that either raise or lower blood glucose levels. Glucose homeostasis depends on a balance between glucose production by the liver and glucose utilization by both insulin-dependent tissues (mainly fat and muscle) and insulin-independent tissues (such as brain and kidney). In normal individuals, this balance helps to keep the blood glucose concentration in a narrow range between 3.9 and 6.1 mmol/L.

Glucose is the primary fuel for the central nervous system (CNS). A constant supply of glucose at sufficient levels is critical for normal functioning of the CNS. On the other hand, the prevention of hyperglycemia is important to avoid loss of calories that would occur when excess glucose is spilled into the urine (the glucose concentration at which proximal tubular glucose transporters are saturated and excess glucose begins to be spilled into the urine is about 10 mmol/L) and excess glycation of proteins.

Plasma glucose concentrations are deter-

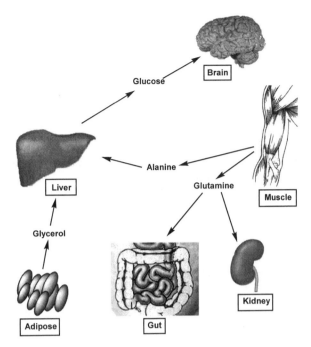

Figure 32-3. Schematic representation of fuel mobilization during fasting. Catabolism of muscle proteins provides alanine for gluconeogenesis and glutamine for utilization by the gut and kidney, while branched chain amino acids are primarily oxidized within the muscle. Breakdown of adipocyte triacylglycerols provides glycerol and free fatty acids (not shown); the free fatty acids provide fuel for liver, muscle and most other peripheral tissues. The liver utilizes both alanine and glycerol to synthesize glucose which is required for the brain and for red blood cells (not shown). Adapted from Besser and Thirner (2002).

mined by a net balance between glucose released into the circulation and glucose taken up from plasma. Normal regulation of glucose levels depends largely on three factors: (1) the ability of the pancreatic β-cell to secrete insulin both acutely and in a sustained fashion; (2) the ability of insulin to inhibit hepatic glucose production and promote glucose utilization in muscle and other tissues; and (3) the ability of glucose to enter cells in the absence of insulin (glucose effectiveness).

In the fasting state, approximately 80% of glucose uptake by tissues is non-insulin mediated, with the CNS the main consumer of glucose. In the setting of reduced insulin levels, pyruvate dehydrogenase activity in muscle is decreased, thus limiting glucose oxidation. At the same time, lack of insulin promotes catabolism of muscle protein and the release of alanine and glutamine. The alanine is taken up by the liver and provides a major substrate for gluconeogenesis, thus ensuring a constant supply

of glucose to the brain during periods of caloric deprivation (Figure 32-3). The glutamine is metabolized by the gut and kidney, and in the latter organ, also serves to provide ammonium ions to buffer the metabolic acids produced during ketogenesis.

The roles of hepatic glycogen metabolism and gluconeogenesis in the regulation of blood glucose are best illustrated by a description of normal glucose homeostasis in fed and fasted states. It can be divided into five phases, as depicted in Figure 32-4. Glucose utilization is plotted against time in a person who ingests 100 g of glucose and then fasts for 40 days (Ruderman, 1975).

- Phase 1, Absorptive Phase: For 3–4 h after glucose ingestion, blood glucose is derived principally from exogenous carbohydrate. Concentrations of insulin and glucose are increased, and glucagon is depressed. Excess glucose is stored in liver and muscle

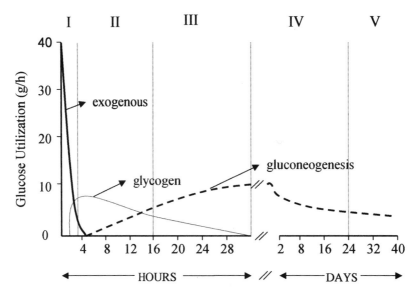

Figure 32-4. Phases of glucose homeostasis in a normal human during a prolonged fast. Adapted from Ruderman et al. (1975).

as glycogen or is converted to lipid. The absorptive phase is the only phase in which the liver is a net glucose sink.

- Phase 2, Postabsorptive Phase: By approximately 4 h after feeding, insulin and glucose return to their basal states and the liver produces glucose from stored glycogen. The brain is the major user of glucose during the postabsorptive phase, while muscle and adipose tissue use glucose at a reduced rate. There is an increase in the release of alanine which is used as substrates for gluconeogenesis.

- Phases 3 and 4, After 12–14 h of starvation, the ability of the liver to carry out gluconeogenesis is enhanced secondary to a decrease in insulin and an increase in glucagon. In addition, the release of amino acids from muscle continues to be increased. At this point, liver glycogen is depleted, but the brain is not yet using ketone bodies, and the demand for gluconeogenesis is at its peak. Thus, this is the time of greatest susceptibility for hypoglycemia because of impaired gluconeogenesis.

- Phase 5, Prolonged Starvation: In the later part of phase 4 and in phase five, plasma levels of ketone bodies increase and ketone bodies partially replace glucose as a fuel supply for the brain. This, in turn, decreases the demand for hepatic gluconeogenesis and acts to conserve muscle protein.

Fatty Acid and Ketone Body Metabolism

Most peripheral tissues can use ketone bodies (acetoacetate and β-hydroxybutyrate) as well as nonesterified fatty acids and glucose for metabolic fuel. Ketone bodies are produced by the liver during gluconeogenesis. They are an important fuel for the brain during starvation, and are thus crucial for protein conservation during prolonged fasting. A near-total deficiency of insulin, such as occurs in untreated type 1 diabetes, can, however, yield dangerously high concentrations of ketone bodies secondary to an imbalance between their hepatic production and peripheral utilization. This pathologic ketosis causes severe metabolic acidosis due to the marked excess of the weak organic acids, acetoacetate, and β-hydroxybutyrate, which can be fatal if not treated promptly.

A schematic depiction of the intracellular pathway for β-oxidation of long-chain fatty acids and, ultimately, ketogenesis is shown in Figure 32-5. Long-chain fatty acids are activated prior to entering the mitochondria by converting them to acyl-CoA derivatives. Because the mitochondrial membrane is impermeable to CoA and its derivatives, a specific transport system is required. As shown in Figure 32-5, this system has three components: (1) the enzyme carnitine acyltransferase I (CAT I), which transfers the activated acyl unit from fatty acyl-CoA

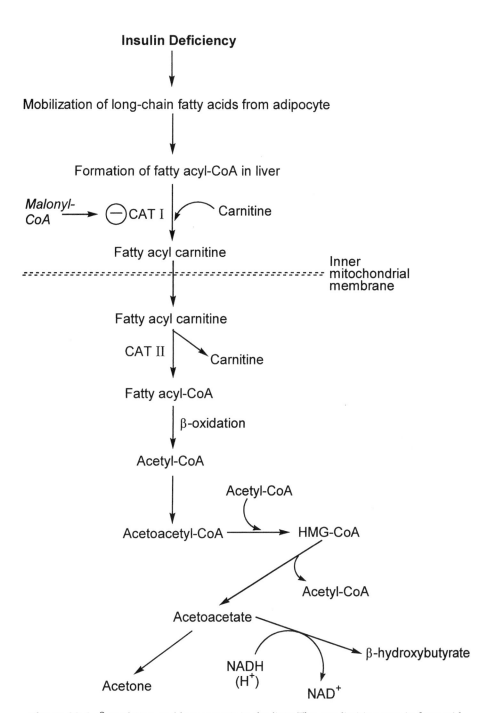

Figure 32-5. β-oxidation and ketogenesis in the liver. The rate-limiting step in fatty acid oxidation and subsequent ketone body production is the activity of carnitine acyltransferase I (CAT I). The activity of CAT I is inhibited by malonyl-CoA. Insulin deficiency results in inhibition of acetyl-CoA carboxylase, decreased levels of maloyl-CoA, and thus increased activity of CAT-I. Adapted from Foster and McGarry (1983).

Table 32-4. Physiological Consequences of the Action of Insulin

Variable	Action	Tissue
Carbohydrate Metabolism		
Glucose transport	Increase	Muscle, adipose tissue
Glycolysis	Increase	Muscle, adipose tissue
Glycogen synthesis	Increase	Liver, muscle, adipose tissue
Glycogen degradation	Decrease	Liver, muscle, adipose tissue
Gluconeogenesis	Decrease	Liver & kidney
Lipid Metabolism		
Lipolysis	Decrease	Adipose tissue
Synthesis of fatty acids and triglycerides	Increase	Liver, adipose tissue
Synthesis of very low density lipoprotein	Increase	Liver
Lipoprotein lipase activity	Increase	Adipose tissue
Fatty acid oxidation	Decrease	Muscle, liver
Cholesterol formation	Increase	Liver
Protein Metabolism		
Amino acid transport	Increase	Muscle, liver, adipose tissue
Protein synthesis	Increase	Muscle, liver, adipose tissue
Protein degradation	Decrease	Muscle
Urea synthesis	Decrease	Liver

to carnitine; (2) a translocase system for facilitating the exchange diffusion of fatty acyl-carnitine into the mitochondrial matrix in exchange for carnitine; and (3) a second transferase called carnitine acyltransferase II (CAT II), which catalyzes the transfer of the fatty acyl unit from fatty acyl-carnitine back to CoA prior to β-oxidation. The fatty acylation of carnitine by CPT 1 is the rate-limiting intracellular event of fatty acid oxidation and is inhibited by malonyl-CoA.

Most tissues oxidize the acetyl-CoA produced during β-oxidation to CO_2 and water via the TCA cycle. During fasting, however, the liver utilizes the intermediates of the TCA cycle as gluconeogenic substrates. Under these conditions, the liver converts acetyl-CoA to ketone bodies (acetoacetate and β-hydroxybutyrate) (Figure 32-5). Most other peripheral tissues can oxidize ketone bodies by the pathway shown in the figure. After entering the mitochondria, acetoacetate reacts with succinyl-CoA to form acetoacetyl-CoA, a reaction that is catalyzed by 3-oxoacid-CoA transferase. Alternatively, acetoacetyl-CoA is formed by direct activation of acetoacetate by the enzyme acetoacetyl-CoA synthetase. Acetoacetyl-CoA is then cleaved to form two molecules of acetyl-CoA by acetoacetyl-CoA thiolase. As noted earlier in

the discussion of phases of glucose metabolism, ketone bodies are only utilized by the brain during prolonged fasting and starvation.

Type 1 Diabetes Mellitus

Type 1 diabetes (formerly referred to as juvenile-onset diabetes mellitus and insulin-dependent diabetes mellitus) results from destruction of beta cells and a complete or near total absence of insulin synthesis. Insulin is the primary hormone responsible for regulating glucose metabolism and in signaling for the utilization and storage of basic nutrients. As shown in Table 32-4, insulin acts as a powerful anabolic hormone, and it is also a potent inhibitor of the catabolic processes evoked by the counterregulatory hormones (i.e., glucagon, epinephrine, cortisol, and growth hormone). Although the important target tissues for insulin are liver, muscle, and fat, insulin has pleiotropic effects on cell growth and metabolism in many tissues (Kahn, 2001).

The development of type 1 diabetes is the culmination of a chronic autoimmune destruction of the pancreatic β-cells that occurs over many years. This process results in severe, and ultimately complete, insulin deficiency. In the absence of insulin, fasting hyperglycemia is primarily due to an unrestricted increase in hepatic glucose production. Gluconeogenic precursors are elevated to supply the necessary substrate to support gluconeogenesis. In addition, insulin deficiency results in the unrestrained lipolysis and increased ketogenesis that leads to diabetic ketoacidosis.

Type 1 diabetes accounts for approximately 10% of all patients diagnosed with diabetes mellitus. It is a major chronic disease of children and is now being recognized with increasing frequency in adults. In the absence of insulin, the resulting metabolic derangements in acute diabetic ketoacidosis eventually lead to coma and death.

Approximately 90% of diabetics have type 2 diabetes mellitus rather than type 1. Type 2 diabetes (previously called maturity-onset diabetes), is characterized by insulin resistance. These patients initially exhibit impaired glucose uptake into tissues and a compensatory increase in insulin secretion. Although type 2 diabetes usually occurs in people over 40 years of age, its incidence has been increasing markedly in younger individuals over the past decade. Type 2 diabetes is often accompanied by hypertension and dyslipidemia (abnormalities in blood lipoproteins) and most of these patients are obese. Long term compensatory increase in insulin secretion frequently leads to pancreatic failure and most patients with type 2 diabetes eventually require insulin. Certain ethnic groups currently exhibit higher rates of type 2 diabetes than the general population. For example, half of the adult Pima Native Americans in the U.S. Southwest are now diabetic. Overall, the rate of diabetes for American Indians and Alaska Natives is more than twice the rate for the U.S. population as a whole.

The typical pancreatic lesion of type 1 diabetes is the selective loss of almost all β-cells, whereas other islet cell types (α, δ, and pancreatic polypeptide cells) remain intact. The most common mechanism for β-cell destruction is thought to be autoimmune-mediated inflammatory damage. Prospective family studies strongly support a genetic basis for susceptibility to this autoimmune process and suggest that the underlying immune abnormalities precede clinical insulin deficiency by many years. However, not all spontaneous type 1 diabetes is the result of autoimmune mechanisms.

It has been long-recognized that heredity is a major factor in diabetes. Identical twins who share all the same genes have a much greater risk of diabetes than fraternal twins who may share only 50% of the same genes: concordance in identical twins is about 25–50% for type 1 diabetes. The lack of complete concordance strongly suggests that environmental factors also play a role in the development of clinical diabetes. Environmental factors that have been implicated include certain foods (including cow's milk), common viruses, and vaccines, but there is little evidence for any specific association. The exception is exposure to wild-type rubella virus during the first trimester of pregnancy. As many as 20% of the children born after prenatal exposure to rubella later develop type 1 diabetes.

Islet Cell Antibodies and Other Immunological Markers

Circulating IgG antibodies specific for islet cell antigens are found in 70%–80% of individuals with type 1 diabetes at the time of diagnosis. These antibodies do not appear to play a role in β-cell destruction, but they serve as useful markers for immunological autoreactivity. Some of the specific targets for these antibodies include insulin and glutamic acid decarboxylase. Islet cell antibodies are detectable from infancy or early childhood in 3%–8% of the first-degree relatives of patients with type 1 diabetes. About of half of these individuals will eventually develop clinical diabetes. The lifetime risk of developing type 1 diabetes in these individuals is related to the titer of islet cell antibodies, but antibody screening is currently used only in the research settings to define risk among the relatives of affected individuals.

Two rodent models of genetically determined autoimmune β-cell destruction and diabetes are available to provide some insight to the human disease. The disease process has several discrete steps, each of which may be subject to genetic or pharmacological control in the future. The process is thought to be initiated by release of antigens from the β-cells. This could be the result of genetic defects, infectious agents, or β-cell toxins. These antigens are then presented to the immune system, resulting in lymphocytic activation. Normal mice react to the antigen exposure with a self-limited immune response, but, in diabetes-prone rodents, this exposure results in self-perpetuating autoimmune destruction. Once initiated, proinflammatory cytokines, highly reactive oxygen radicals and nitric oxide are released, causing direct cellular damage.

Clinical Manifestations

The clinical manifestations of type 1 diabetes are the end result of persistent hyperglycemia. Sustained glucose levels above the renal threshold (approximately 10 mmol/L) leads to an osmotic diuresis and polyuria, which in turn leads to dehydration and a hyperosmolar state. Weight loss is universally present due to a combination of fluid loss and catabolism of muscle and fat stores. Excessive production of ketoacids consumes buffer (i.e., HCO_3^-) and lowers the serum pH. The combination of energy deprivation, dehydration, and sleep deprivation due to nocturia leads to fatigue and malaise. Vision is often affected, with patients complaining of blurry vision or inability to focus. This sign is attributable to the deposition of excess glucose and sorbitol in the lens, which results in osmotic swelling and a distortion of light refraction. Sorbitol arises from the action of nearly ubiquitous enzymes, known as aldose reductases, that have a low affinity for glucose but that convert glucose to sorbitol when glucose concentrations are elevated. These symptoms eventually resolve with treatment.

At diagnosis, new patients with type 1 diabetes may exhibit ketoacidosis with resultant acid-base and electrolyte disturbances. The most common abnormality is hyponatremia, which is often due to the movement of water to the extravascular space. Volume contraction may lead to elevations in blood urea nitrogen (BUN) and creatinine, as well as mild erythrocytosis. Leukocytosis may also exist in the absence of infection, and serum triglycerides and urine glucose are almost universally elevated.

Newly diagnosed patients with type 1 diabetes may present with acute metabolic decompensations, ketone production, and metabolic acidosis, a condition known as diabetic ketoacidosis (DKA). Although β-cell destruction occurs gradually, acute physical or emotional stress can acutely create a demand for increased insulin production.

The pathophysiology of DKA is as follows. Severe insulin deficiency leads to hyperglycemia and hyperosmolality. Unopposed glucagon action then leads to accelerated glycogenolysis, gluconeogenesis, and lipolysis (Figure 32-3). During gluconeogenesis, the acetyl-CoA produced from during oxidation of fatty acids in the liver is converted to acetoacetate and β-hydroxybutyrate. Ketones are weak organic acids, and their accumulation in the serum leads to metabolic acidosis. The combination of dehydration and acid-base abnormalities ultimately leads to severe electrolyte disturbances.

Most patients with DKA appear ill and weak. They are usually hypotensive and have poor skin turgor, indicating severe dehydration. If the patient is able to give a history, symptoms of polyuria, polydipsia, and weight loss are invariably present. The breath may have a classic "fruity odor" due to the excretion of acetone in expired breath. Acetone arises from the spontaneous, nonenzymatic decarboxylation of acetoacetate:

$$CH_3\text{-}\overset{\overset{\displaystyle O}{\|}}{C}\text{-}CH_2\text{-}COOH \rightarrow CH_3\text{-}\overset{\overset{\displaystyle O}{\|}}{C}\text{-}CH_3 + CO_2$$

Tachycardia is usually present, and breathing can be deep and labored (Kussmaul breathing). Anorexia, nausea, and vomiting may also be present. Abdominal pain may be severe without underlying pathology. Patients are generally lethargic, but the level of consciousness can range from alert to coma.

Diabetics are prone to many long-term complications. Chronic hyperglycemia (even if partially controlled) affects many different organ systems. Individuals with diabetes are at increased risk of heart attack, stroke and complications related to poor circulation. Neuropathy is one of the most common complications of diabetes. The combination of nerve damage and poor blood flow can result in foot complications so severe as to lead to amputation. Diabetes can also damage the kidneys (nephropathy), resulting in kidney failure or a reduced ability to carry out their normal filtration function. This complication develops in 20–30% of people with type 2 diabetes, and in the U.S. accounts for more than 50% of cases of end-stage renal disease. Retinopathy (eye disease) is another complication of diabetes. It is caused by narrowing, hardening, swelling, hemorrhaging or severing of the capillaries of the retina and can lead to blindness. Gastroparesis (delayed gastric emptying) is also common in individuals with both type 1 and type 2 diabetes.

THERAPY

While insulin replacement will be the primarily aspect of long-term management of this patient, the acute problem is the diabetic keto-

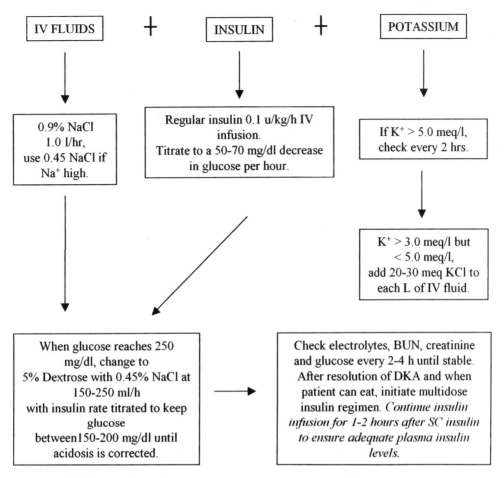

Figure 32-6. Summary of the critical components in the medical management of diabetic ketoacidosis.

acidosis. Correction of hyperglycemia is not the primary therapeutic approach to the medical management of DKA, although such treatment will ultimately result in a reduction in osmotic diuresis and dehydration. Fluid replacement, restoration of tissue perfusion, and correction of electrolyte imbalance are the primary goals of DKA management. The critical components in the medical management of DKA are summarized in Figure 32-6.

Fluid Replacement

The patient discussed in the illustrative case presented with orthostatic hypotension, poor skin turgor, dry mucous membrane, a ketotic odor to the breath, elevations in BUN and creatinine, and ketoacidosis. She had severe extracellular volume depletion, which can be estimated using the following clinical criteria:

1. Loss of greater than 10% of extracellular fluid (ECF) volume results in an orthostatic increase in pulse without a change in blood pressure.
2. A 15%–20% loss of ECF volume manifests as an orthostatic drop in blood pressure of more than 15 mm Hg systolic and more than 10 mm Hg diastolic. This amounts to approximately 3–4 L of fluid loss.
3. A greater than 20% loss of ECF volume causes supine hypotension, usually after losing more than 4 L of fluid.

The intravenous administration of isotonic saline (0.9% NaCl) should be used to restore ECF and intracellular fluid volumes. Infusion of isotonic saline restores the extracellular volume deficit. Isotonic saline also restore intracellular volume deficits in patients with DKA and hypotonicity. Aggressive hydration itself causes reduction in counterregulatory hormone concentrations and in blood glucose, and this remains the cornerstone of DKA therapy. Once the patient has been stabilized, rehydration should be gradual over a period of 36–48 h order to prevent cerebral edema. An accurate record of fluid input and output should be maintained to help assess volume status. Oral rehydration should be avoided until the patient is hemodynamically stable and vomiting has stopped (Foster and McGarry, 1983; Waldhausl et al., 1979).

Insulin Administration and Correction of Ketoacidosis

DKA is a positive anion gap metabolic acidosis associated with the accumulation of β-hydroxybutyrate and acetoacetate. Lactic acidosis secondary to cardiac or renal failure, hypoxia, poor tissue perfusion, shock, or sepsis may also contribute to the anion gap in DKA. A normal anion gap (AG) is 12 ± 2 mEq/L. The anion gap (AG) is calculated using the following formula: AG = $([Na^+ + K^+] - [Cl^- + HCO_3^-])$. In our illustrative case, the anion gap was 28, indicating severe metabolic acidosis.

As ketoacidosis is corrected, the anion gap will normalize. Although fluid replenishment improves insulin sensitivity and promotes tissue perfusion, simultaneous administration of a low-dose insulin infusion is shown to cause a faster decline in ketonemia. Regular insulin should be initially infused at a rate of 0.1 U/kg/h intravenously. Intravenous insulin boluses are not recommended in an effort to avoid hypokalemia, hypoglycemia, and cerebral edema. With a low-dose insulin infusion, steady-state insulin concentrations are achieved within 20 to 30 min. Insulin infusion should not be terminated prematurely because of falling blood glucose levels approaching hypoglycemia. Since hyperglycemia is corrected more rapidly than ketoacidosis, dextrose should be added to fluids once the blood glucose concentration is less than 13.9 mmol/L, continued insulin administration will help clear the ketonemia, and dextrose infusion will help maintain plasma glucose concentrations in the ideal range of 6.1–13.9 mmol/L. Once the ketoacidosis has resolved and the patient is eating, intravenous insulin can be safely switched to subcutaneous insulin (Wagner et al., 1999).

Correction of Electrolyte Imbalances

Sodium: When patients present with hypernatremia and elevated serum osmolality, they are suffering from severe fluid deficits. Depending on the patient's hemodynamic stability, fluid therapy should generally be instituted as a moderate-to-slow intravenous infusion of 0.9% normal saline over a period of 48–72 h to avoid cerebral edema. Patients with evidence of circulatory compromise will require more aggressive fluid resuscitation. Estimated plasma osmolality and corrected serum sodium concentrations are calculated using the following formulas:

Estimated plasma osmolality
= 2(Measured Na$^+$ mEq/L)
+ (Glucose mg/dL/18)
+ (BUN mg/dL/2.8)

Normal serum osmolality
= 280–290 mOsm/kg H$_2$O.

Corrected serum sodium
= Measured Na$^+$
+ [(Glucose in mg/dL
− 100)/100] × 1.6

Normal serum sodium = 135–145 mEq/L

Using these formulas, our illustrative case had an estimated serum osmolality of (256 + 28.4 + 8.9 = 293.3 mOsm/kg H$_2$O) and a corrected serum sodium of (128 + [4.12 × 1.6] = 135 meq/L), suggesting that the losses of fluid were isotonic.

Potassium: Hyperglycemia shifts water and potassium from the intracellular to the extracellular compartment, and this shift is augmented by acidosis and protein breakdown. Loss of potassium occurs during osmotic diuresis and is amplified by the secondary hyperaldosteronism resulting from volume contraction. Aldosterone, a steroid hormone produced by the adrenal cortex, regulates fluid volume by causing the renal retention of sodium (and the consequent excretion of potassium) as a result of increased angiotensin II availability. Most DKA subjects actually have a total body potassium deficit of 500–700 meq/L. Once fluid replacement and insulin infusions have commenced, there is a shift of potassium back into the intracellular compartment, resulting in a rapid fall in serum potassium. Intravenous potassium administration should usually begin with insulin infusions but should not exceed 40 mEq/L in the first hour and 20–30 meq/L/h thereafter. For rare patients who present with hypokalemia (<3.3 mEq/L), insulin administration should be withheld until the potassium level is greater than 3.3 mEq/L (Kitabchi et al., 2001; White, 2003).

Phosphate: An intracellular shift of phosphate occurs along with potassium as fluid rehydration commences. The phosphate deficit can also be worsened with correction of the metabolic acidosis. Controlled, randomized studies have shown that routine phosphate repletion is not necessary, but some practitioners think it prudent to provide supplemental phosphate if serum phosphate levels are less than 1 mEq/L, potentially reducing the risk of seizure or tissue ischemia. During intravenous phosphate administration, serum calcium concentrations should be monitored carefully to avoid hypocalcemia and tetany (Fisher and Kitabchi, 1983).

Bicarbonate: Current guidelines state that acidosis need not be corrected using exogenous bicarbonate therapy. Intravenous administration of fluids and insulin are sufficient to correct the metabolic acidosis and to regenerate bicarbonate. Some practitioners believe, however, that bicarbonate repletion should be provided in the setting of severe acidosis with pH less than 6.9.

Management of Type 1 Diabetes Mellitus

Effective management of type 1 diabetes involves a team approach in which physicians collaborate with certified diabetes educators, nutritionists, and other health care professionals (such as psychologists and social workers) to achieve the therapeutic goals of acceptable glycemic control and prevention of complications. The requirements for effective management of type 1 diabetes are shown in Table 32-5. Apart from diet and exercise, instituting intensive diabetes therapy using either multiple daily insulin injections or continuous subcutaneous insulin infusion (insulin pump) therapy may help in achieving these goals.

Human recombinant insulins and their analogues are classified as long- or short-acting insulins based on their pharmacokinetic characteristics. The pharmacokinetic properties of the common insulin preparations are given in Table 32-6. Possible approaches include (1) injection

Table 32-5. Requirements for Intensive Insulin Therapy

Patient motivation and interest

Diet compliance and carbohydrate counting

Frequent home blood glucose monitoring (generally four to six times per day)

Establishment of target blood glucose levels

Management of hypo- and hyperglycemia

Regular contact and support from diabetes team, including physician, diabetes educator, and dietitian

Family and social support

---

of rapid-acting insulins at mealtime combined with intermediate-acting insulin at breakfast and dinner or at bedtime, (2) injection of rapid-acting insulin with meals combined with a long-acting insulin once a day, or (3) continuous subcutaneous insulin infusion administration using an external insulin pump. All of these insulin regimens depend on routine home blood glucose monitoring and the application of rational insulin algorithms for effectiveness.

The Diabetes Control and Complications Trial (DCCT) has shown that intensified diabetes therapy resulted in HbA_{1C} reductions of approximately 2% compared to conventional therapy, and that patients practicing intensified diabetes therapy enjoyed significant reductions in the feared microvascular complications of diabetes (DCCT Research Group, 1993). As such, the current aim of diabetes therapy is to achieve glycemic control that is as close to normal as possible while maintaining an acceptable quality of life for those patients for whom the therapy is prescribed. The DCCT also demon-

Table 32-6. Insulin Preparations and Their Pharmocokinetic Properties

Preparation	Onset	Peak	Duration
Rapid Acting			
Regular	0.5–1 h	2–4 h	6–8 h
Insulin lispro	15 min	1 h	3–4 h
Insulin aspart	15 min	1 h	3–4 h
Intermediate acting			
NPH	1–3 h	6–8 h	12–16 h
Lente	1–4 h	6–10 h	14–18 h
Long acting			
Ultralente	1 h	8–10 h	16–24 h
Glargine	1–2 h	No peak	24 h

NPH, neutral protamine Hagedon.

strated, however, that patients using intensified diabetes therapy experienced hypoglycemia at a rate that was three times greater than patients employing conventional therapy. Thus, hypoglycemia is the single most important limiting factor in the glycemic management of type 1 diabetes.

Prevention of Diabetic Ketoacidosis

Individuals with type 1 diabetes are also at risk of subsequent ketoacidotic crises. One common cause of DKA is noncompliance with insulin therapy. Infections, (including subclinical infections) and physiological stressors (such as myocardial infarction) can also precipitate DKA. Since the mortality rate associated with DKA can be as high as 10%, successfully educating patients about the early warning signs of the condition and providing a plan for early intervention is crucial to its effective prevention.

Case Resolution

At presentation, the patient was hemodynamically unstable. She had a rapid heart rate and exhibited orthostatic hypotension (a fall in blood pressure on assuming an upright posture) and slow mentation. Her fluid deficit was greater than 4 L. Her lab work revealed hyponatremia (low serum sodium), hyperkalemia (high serum potassium), and a severe anion gap metabolic acidosis with dehydration. Her anion gap was 28, and her corrected serum Na^+ was 135 mEq/L.

The patient was treated with 0.9% NaCl at a rate of 1L/h. Orders were given to sample for serum electrolytes, glucose, BUN, Cr, and pH every 2 h initially and then every 4 h thereafter. Intravenous insulin was started at the rate of 0.1 µ/kg/h, and 20 mEq of KCl were added to each liter of intravenous fluid. The rate was adjusted so that plasma glucose declined at a rate of 2.8–3.9 mmol/L/h. Once the patient's blood glucose was less than 13.9 mmol/L, she was switched to intravenous fluids containing 5% dextrose with 0.45% NaCl to maintain her blood glucose concentration between 8.3 and 11.1 mmol/L. Blood and urine cultures were also obtained but failed to reveal an underlying infection.

Once the patient was clinically stable and the acidosis had resolved, the insulin infusion was changed to subcutaneous insulin, and she was discharged home after 4 days in the hospital and plenty of diabetes home care training.

She is currently doing well with a HbA_{1C} of 6.9% on a regimen of insulin glargine at bedtime and insulin lispro at meals, and she is beginning to develop an interest in obtaining an insulin pump. She looks forward to a long and healthy life with type 1 diabetes.

QUESTIONS

1. Why was the patient tachycardic?
2. What is the main reason for administering insulin in the treatment of diabetic ketoacidosis (DKA)?
3. List three serious adverse events that may result from the over zealous administration of insulin during the treatment of DKA?
4. Why is volume resuscitation the mainstay of DKA therapy?
5. What is the best way to avoid life-threatening hypokalemia during the treatment of DKA?
6. What is the single most important factor for this patient's health as she attempts to avoid diabetes-related organ damage over the decades to come?
7. What would the blood levels of glucose and ketones be after 48 h of fasting in a person who was carnitine deficient? Explain your reasoning.
8. Name another disease of sugar metabolism, aside from diabetes mellitus, that involves a glycation reaction as a component of the pathophysiology.

BIBLIOGRAPHY

American Diabetes Association: Clinical practice recommendations. Diagnosis and classification of diabetes mellitus. *Diabetes Care* **27**:S5–S10, 2004a.

American Diabetes Association: Clinical practice recommendations. Standards of medical care in diabetes. *Diabetes Care* **27**:S15–S35, 2004b.

Besser GM, Thorner MO (eds): *Comprehensive Clinical Endocrinology*. 3rd ed. Mosby, St. Louis, MO, 2002.

Brownlee M: Glycation products and the pathogenesis of diabetes complications. *Diabetes Care* **15**:1835–1843, 1992.

DCCT Research Group: The effect of intensive treatment of diabetes on the development and progression of long-term complications in insulin-dependent diabetes mellitus. *N Engl J Med* **329**:977–986, 1993.

Eisenbarth GS: Classification, diagnostic tests, and pathogenesis of Type I Diabetes Mellitus, in Becker KL (ed): *Principles and Practice of Endocrinology and Metabolism*. 3rd ed. Lippincott Williams and Wilkins, 2001, pp. 1307–1314.

Fein IA, Rackow EC, Sprung CL, Grodman R: Relation of colloid osmotic pressure to arterial hypoxemia and cerebral edema during crystalloid volume loading of patients with diabetic ketoacidosis. *Ann Intern Med* **96:**570–575, 1982.

Fisher JN, Kitabchi AE: A randomized study of phosphate therapy in the treatment of diabetic ketoacidosis. *J Clin Endocrinol Metab* **57:** 177–180, 1983.

Foster DW, McGarry JD: The metabolic derangements and treatment of diabetic ketoacidosis. *N Engl J Med* **309:**159–169, 1983.

Kahn CR: Glucose homeostasis and insulin action, in Becker KL (ed): *Principles and Practice of Endocrinology and Metabolism*. 3rd ed. Lippincott Williams and Wilkins, 2001, pp. 1303–1306.

Kitabchi AE, Umpierrez GE, Murphy MB, et al.: Management of hyperglycemic crises in patients with diabetes (technical review). *Diabetes Care* **24**(suppl 1):131–153, 2004.

Morris LR, Murphy MB, Kitabchi AE: Bicarbonate therapy in severe diabetic ketoacidosis. *Ann Intern Med* **105:**836–840, 1986.

Position Statement of the American Diabetes Association. Hyperglycemic crises in diabetes. *Diabetes Care* **27**(suppl 1):S94–S102, 2004.

Ruderman NB, Aoki TT, Cahill GF: Gluconeogenesis and its disorders in man, *in* Hanson R, Mehlman M (eds): *Gluconeogenesis*. Wiley, New York, 1975, p. 515.

Wagner A, Risse A, Brill HL, et al.: Therapy of severe diabetic ketoacidosis: zero-mortality under very-low-dose insulin application. *Diabetes Care* **22:**674–677, 1999.

Waldhausl W, Kleinberger G, Korn A, Dudcza R, Bratusch-Marrain P, Nowatny P: Severe hyperglycemia: effects of rehydration on endocrine derangements and blood glucose concentration. *Diabetes* **28:**577–584, 1979.

White NH: Management of diabetic ketoacidosis. *Endocrinol Metabol Dis* **4:**343–353, 2003.

33

Congenital Adrenal Hyperplasia: P450c21 Steroid Hydroxylase Deficiency

GERALD J. PEPE and MIRIAM D. ROSENTHAL

CASE REPORTS

Patient 1

A 2-day-old neonate was referred to the pediatric endocrinology team with ambiguous external genitalia, including clitoral hypertrophy and fusion of the labia. The baby had been delivered spontaneously at 38 weeks of gestation after an uneventful pregnancy and presented with no obvious clinical manifestations other than apparent masculinization of the external genitalia/genital ambiguity. A sample was obtained for genetic testing, which subsequently confirmed a 46XX chromosomal makeup. Examination of serum electrolytes indicated mild hyponatremia (decreased sodium concentration) and hyperkalemia (elevated potassium). A blood sample was also sent to a central laboratory for hormone analyses. The results, obtained 5 days after the patient was sent home, showed that blood levels of cortisol (hydrocortisone) and aldosterone were well (<4 fold) below normal, whereas levels of androgens, including dehydroepiandrosterone (DHEA), DHEA-sulfate (DHEAS), androstenedione, and testosterone, were elevated more than 5-fold. Serum levels of 17-hydroxyprogesterone (17-OHP) exceeded 10,000 ng/mL (>100-fold above normal), while estradiol and estrone were barely detectable and thus normal for age. Plasma levels of renin were also elevated.

Four days later, the neonate was brought by ambulance to the emergency room barely conscious, severely dehydrated, and apparently in hypovolemic (abnormally low plasma fluid volume) shock, signs consistent with "adrenal crisis." Laboratory tests revealed severe hyponatremia and hyperkalemia. Serum levels of cortisol and aldosterone were well below normal, while those of DHEAS, renin, and 17-hydroxyprogesterone were markedly elevated. The patient was diagnosed with classic (severe) 21-hydroxylase (P450c21) deficiency congenital adrenal hyperplasia (CAH). After restoration of fluids and electrolytes, the patient was treated with cortisol (hydrocortisone) at doses that restored levels of DHEA, DHEAS, androstenedione, testosterone, and 17-OHP to within the normal range.

Surgery was subsequently performed to correct the labial fusion and clitoral hypertrophy. The child has developed normally and is being closely monitored for hormone replacement dose requirements to avoid either iatrogenic Cushing's syndrome from excess glucocorticoid or premature epiphyseal closure and short stature from unsuppressed adrenal androgen production.

Patient 2

The patient, a 7-year-old male, was brought to the clinic by his parents, who were concerned about apparent precocious puberty, including onset of maturation of secondary sex characteristics (e.g., increased pubic hair, penile development). The boy's height was greater than expected (51 inches, three standard deviations above mean for chronological age based on standardized growth curves), and he appeared to be rather husky, consistent with increased somatic maturation.

Blood pressure and other vital signs were normal. Although serum electrolytes were also normal, blood levels of DHEA, DHEAS, androstenedione, and testosterone were elevated threefold, while cortisol levels were twofold lower than normal. Serum levels of aldosterone were normal and those of were renin only slightly elevated. As in patient 1, however, the blood levels of 17-hydroxyprogesterone (>10,000 ng/mL) were extremely elevated compared to normal (<100 ng/mL). Blood levels of leuteinizing hormone were low and were only slightly increased following injection of gonadotropin-releasing hormone, thus indicating that the patient was truly prepubertal, and that the elevated androgens were not gonadal but more likely adrenal in origin. The patient was diagnosed with CAH due to classic P450c21 hydroxylase deficiency and subsequently treated with exogenous glucocorticoid (hydrocortisone), which suppressed excess adrenal 17-OHP and androgen production.

DIAGNOSIS

Sexual differentiation is initiated very early in fetal development (for review, George and Wilson, 1994; Jost, 1972). Although genetic sex determines whether the fetal bipotential gonad will develop into an ovary (46XX) or testes (46XY), sexual differentiation of internal duct systems and external genitalia is markedly influenced by hormones (Fig. 33-1). In the male, production of testosterone by the fetal testes is required to induce development of the Wolffian duct into epididymis, ductus deferens, ejaculatory ducts, and seminiferous tubules and differentiation of the primordia of the external genitalia as male. Differentiation of the primordia of the external genitalia as female and of the internal duct system (i.e., Müllerian ducts) into fallopian tubes, uterus, and cervix is thought to occur by a default mechanism and thus spontaneously without a requirement for steroid hormones. In females, the Wolffian duct will spontaneously regress in the absence of high concentrations of testosterone, whereas in males the production of anti-Müllerian hormone by the fetal testes induces regression of the Müllerian ducts. In genetic female fetuses,

therefore, exposure to elevated levels of androgens *in utero* can result in various degrees of masculinization of the primordia of the external genitalia as was noted in patient 1.

The most common cause of genital ambiguity is virilizing congenital adrenal hyperplasia (CAH), a group of autosomal recessive disorders caused by deficiency of enzymes essential for steroid hormone synthesis. It is now well established that 90%–95% of CAH cases are caused by a deficiency of the steroidogenic enzyme 21-hydroxylase (P450c21, CYP21). First described in the mid-19th century by De Crecchio (1865), our understanding of this disease was not forthcoming until the mid-20th century, when the recessive nature of the genetic trait and identification of the hormonal abnormalities were recognized (Speiser and New, 1987). The underlying defect among patients with CAH due to 21-hydroxylase deficiency is failure of the adrenal gland to synthesize cortisol efficiently. Reduced blood levels of cortisol lead to activation of the hypothalamic-pituitary axis and thus subsequent increased secretion of corticotropin-releasing hormone and corticotropin (ACTH) (Fig. 33-2).

In classic salt-wasting patients (such as patient 1), deficiency of 21-hydroxylase also precludes adequate production of the physiologically important mineralocorticoid aldosterone. Patients with classic simple virilization (such as patient 2) have a milder form of the enzyme deficiency and are able to produce aldosterone in levels sufficient to maintain electrolyte balance. In both forms of CAH, levels of 17-hydroxyprogesterone, the substrate for 21-hydroxylase, is markedly elevated. The adrenal responds to the buildup of 17-OHP by increasing synthesis of steroid hormones that lack a 21-OH group, namely, the androgens DHEA and DHEAS, which on secretion are further metabolized to the more active androgenic hormones testosterone and dihydrotestosterone. The net effect of increased androgen production is thus prenatal virilization of females and rapid somatic growth, with early closure of epiphyseal plates in both sexes.

The incidence of classic CAH-P450c21 in the United States ranges from 1:10,000 to 1:18,000, with approximately 75% of patients with CAH-P450c21 exhibiting classic salt wasting (White and Speiser, 2000). Aldosterone is essential for normal sodium homeostasis and acts to enhance sodium absorption and potassium excretion (Fig. 33-3). In the relative absence of aldosterone, there is an increase in sodium loss

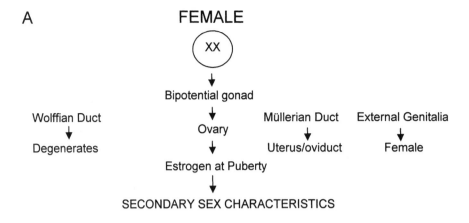

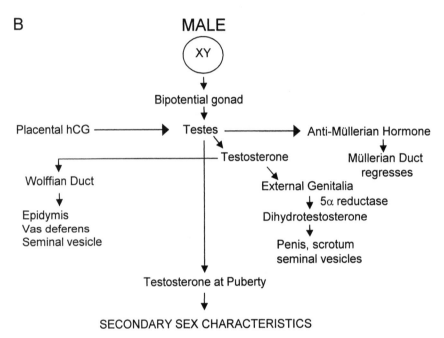

Figure 33-1. Summary of sexual differentiation: impact of genetic sex on differentiation of the bipotential gonad and role of the hormonal milieu on development of the primordia of the internal duct system and external genitalia *in utero*.

via the kidney as well as other organ systems (colon, sweat glands), which can compromise maintenance of adequate blood pressure (Bondy, 1985). Moreover, because salt-wasting patients also have a more marked deficiency in cortisol synthesis, they are more prone to crises that can be life-threatening. For example, in the absence of glucocorticoids, cardiac output can decrease, leading to a decrease in glomerular filtration, inability to excrete water, and, consequently, hyponatremia. Salt-wasting CAH is often more difficult to diagnose in males since the external genitalia are normal, and there is

usually no suspicion of adrenal insufficiency prior to the initial presenting crisis.

In addition to the two classic forms of P450c21 deficiency (salt wasting and simple virilizing), there is another more common form (occurrence 1:500 to 1:1000), which is termed nonclassic P450c21 CAH. This form is much less problematic physiologically, with patients asymptomatic at birth but exhibiting various degrees of problems associated with androgen excess later in life, including acne, hirsutism, oligomenorrhea, and perhaps infertility. In women, these symptoms and signs can

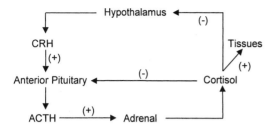

Figure 33-2. Hypothalamic-pituitary-adrenal axis. Corticotropin-releasing hormone (CRH) acts to increase pituitary ACTH secretion, which enhances steroid hormone synthesis by the adrenal, including production of cortisol (hydrocortisone), which controls CRH/ACTH secretion via negative feedback.

be confused with the more common polycystic ovarian syndrome.

Other, more rare, forms of congenital adrenal hyperplasia are the result of deficiencies of other steroidogenic enzymes, particularly 17-hydroxylase (P450c17) and 11β-hydroxylase (Bondy, 1985; White and Speiser, 2000). As with P450c21 deficiency, impaired activity of either of these other enzymes also results in decreased cortisol production, enhanced ACTH secretion, and thus increased tropic drive to the adrenal. Deficiency of 11β-hydroxylase is characterized by increased production of adrenal mineralocorticoids (e.g., corticosterone, aldosterone), resulting in sodium retention, potassium excretion, and increased blood pressure. In addition, adrenal androgens are produced in

excess, and genital ambiguity is often seen in affected females.

By contrast, deficiency of 17-hydroxylase results in impaired ability of the gonads (as well as the adrenals) to synthesize androgens (males) or estrogen (females); patients subsequently manifest with problems typically associated with primary hypogonadism. Deficiency of 17-hydroxylase is similar to that of 11β-hydroxylase in that there is adrenal overproduction of mineralocorticoids, resulting in sodium retention and high blood pressure. Differential diagnosis is usually facilitated by examination of the complete profile of adrenocortical steroid hormones.

BIOCHEMICAL PERSPECTIVES

Steroid Biosynthesis

Steroid hormones are members of a group of compounds having in common the cyclopentanoperhydrophenanthrene nucleus, a hydrated four-ring system in which the five-sided ring D is attached to three six-sided rings of phenanthrene (Fig. 33-4). The carbon atoms of the ring structure are numbered 1-17, while the additional carbons atoms are 18-21. Compounds having 21 carbons are derivatives of pregnane, and their biological activity is progestational, glucocorticoid, or mineralocorticoid. Progestins such as progesterone are involved in the support of pregnancy. Glucocorticoids provide the response to stress and are involved in carbohydrate

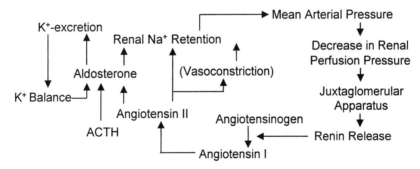

Figure 33-3. Summary of the renin-angiotensin-aldosterone system. Aldosterone secretion is controlled by several factors, including increased K^+, ACTH, or angiotensin II. Aldosterone acts to increase Na^+ retention by both the kidney and colon. Aldosterone also promotes renal K^+ excretion, which contributes to maintenance of Na^+/K^+ balance. In the absence of aldosterone, Na^+ is lost, K^+ is enhanced, the extracellular fluid volume is reduced, and mean arterial pressure and renal perfusion pressure are decreased. As a result, renin secretion is increased, leading to increased formation of angiotensin II, which promotes vasoconstriction and aldosterone secretion.

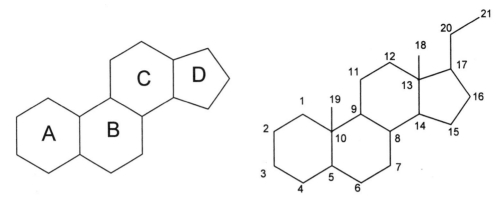

Figure 33-4. The four-ring cyclopentanoperhydrophenanthrene nucleus identifying the four rings and the numbering of the carbon atoms of a 21-carbon steroid such as cortisol. The ring carbons are numbered 1–17, while those of the side chain are 18–21.

metabolism by promoting gluconeogenesis. Mineralocorticoids are involved in regulation of electrolyte and water balance through their effect on ion transport in the renal tubules. Compounds having 19 carbon atoms are derivatives of androstane and biological activity is androgenic (producing masculine characteristics), whereas steroids with 18 carbons are derivatives of estrane and exhibit estrogenic (female sex hormone) activity.

All steroid hormones are derived from cholesterol, a sterol molecule comprised of 27 carbon atoms (Fig. 33-5). Cholesterol can be synthesized in the steroid-producing glands (adrenal, gonads) or brought to these glands bound to low-density lipoprotein (LDL) following synthesis in the liver (see Chapter 14, this volume). To serve as a substrate, cholesterol in the cytosol must be transported to the inner mitochondrial membrane where the P450 cholesterol–side-chain cleavage enzyme complex (CYP11A, cholesterol desmolase, side-chain cleavage enzyme, P450scc) is located. Recent studies indicated that steroid acute regulatory protein (StAR) transports cholesterol to the inner mitochondrial membrane (Lin et al., 1995; Tuckey et al., 2002). In the mitochondria, cholesterol is converted by P450scc to the 21-carbon molecule pregnenolone (Fig. 33-5), which is the common precursor for all other steroid hormones.

Within the adrenal gland, steroids are synthesized by the outer layer of cortical cells, while the central core of medullary cells is innervated by sympathetic preganglionic neurons, which stimulate it to produce and release epinephrine. The adrenal cortex is comprised of three histologically and metabolically distinct zones of cells, including an outer glomerulosa, an intermediate zone known as the fasciculata, and an internal layer termed the reticularis. In the adrenal, StAR is synthesized in response to ACTH (zona fasciculata) or calcium (zona glomerulosa).

Synthesis of cortisol (also known as 11,17,21-hydroxyprogesterone) occurs in the zona fasciculata of the adrenal. Pregnenolone is first converted by the enzyme 17-hydroxylase to 17-hydroxypregnenolone; the latter is converted by the enzyme 3β-hydroxysteroid dehydrogenase (3βHSD) to 17-hydroxyprogesterone (17-OHP) which is then hydroxylated sequentially at carbon 21 (P450c21) and then carbon 11 (P450c11) (Fig. 33-2). Since patients with P450c21 deficiency cannot utilize 17-OHP for cortisol synthesis, the levels of this metabolic intermediate increase dramatically. The inability to form cortisol results in increased release of pituitary ACTH, increased synthesis/uptake of cholesterol, and, consequently, continued production of 17-OHP (Figs. 33-2 and 33-5).

Aldosterone production is initiated by 21-hydroxylation of pregnenolone in the adrenal glomerulosa, where there is no 17-hydroxylase activity. The product of hydroxylation of pregnenolone by P450c21 is 21-hydroxyprogesterone, also known as deoxycorticosterone (DOC). The quantity of aldosterone produced by the adrenal is only 1% of that of cortisol; for this reason, not all patients with classic P450c21 deficiency manifest with salt wasting.

Androgens produced by the adrenal gland are synthesized in the inner zone of cortical

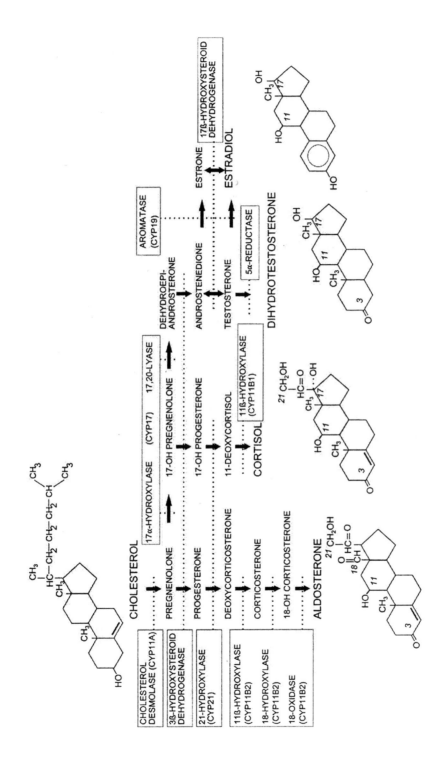

Figure 33-5. Summary of the pathway and enzymes catalyzing steroid hormone synthesis from precursor cholesterol. Reproduced with permission from White and Speiser (2000). Copyright 2000, The Endocrine Society

cells, known as the reticularis, which lack 3βHSD. In these cells, 17-hydroxypregnenolone is converted to DHEA by P450c17, an enzyme that, in the reticularis, also exhibits a lyase function which produces a C_{19} steroid by cleavage of two carbons. Thus, in patients with classic P450c21 deficiency and increased ACTH drive to the adrenal, levels of DHEA (and its sulfate DHEAS) are increased. Importantly, the C19 steroid DHEA can be hydroxylated by 3βHSD in other regions of the adrenal to more active androgens, including androstenedione. In the gonads, androstenedione can be converted to testosterone by 17-hydroxysteroid dehydrogenase and then to the very active androgen dihydrotestosterone by the enzyme 5α-reductase. The presence of such active androgens, normally not secreted in a female (genetic sex 46XX) fetus, during the period when the external genitalia are developing is responsible for the masculinization observed in patients with classic P450c21 deficiency.

P450c21 Hydroxylase

The human P450c21 protein is composed of 494 amino acid residues and exhibits a molecular mass of 52 kd (Higashi et al., 1986). It is a member of the cytochrome P450 (CYP) superfamily of proteins, all of which are monooxygenases in that they incorporate one of two atoms of molecular oxygen into the lipophilic substrate. The name P450 is derived from the absorbance maximum at approximately 450 nm of the reduced form of the heme prosthetic group. In addition to characterizing many of the reactions of steroidogenesis, mammalian cytochrome P450 enzymes are involved in catalysis of numerous other reactions, including oxidation of xenobiotics (exogenous substrates) such as drugs. Some cytochrome P450 enzymes, including P450scc and 17-hydroxylase, are mitochondrial enzymes; others, including P450c21 and the 17α-hydroxylase/17,20 lyase (P450c17), are localized on the endoplasmic reticulum.

The P450c21 gene (CYP21) is located in the HLA major histocompatibility complex on the short arm of chromosome 6 (6p21.3) and is comprised of 10 exons spaced over 3.1 kb (Carroll et al., 1985). CAH due to P450c21 deficiency is inherited as a monogenic autosomal recessive trait closely linked to the HLA complex. Thus, siblings with 21-hydroxylase deficiency are almost always HLA identical. Indeed, before cloning of CYP21, HLA typing was a major means to perform prenatal diagnosis.

The 6p21.3 region of chromosome 6 also contains a pseudogene (CYP21P), a nonfunctional DNA sequence approximately 30 kb from CYP21P. The exon and intron nucleotide sequences of CYP21 and CYP21P are 98% and 96% identical, respectively. Some 40–50 distinct mutations that cause 21-hydroxylase deficiency have been characterized (New and Wilson, 1999; White and Speiser, 2000). More than 90% of them appear to be the result of two types of meiotic interactions between CYP21 and CYP21P. One type of interaction involves misalignment and unequal crossing over, resulting in large-scale DNA deletions. The other type of interaction, called gene conversion, results in the transfer of deleterious mutations from CYP21P to CYP21. CAH is unusual among genetic diseases in the high proportion of mutant alleles generated by intergenic recombination (White and Speiser, 2000). Indeed, the high rate of *de novo* mutations in CYP21 may explain the high carrier frequency (1%–2%) of CAH despite the fact that classic CAH is potentially lethal if untreated.

The various CAH phenotypes (salt wasting, simple virilizing, and nonclassic) represent a spectrum of severe to moderate to mild loss of CYP21 enzymatic activity. Attempts have been made to correlate the genotype of the individual (specific mutations) with this CAH phenotype. As described by White and Speiser (2000), patients are usually compound heterozygotes for two different mutations, and the phenotype of each patient correlates quite well with the nature of the less severely impaired allele. Factors other than 21-hydroxylase activity may also influence phenotype. Genetic variations in androgen biosynthesis or sensitivity may influence clinical expression of androgen excess. Similarly, both genetic and nongenetic factors may contribute to the expression of salt wasting.

THERAPY

Glucocorticoid Replacement

Patients with CAH require lifelong glucocorticoid replacement therapy to correct the deficiency in cortisol secretion. This in turn suppresses ACTH production, excess adrenal 17-hydryoxyprogesterone, and excess androgen production. Hydrocortisone is the corticosteroid of choice for children with CAH because of its short half-life and easy dose adjustment (Marshall and New, 2003). Older individuals may be treated with synthetic glucocorticoids such as prednisone or dexamethasone. Treatment efficacy is determined by monitoring of 17-hydroxyprogesterone and androstenedione levels.

The therapeutic goal is to provide the minimum dosage that will effectively suppress excess adrenal function. Excess glucocorticoid treatment can be detrimental in children, resulting in growth suppression. Excess glucocorticoids can also result in Cushing's syndrome, which is characterized by a cluster of symptoms including so-called moon face, weight gain, central obesity, fatigue, muscle atrophy, osteoporosis, increased thirst and urination, hyperglycemia, and changes in mental status.

Stress Dosing and Medical Alerts

Patients with classic CAH do not adequately increase endogenous cortisol production in response to stress and thus require additional exogenous glucocorticoid in a number of situations, including febrile illnesses and surgery under general anesthesia. Increased requirements can be 2–3 times normal dosage during physiological stress and as much as 5–10 times normal dosage for the first 24–48 h during and after a surgical procedure. Families should be given injection kits with age-appropriate dosages of hydrocortisone for emergency use and trained in their appropriate use. In addition, patients with CAH, like others who are receiving corticosteroid replacement therapy, should wear a Medic-Alert identifying bracelet to alert health care providers in an emergency situation.

Mineralocorticoid Replacement

Infants with salt-wasting CAH require mineralocorticoid replacement therapy, usually with fludrocortisone (9α-fluorohydrocortisone). In addition, they require sodium chloride (1–2 g/day) since the sodium content of both breast milk and common infant formulas is only sufficient to meet the requirements of healthy infants (White and Speiser, 2000). Older children often acquire a taste for salty foods and do not require daily sodium chloride tablets. Plasma renin activity may be used to monitor mineralocorticoid and sodium replacement.

Other Therapeutic Approaches

Several additional pharmacological approaches, currently still considered experimental, were reviewed by White and Speiser (2000). In addition, these authors reviewed the corrective surgical procedures that have been used for newborns with ambiguous genitalia. They also discussed the need for appropriate psychological counseling for families of genetic females born with virilized external genitalia.

Prenatal Treatment and Diagnosis

In pregnancies at risk for a child affected with classic P450c21 deficiency, prenatal hormone therapy can be used to eliminate the virilizing effects of excess androgen *in utero* (David and Forest, 1984; Mercado et al., 1995). As reviewed by New and Wilson (1999), prenatal maternal treatment with dexamethasone (a potent synthetic glucocorticoid) has been shown to prevent or significantly reduce virilization of genitalia in female neonates with CAH and preclude the need for genitoplasty. Dexamethasone is used because it can cross the placenta and, unlike cortisol itself, is not metabolized to less-active forms by the enzyme 11β-hydroxysteroid dehydrogenase (Pepe and Albrecht, 1995). To be effective, treatment must be initiated on or before the ninth week of pregnancy.

Because of the need to initiate therapy early in fetal development, dexamethasone treatment of at-risk pregnancies must be initiated prior to prenatal diagnosis. Amniocentesis cannot be performed until after week 15; chorionic villus sampling can be performed earlier (weeks 10–12) but has a higher pregnancy loss rate (1%–2%). In either case, initial karyotyping is performed; if the fetus is male, then the dexamethasone treatment is discontinued (Mercado et al., 1995). If the fetus is female, then DNA analysis is required; hydroxyprogesterone levels will be uninformative since the dexamethasone treatment suppresses amniotic fluid adrenocortical hormones. As reviewed by White and Speiser (2000), the molecular analysis is complicated by need to amplify PCR without amplifying the highly homologous CYP21P pseudogene, which already carries most of the mutations of interest.

Although studies to date have not identified untoward effects of the dexamethasone treatment on either the mother or the fetus, there is a potential for long-term/long-lasting effects of glucocorticoid treatment (e.g., programming fetal organ system development/function) and thus increasing risk for development of diseases in adulthood. For this reason, current protocols for prenatal therapy include prenatal diagnosis and discontinuation of treatment as soon as the fetus can be identified as male or unaffected female.

QUESTIONS

1. Why do severe forms of CAH affect synthesis of both cortisol and aldosterone?
2. Why are males with classic P450c21 deficiency at more risk than females?
3. What is the mechanism by which impaired synthesis of cortisol actually enhances synthesis of 17-hydroxyprogesterone (17-OHP)?
4. Why does a deficiency of 21-hydroxylase result in increased fetal synthesis of androgens?
5. Why is it important to initiate prenatal therapy for CAH early in pregnancy?
6. Why does excess hydrocortisone treatment increase blood glucose?
7. Why do patients with 21-hydroxylase deficiency exhibit low blood pressure whereas those with 17α-hydroxylase deficiency exhibit high blood pressure?
8. Why are ACTH levels elevated in patients with P450c21, P450c17, and P45011β steroid hydroxylase deficiency?
9. Why are deficiencies in adrenal steroid enzymes collectively termed congenital adrenal hyperplasia?

BIBLIOGRAPHY

Bondy PK: Disorders of the adrenal cortex, *in* Wilson JD, Foster DW (eds): *Textbook of Endocrinology.* Saunders, New York, 1985, pp. 816–890.

Carroll MC, Campbell RD, Porter RR: Mapping of steroid 21-hydroxylase genes adjacent to complement component C4 genes in HLA, the major histocompatibility complex in man. *Proc Natl Acad Sci USA* **82:**521–525, 1985.

David M, Forest MG: Prenatal treatment of congenital adrenal hyperplasia resulting from 21-hydroxylase deficiency. *J Pediatr* **105:**799–803, 1984.

De Crecchio L: Sopra un caso di apparenz virile in una donna *Morgagni* **7:**154–188, 1865.

George FW, Wilson JD: Sex determination and differentiation, *in* Knobil E, Neill JD (eds): *The Physiology of Reproduction.* 2nd ed. Raven Press, New York, 1994, pp. 3–28.

Higashi Y, Yoshioka H, Yamane M, et al.: Complete nucleotide sequence of two steroid 21-hydroxylase genes tandemly arranged in human chromosome: a pseudogene and a genuine gene. *Proc Natl Acad Sci USA* **83:**2841–2845, 1986.

Jost A: A new look at the mechanisms controlling sex differentiation in mammals. *Johns Hopkins Med J* **130:**38–53, 1972.

Lin D, Sugawara T, Strauss JF 3rd, et al.: Role of steroidogenic acute regulatory protein in adrenal and gonadal steroidogenesis. *Science* **267:**1821–1831, 1995.

Marshall I, New MI: Adrenal disorders, *in* New M (ed.): *Pediatric Endocrinology.* Endotext.org, 2003, Chapter 8. Available at: http://www.endotext.com/pediatrics/pediatrics8/pediatrics-frame8.htm.

Mercado AB, Wilson RC, Cheng KC, et al.: Prenatal treatment and diagnosis of congenital adrenal hyperplasia owing to steroid 21-hydroxylase deficiency. *J Clin Endocrinol Metab* **80:**2014–2020, 1995.

Migeon CJ: Editorial: comments about the need for prenatal treatment of congenital adrenal hyperplasia due to 21 hydroxylase deficiency. *J Clin Endocrinol Metab* **70:**836–837, 1990.

New MI, White PC: Genetic disorders of steroid hormone synthesis and metabolism. *Baillieres Clin Endocrinol Metab* **9:**525–554, 1995.

New MI, Wilson RC: Steroid disorders in children: congenital adrenal hyperplasia and apparent mineralocorticoid excess. *Proc Natl Acad Sci USA* **96:**12790–12797, 1999.

Pepe GJ, Albrecht ED: Actions of placental and fetal adrenal steroid hormones in primate pregnancy. *Endocr Rev* **16:**608–648, 1995.

Speiser PW, New MI: Genotype and hormonal phenotype in nonclassical 21-hydroxylase deficiency. *J Clin Endocrinol Metab* **64:**86–91, 1987.

Tuckey RC, Headlam MJ, Bose HS, Miller WL: Transfer of cholesterol between phospholipid vesicles mediated by the steroidogenic acute regulatory protein (StAR). *J Biol Chem* **277:** 47123–47128, 2002.

White PC: Genetic diseases of steroid metabolism. *Vitam Horm* **49:**131–195, 1994.

White PC, Speiser PW: Congenital adrenal hyperplasia due to 21-hydroxylase deficiency. *Endocr Rev* **21:**245–291, 2000.

Index